Biochemical Basis of Pediatric Disease

EDITED BY

Steven J. Soldin

Nader Rifai

Jocelyn M.B. Hicks

AACC Press   2029 K Street, N.W.   Washington, D.C. 20006

Library of Congress Cataloging-in-Publication Data

Biochemical basis of pediatric disease / edited by Steven J. Soldin,
  Nader Rifai, Jocelyn M.B. Hicks.
       p.   cm..
    Includes index.
    ISBN 0-915274-60-4
    1. Pediatric pathology. 2. Physiology, Pathological. 3. Clinical
biochemistry. 4. Clinical chemistry. I. Soldin, Steven J.
II. Rifai, Nader. III. Hicks, Jocelyn M.
    [DNLM: 1. Chemistry,Clinical--in infancy & childhood.
2. Diagnosis, Laboratory--in infancy & childhood.   WS 141   B615]
RJ49.B56   1992
618.92'007--dc20
DNLM/DLC   92-17731
for Library of Congress   CIP

Production and typography by Sterling Editorial Services, Albuquerque, NM
Cover design by Carol Conway

ISBN 0–915274–60–4

Printed in the United States of America.

Contents

Frank A. Oski, M.D.
Director, Department of Pediatrics
Given Professor of Pediatrics
The Johns Hopkins University School of Medicine
Baltimore, MD

Gillian Lockitch, M.B., Ch.B., M.D., F.R.C.P.(C)
Associate Professor, Department of Pathology
University of British Columbia
Program Head, Division of Clinical Biochemistry
British Columbia's Children's Hospital
Vancouver, British Columbia

Anne Catherine Halstead, M.D., F.R.C.P.(C)
Clinical Associate Professor, Department of Pathology
University of British Columbia
Medical Biochemist, Division of Clinical Biochemistry
British Columbia's Children's Hospital
Vancouver, British Columbia

Michele C. Walsh-Sukys, M.D.
Assistant Professor, Department of Pediatrics
Case Western Reserve University School of Medicine
Associate Director, ECMO Center, and Co-Director,
 Neonatal Intensive Care Unit
Rainbow Babies' & Children's Hospital
Cleveland, OH

L. Kyle Walker, M.D.
Assistant Professor, Department of Anesthesiology
 and Critical Care Medicine
The Johns Hopkins Medical Institutions
Director, ECMO Program
The Johns Hopkins University Hospital
Baltimore, MD

Billie Lou Short, M.D.
Professor, Department of Pediatrics
George Washington University School of Medicine
Director, ECMO Program
Children's National Medical Center
Washington, DC

Elizabeth A. Harvey, M.D., F.R.C.P.(C)
Assistant Professor, Pediatrics
University of Toronto
Staff Nephrologist, Division of Nephrology
The Hospital for Sick Children
Toronto, Ontario, Canada

John Williamson Balfe, M.D., F.R.C.P.(C)
Professor, Department of Pediatrics
University of Toronto
Clinical Director, Division of Nephrology
The Hospital for Sick Children
Toronto, Ontario, Canada

Robert M. Gow, M.B., B.S.

Assistant Professor of Pediatrics
The University of Toronto Faculty of Medicine
Director, Section of Electrophysiology, Division of Cardiology
The Hospital for Sick Children
Toronto, Canada

John Dyck, M.D.

Assistant Professor of Pediatrics
The University of Toronto Faculty of Medicine
Staff Physician, Division of Cardiology
The Hospital for Sick Children
Toronto, Canada

Ivan M. Rebeyka, M.D.

Assistant Professor of Surgery
The University of Toronto Faculty of Medicine
Staff Surgeon, Division of Cardiovascular Surgery
The Hospital for Sick Children
Toronto, Canada

Vera Rose, M.D.

Professor of Pediatrics
The University of Toronto Faculty of Medicine
Director, Lipid Disorder and Vascular Disease Prevention Clinic
Division of Cardiology
The Hospital for Sick Children
Toronto, Canada

Robert M. Freedom, M.D.

Professor of Pediatrics and Pathology
The University of Toronto Faculty of Medicine
Head, Division of Cardiology
The Hospital for Sick Children
Toronto, Canada

Raphaël Rappaport, M.D.

Professor of Developmental Biology
University René Descartes, Paris
Head of Pediatric Endocrinology
Hôpital Necker Enfants Malades
Paris, France

Jean-Claude Souberbielle, Ph.D.

Assistant Director, Radioimmunology Laboratory
Department of Physiology
University René Descartes, Paris
Hôpital Necker Enfants Malades
Paris, France

Claude J. Migeon, M.D.

Professor, Department of Pediatrics
The Johns Hopkins University School of Medicine
Director, Pediatric Endocrine Clinic
Johns Hopkins Hospital
Baltimore, MD

Gary D. Berkovitz, M.D.

Associate Professor, Department of Pediatrics
Division of Pediatric Endocrinology
The Johns Hopkins University School of Medicine
Johns Hopkins Hospital
Baltimore, MD

Patricia Y. Fechner, M.D.

Fellow, Department of Pediatrics
Division of Pediatric Endocrinology
The Johns Hopkins University School of Medicine
Baltimore, MD

Wellington Hung, M.D., Ph.D. F.A.A.P., F.A.C.P.

Professor, Department of Pediatrics
The Georgetown University School of Medicine
Washington, DC
Senior Clinical Investigator, Developmental Endocrinology Branch
National Institute of Child Health and Human Development
National Institutes of Health
Bethesda, MD

G. Michael Addison, M.A., M.B., B.Chir., M.Sc., Ph.D.

Consultant, Department of Chemical Pathology
Royal Manchester Children's Hospital
(University of Manchester School of Medicine)
Manchester, United Kingdom

Maria Lourdes A. Cruz, M.D.
Senior Fellow, Neonatology
University of Cincinnati College of Medicine
Cincinnati, OH

Ronald Bainbridge, M.D.
Former Fellow, Neonatology
University of Cincinnati College of Medicine
Cincinnati, OH

Reginald C. Tsang, M.D.
Professor, Pediatrics, Obstetrics and Gynecology
University of Cincinnati College of Medicine
Executive Director, Perinatal Research Center
Children's Hospital Medical Center
Cincinnati, OH

Denis Daneman, M.B., B.Ch., F.R.C.P.(C)
Associate Professor, Department of Pediatrics
University of Toronto
Chief, Division of Endocrinology
The Hospital for Sick Children
Toronto, Ontario, Canada

Roger J. Packer, M.D.
Professor of Neurology and Pediatrics
The George Washington University School of Medicine
Chairman, Department of Neurology
Children's National Medical Center
Washington, DC

Stephen I. Deutsch, M.D., Ph.D.
Professor of Psychiatry
Associate Chairman for Clinical Neurosciences
Department of Psychiatry
Georgetown University School of Medicine
Chief, Psychiatry Service
Department of Veteran Affairs Medical Center
Washington, DC

Preface

Frank A. Oski, M.D.

Biochemical Basis of Pediatric Disease contains all the important information that the traditional textbooks of pediatrics did not include.

The underpinnings of much of what we expect and order from the laboratory are explained clearly here. A reading of this book can assist both clinicians and investigators in selecting the appropriate diagnostic tests for their patients.

At a time when physician requests for laboratory tests often seem to be nothing more than a sampling from a large and expensive menu, a book that provides a discussion of the tests and the information they do and don't provide, as well as the factors that confound or interfere with interpretation, is a most welcome addition to any library.

Drs. Soldin, Rifai, and Hicks have provided the reader with a well-ordered treatise which explains everything from the why, where, when, and how much of blood drawing, to lucid discussions of the laboratory findings in patients with a vast array of disorders, such as disturbances of porphyrin metabolism, thyroid disease, and growth.

Once you examine this book, you will recognize that it would be difficult to practice good, economically sensible pediatric medicine without it, and you will wonder why a book like this wasn't made available to you a long time ago.

Pediatric Nutrition

Gillian Lockitch, M.B. Ch.B., M.D., F.R.C.P.(C)
Anne Catherine Halstead, M.D., F.R.C.P.(C)

INTRODUCTION

Nutrition of infants and children influences growth, physical and mental development, and the capability to respond to disease. Recognition of this fact has led to increased use of laboratory tests as part of the assessment of nutritional status in these age groups. However, lack of appropriate reference ranges for many analytes remains a major problem. In this chapter, the biochemistry and metabolism of proteins, fatty acids, essential trace elements, and vitamins are outlined from a nutritional perspective, and clinical presentations of deficiency, selected inherited metabolic defects, and toxicity are described. Strategies for laboratory investigation of specific nutrient abnormalities are presented, with discussion of the limitations of tests and factors that can affect the results. Complications of total parenteral nutrition illustrate the difficulties of supplying appropriate nutritional supplements to infants and children and of monitoring their nutritional status.

LABORATORY ASSESSMENT OF NUTRITIONAL STATUS IN PEDIATRICS

The use of laboratory tests in assessment of nutritional status in children has become increasingly important with the recognition that marginal or subclinical nutrient deficiencies may contribute to increased mortality and morbidity.[1, 2] As many as 45% of children admitted to hospital may be malnourished on admission,[3] and chemotherapy, radiation, surgery, dialysis, and specialized metabolic formulas may result in both specific and generalized nutrient depletion.[4, 5] As parenteral and enteral nutrition support have evolved, previously unsuspected micronutrient deficiencies have been recognized.[6-8]

Nutritional assessment in children is more complex than in adults, for several reasons. A child's healthy growth and development require a greater intake of protein, energy, and many other nutrients relative to body weight than for the adult. Particularly in the very premature infant, physiological immaturity of metabolic systems may alter both nutrient requirements and the ability to process them.[9] Laboratory reference ranges for many analytes are influenced by age, and a laboratory providing tests for a pediatric population must have age-specific reference ranges for the methods used in that laboratory. Pediatric reference ranges derived from a variety of sources can be found in a recent reference handbook.[10]

The laboratory investigation of nutritional status is complementary to a careful clinical evaluation by history, physical examination, and anthropometry. In choosing components of a nutritional test panel, the specific objectives of laboratory testing must be clear. These objectives may include detection of subclinical or preclinical generalized or specific nutrient deficiencies, confirmation of a generalized or specific overt nutritional deficiency, or monitoring the efficacy of nutritional therapy support. Testing therefore may be nutrient specific or utilize nutritional panels.[11]

Several caveats must be borne in mind. For practical purposes, most tests are performed on readily accessible, relatively non-invasive specimens, such as blood or urine. A single blood analysis does not always accurately reflect the state of body stores, for a number of reasons[11] (Table 1–1).

TABLE 1–1. Factors Affecting Nutrient Concentrations in Plasma

Factor	Nutrient
Recent dietary intake	Water-soluble vitamins
Acute phase response	Proteins, iron, zinc, copper
Diurnal variation	Iron, zinc
Protein binding	Zinc, copper, retinol, folate, B12, 25-hydroxyvitamin D
Lipid association	Vitamin E, vitamin K, carotene
pH	Ionized calcium
Homeostatic regulation	1,25-dihydroxyvitamin D, calcium
Plasma enzyme activity	Pyridoxal-5-phosphate
Acute tissue uptake	Folate, vitamin B12
Acute tissue release	Pyridoxal-5-phosphate, zinc, copper

The acute phase response is characterized by short-term alteration in plasma concentrations of several trace elements and proteins.[12] Diurnal variation is important for iron and zinc,[13] among others. Homeostatic regulation of blood concentrations may mask deficiency of body stores, as for calcium, which remains within normal limits despite advanced bone demineralization in rickets or osteomalacia. The effect of pH on protein-binding activity of free versus bound analyte and cellular redistribution of elements with altered acid-base status may influence interpretation of blood analyses. Low concentrations of transport proteins may imply low concentrations of a nutrient despite adequacy of nutrient stores; for example, low transthyretin may suggest retinol deficiency.[11]

The relative specificity of laboratory testing is both advantageous and disadvantageous. Compared to a clinical sign or symptom which may raise the possibility of one of several nutritional deficiencies (Table 1-2), a laboratory test is specific for a single nutrient. Conversely, however, this means that assessment of multiple deficiencies requires multi-test panels. This is expensive and may require a large blood specimen, limiting such investigations in pediatrics, especially in very premature or low-birth-weight infants.

Functional testing has been proposed as an alternative to static indices of nutritional status. Many of these tests have been developed for testing of pediatric populations, but changes in methodology and specimen size may be required to adapt these tests to smaller infants.[11] Growth velocity, in fact, represents a good overall functional test of nutritional status in children.

PROTEIN-ENERGY NUTRITION

Pathophysiology of Protein Energy Malnutrition

Protein-energy nutritional deficiency remains a major problem among children of the third world[14] but is also found in 15–40% of children admitted to pediatric hospitals.[3] The syndrome may range from malnutrition, characterized by a decrease in weight and/or height for age, to severe marasmus or kwashiorkor.[15]

The protein component of the body is distributed between noncellular structural proteins, such as cartilage and fibrous and skeletal tissues, and the metabolically active lean body mass. Somatic protein or skeletal muscle comprises 30–50% of total body protein. The visceral protein pool is comprised of serum proteins, the cellular blood components, and the solid tissue organs, such as liver, kidney, and heart.

Chronic protein-energy deficiency results in slowing of growth and development, depletion of available fat stores, catabolism of muscle tissue, and finally depletion of the visceral protein pool, including plasma

TABLE 1–2. Clinical Findings Suggestive of Nutritional Disorders

Clinical Finding	Possible Deficiency	Possible Toxicity
Dermatitis	Zinc, manganese, essential fatty acids, riboflavin, pyridoxine, biotin	Selenium, vitamin A (chronic)
Alopecia	Zinc, essential fatty acids, biotin, protein	Selenium, vitamin A (chronic)
Other hair changes, e.g., pigment, structure	Selenium, manganese, Menkes	Selenium
Glossitis, stomatitis	Riboflavin, niacin, pyridoxine	
Hemorrhage, bruising	Manganese, vitamin K, vitamin C	
Skeletal changes	Copper, manganese, vitamin D, vitamin C, calcium, phosphate	Vitamin A (chronic)
Peripheral neuropathy	Chromium, vitamin E, thiamin, niacin, vitamin B12, pantothenic acid	Pyridoxine
Other neurological findings	Menkes, Wilson's, vitamin E, thiamin, niacin, pyridoxine, folate, vitamin B12	Manganese, vitamin A (acute)
Myopathy, muscle tenderness	Selenium, vitamin E, vitamin C	Zinc
Cardiac failure	Selenium, iron, thiamin	Hemochromatosis
Anemia	Iron, copper, selenium folate, vitamin B12, sometimes vitamin E, thiamin, pyridoxine	Lead
Jaundice	Wilson's disease	Hemochromatosis, niacin, menadiol
Night blindness	Zinc, molybdenum, vitamin A	
Gastrointestinal disturbance	Iron, zinc, vitamin A, niacin, folate, vitamin B12	Iron, zinc

proteins. Marasmic protein-energy malnutrition, following prolonged depletion, is characterized by extreme loss of adipose tissue and muscle mass. Acute superimposed protein loss due to recurrent infections, acute stress as in trauma, or gastrointestinal losses causes depletion of the visceral protein pool, and the edema of kwashiorkor results.[15] Marasmus and kwashiorkor represent different manifestations of severe protein-energy malnutrition; features of both are seen in infants with marasmic-kwashiorkor.

Evaluation of Protein-Calorie Malnutrition

Nitrogen balance measures the net change in total body protein. Measures used in assessment of the skeletal muscle or somatic protein compartment include creatinine-height index or 3-methylhistidine urine excretion, whereas specific measurement of hepatosecretory plasma proteins is used to assess changes in the visceral protein compartment.

Nitrogen Balance

Nitrogen balance exists when nitrogen intake is adequate to replace endogenous nitrogen losses. Growing children should be in positive nitrogen balance. A negative nitrogen balance may result from protein-energy insufficiency, excess protein loss, or protein catabolism, as in sepsis or severe burns. Assessment of nitrogen balance is dependent on adequacy of 24 h urine collections, and a minimum of three collections should be made.

Assessment of Plasma Proteins

With the basic assumption that plasma protein concentration will be decreased in protein deficiency and normalize with protein adequacy, several plasma proteins of hepatic origin have been used in the assessment of protein status (Table 1–3). The concentration of a given plasma protein at any time depends on interrelated components: protein synthesis, protein catabolism, and protein pool size or volume of distribution. Several other factors affect plasma protein concentration independent of dietary protein intake.

The acute phase reaction is characterized by an increase in positive acute reactants (C-reactive protein, ceruloplasmin, α-1-antitrypsin, α-1-acid glycoprotein) and a decrease in negative acute phase reactants (albumin, prealbumin, retinol-binding protein).[12] Quantitation of serum proteins during an acute stress, surgery or trauma, may be misleading.

Hepatic protein synthesis may decrease in dietary protein deficiency, zinc deficiency, hepatic disease, hypothyroidism, hypercortisolism, or stress states. Conversely, increases in ambient temperature or decreased plasma oncotic pressure can stimulate protein synthesis.[16]

Along with the usual protein catabolism or degradation, protein loss can be increased by renal disease with increased glomerular loss or decreased tubular reabsorption, in protein-losing enteropathies, or

TABLE 1–3. Plasma Proteins Used in Assessment of Protein Nutrition

Protein (half life)	Non-protein Factors Altering Plasma Concentrations	
	Increased	Decreased
Albumin (21 d)	Hemoconcentration	Liver disease Nephrotic syndrome Protein-losing enteropathy Analbuminemia Acute phase response
Transferrin (8 d)	Iron deficiency	Acute phase response
Fibronectin (0.5–1 d)		Sepsis, trauma, burns Post-surgery disseminated intra-vascular coagulation
Prealbumin (2 d)		Acute phase response Zinc deficiency
Retinol-binding protein (0.5 d)	Renal failure	Zinc deficiency Vitamin A deficiency Liver disease Nephrotic syndrome Tubular proteinuria Acute phase response

by rapid blood loss. Fluid shifts and loss into edema compartments may alter the apparent volume of distribution of the protein pool.

Albumin is still most commonly used to assess protein status because it can be measured in most laboratories. The relatively long half-life of 21 days and change with state of hydration reduce the sensitivity of serum albumin in diagnosis of acute protein deficiency. However, if renal, hepatic, and enteropathic causes of hypoalbuminemia are excluded, a low albumin indicates severe protein deficiency. In view of the relative insensitivity of albumin to acute protein deprivation, the measurement of other "rapid turnover" proteins has been recommended.

Prealbumin or transthyretin, synthesized in the liver, binds both retinol-binding protein and thyroid hormone. Prealbumin is a sensitive indicator of acute protein or energy deprivation and repletion in older subjects,[17] but its usefulness in premature infants has yet to be confirmed.[18, 19]

Retinol-binding protein (RBP) is stabilized by binding to prealbumin, and concentrations correlate closely with prealbumin in protein-energy deprivation and repletion. However, the very short half-life and low plasma reference concentrations make it less useful than prealbumin. RBP may be very low in vitamin A or zinc deficiency.[18]

Fibronectin, an opsonic protein involved in cell adhesion and wound healing, has a short half-life and is very sensitive to acute protein-calorie deprivation and repletion.[19, 20] However, it is greatly influenced by the acute phase process. Concentrations are normally lower in preterm than in full-term neonates.[20] Wider use in pediatric nutritional evaluation awaits the delineation of age-specific reference values.

Transferrin has been extensively studied as an indicator of protein-energy deprivation because it has a shorter half-life than albumin. However, both iron status and the acute phase response influence transferrin concentrations and decrease its utility as an indicator of protein deficiency.[16]

Overall, the most useful indicator appears to be prealbumin, but its value in small infants and children requires further study.

Assessment of Somatic Protein Status

Urinary Creatinine and the Creatinine-Height Index

Assessment of lean cell mass by use of the creatinine-height index is based on the principle that the creatine content of muscle is constant and that urine creatinine excretion is proportional to total body creatine content and directly reflects muscle mass. However, diet, age, gender, physical activity, metabolic state, and disease may alter urine creatinine, and there is day-to-day variability in urine 24 h creatinine collection even under the most careful conditions.[15]

The creatinine-height index is calculated by dividing actual 24 h urine creatinine by expected 24 h urine creatinine for height. An index of 60–80% indicates moderate deficit in muscle mass, whereas < 60% indicates a severe deficit.[21] However, incomplete urine collections invalidate the results; therefore, at least three 24 h urine collections should be performed. This index also does not correct for the metabolic consequences of disease, the rate of muscle protein turnover, or the initial muscle mass prior to acute protein deprivation.

Urinary 3-methylhistidine

This amino acid is formed by methylation of histidine in the actin and myosin components of muscle fibers. On catabolism of muscle, 3-methylhistidine is released and excreted, without further metabolism, in the urine. If exogenous sources of 3-methylhistidine such as meat are eliminated and muscle anabolism and catabolism are in relative equilibrium, the urine 3-methylhistidine excretion should provide an index of muscle mass.[22] However, limited data on the effect of age, hormonal status, exercise, stress, and various other factors on 3-methylhistidine excretion restricts the usefulness of the test. The requirement for complete 24 h urine collections and the anabolic state of the growing child further limit its usefulness in pediatrics.

Amino-Acid Profiles

Amino acid profiles (aminograms) have been studied in various disease states as a predictor of outcome. One application is use of the ratio of non-essential amino acids (glycine, serine, glutamine, taurine) to essential amino acids (leucine, isoleucine, valine, methionine) in differentiating kwashiorkor and marasmus. A ratio > 3 occurs in kwashiorkor.[21] The plasma aminogram in both parenterally and orally fed infants has been used to modify composition of infant formula and parenteral nutrition formulations.[23]

LIPIDS

Lipids are the major energy store, utilized once the short-term carbohydrate stores such as glycogen are used. Altered lipid metabolism may be seen in a variety of disease states, including hereditary and secondary dyslipoproteinemias (Chapter 15). Deficiency of lipid-soluble nutrients such as vitamins A, D, E, and K may occur in disorders of digestion and absorption such as cystic fibrosis or Crohn's disease.[24, 25] The use of parenteral nutrition with inadequate lipid supplementation results in essential fatty acid deficiency (EFA).[26]

Essential Fatty Acid Deficiency

Linoleic acid, the principal essential fatty acid required for synthesis of arachidonic acid and prostaglandins, cannot be synthesized by humans and must be obtained from dietary sources. Essential fatty acid deficiency has been described in infants and children maintained on a fat-free diet,[27] on fat-free total parenteral nutrition,[26] and in malnourished infants.[28] Premature infants may develop biochemical signs of EFA deficiency within days of birth.[29] Children with chronic cholestasis maintained on formula with medium-chain triglyceride as the major lipid source developed essential fatty acid and vitamin E deficiency.[30] One child developed a photosensitive dermatitis resembling that seen in porphyria.[31]

The clinical syndrome of essential fatty acid deficiency is characterized by skin lesions (a dry, scaly seborrhoeic dermatitis with desquamation and thickening), impaired growth, sparse hair, poor wound healing, and increased susceptibility to infection. However, biochemical evidence of EFA deficiency may be present in the absence of clinical signs.

Essential fatty acid deficiency may be diagnosed by low plasma linoleic acid, presence of eicosatrienoic acid, and an increased triene:tetraene ratio.[29]

Fatty acid composition in plasma total lipid extracts may be quantitated by gas chromatography.[29] The distribution of fatty acids in normal older infants and children is approximately 36% linoleic, 20% palmitic, and 8% arachidonic, while no eicosatrienoic acid is expected. In contrast, cord blood fatty acids from infants of < 37 weeks gestation were comprised of approximately 10% linoleic, 26% palmitic, 16% arachidonic, and 1% eicosatrienoic. It was suggested that the high arachidonic acid in the face of low linoleic acid in cord blood could reflect placental metabolism.

A *triene:tetraene ratio* > 0.2 due to increased concentrations of the non-essential fatty acid, eicosatrienoic acid, relative to arachidonic acid is considered indicative of essential fatty acid deficiency. By 10 days of postnatal age, 43% of premature infants had an increased triene:tetraene ratio, indicating the extreme susceptibility of this group to essential fatty acid deficiency.[29]

TRACE ELEMENTS

Ten trace elements—copper, cobalt, chromium, iodine, iron, fluoride, manganese, molybdenum, selenium, and zinc—are considered essential for growth and development.[32, 33] Clinical disorders resulting from acquired nutrient deficiency[6, 7, 34-37] and deficiency resulting from inherited metabolic disorders[38-40] have been described. Similarly, toxicity states have resulted from trace element excess, acquired[41-43] or in association with genetic disease.[44, 45]

Trace element deficiencies may result from several therapeutic modalities or may be anticipated in a variety of disease states (Table 1–4). Currently, evaluation of iron, copper, zinc, and selenium status has clinical application.[32, 33]

Much less is known about pediatric, and indeed adult nutritional requirements, for the remaining six elements.[46, 47]

Analytical limitations for assessing these ultra-trace elements in biological matrices constrain clinical research on their nutritional requirements.[32, 33]

Iron

Iron is a component of heme proteins, including hemoglobin, myoglobin, and other heme enzymes, as well as cytochromes. Of total body iron, about 66% is found in hemoglobin, about 3% in myoglobin, and < 1% in other enzymes. Approximately 30% is stored within ferritin and hemosiderin, predominantly in the liver, spleen, and bone marrow.

TABLE 1–4. Clinical Situations in which Trace Element or Vitamin Deficiency Should be Suspected

Iatrogenic Causes	Disease States
Parenteral nutrition	Prematurity
Special metabolic formulas (PKU)	Infants of malnourished mothers
Soy-based infant formulas	Gastritis
Enteral formulas	Intestinal malabsorption
Elimination diets for allergies	Celiac disease
Dialysis	Short bowel syndrome
Chemotherapeutics	Inflammatory bowel disease
Anticonvulsants	Small bowel bacterial overgrowth
Antitubercular agents	Chronic diarrhea
	Cystic fibrosis
	Cholestatic liver disease
	Cancer
	Renal disease

The main transport protein for iron is transferrin, which is also capable of binding copper and manganese.[48]

Disorders of Iron Metabolism

Iron Deficiency

The major clinical disorder resulting from severe iron deficiency is anemia.[34] However, it is now recognized that at lesser degrees of deficiency—identifiable by decreased concentrations of storage or transport iron and prior to the development of frank anemia—impaired growth, decreased muscle function and poor work performance, altered response to infection, and behavioral changes can be identified.[49]

Iron deficiency provides a model for the use of laboratory testing in identifying preclinical stages of a developing nutritional disorder. Thus, three stages of developing iron deficiency have been defined (Table 1–5),[34] with hypochromic microcytic anemia apparent only in the final stage.

Iron Toxicity

Although iron is an essential element, excess iron is toxic.[48] Iron overload may be acute, from accidental or intentional iron ingestion,[50, 51] or chronic, resulting from dietary overload[48] or an inherited disorder, hemochromatosis.[48, 52, 53]

Iron poisoning by iron preparations or iron-containing multivitamin preparations[50] is still extremely common, although fatality is now unusual.[51] (See Chapter 19.)

TABLE 1–5. Progression of Nutritional Iron Deficiency

Stage of Adequacy/Deficiency	Biochemical Findings
Normal iron stores	No biochemical abnormality detected
Depletion of iron stores	Serum ferritin decreased
Iron deficient erythropoiesis	Low ferritin
	Low transferrin saturation
	Increased erythrocyte protoporphyrin
Iron deficiency anemia	Low ferritin
	Low transferrin saturation
	Increased erythrocyte protoporphyrin
	Decreased hemoglobin

The laboratory assessment should include serum iron, iron-binding capacity, and transferrin saturation. High concentrations of non-transferrin-bound iron (serum iron / iron binding capacity) suggest severe toxicity.

Chronic iron overload can result from multiple transfusions, as in thalassemia, or from dietary iron overload.[48] Excessive accumulation of iron in tissues is seen in disorders of iron metabolism which are of presumed genetic origin but for which the specific defects are not known. Classical hemochromatosis presents in mid to late adulthood,[48] but juvenile forms have also been described.[52] Infantile hemochromatosis or neonatal iron storage disease appears to be a different entity.[53]

Hemochromatosis in the adult is characterized by the classical triad of cirrhosis, diabetes mellitus, and skin pigmentation, but excessive iron accumulation also affects the heart, kidney, and other endocrine organs. The neonatal form of hemochromatosis is a rapidly lethal form of cirrhosis, leading to death within days to weeks after birth.[53] Hepatic fibrosis is associated with massive iron accumulation in hepatocytes, with little iron in the cells of the reticuloendothelial system.

The biochemical findings in hemochromatosis include very high serum iron with transferrin saturation usually > 62 %, ferritin raised 2–20 times the normal upper limit, and extremely high hepatic iron concentrations.[48]

Assessment of Iron Status

In uncomplicated iron deficiency, plasma iron decreases, transferrin and iron binding capacity increase, and the percentage of saturation decreases. However, other factors, such as diurnal variation, may alter plasma iron.[13] The acute phase response is associated with decreased plasma iron[54] as iron is sequestered in the liver, and changes in transferrin saturation can occur within hours. Transferrin synthesis is decreased in dietary protein deficiency and chronic inflammation or infection but increased in iron deficiency. Iron deficiency with low iron, high binding capacity, and low saturation can thus be distinguished from the anemia of chronic disease with low iron and low binding capacity but saturation at the low end of the normal range.

Plasma ferritin concentrations correlate well with tissue iron ferritin stores and increase with iron therapy or repeated transfusions.[34, 48] Ferritin is an acute phase reactant which increases greatly in infection and malignancy. Ferritin is also useful in differentiating iron deficiency anemia (ferritin low) and anemia of chronic infection (ferritin normal or high).[34]

Erythrocyte protoporphyrin increases in iron deficiency.[34] The final stage of heme synthesis involves incorporation of iron into protoporphyrin IX. In iron deficiency, free protoporphyrin increases in erythrocytes. Other cations such as zinc may complex with protoporphyrin to form zinc protoporphyrin. Erythrocyte protoporphyrin provides an indication of long-term iron deficiency, as changes occur slowly, reflecting weeks of iron deprivation.[34] However, concentrations also decrease slowly on iron therapy, so this is not a sensitive monitor of response to therapy.[34] An increase of erythrocyte protoporphyrin also occurs in lead poisoning.[34]

Zinc

Zinc is a component of over 70 metalloenzymes, including alkaline phosphatase, carbonic anhydrase, alcohol dehydrogenase, thymidine kinase, and DNA polymerase.[41] Zinc is required for cellular proliferation, maintains cellular immunity and delayed hypersensitivity response, and forms an integral component of pancreatic insulin and muscle tissue.[41]

Disorders of Zinc Metabolism

Zinc Deficiency

Primary (dietary) and secondary (conditioned) causes of acquired zinc deficiency have been comprehensively reviewed.[41] Common causes of nutritional zinc deficiency include protein-calorie malnutrition, malabsorption, and inadequately supplemented parenteral nutrition (Table 1–4). The syndrome of zinc deficiency is characterized by impaired growth; poor wound healing; bullous dermatitis; immune defects, particularly T-cell function with increased susceptibility to infection; alopecia; night blindness; gastrointestinal disturbances; nervous system disorder; and impaired carbohydrate metabolism.[55]

Acquired acrodermatitis, with erythematous scaly skin lesions and candida albicans superinfections, occurs in premature neonates on parenteral nutrition with insufficient zinc supplement.[36]

The genetic disorder of zinc deficiency, acrodermatitis entero-pathica, is believed to be related to impaired zinc absorption due to a defective or absent ligand which normally facilitates zinc absorption in the gut. The exact defect is not known. This condition presents shortly after weaning with gastrointestinal symptoms, failure to thrive, infections, and other characteristics of zinc deficiency.[39]

Zinc Toxicity

Acute zinc poisoning causes gastrointestinal disturbances, while chronic zinc excess interferes with absorption of other essential elements such as copper.[45] Accidental acute zinc toxicity has occurred by ingestion, intravenous infusion, and by intravenous contamination during hemodialysis. Symptoms include diarrhea, nausea and vomiting, muscle pain, and fever.[41] Oral zinc taken at therapeutic doses may cause nausea and gastrointestinal distress and induce gastric ulceration. Zinc competes with copper for intestinal absorption and transport proteins. Zinc supplements from 150–5000 mg/d have resulted in copper-deficiency-induced anemia.[41]

Assessment of Zinc Status

Serum zinc analysis is most commonly used to assess zinc status and can provide a good indication of zinc nutriture if several factors are borne in mind. Low concentrations of serum or plasma zinc may occur for many reasons other than depletion of body stores. Serum zinc is about 65% albumin bound, and in severe hypoalbuminemia, similarly to total calcium, total plasma zinc concentration may be low.[56] Zinc concentrations may change with diurnal variation by as much as 40%.[13] Serum or plasma zinc is transiently decreased in the acute phase response with uptake of zinc into tissues;[54] therefore, a single serum zinc concentration measured in an acute situation may be misleading. Monitoring of zinc status by serum zinc requires sequential sampling in the fasting state and at the same time of day.[41]

Daily urine zinc excretion is about 400–600 μg, or about 5% of total daily zinc excretion.[41] Urine zinc excretion decreases rapidly in clinical zinc depletion,[57] suggesting that this might be a useful index of deficiency. However, urine zinc excretion is also greatly increased in catabolic states such as starvation and in cirrhosis,[41] even though total body zinc may be depleted.

Measurement of leucocyte zinc has been suggested as a alternative to serum[58] but is still largely a research tool. Confirmation of functional zinc deficiency is best established by the response of clinical symptoms to zinc supplementation.[41] Zinc tolerance testing has been used to assess zinc absorption.[41] After a fasting zinc concentration is obtained, 5–50 mg of elemental zinc is administered orally, and serum zinc measurements are obtained hourly up to 6 hours. In zinc malabsorption, the absorption curve is flatter, with a lower peak concentration and more rapid return to baseline than in controls.

Copper

Copper is an essential trace element which forms several important metalloenzymes. *Dopamine-β-hydroxylase* is required for catecholamine synthesis, *lysyl oxidase* is necessary for collagen synthesis, mitochondrial *cytochrome c oxidase* is important in energy transfer, superoxide dismutase is an antioxidant enzyme, *tyrosinase* is required for skin and hair pigmentation, and *ceruloplasmin*, the major copper-carrying protein in plasma, is important in iron metabolism.

Disorders of Copper Metabolism

Copper Deficiency

Nutritional copper deficiency, once considered to be uncommon,[35] is now increasingly recognized in infants.[59, 60] Although uncommon in infants born at term, copper deficiency has been described in infants recovering from diarrheal illness and fed cow's milk formulas.[35, 61] It is much more common in premature infants, particularly after parenteral nutrition.[59] The syndrome includes a hypochromic normocytic anemia, neutropenia, neurological and cardiac problems, skeletal abnormalities, osteoporosis, and metaphyseal irregularity resulting from defective collagen and elastin synthesis.[59, 60]

In very-low-birth-weight infants, copper deficiency may result in fractures, although the use of this possibility as a legal defense in suspected non-accidental injury in infants has aroused intense controversy.[59, 60] The diagnosis of true copper deficiency requires a plasma copper less than 6.8 μmol/L (43 μg/dL) in a term infant after 4 months of age, or 5.2 μmol/L (33 μg/dL) in a premature infant, concurrent sideroblastic anemia and neutropenia, and a prompt response to copper supplementation.[60]

Menkes' steely hair syndrome, an X-linked recessive disorder which results in a syndrome of severe copper deficiency, is clinically well defined, although the exact defect is not yet determined.[38] This disorder of copper metabolism is usually recognized in the neonatal period and is frequently fatal by early childhood. The clinical presentation is of severe psychomotor retardation, seizures, hypertonia, temperature instability, superficial vascular dilatation, skeletal abnormalities, and a characteristic grey steel-wool appearance to the hair.[38] Liver and brain are copper deficient, while high concentrations of copper are found in extra hepatic tissues, including the placenta.[62] The genetic defect remains unidentified. Laboratory findings include very low serum copper and ceruloplasmin, abnormal *in vitro* tissue copper binding, and increased copper uptake in cultured fibroblast cells.[62]

Copper Toxicity

Like iron, chronic excess of copper can cause severe tissue damage, and both nutritional and genetic disorders of copper toxicity are recognized.[44, 45]

Wilson's disease, an autosomal recessive disorder of copper toxicity, is characterized by accumulation of copper in tissues, particularly liver, brain, and kidneys, resulting in structural and functional damage.[45] Wilson's disease commonly presents at 10–15 years (range 5–40 years) with symptoms of liver disease or neurological disease. Hepatic symptoms include jaundice, anorexia, nausea and weight loss, fluid retention, bruising, and bleeding. Neurological manifestations include dysarthria, drooling, movement disorders or tremors, rigidity, ataxia, dystonia, and bradykinesia. Children may also present with school problems or behavior and personality disorders. A less common presentation is with an acute hemolytic crisis. The Kayser-Fleischer ring (corneal pigmentation due to copper) is indicative of central nervous system copper deposition. Wilson's disease is a critical diagnosis to establish, as early treatment can prevent progression of the disorder.[45]

Ceruloplasmin and copper concentrations are also low in this condition, and an increase in the proportion of non-ceruloplasmin bound copper is seen. Urine copper excretion is increased and increases further after a penicillamine load.

Chronic nutritional copper toxicity has not been confirmed as a clinical problem, although excess copper from milk or water contaminated by storage in brass containers has been proposed as the etiology of Indian childhood cirrhosis.[43] Sporadic episodes of acute copper poisoning from water mains[63] or other unusual sources[64] usually have been recognized by acute onset of gastrointestinal symptoms, such as nausea and vomiting.

Assessment of Copper Status

Serum or plasma copper is low at birth but increases to adult concentrations by 4–6 months of age. Moderately higher concentrations are found in girls than in boys after puberty.[10]

Ceruloplasmin, to which most serum copper is bound, follows a similar pattern. Copper and ceruloplasmin increase with oral contraceptive use, in pregnancy, and in malignancy. Hypercupremia with elevated ceruloplasmin also occurs in primary biliary cirrhosis and other cholestatic syndromes.[65]

Non-nutritional causes of low serum copper and ceruloplasmin are Menkes' syndrome and Wilson's disease. Liver copper is high in Wilson's disease, but since copper is not evenly distributed throughout the liver, copper assays must be interpreted with caution.[66] Extremely high concentrations may also be seen in Indian childhood cirrhosis[43] and primary biliary cirrhosis. High liver copper occurs physiologically in the term newborn.

Selenium

Selenium is an essential component of glutathione peroxidase, which detoxifies hydrogen peroxide and other organic peroxides.[67, 68] Other selenoproteins have been identified in blood and tissues, but their function in human physiology is not yet established.[67, 68]

Assessment of selenium nutritional status is increasingly important, as selenium deficiency has been identified in patients on unsupplemented parenteral nutrition[37, 69, 70] and in infants fed formulas, both milk and soy based.[71]

The natural occurrence of areas in China which have both the highest and the lowest known dietary selenium intakes has provided much of the currently known data on human selenium deficiency and toxicity, and clinical syndromes of nutritional deficiency and toxicity have both been described from China.[72]

Disorders of Selenium Metabolism

Selenium Deficiency

Keshan Disease, a multifocal cardiomyopathy predominantly affecting young children in selenium-deficient areas of China, was virtually eradicated from endemic areas by oral supplementation with sodium selenite.[72] Other low-selenium areas such as New Zealand and Finland, where selenium intake is low but not as extreme as in China, have not been similarly affected.[73] However, there is ongoing concern about the relationship between low environmental selenium and long-term population effects, such as death rates from atherosclerotic heart disease and cancer.[74]

Acquired selenium deficiency should be suspected or anticipated in several clinical situations.[75] Severe acquired selenium deficiency has been described in adults,[69] adolescents,[76] children,[37] and infants[70, 77] on parenteral nutrition. Severe deficiency may develop very rapidly after parenteral nutrition is begun in already malnourished infants[77] or premature infants.[70]

Infant formulas have not been supplemented with selenium until now, and selenium deficiency can occur in babies fed soy-based formulas or special metabolic formulas, such as those for phenylketonuria, or in children on enteral formulas.[5] The development of selenium deficiency should also be anticipated in children with malabsorption as in cystic fibrosis, inflammatory bowel disease, or celiac disease.[75]

Symptoms and signs of selenium deficiency include muscle tenderness, pain and weakness, depigmentation of hair and nails, and, in prolonged severe deficiency, cardiomyopathy and death.[75] Plasma selenium concentrations may be extremely low for a long time before symptoms of skeletal myopathy[37] or cardiomyopathy[69, 76] become apparent. Thinning of hair, loss of skin and hair pigmentation, and macrocytosis may be present earlier.[75] Laboratory findings include very low, often undetectable selenium concentrations in plasma, erythrocytes, or whole blood; decreased glutathione peroxidase activity; macrocytosis and erythrocyte fragility; and altered leucocyte metabolism.[75]

Because of the extreme range of reference values found in healthy, free-living populations in different countries, assessment of selenium status must be based on laboratory-specific, locally derived population reference intervals.[75]

Selenium Toxicity

Chronic selenosis (loss of hair and nails; blistering skin lesions; mottled, pitted teeth) was described from a region of very high environmental selenium in China.[72] These extreme effects have never been well documented in other high-selenium areas where animals manifested selenosis.[75]

Accidental chronic ingestion of excess selenium resulted in a similar clinical syndrome characterized by loss of hair and fingernails, fatigue, and breath odor, which was alleviated when selenium intake was discontinued.[42] Acute selenium poisoning may be suspected by a strong garlic breath odor due to dimethylselenide in the expired air.[75]

Assessment of Selenium Status

Selenium may be measured in serum or plasma, erythrocytes, or whole blood. Generally, plasma selenium is most sensitive to selenium depletion and responds most quickly to repletion. Activity of glutathione peroxidase in plasma also reflects recent changes in selenium nutrition more rapidly than the erythrocyte glutathione peroxidase assay.[75]

OTHER ULTRA-TRACE ELEMENTS

There is little clinical information about the other essential ultra-trace elements in pediatrics. Many earlier estimates of reference blood intervals are now recognized to be erroneously high.[32, 33] This is due to previously unrecognized sampling or analytical contamination, as well as technical difficulty of analysis resulting from the extremely low concentrations in biological specimens and the complexity of many biological matrices.[32, 33] A brief review of manganese, molybdenum, and chromium follows.

Manganese

Manganese is an essential element which is a cofactor for numerous enzymes. Manganese appears to be a specific cofactor for mucopolysaccharide glycosyl-transferases, required for mucopolysaccharide synthesis.[78] Prenatal deficiency results in defective chondrogenesis with bone and tendon abnormalities in several animal species.[78]

Disorders of Manganese Metabolism

Clinical manganese deficiency has not been documented in a pediatric population. One case of accidentally induced manganese deficiency in an adult has been described. Symptoms included loss of weight, dermatitis, pigmentary changes of hair, nausea and vomiting, prolonged clotting time and hypocholesterolemia.[78] Manganese deficiency has been associated with epilepsy,[79] but whole blood manganese concentrations in epileptics[79] were higher than concentrations in healthy subjects studied more recently.[80]

Occupational manganese toxicity in miners or dry-cell battery workers is characterized by a severe psychiatric disturbance and a Parkinson-like syndrome.[78] No clinical manganese toxicity has been identified in children, but plasma manganese has been reported to be almost three times normal in parenterally fed patients with cholestasis[81] and to decrease on removal of supplemental manganese from parenteral infusates.

Assessment of Manganese Status

Adult concentrations of manganese in whole blood approximate 10 µg/L and in plasma, 1 µg/L.[80] Serum concentrations in healthy Swedish children were 0.43 µg/L.[82] Manganese assays are not generally available, and laboratory assessment of manganese status remains a research area at present.

Molybdenum

Molybdenum is an integral component of molybdopterin, a cofactor required for normal function of molybdoenzymes.[83] Xanthine dehydrogenase or oxidase is deficient in the autosomal recessive disorder, xanthinuria. Deficiency of sulfite oxidase, which detoxifies sulfite by converting it to sulfate, results in a congenital syndrome characterized by severe neurological disease.[83]

Molybdenum cofactor deficiency, an inherited disorder, has been described in 15 cases.[40] The clinical syndrome and biochemical findings combine features of both xanthinuria and sulfite oxidase deficiency. The infants may have brain atrophy, hydrocephalus, and bilateral lens ectopia, and present with hypertonia, seizures, and severe psychomotor retardation.

Disorders of Molybdenum Metabolism

Nutritional molybdenum deficiency has not been recognized in infants or children. Acquired molybdenum deficiency was described in an adult on long-term total parenteral nutrition who developed headaches and night blindness and progressed from lethargy to coma after about 18 months of total parenteral nutrition.[7] The biochemical findings suggested deficient functioning of both xanthine oxidase and sulfite oxidase enzymes. The laboratory results included hypouricemia, hypouricosuria, increased serum methionine, and excess urinary thiosulfate and sulfite. Infusion of ammonium molybdate reversed these findings.

Assessment of Molybdenum Status

There is little reference data for molybdenum in serum or blood. Serum molybdenum in maternal and cord serum was reported to approximate 1.44 µg/L.[84] Diagnosis of molybdenum deficiency requires demonstration of decreased xanthine oxidase and sulfite oxidase activity, shown by hypouricemia, hypouricosuria, increased serum methionine, and excess urinary thiosulfate and sulfite, which improves on molybdenum supplementation.[7]

Chromium

Trivalent chromium is a component of a biologically active factor which is thought to potentiate the action of insulin.[85] Although chromium deficiency has not been confirmed in pediatrics, acquired chromium deficiency has been reported in three adults on long-term total parenteral nutrition.[6, 86, 87] These patients developed hyperglycemia with abnormally high insulin requirements, weight loss, and peripheral neuropathy. Supplemental chromium improved the symptoms. However, in a young boy on long-term, unsupplemented total parenteral nutrition, no symptoms of chromium deficiency were found.[88]

Improvement of glucose tolerance after chromium supplementation has been reported in malnourished children.[89]

Assessment of Chromium Status

Chromium assays in blood and urine are not generally available, and laboratory assessment of chromium status remains a research area at present.

VITAMINS

Vitamins are trace organic compounds that are needed in adequate amounts in the diet to allow normal metabolism and prevent deficiency diseases. The 13 substances usually considered as vitamins are the fat-soluble vitamins—A (retinol), D (cholecalciferol), E (tocopherol), and K—and the water-soluble vitamins—thiamin (B_1), riboflavin (B_2), niacin (B_3), pyridoxine (B_6), cobalamin (B_{12}), folic acid, ascorbic acid (vitamin C), biotin, and pantothenic acid.[90]

The most common vitamin nutritional problem is deficiency, but toxicity is of increasing concern in affluent populations with widespread use of vitamin supplements, occasional accidental ingestion, and unusual diets.[91] In children, inborn errors of metabolism may cause vitamin dependency states that respond to high-dose supplementation with the appropriate cofactor vitamin.[92]

Vitamin A

Vitamin A (retinol) is obtained from plant carotenoids or retinyl esters in animal tissues. Retinol is absorbed after cleavage of β-carotene or hydrolysis of the esters in the intestinal lumen, re-esterified in the mucosal cell, and transported via chylomicrons to the liver. Hydrolysis and re-esterification occur again in the liver prior to storage. Retinol is cycled from the main body store in the liver to the tissues, where it is required for vision, spermatogenesis, maintenance of epithelial tissues and the immune system, and promotion of cell growth and differentiation.

Retinol circulates bound in a 1 : 1 complex with retinol binding protein (RBP). RBP secretion requires adequate retinol, and serum retinol concentration depends on RBP concentrations. In deficiency, both are low. Toxicity is thought to occur when retinol exceeds the binding capacity of RBP and liver and unbound retinol or retinyl esters damage cell membranes.[93]

Disorders of Retinol Metabolism

Retinol Deficiency

Vitamin A deficiency is a major nutritional problem in much of the world, with peak incidence in preschool children. Clinical signs progress from abnormal dark adaptation due to impaired regeneration of rhodopsin, to xerophthalmia, and culminate in keratomalacia or corneal ulceration and blindness. In severe deficiency, epithelia of genitourinary, gastrointestinal, and respiratory tracts also become abnormal. Deficiency predisposes to infection and increased mortality, and infection or protein energy malnutrition can precipitate clinical signs of deficiency.[2]

In better nourished populations, risk factors for deficiency include prematurity,[94] food faddism, parenteral nutrition, and fat malabsorption.

Inherited Metabolic Defects

There is a rare inherited defect in the ability to convert carotene to retinol. When carotenoids are the main dietary source of retinol, these patients develop carotenemia and vitamin A deficiency.[95, 96]

Retinol Toxicity

Acute toxicity causes anorexia, vomiting, irritability, drowsiness, and increased intracranial pressure (bulging fontanelles in infants). In chronic toxicity, hepatomegaly, hyperostosis and premature closure of epiphyses, photophobia, alopecia, pruritus, and skin erythema and desquamation also develop. Liver disease or protein energy malnutrition increase the risk of toxicity. Intake of more than 15,000–20,000 IU retinol or therapeutic doses of retinoids in pregnancy can cause congenital anomalies. Lower doses in animal models have caused learning disabilities or behavioral defects.[95] β-carotene is not known to be toxic. Only a portion of the carotene is converted to retinol in the gut; some is absorbed intact, circulates bound to lipids, and is stored in adipose tissue and skin, giving a characteristic yellow skin with white sclerae. Carotenemia is often due to excessive dietary intake but also has been found in diabetes mellitus, hypothyroidism, hypopituitarism, anorexia nervosa or rapid weight loss, castration, liver disease, chronic glomerulonephritis, nephrotic syndrome, and malaria.[96] Retinol concentrations in dietary carotenemia are usually in the upper part of the reference range.[96]

Assessment of Retinol Status

Tests of vitamin A status recently have been reviewed.[97, 98] Serum retinol or vitamin A concentrations are the usual index of vitamin A status. Values less than 0.7 μmol/L (20 μg/dL) are considered low, and concentrations less than 0.35 μmol/L (10 μg/dL) deficient. Interpretation must take into account the dependence of retinol concentrations on RBP and the factors that affect RBP (Table 1–3).

Retinol concentrations tend to plateau in toxicity because of the association with RBP, but retinyl esters increase. Thus, non-specific vitamin A methods or measurement of retinyl esters may be useful in this situation. Fasting specimens are required for measurement of retinyl esters, but not retinol.

Serum RBP has been suggested as a substitute for vitamin A measurement, with the limitations above. It is not altered in toxicity.

Serum carotene reflects vitamin A status only when carotenoids are the main dietary source of vitamin A.[98] Serum carotene is increased in carotenemia. Low concentrations suggest poor dietary intake or fat malabsorption. Further investigation of these conditions has been outlined elsewhere.[96]

Tests of dark adaptation and the histological test, conjunctival impression cytology,[97, 98] are not described here.

The Relative Dose Response (RDR) test is a biochemical loading test that may be more sensitive for marginal vitamin A deficiency than serum retinol concentrations. It involves sampling for serum retinol while fasting, again 5 hours after administration of an oral vitamin A load, and calculating the percentage increase in serum retinol relative to the 5 hour concentration. Since RBP secretion is decreased in vitamin A deficiency, RBP accumulates and is then mobilized by the test vitamin A dose, resulting in a RDR greater than 20%.[97, 98]

Hepatic vitamin A is considered the best index of vitamin A status, but specimens are seldom available. Isotope dilution also has been used to estimate vitamin A reserves.[97, 98]

Vitamin D

Vitamin D is now considered a prohormone. All of the human requirement can be produced in the skin. When 7-dehydrocholesterol in the epidermis is exposed to sunlight or UVB radiation, it forms a pre-vitamin that isomerizes to vitamin D_3 (cholecalciferol). The supply of endogenous vitamin D_3 depends on season, latitude, length of sun exposure, use of sunscreens, skin pigmentation, and age.[99] Vitamin D is also obtained from the diet, either as vitamin D_3 from fish oils, or vitamin D_2 (ergocalciferol) from plant sources. They are equally effective as supplements.

Vitamin D is metabolized to the active hormone, 1,25-dihydroxy vitamin D, by 25-hydroxylation in the liver followed by 1-hydroxylation in the kidney. Concentrations of 1,25-dihydroxy vitamin D are tightly regulated and vary with concentrations of parathyroid hormone, calcium, phosphate, calcitonin, estrogens, and possibly other hormones. The hormone acts by stimulating DNA transcription and synthesis of vitamin D-dependent proteins. The main effects of 1,25-dihydroxy vitamin D are to increase intestinal absorption of calcium and phosphate, stimulate osteoclast and osteoblast activity and synthesis of calcium binding proteins in bone, modify renal calcium and phosphorus excretion, and regulate its own metabolism. Effects on polyamine synthesis, insulin secretion, and differentiation of bone marrow and skin also have been discovered.[100, 101]

Disorders of Vitamin D Metabolism

Vitamin D Deficiency

Vitamin D deficiency results in muscle weakness, hypotonia, and bone deformities and fractures (rickets in children and osteomalacia in adults). It occurs only when exposure to sunlight and vitamin D intake and absorption are insufficient, or when metabolic activation of vitamin D is impaired.[99]

Vitamin D deficiency may occur in children with fat malabsorption, chronic hepatic or renal disease, or altered vitamin D metabolism. In chronic liver disease, low 25-hydroxy vitamin D concentrations may reflect decreased synthesis of D-binding protein (low total but normal free concentrations) rather than a true deficiency.[102] True deficiency in advanced liver disease is due to vitamin D malabsorption or decreased 25-hydroxylation. 1-hydroxylation is decreased in chronic renal failure, and there may be peripheral resistance to vitamin D. Supplementation with 1,25-dihydroxy vitamin D or analogues prevents bone disease. Vitamin D metabolism is altered in children with abnormal parathyroid function, and possibly in those receiving anticonvulsants. Target organ effects of anticonvulsants also have been postulated.[103]

Newborns, especially premature infants, may have a low vitamin D supply from the mother and seem to have high vitamin D requirements, possibly due to decreased absorption, altered metabolism, or immature intestinal response to 1,25-dihydroxy vitamin D. Vitamin D supplementation is recommended, in combination with adequate phosphorus and calcium intake to prevent rickets.[104, 105]

Inherited Metabolic Defects

Inherited defects in vitamin D metabolism recently have been renamed to more accurately reflect current knowledge of their pathogenesis.[106]

Pseudo vitamin D deficiency (formerly vitamin D dependent rickets) occurs in two forms, Type I and Type II. These autosomal recessive disorders present at 2 months to 2 years of age with clinical features of dietary vitamin D deficiency unresponsive to usual doses of vitamin D. Some patients with Type II have alopecia. Type I is due to defective renal 1-hydroxylase, resulting in low or undetectable 1,25-dihydroxy vitamin D, despite normal or increased 25-hydroxy vitamin D. In Type II, 1,25-dihydroxy vitamin D concentrations are increased rather than decreased, suggesting a vitamin D receptor defect. Five types of vitamin D receptor abnormalities have been identified in different kindreds.[106]

Hypophosphatemic (vitamin D resistant) rickets is caused by renal tubular defects in phosphate reabsorption that lead to phosphate wasting and secondary hyperparathyroidism. The defect in the most common form, X-linked dominant familial hypophosphatemic rickets, also involves renal 25-hydroxy vitamin D 1-hydroxylase. 1,25-dihydroxy vitamin D concentrations are inappropriately low for the hypophosphatemia.[101]

A defect in vitamin D metabolism has been considered in idiopathic infantile hypercalcemia (Williams-Beuren syndrome). Patients have elfin facies, failure to thrive, and sometimes supravalvular aortic stenosis and mental handicap. Calcium absorption during the first two years of life is increased despite hypercalcemia, suggesting possible increased sensitivity to vitamin D. Measurements of vitamin D metabolites have been inconclusive.[105, 106]

Vitamin D Toxicity

Vitamin D toxicity is due to increased intestinal absorption of calcium and hypercalcemia. Toxicity is less severe if dietary calcium and phosphorus are low. Symptoms include feeding difficulties, poor weight gain, polydipsia, polyuria, dehydration, and hyperreflexia. Chronic hypercalcemia leads to renal tubular damage, renal stones, ectopic calcification, arterial damage and hypertension.[105, 107]

Toxicity is caused by excessive enteral or parenteral vitamin D intake or increased synthesis of 1,25-dihydroxy vitamin D as in primary hyperparathyroidism, sarcoidosis, and other granulomatous diseases (unregulated 1-hydroxylation by macrophages) and lymphoma. High doses of vitamin D are used in hypoparathyroidism, pseudohypoparathyroidism, renal osteodystrophy, inherited defects of vitamin D or phosphate metabolism, and psoriasis. These patients must be monitored carefully.[107] High-dose vitamin D in pregnancy has minimal effect on the fetus.[105]

Assessment of Vitamin D Status

Analyses of vitamin D metabolites are not always available, and indirect tests are usually the first approach. Radiographic evidence of decreased bone mineralization may suggest a deficiency. Serum calcium and phosphorus are often low in children with vitamin D deficiency, but are not specific. Vitamin D toxicity should always be considered as a possible cause of hypercalcemia.[98]

Alkaline phosphatase increases early in rickets, but it is particularly difficult to interpret in children because of variation in reference ranges with sex and age[10] and sporadic unexplained high values, as in transient benign hyperphosphatasemia.

Serum total 25-hydroxy vitamin D is the best test of vitamin D status in the absence of liver damage.[104, 108] The method chosen must measure 25-hydroxylated forms of both vitamin D_2 and D_3 to detect dietary supplements. Reference ranges vary with season and location. Rickets is usually present when concentrations are below 7.5 nmol/L (3 µg/L); concentrations from 7.5–25 nmol/L (3–10 µg/L) are considered at risk.[98] Measurement of free 25-hydroxy vitamin D eliminates variations due to D-binding protein, but it is not routine.[102] D-binding protein decreases in newborns and liver disease and increases in pregnancy.

Serum 1,25-dihydroxy vitamin D is a poor indicator of vitamin D status because of the tight hormonal regulation, but it should be measured when abnormal metabolism is suspected. Assays are complex because of the low concentration and similarity to other, more plentiful vitamin D metabolites. Plasma concentrations are 40–140 pmol/L (25–65 ng/L) in adults[99,108] and higher in children.[106] Methods for measuring vitamin D metabolites have been reviewed.[108]

Vitamin E

Metabolism and clinical effects of vitamin E have been reviewed recently.[109] Vitamin E refers to tocopherols and tocotrienols, of which α-tocopherol is the most bioactive. Tocopherols are incorporated into bile salt-lipid micelles for intestinal absorption. In the mucosal cell, absorbed tocopherol is secreted with chylomicrons and taken up by the liver. α-tocopherol is preferentially resecreted in VLDL particles, remaining with the particle as VLDL are catabolized to LDL and HDL. Plasma or serum tocopherol is associated mainly with LDL and HDL, according to the distribution of total lipids.[110]

Cells take up tocopherols released by lipoprotein lipase action on chylomicrons or VLDL, or with LDL via the LDL receptor pathway. Tocopherol is incorporated into cell membranes, where it interrupts free-radical-catalyzed lipid peroxidation, protecting against oxidative damage. It is regenerated by other antioxidant systems, such as ascorbic acid or reduced glutathione.

Disorders of Vitamin E Metabolism

Vitamin E Deficiency

Vitamin E deficiency causes neural and muscular degeneration presenting as spinocerebellar ataxia, loss of proprioception and vibration sense and deep tendon reflexes, myopathy, ophthalmoplegia, and retinopathy.[109] Overt neurological signs develop only after several years of deficiency. In the neonate, vitamin E deficiency may cause hemolytic anemia. Symptomatic deficiency is rarely due to diet alone, because vitamin E is abundant in vegetable oils, cereal grains, animal fats, and liver. Except for inherited conditions, it is always related to chronic fat malabsorption as in chronic cholestasis, abetalipoproteinemia, short bowel syndrome, or cystic fibrosis. Neurologic findings occur earliest (2–3 y) and are most severe in unsupplemented children with neonatal cholestatic disorders because of low stores at birth, severe fat malabsorption, and possibly increased oxidative stresses secondary to liver disease. Symptoms develop in 5–10 y in other congenital disorders, and in 10–20 y in cystic fibrosis or later-onset malabsorptive disorders.[109]

Inherited Metabolic Defects

Clinical signs of vitamin E deficiency were first recognized in abetalipoproteinemia. Vitamin E deficiency in this and related disorders is a result of impaired absorption of fat and fat-soluble vitamins and impaired transport due to lack of apolipoprotein-B containing lipoproteins.[109]

An inherited defect specific for vitamin E has been described in the last decade. Familial isolated vitamin E deficiency is characterized by development of neurological findings of vitamin E deficiency in children or young adults with otherwise normal intestinal absorption. Incorporation of tocopherol into VLDL in hepatocytes is thought to be impaired. Patients respond to oral vitamin E supplementation.[109, 111]

Vitamin E Toxicity

The toxicity of oral vitamin E in adults appears to be low. High doses may worsen coagulation defects in vitamin K deficient individuals, and caution has been advised when replacing vitamin E in patients with malabsorption or on anticoagulants.[112]

The situation in low-birth-weight infants is unclear. Tocopherol seems to decrease the incidence of serious peri- and intraventricular hemorrhage, but the amount required is unknown.[113] Concentrations above 35-45 mg/L (80–100 µmol/L) have been associated with an increased incidence of necrotizing enterocolitis.[114] Toxicity could be due to factors other than tocopherol in the administered preparations, as in the case of the parenteral preparation, E-Ferol, which also contained polysorbates.[115]

Assessment of Vitamin E Status

α-tocopherol (or total tocopherol) can be quantitated in plasma or serum. Reference ranges are approximately 4–11 mg/L (10–25 µmol/L). Interpretation is complicated by the association of tocopherol with lipoproteins. In hyperlipidemia, as in cholestasis or pregnancy, increased tocopherol in the circulation may mask a deficiency. Conversely, when lipoproteins are low, as in newborns or in abetalipoproteinemia, little tocopherol can be carried in plasma and concentrations do not reflect body stores. The effect of hyperlipidemia is diminished by calculating the ratio of tocopherol to total lipids or to cholesterol.[116]

Tocopherol in red blood cells, leukocytes, buccal mucosal cells,[117] and in adipose, neural, and other tissues are currently being researched. Adipose tissue obtained by needle biopsy is used for definitive assessment of tocopherol status.[109] Hepatic tocopherol does not reflect stores because the liver contains tocopherols for biliary excretion.

Tests of vitamin E function are used when tocopherol concentrations are unavailable or interpretation is problematic, as in hypolipidemia. Red blood cell response to *in vitro* oxidation is measured in the hydrogen peroxide hemolysis test or its more sensitive variation, peroxide-induced release of thiobarbituric acid-reactive substances from red blood cells.[118] A new research technique, determination of exhaled pentane, reflects *in vivo* oxidation.[119]

Vitamin K

Vitamin K is a coenzyme for the activation of a number of proteins by post-translational gamma-carboxylation of glutamic acid residues. Proteins involved include the coagulation factors II (prothrombin), VII, IX, and X; plasma proteins C, S, and Z; and the vitamin D-dependent bone proteins, bone Gla-protein (osteocalcin) and bone matrix Gla-protein.[120-122]

Vitamin K occurs in two forms: vitamin K_1 (phylloquinone) from green plants, and vitamin K_2 (menaquinones) synthesized by intestinal bacteria. (Vitamin K_3, menadione, does not occur naturally but can be alkylated to menaquinones *in vivo*.) The body pool of vitamin K is small compared to other fat-soluble vitamins, and the requirement is unexpectedly low because of efficient regeneration of vitamin K hydroquinone after its oxidation during gamma-carboxylation. This process has been reviewed in detail.[120, 121, 123] The three-step vitamin K cycle is blocked by coumarin anticoagulants and other drugs but can be bypassed by large doses of vitamin K.

Disorders of Vitamin K Metabolism

Vitamin K Deficiency

Newborn infants are at high risk for vitamin K deficiency because of poor placental transfer, low hepatic stores, low content in human milk, questionable absorption, and lack of intestinal flora. This causes hemorrhagic disease of the newborn (HDN). The classical type presents at 1–7 d with gastrointestinal or skin bleeding or bruising and is prevented by administration of vitamin K at birth. The other two types of HDN are more serious because of the risk of intracranial hemorrhage. Early HDN (in the first day of life) is related to poor maternal nutrition or use of coumarins, anticonvulsants, or antitubercular drugs during pregnancy. Antepartum vitamin K supplementation of pregnant women at risk is preventative. Late HDN occurs between 2 w – 3 m in breast-fed infants not given prophylactic vitamin K, or in infants with fat malabsorption. Idiopathic cases might be due to transient subclinical hepatic dysfunction.[124, 125]

Vitamin K deficiency is much less common after the newborn period but can occur with severely restricted diet or intravenous nutrition, usually in combination with bowel-sterilizing antibiotics, or with fat malabsorption. In liver disease, coagulation defects may be due only partly to vitamin K deficiency; non-vitamin-K-dependent synthesis of coagulation factors is often impaired as well.[25] Coumarin anticoagulants, certain cephalosporins, salicylate, and other drugs interfere with the vitamin K cycle, causing functional deficiency.[122] High doses of vitamins A and E also antagonize vitamin K; the former by decreasing absorption, the latter probably on a metabolic basis.[121]

Inherited Metabolic Defects

Variable requirements for vitamin K in the neonate and abnormal responses to vitamin K and warfarin may be manifestations of inherited defects in vitamin K metabolism. Familial deficiency of protein C, a vitamin K-dependent anticoagulant and fibrinolytic protein, responds in some cases to vitamin K.[92] Congenital deficiency of vitamin K epoxide has features similar to fetal warfarin syndrome.[122]

Vitamin K Toxicity

The toxicity of oral phylloquinone has not been well documented.[126] High doses of oral vitamin K block the effect of oral anticoagulants.[127] Parenteral phylloquinone may rarely cause skin lesions, probably due to delayed hypersensitivity.[128] Menadiol in high doses may cause hemolysis and contribute to neonatal jaundice and kernicterus.[92]

Assessment of Vitamin K Status

Methods for the assessment of vitamin K status are rapidly evolving. At present, functional tests usually are used. The traditional index of deficiency, prolongation of the one-stage prothrombin time (with prolonged partial thromboplastin time and normal thrombin time) is convenient but not very sensitive. Concentrations of individual clotting factors, particularly factor VII, which has the shortest half-life, may be better.[123]

Immunoassays for incompletely gamma-carboxylated clotting factors (Proteins Induced by Vitamin K Absence or Antagonism, PIVKA) are the most promising tests at present.[122] PIVKA-II, abnormal prothrombin, is usually measured. Concentrations are very low or undetectable in normal individuals but increase dramatically in vitamin K deficiency and remain so for a few days after supplementation, allowing later documentation of a deficiency. Advantages include sensitivity, stability, and use of serum as a sample. Specificity for vitamin K deficiency must be determined.

Phylloquinones and menaquinones can be measured by HPLC, but methods are difficult. Low plasma concentrations reflect reduced liver reserves. As for vitamin E, plasma lipids affect the values. An interesting finding is a transient decrease after fractures.[122] More study of various parameters of vitamin K status is needed to establish interpretive guidelines for these assays.

Thiamin

Thiamin (vitamin B_1) is found in whole grain or enriched cereals, meat, vegetables, and dairy products. Requirements increase with diets high in carbohydrate and calories. Raw fish, shellfish, tea leaves, betel nuts, ferns, and some microorganisms contain thiaminases that inactivate thiamin.[129, 130]

Thiamin is absorbed in jejunum and ileum by a saturable carrier-mediated transport process. It circulates bound to albumin, is taken up by cells, phosphorylated, and retained mainly as the diphosphate. There is no significant storage. Deficiency develops after about 2–3 w inadequate intake. Thiamin diphosphate is a coenzyme for oxidative decarboxylation in the pyruvate, α-ketoglutarate and branched-chain ketoacid dehydrogenase complexes and for transketolase reactions in the pentose phosphate pathway. Deficiency disrupts oxidative metabolism of glucose, and tissue damage results from energy depletion.[129] The physiology and pathology of thiamin have been reviewed.[129, 130]

Disorders of Thiamin Metabolism

Thiamin Deficiency

The clinical presentation of thiamin deficiency depends on age, caloric intake and physical activity, as well as the chronicity of thiamin depletion.

Beriberi is caused by chronic dietary deficiency of thiamin. It is endemic where the diet consists of refined cereals (polished rice), or thiaminase-containing foods. Peripheral polyneuropathy (dry beriberi) predominates when total caloric intake is low. High physical activity and high caloric intake predispose to wet beriberi, so called because of high output cardiac failure and peripheral edema. Occasionally, cardiac failure is acute and fulminant.[129, 130]

Infantile beriberi develops in infants receiving inadequate thiamin from breast milk of deficient mothers or from deficient formulas. Clinical signs include transient gastrointestinal disturbances followed by fairly acute neurological or cardiac deterioration and death. Aphonia or meningismus sometimes occur.[131]

Wernicke's encephalopathy is characterized by confusion, nystagmus, ophthalmoplegia, ataxia and peripheral neuropathy, and Korsakoff's psychosis by memory impairment. Administration of carbohydrate without thiamin often precipitates encephalopathy. It responds to thiamin, but Korsakoff's psychosis often persists. The syndrome is most common in adult alcoholics, but has been described in adults with malnutrition or vomiting (dietary deficiency, anorexia nervosa, parenteral nutrition, hyperemesis gravidarum, gastric disorders, lymphoma).[129, 132, 133] Wernicke's encephalopathy can also occur in children on parenteral or enteral feedings that contain inadequate thiamin to meet their requirements.[134]

Inherited Metabolic Defects

The inherited disorder, thiamin responsive megaloblastic anemia with diabetes mellitus and sensorineural deafness, is thought to be a disorder of thiamin transport. Thiamin concentrations in plasma and red blood cells are low, despite normal dietary thiamin intake, but values increase and clinical symptoms improve after thiamin supplementation.[135]

Some cases of maple syrup urine disease respond to thiamin. In these patients, thiamin appears to stabilize the defective branched-chain ketoacid dehydrogenase enzyme complex, thereby improving its activity.[129, 130]

Thiamin Toxicity

Toxicity of oral thiamin is not expected because of limited intestinal transport. Hypersensitivity reactions, possibly due to impurities in the formulations, have occasionally occurred.[126]

Thiamin toxicity was postulated to contribute to Sudden Infant Death Syndrome, but altered thiamin concentrations in postmortem specimens were probably artifactual.[136]

Assessment of Thiamin Status

Techniques for assessing thiamin status have been reviewed.[130, 137] Transketolase is convenient to measure because it is present in erythrocytes. Activity decreases in thiamin deficiency due to cofactor depletion, but in more severe deficiency or liver disease, apoenzyme also decreases. Basal activity and response to addition of excess thiamin diphosphate (TPP) are measured. Increased percent stimulation by TPP is characteristic of deficiency. Problems with this index of thiamin deficiency include alterations in disease, instability of the enzyme, analytical variability, and the possibility of enzyme variants with different activities.[137-139]

Total thiamin and thiamin phosphate esters can be measured in blood, urine, or cells. Erythrocyte thiamin diphosphate may be a better predictor of thiamin status than transketolase.[139] Urinary thiamin or excretion of a thiamin load have been used to detect deficiency in population studies.

Riboflavin

Recent reviews of riboflavin metabolism[140] and clinical significance[141] are available. Riboflavin is found in dairy products, meat, yeast, eggs, and plants. Bound and coenzyme forms in the diet are hydrolyzed to free riboflavin, which is absorbed by a saturable transport process. Bile acids are required. Riboflavin circulates in plasma bound mainly to immunoglobulins. Additional plasma and placental riboflavin-binding proteins appear during pregnancy, presumably to enhance riboflavin delivery to the fetus.[140]

Riboflavin is converted in cells to its active coenzyme forms, riboflavin-5'-phosphate (flavin mononucleotide, FMN) and flavin adenine dinucleotide (FAD).[140] These coenzymes are essential for the numerous electron transfer reactions involved in metabolism of glucose, fatty acids, and amino acids and formation of pyridoxine and folic acid coenzymes.

Disorders of Riboflavin Metabolism

Riboflavin Deficiency

Clinical signs of riboflavin deficiency are not specific. They include angular stomatitis, cheilosis, glossitis, and seborrheic dermatitis.[141] Deficiency syndromes of riboflavin, pyridoxine, and niacin overlap because FMN is required for activation of pyridoxine, and coenzymes of riboflavin and pyridoxine are necessary for conversion of tryptophan to niacin.[140]

Inadequate diet is the main cause of riboflavin deficiency worldwide. Pregnant women and neonates are at increased risk.[141] Riboflavin is light sensitive and decreases in infant feeds exposed to light, or in infants themselves during phototherapy for hyperbilirubinemia.[142] Deficiency also occurs in alcoholics, due to dietary deficiency and altered metabolism, and in anorexia nervosa,[138] biliary atresia, liver disease, and diabetes mellitus.[143] Chlorpromazine, other phenothiazines, and tricyclic antidepressants inhibit riboflavin conversion to FAD, and supplementation is recommended. Boric acid intoxication also requires riboflavin replacement.[141]

Inherited Metabolic Defects

A number of metabolic defects involving flavoenzymes have shown a response to riboflavin. These include various defects in fatty acyl-CoA dehydrogenase flavoenzymes, defective NADH-CoQ reductase, congenital methemoglobinemia, and one case of pyruvate kinase deficiency.[141, 144]

Riboflavin Toxicity

There is no known toxicity associated with oral riboflavin.[126]

Assessment of Riboflavin Status

Erythrocyte glutathione reductase, with and without *in vitro* stimulation by excess flavin adenine dinucleotide, is the most common procedure for assessing riboflavin status. The relative response to stimulation by FAD increases in deficiency. Reference ranges are method-dependent.[141, 143] This enzyme is more stable *in vitro* than transketolase.[138] Activity varies with the age of the patient and the age of the erythrocytes.[137] Values are not reliable in glucose-6-phosphate dehydrogenase deficiency because FAD is not lost with riboflavin depletion, giving a falsely normal activation coefficient.[141]

Riboflavin can be measured in blood, urine, and other specimens.[137] Plasma riboflavin responds rapidly to dietary intake and is not a useful index of riboflavin status. Flavins in red blood cells are in the cofactor forms, and more closely reflect tissue concentrations.[141]

Urine excretion and fractional excretion of a test dose of riboflavin are useful for monitoring riboflavin status. Differences between normal and deficient individuals are greater for urine than for blood values.[141] Reference ranges are age-dependent.[143]

Niacin

Niacin is a descriptive term for pyridine-3-carboxylic acid (nicotinic acid) and its derivatives with similar biological activity.[145] Niacin is essential for the formation of the coenzymes nicotinamide adenine dinucleotide (NAD) and nicotinamide adenine dinucleotide phosphate (NADP). It can be obtained from the diet or synthesized from tryptophan.

Disorders of Niacin Metabolism

Niacin Deficiency

Niacin deficiency (pellagra) is characterized by dermatitis (skin sensitivity, desquamation, hyperpigmentation, and hyperkeratosis), diarrhea with atrophy and inflammation of small intestinal, gastric (achlorhydria) and oral mucosa (glossitis, cheilitis, angular stomatitis), dementia (depression, psychosis, encephalopathy, seizures), and ultimately death. Other findings include peripheral neuropathy and ataxia, failure to grow, and anemia.

Pellagra occurs when dietary niacin and tryptophan are inadequate, poorly available, or not absorbed; when synthesis from tryptophan is impaired; or when losses are excessive. Risk factors include famine, maize diets, malabsorption, chronic diarrhea, cirrhosis, cancer, diabetes mellitus, hemodialysis, pyridoxine or riboflavin deficiencies, and excess dietary leucine (millet diet). The last three may interfere with niacin synthesis from tryptophan, but this is controversial.[145, 146]

Niacin Toxicity

Megadose niacin has been tried in schizophrenia, depression, and other disorders,[146] but its only use at present is in the management of hyperlipidemia. Complications of nicotinic acid include flushing, gastrointestinal upset, cutaneous problems, hypertension, headache, hyperuricemia, gout, and impaired glucose tolerance.[147] Occasional patients develop dose-related cholestasis and acute hepatocellular damage.[148]

Assessment of Niacin Status

Laboratory assessment of niacin status has been controversial. The traditional approach is to measure urinary metabolites N′-methyl-nicotinamide (NMN) and N′-methyl-2-pyridone-5-carboxylamide (2-pyridone). Decreased NMN or a ratio of NMN : 2-pyridone less than one suggest latent deficiency.[143] Recent depletion studies show that NMN tracks dietary intake, but erythrocyte NAD and NAD : NADP ratio are better indices of body supply. In severe deficiency, plasma tryptophan is also low.[149] Vitamin indices have not been studied in toxicity, but bilirubin, hepatocellular enzymes, and uric acid should be monitored.

Vitamin B$_6$

Vitamin B$_6$ occurs naturally as pyridoxine (PN), pyridoxal (PL), pyridoxamine (PM), and their phosphorylated forms. In humans, pyridox-al-5-phosphate (PLP) and pyridoxamine-5-phosphate (PMP) act as coenzymes in reactions involved in amino acid metabolism: transamination, deamination, desulfhydration, and nonoxidative decarboxylation. The physiology, pathology, and functions of vitamin B$_6$ have been reviewed recently.[150, 151]

Dietary vitamin B$_6$ is absorbed mainly in the jejunum, phosphorylated in the liver, and largely stored in muscle. In plasma, PL and PLP are bound to albumin; PL is also taken up by red blood cells and bound to hemoglobin. Clearance of PLP from plasma is inversely related to alkaline phosphatase activity. The main excretory product is urinary 4-pyridoxic acid.[140, 150]

Disorders of Vitamin B$_6$ Metabolism

Vitamin B$_6$ Deficiency

Florid vitamin B$_6$ deficiency is rare in humans, but has been described in infants fed formula in which the vitamin was destroyed by autoclaving. Deficiency is characterized by hypochromic microcytic anemia, weight loss, vomiting, and central nervous system abnormalities, including electroencephalogram changes, hyperirritability, depression, confusion, and convulsions. Some patients have had dermatitis, glossitis, stomatitis, cheilosis, kidney stones, dental caries, or immunological abnormalities.[152]

Pediatric patients at risk for vitamin B_6 deficiency include those with inadequate dietary intake (particularly infants who require relatively large amounts for deposition in rapidly growing muscle); malabsorption (celiac disease); ingestion of carbonyl compounds such as isoniazid, hydrazine, penicillamine, and mushrooms; phototherapy for hyperbilirubinemia; chronic renal failure with dialysis or renal transplant; oral contraceptive use; and pregnancy or lactation.[151]

Inherited Metabolic Defects

Pyridoxine dependency refers to an inherited condition characterized by infantile convulsions responsive to pharmacological doses of pyridoxine. The mechanism is thought to involve deficient synthesis of GABA because of either defective binding of PLP to apoenzyme or instability of the PLP-albumin complex in plasma.[153]

Metabolic diseases such as sideroblastic anemia, homocystinuria, cystathioninuria, xanthurenic aciduria, ornithinemia, and primary hyperoxaluria may improve when high-dose pyridoxine is given.[151, 154] In other pediatric conditions, such as attention deficit disorder, autism, mental retardation, and Down's syndrome, megadose vitamin B_6 has been tried, but its efficacy is not proven.

Vitamin B_6 Toxicity

Pyridoxine toxicity is suspected clinically when peripheral sensory neuropathy occurs in a patient supplemented with high doses of the vitamin. Pyridoxine doses above 200 mg/d or cumulative doses of 1 g in adults may be toxic.[126, 155] The toxic dose in children is not known. Neonates treated for seizures occasionally collapse and may require ventilation.[156]

Assessment of Vitamin B_6 Status

Either of the pyridoxine-dependent enzymes, erythrocyte alanine aminotransferase (EALT) or aspartate aminotransferase (EAST), can be assayed. Basal enzyme activity and the increase in activity after addition of exogenous PLP are measured. Low basal activity and increased stimulation index reflect deficiency. Interpretation of basal EALT activity is complicated by genetic polymorphism affecting enzyme structure and activity. Only the EALT stimulation index is independent of phenotype.[157] EAST is not subject to genetic variation, so a population reference range can be used.

Plasma PLP concentrations parallel intake if taken at steady state 10 days after a change in diet. Concentrations do not reflect vitamin status in hypophosphatasia or cirrhosis (altered PLP clearance) or in acute hepatic failure, including Reye's syndrome (high concentrations due to release from liver). Erythrocyte PLP may be more useful.[158]

Urinary 4-pyridoxic acid excretion parallels steady state intake of vitamin B_6. Xanthurenic acid excretion after a tryptophan load has been used in population studies but may be misleading when the pathway is disturbed for other reasons, as in women taking estrogens. The kynurenine load test or methionine load test have been used in this situation.[137, 158] Standard problems of timed urine collections and creatinine excretions limit the usefulness of loading tests in children. Literature reference values for tests of vitamin B_6 status have been compiled.[150]

Vitamin B_{12} and Folate

The metabolic actions of vitamin B_{12} and folate are interdependent, so these vitamins are discussed together. Vitamin B_{12} (cobalamin) is required to form the coenzymes (methylcobalamin and adenosyl-cobalamin) necessary for synthesis of methionine from homocysteine (a reaction also involving methyltetrahydrofolate) and for the conversion of methylmalonyl-CoA to succinyl-CoA. Folate, usually as a polyglutamate, is involved in a number of single carbon transfer reactions that are important for the synthesis of purines, pyrimidine nucleotides, and methionine (see discussion above), and for the catabolism of histidine. Synthesis of folate polyglutamates requires adequate cobalamin and methionine.[159]

Absorption of vitamin B_{12} involves a series of binding proteins and receptors. Dietary cobalamin is released from proteins in the stomach and binds to haptocorrin (R proteins) from saliva and gastric secretions. In the duodenum, alkaline pH, haptocorrin degradation, and other factors cause dissociation of that complex and binding to intrinsic factor, a highly specific cobalamin binding protein secreted by gastric parietal cells. Cobalamin from stomach or bile is thus delivered to ileal mucosal receptors. In the blood, cobalamin binds to transcobalamin II or haptocorrins (transcobalamin I), but only that bound to transcobalamin II is taken up by cells. Liver stores are sufficient to last for several years—20 years if enterohepatic recycling and absorption are not impaired.[160]

Folate absorption occurs after deconjugation of dietary polyglutamates in the jejunum. It is converted to 5-methyltetrahydrofolate in the intestinal mucosal cell, passes to the liver, is secreted into bile, and reabsorbed unchanged. The reabsorbed 5-methyltetrahydrofolate is bound to albumin and distributed to tissues. Special binding proteins in placenta, cord serum, and milk usually protect the fetus from effects of maternal deficiency.[159]

Disorders of Vitamin B₁₂ and Folate Metabolism

Deficiency

Deficiency of either folate or vitamin B_{12} leads to inhibition of folate-dependent metabolic pathways, with a characteristic decrease in synthesis of thymidine deoxyribonucleotide, slower replication of DNA, and megaloblastic anemia. The same process in the small bowel exacerbates malabsorption. Neurological complications are unpredictable. Low body reserves of vitamin B_{12} are associated with subacute combined degeneration of the spinal cord, peripheral neuropathy, optic neuritis, and/or dementia that are often refractory to vitamin B_{12} treatment. In folate deficiency, depression or dementia are more common, but subacute combined degeneration or peripheral neuropathy sometimes occur. Fortunately, they respond to folate supplementation.[161]

Vitamin B₁₂ Deficiency

Deficiency of vitamin B_{12} in children can be caused by dietary insufficiency (as in strict vegetarians [vegans] and in breast-feeding infants of such mothers), generalized malabsorption, or abnormalities of binding proteins or receptors specific for vitamin B_{12}. Generalized malabsorption may be due to ileal resection or disease (Crohn's disease, tuberculosis, lymphoma, etc.) or drugs (neomycin, cholestyramine, H2 receptor blockers). Absorption is also decreased in cystic fibrosis, but this seldom causes deficiency.

Juvenile pernicious anemia is similar to the adult form, with atrophic gastritis, achlorhydria, and antibodies to intrinsic factor. It is often associated with other endocrinopathies and sometimes with moniliasis, immunoglobulin A deficiency, or hypogammaglobulinemia.[162]

Folate Deficiency

As most folate is stored in the fetus in the last month of gestation, premature and small-for-gestational-age infants and those with erythroblastosis or sickle cell anemia may have low folate stores at birth. Other causes of deficiency in infancy include inherited defects of intestinal folate absorption and goat milk feeding.[159, 163]

As with other nutrients, folate deficiency is due to decreased intake, decreased absorption, or increased utilization. Nutritional deficiency of folate is common in underdeveloped countries and in lower socioeconomic groups. Malabsorption is seen with tropical sprue, gluten-sensitive enteropathy, and giant hypertrophic gastritis. Folate requirements are increased in hemolytic disorders, thalassemia, sickle cell anemia, malaria, pregnancy, prolonged lactation, critical illness (serious infections, trauma, surgery), and parenteral nutrition. Anticonvulsants (phenytoin, phenobarbital, primidone) decrease serum folate by an unknown mechanism but rarely cause megaloblastic anemia.

Inherited Defects in Vitamin B_{12} Metabolism

Inherited abnormalities of cobalamin metabolism recently have been reviewed in detail.[162] Any step of the complex vitamin B_{12} utilization pathway may be affected, from absorption to plasma transport to coenzyme formation or function. Megaloblastic anemia in infancy or early childhood, asymptomatic low serum B_{12}, or methylmalonic aciduria may be clues to one of these defects.

Inherited Defects in Folate Metabolism

The inherited abnormality of intestinal folate transport is discussed above. Disorders of intracellular folate metabolism include deficiencies of methylene tetrahydrofolate reductase, glutamate formiminotransferase (for histidine metabolism), methionine synthase (also affecting vitamin B_{12}), and dihydrofolate reductase (also blocked by methotrexate). These conditions and other enzymes involved in folate metabolism have been reviewed recently.[163]

Assessment of Vitamin B_{12} and Folate Status

Megaloblastic anemia is diagnosed by increased mean corpuscular volume, pancytopenia, and hypersegmented neutrophils. Red blood cell abnormalities are less obvious if iron deficiency (common in young children and pregnancy) or hemoglobinopathy is also present, or if the depletion is rapid. The bone marrow aspirate is usually diagnostic.

Vitamin measurements must be included in the investigation of megaloblastic anemia. In children, serum transcobalamin II and urine methylmalonic acid, homocystine, and orotic acid should be measured to rule out inherited disorders. Vitamin B_{12} is measured in serum using microbiological assays or immunoassays with intrinsic factor as the binding protein. Concentrations may be falsely increased due to chloral hydrate (method-dependent); increased transcobalamin I, as in chronic myelogenous leukemia; or in some inborn errors of cobalamin metabolism. Non-diagnostic low values occur in folate deficiency, pregnancy, oral contraceptive use, some hematologic conditions, haptocorrin deficiency, and with method-dependent analytical interferences such as ascorbic acid or radiolabelled dyes.[164]

Diagnosis of vitamin B_{12} deficiency must be followed by a search for the cause. This usually involves one or more Schilling tests and modifications that test absorption of B_{12} or protein-bound B_{12} combined with intrinsic factor, antibiotics, pancreatic enzymes, or bicarbonate. Intact renal function and complete urine collection are crucial for valid Schilling test results. Anti-intrinsic factor antibodies, intrinsic factor and acidity in gastric fluid, and gastrin concentrations may provide additional evidence for pernicious anemia. Pancreatic or intestinal malabsorption can be diagnosed by usual tests.[160, 164]

Folate should be measured in serum and red blood cells. Serum concentrations < 3 µg/L suggest deficiency. Serum folate decreases within days of decreased intake and does not reflect body stores. Values may be falsely low due to abnormal protein binding, as in renal failure or salicylate ingestion; with long specimen storage; or with acute ethanol ingestion. Low values in sickle cell anemia or hemolysis do not always indicate deficiency. Values are high in pernicious anemia. Red blood cell folate, because it reflects the folate status at the time the cells were made, is a better indicator of stores. However, cobalamin deficiency can cause low concentrations and reticulocytosis or iron deficiency can cause higher concentrations. Tests of folate absorption analogous to the Schilling test are of research use only.

Because of the limitations of serum and red blood cell vitamin measurements, various tests of metabolic status have been proposed. The most promising is the deoxyuridine suppression test, which assesses the suppression of radioactive thymidine uptake when cells are incubated with deoxyuridine. Utilization of deoxyuridine requires methyltetrahydrofolate, and suppression is less than normal in either folate or B_{12} deficiency. The specific deficiency or metabolic block can be diagnosed by the response to vitamin or metabolites. This test, performed on bone marrow cells, is sensitive to subclinical deficiencies of folate or B_{12}.[164]

Vitamin C

Vitamin C (ascorbic acid) is an effective reducing agent that enhances a variety of hydroxylation/oxidation reactions, probably by keeping the prosthetic metal ions in the reduced form. Reactions include synthesis of collagen, carnitine, and catecholamines, hormone activation by α-amidation and tyrosine metabolism. Free-radical scavenging is another important function. Other physiological effects also have been described.[165, 166]

Vitamin C is absorbed in the intestine by active carrier-mediated transport, with a peak daily absorption of about 3 g. With recommended intakes, ascorbic acid is largely metabolized to oxalate, but as intake increases, excess ascorbic acid is excreted unchanged.[167]

Disorders of Vitamin C Metabolism

Vitamin C Deficiency

Deficiency is always due to insufficient intake of foods containing vitamin C. Classical signs of severe deficiency—scurvy—include fatigue, anorexia, anemia, swollen and bleeding gums, loss of teeth, capillary fragility with bruising and mucosal hemorrhages, joint and muscle pains, skin lesions, increased susceptibility to infection or stress, and neuropsychiatric problems.[166] In recent deprivation studies, gingivitis and bleeding occurred after relatively short periods on a vitamin C deficient diet.[168]

Vitamin C Toxicity

Vitamin C, even in megadoses, is probably not toxic in most individuals because of limits on intestinal absorption and on metabolism to oxalate. High intakes may be a risk in recurrent renal stone formers (possible worsening of hyperoxaluria), patients with renal failure or on hemodialysis (impaired excretion), or in hemochromatosis (possible increase in iron absorption).[167]

Assessment of Vitamin C Status

There is currently no good, functional test of vitamin C status, although various tests such as assessment of gingival integrity, urinary hydroxyproline, or urinary carnitine have been tried. Measurement of ascorbic acid in serum or plasma and in leukocyte fractions are the only approaches validated to date.[169]

Plasma ascorbic acid concentrations reflect recent intake rather than body stores.[170] HPLC methods minimize interferences from dietary substances such as erythorbic acid. It is sufficient to measure ascorbic acid since the oxidized form, dehydroascorbic acid, makes up a fairly constant 5% of the total ascorbic acid in plasma. Concentrations < 0.2 mg/dL (11 µmol/L) are deficient; from 0.2–0.4 mg/dL (11–23 µmol/L) marginal; and > 0.5 mg/dL (28 µmol/L) normal.[169]

Leukocyte ascorbic acid measurement requires a large blood specimen. Leukocyte fractions should be analyzed individually.[170] The highest content is in mononuclear leukocytes, and this pool is less readily available, so depletion reflects more serious deficiency. Dehydroascorbic acid may comprise up to 50% of the total cellular ascorbic acid, but the significance of this is unknown. Interpretation of ascorbic acid concentrations in leukocytes requires more study.[169]

Urinary ascorbic acid indicates only that intake is adequate to high. When the body pool decreases to slightly below normal, ascorbic acid is metabolized and does not appear in urine.[170]

Biotin

Biotin functions as a carboxyl carrier in four human enzymes: pyruvate carboxylase, acetyl-CoA carboxylase, propionyl-CoA carboxylase, and 3-methylcrotonyl-CoA carboxylase. Biotin is covalently linked to a lysine residue in the inactive apoenzymes by the enzyme holocarboxylase synthetase. Reutilization of biotin requires another enzyme, biotinidase, to break this bond.

Biotin is obtained from the diet and from limited synthesis by intestinal bacteria. Raw egg white contains avidin, which binds biotin and makes it unavailable.[171]

Disorders of Biotin Metabolism

Biotin deficiency is rare but has occurred in children on diets rich in raw egg white[172] and in a child receiving total parenteral nutrition.[173] Multiple carboxylase deficiency is the metabolic consequence of biotin deficiency, but it is more commonly caused by inherited defects in holocarboxylase synthetase or biotinidase.[174] Children with inherited deficiencies of propionyl-CoA carboxylase, pyruvate carboxylase, or 3-methylcrotonyl-CoA carboxylase have similar clinical presentations but may not respond to biotin.[171]

The most characteristic sign of deficiency is dermatitis with skin desquamation and generalized hair loss. Neurological findings vary. Infants with inherited enzyme abnormalities often have episodes of ketosis and acidosis leading to dehydration, coma, and death.

Assessment of Biotin Status

Biotin deficiency is suspected by clinical history and physical findings and diagnosed by rapid response to supplementation. Inherited enzyme deficiencies are investigated by quantitative analysis of urine organic acids. The enzyme defect suggested by the pattern of organic acid excretion can be confirmed by enzyme assay. Biotinidase probably should be measured in any suspected cases, as organic acids may be normal.

Biotin assays are not widely available. Urine or plasma concentrations reflect dietary intake. Values are low in biotinidase deficiency and high in holocarboxylase synthetase deficiency. Reference ranges are assay specific.[171, 174]

Pantothenic Acid

Pantothenic acid forms an integral part of coenzyme A and acyl-carrier protein. Coenzyme A is essential for acetylation reactions, acyl-carrier protein for fatty acid synthesis. Pantothenic acid is readily available in the diet, and deficiency is rare.[175]

Disorders of Pantothenic Acid Metabolism

Dietary restriction or administration of a pantothenic acid antagonist leads to fatigue, weakness, personality changes, impaired coordination, paraesthesia ("burning" feet), muscle spasm, and sleep disturbance. Metabolic changes include loss of eosinopenic response to ACTH and insulin sensitivity. Toxicity has not been described in humans.[175]

Assessment of Pantothenic Acid Status

As with other water-soluble vitamins, urinary excretion of pantothenic acid parallels intake.[175] Pantothenic acid also has been measured in serum, plasma, whole blood, and erythrocytes. Concentrations in whole blood or erythrocytes seem to reflect dietary status, [176] but standardization of the assay is a major problem and reference ranges vary greatly.[177]

METABOLIC COMPLICATIONS OF PARENTERAL NUTRITION

Parenteral nutrition provides essential requirements such as water, amino acids, energy (glucose, lipid), minerals, and micronutrients intravenously via central or peripheral veins. Indications for parenteral nutrition in infants include extreme prematurity, severe respiratory disease or necrotizing enterocolitis, and congenital gastrointestinal anomalies or short bowel syndrome. In older children with inflammatory bowel disease, cystic fibrosis, cancer, burns, and severe trauma, parenteral nutrition support has proven an important therapeutic adjunct.

As parenteral nutrition became widely used in the very young and the very ill and as patients were maintained on total parenteral nutrition for extended periods, deficiency states of many micronutrients became evident[6, 26, 36, 55, 70, 173] and many metabolic complications were seen.[178, 179] As a result, the initial glucose and protein-hydrolysate preparations have evolved to the present-day formulations which provide carbohydrate, crystalline amino acids, lipid emulsions, minerals, essential trace elements, and vitamins.[179, 180]

Disorders of Fluid, Electrolytes, and Minerals

Fluid balance requires delicate adjustment in the neonate and particularly in the preterm infant. Proportionally large surface area for body weight and high transcutaneous insensible losses necessitate relatively higher fluid intake than in the adult. Immaturity of renal function and glycosuria may increase urinary loss of fluid and electrolytes.[181] Phototherapy further increases the requirement for fluid. However, bronchopulmonary dysplasia, necrotizing enterocolitis, intraventricular hemorrhage, and patent ductus arteriosus have all been associated with excessive fluid volumes in preterm infants.[181] Hypokalemia and hypocalcemia can complicate diuretic use in these babies.[114] Since both excess or deficiency of calcium, phosphate, and magnesium also may be seen in these infants, careful monitoring is required.

Hyperammonemia and Acid-Base Disorders

Hyperammonemia occurred frequently with the protein hydrolysate and earlier crystalline amino acid preparations, but is much less common with the present crystalline amino acid preparations.[179] Patients with liver failure and those with inborn errors of metabolism require special adjustment of amino acid intake to prevent hyperammonemia. Replacement of some hydrochloride salts of the amino acids with acetate decreases the occurrence of hyperchloremic metabolic acidosis, and metabolic acidosis is an uncommon complication now.[178, 179]

Excessive protein intake in premature infants can result in both hyperammonemia and azotemia.[181] Abnormal plasma aminograms with high concentrations of phenylalanine, tyrosine, and methionine may occur.[23, 179]

Hyperglycemia and Hypoglycemia

Initial intolerance to high glucose infusion rate occurs frequently in the premature infant. These infants are at risk for hyperosmolar coma and intraventricular hemorrhage. Hyperglycemia may necessitate insulin use.[181] Other frequent precipitants of hyperglycemia are sepsis and severe renal disease. Sudden cessation of the parenteral infusion can result in marked hypoglycemia.

Lipid Emulsions

Intravenous fat emulsions provide a concentrated source of energy and essential fatty acids. Soy or safflower oil is stabilized with phospholipid and glycerol is added to make an isotonic preparation. After the lipid droplets enter the bloodstream, apoprotein C is acquired from other circulating lipoproteins and the droplets are metabolized by lipoprotein lipase similarly to chylomicrons. In parenterally fed infants who receive lipids, a lipoprotein particle is found which is similar to that seen in biliary obstruction or lecithin-cholesterol acyltransferase deficiency, Lp-X. This disappears when lipid infusion is stopped.[182]

Lipids may be poorly tolerated by the very-low-birth-weight, small-for-gestational-age, or septic infant, and serum triglyceride and free fatty acid concentrations may be elevated. When lipids are infused faster than the lipoprotein lipase system can metabolize them, unmetabolized lipids interfere with the function of cellular elements such as neutrophils, platelets, and macrophages.[183] "Fat overload" is thus associated with platelet dysfunction and coagulopathy. Visual turbidity correlates poorly with serum total triglyceride concentrations, as does nephelometry. However, to evaluate tolerance for lipid infusion, nephelometry provides a better index of unmetabolized lipid emulsion triglyceride than visual inspection[183]

Use of carnitine supplements[184] or continuous infusion of heparin[185] have been used to improve the ability of the neonate to tolerate lipids. Carnitine, which is lacking in the immature neonate, facilitates transport of fatty acids across mitochondrial membranes. Heparin increases lipoprotein lipase activity.

The earlier concern that free fatty acids can displace unconjugated bilirubin from albumin binding sites, increasing the risk of kernicterus in the hyperbilirubinemic infant, appears to be unfounded. No effect on unbound bilirubin was noted with lipid and heparin infusion over 24 hours.[185]

The autopsy detection of fat emboli in pulmonary capillaries of infants who had received intravenous lipids was later attributed to postmortem artifact.[186] Moreover, infusion of up to 4 g/Kg/day of lipid over 24 hours did not impair oxygen diffusion.[187]

Dermatitis, Alopecia, and Irritability

Deficiency of one of several nutrients may result in dermatitis or alopecia but should be prevented by adequate supplementation. Neonatal zinc deficiency is characterized by an erythematous, exudative, scaly lesion of the body folds and acral areas of the body, often with superimposed infection with Candida albicans.[36] Poor wound healing, alopecia, and immunodeficiency also result from zinc deficiency.[55] Biotin deficiency (scaly dermatitis, alopecia, pallor, irritability, and lethargy) occurred in children with gastrointestinal abnormalities treated with parenteral nutrition unsupplemented with biotin.[173] Essential fatty acid deficiency similarly results in scaly dermatitis, poor growth, and impaired wound healing.[26]

Cholestatic Liver Disease and Cholelithiasis

Cholestasis is an extremely common complication in infants on prolonged total parenteral nutrition. The incidence is highest in the lower birth weight infants, but total parenteral nutrition associated steatosis and cholestasis also occurs in adults.[188] Increase in conjugated bilirubin is the most reliable indicator of developing liver disease, but alkaline phosphatase and the aminotransferases also increase. Gallbladder sludge was detected by sonography in 44% of neonates after a mean period of only 10 days of total parenteral nutrition, and 5%

developed actual gallstones.[189] Suggested etiological factors include prolonged enteric fasting leading to bile sludging in the liver and gall bladder, furosemide use, taurine deficiency, tryptophan degradation products, glutathione depletion, excessive glucose intake, and bacterial sepsis. It is probable that the condition is multifactorial in origin.[188]

Metabolic Bone Disease

Metabolic bone disease, roentgenographically indistinguishable from rickets, occurs commonly in infants on long-term parenteral nutrition despite supplementation with vitamin D_2, calcium, and phosphate.[190] Other possible etiological factors include copper deficiency[59, 60] and aluminum excess.[191]

Concentrations of alkaline phosphatase are high, but there is overlap with concentrations found in the growing preterm infant with radiologically normal bones.[192]

Evaluation of Parenteral Nutrition Support

Laboratory testing in assessment of total parenteral nutrition is complementary to the daily evaluation of intake and output. It should be noted that the volume of total parenteral nutrition, and therefore the calories, protein, and fat prescribed, is not consistently achieved in the pediatric population. In a recent study, the prescribed volume was achieved on only 62% of the days on parenteral nutrition, while the target nutrient intake was achieved on only 50–60% of the days on which the goal volume was achieved. Adequacy of nutritional support requires daily review of actual intake.[193] However, routine monitoring of infants and children on total parenteral nutrition must be planned to minimize blood loss and the need for subsequent transfusion.

REFERENCES

1. Buzina R, Bates CJ, van der Beek J, et al. Workshop on functional significance of mild to moderate malnutrition. Am J Clin Nutr 1989;50:172-6.
2. Sommer A. Vitamin A status, resistance to infection, and childhood mortality. Ann N Y Acad Sci 1990;587:17-23.
3. Merritt RJ, Suskind RM. Nutritional survey of hospitalized pediatric patients. Am J Clin Nutr 1979;32:1320-5.
4. Holcomb GW, Ziegler MM. Nutrition and cancer in children. Surg Ann 1990;22:129-42.
5. Acosta PB, Stepnick-Gropper S, Clarke-Sheehan N, et al. Trace element status of PKU children ingesting an elemental diet. J Parenter Enteral Nutr 1987;11:287-92.
6. Jeejeebhoy DN, Chu RC, Marliss EB, et al. Chromium deficiency, glucose intolerance, and neuropathy reversed by chromium supplementation in a patient receiving long-term total parenteral nutrition. Am J Clin Nutr 1977;30:531-8.

7.   Abumrad NN, Schneider AJ, Steel D, Rogers LS. Amino acid intolerance during prolonged total parenteral nutrition reversed by molybdate therapy. Am J Clin Nutr 1981;34:2551-9.

8.   Kien CL, Ganther HE. Manifestations of chronic selenium deficiency in a child receiving total parenteral nutrition. Am J Clin Nutr 1983;37:319-28.

9.   Raiha NCR, Boehm G. Protein and nitrogen metabolism in low birth weight infants. In: Stern L, ed. Feeding the sick infant. New York: Vevy/Raven Press, 1987:63-74.

10.   Meites S, ed. Pediatric clinical chemistry: Reference (normal) values. Washington, DC: AACC Press, 1989.

11.   Solomons NW. Assessment of nutritional status: Functional indicators of pediatric nutriture. Pediatr Clin NA 1985;32:319-34.

12.   Heinrich PC, Castell JV, Andus T. Interleukin-6 and the acute phase response. Biochem J 1990;265:621-36.

13.   Morrison B, Shenkin A, McLelland A, et al. Intra-individual variation in commonly analyzed serum constituents. Clin Chem 1979;25:1799-805

14.   Suskind D, Murthy KK, Suskind RM. The malnourished child: An overview. In: Suskind R, Lewinter-Suskind L, eds. The malnourished child. New York: Vevy/Raven Press, 1990;1-22.

15.   Phinney SD. The assessment of protein nutrition in the hospitalized patient. Clin Lab Med 1981;1:767-74.

16.   Benjamin DR. Laboratory tests and nutritional assessment: Protein-energy status. Pediatr Clin NA 1989;36:139-61.

17.   Sachs E, Bernstein LH. Protein markers of nutrition status as related to sex and age. Clin Chem 1986;32:339-41.

18.   Lockitch G, Pendray MR, Godolphin BJ, Quigley G. Serial changes in selected serum constituents in low birth weight infants on peripheral parenteral nutrition with different zinc and copper supplements. Am J Clin Nutr 1985;42:24-30.

19.   Yoder MC, Anderson DC, Gopalakrishna GS, et al. Comparison of serum fibronectin, prealbumin and albumin concentration during nutritional repletion in protein-calorie malnourished infants. J Pediatr Gastroenterol Nutr 1987;6:84-8.

20.   Delpeuch P, Desch G, Hassanaly F, Sautecoeur M. Fibronectin concentrations in plasma of healthy pre-term, full-term and sick full-term neonates. Clin Chem 1988;34:592.

21.   Coward WA, Lunn PG. The biochemistry and physiology of kwashiorkor and marasmus. Brit Med Bull 1981;37:19-24.

22.   Young VR, Munro HN. N-methylhistidine (3-methylhistidine) and muscle protein turnover: An overview. FASEB J 1978;37:2291-300.

23.   Moro G, Fulconis F, Minoli I, et al. Growth and plasma amino acid concentrations in very low birthweight infants fed either human milk protein fortified human milk or a whey-predominant formula. Acta Paediatr Scand 1989;78:18-22.

24.   Solomons NW, Wagonfeld JB, Rieger C, et al. Some biochemical indices of nutrition in treated cystic fibrosis patients. Am J Clin Nutr 1981;34:462-74.

25.   Krasinski SD, Russell RM, Furie BC, et al. The prevalence of Vitamin K deficiency in chronic gastrointestinal disorders. Am J Clin Nutr 1985;41:639-43.

26.   Paulsrud JR, Pensler L, Whitten CF, et al. Essential fatty acid deficiency in infants induced by fat-free intravenous feeding. Am J Clin Nutr 1972;25:897-904.

27.   Friedman Z, Danon A, Stahlman MT, Oates JA. Rapid onset of essential fatty acid deficiency in the newborn. Pediatr 1976;58:640-9.

28.   Holman RT, Johnson SB, Mercuri O, et al. Essential fatty acid deficiency in malnourished children. Am J Clin Nutr 1981;34:1534-9.

29.   Farrell PM, Gutcher GR, Palta M, DeMets D. Essential fatty acid deficiency in premature infants. Am J Clin Nutr 1988;48:220-9.

30.   Pettei MJ, Daftary S, Levine JJ. Essential fatty acid deficiency associated with the use of a medium-chain-triglyceride infant formula in pediatric hepatobiliary disease. Am J Clin Nutr 1991;53:1217-21.

31.   Levy J, DeFelice A, Lepage G. Essential fatty acid deficiency mimicking porphyria cutanea tarda in a patient with chronic cholestasis. J Pediatr Gastroenterol Nutr 1990;10:242-5.

32. Versieck J. Trace elements in human body fluids and tissues. CRC Crit Rev Clin Lab Sci 1985;22:97-181.

33. Delves HT. Assessment of trace element status. Clin Endocrinol Metab 1985;14:725-60.

34. Reeves JD, Vichinsky E, Addiego J, Lubin BH. Iron deficiency in health and disease. Adv Pediatr 1984;31:281-320.

35. Cordano A, Graham GG. Copper deficiency complicating severe chronic intestinal malabsorption. Pediatr 1966;38:596-604.

36. Lockitch G, Johnston MM, Pendray MR, Godolphin WJ. The effect of varying zinc and copper supplementation on the acrodermatitis syndrome in infants on parenteral nutrition. In: Brown SS, Savory J, eds. Chemical toxicology and clinical chemistry of metals. New York: Academic Press, 1983:347-50.

37. Kelly DA, Coe AW, Shenkin A, et al. Symptomatic selenium deficiency in a child on home parenteral nutrition. J Pediatr Gastroenterol Nutr 1988;7:783-6.

38. Menkes JH. Kinky hair disease: Twenty-five years later. Brain Dev 1988;10:77-9.

39. Moynahan EJ. Acrodermatitis enteropathica: A lethal inherited human zinc-deficiency disorder. Lancet 1974;ii:399-400.

40. Johnson J, Wadman SK. Molybdenum cofactor deficiency. In: Scriver CR, Beaudet AL, Sly WS, Valle D, eds. Metabolic basis of inherited disease, 6th ed. New York: McGraw-Hill, 1989:1463-75.

41. Cunnane SC. Zinc: Clinical and biochemical significance. Boca Raton, FL: CRC Press, 1988:1-195

42. Jensen R, Closson W, Rothenberg R. Selenium intoxication. New York: MMWR 1984;33:157-8.

43. Muller-Hocker J, Meyer U, Wiebecke B, et al. Copper storage disease of the liver and chronic dietary copper intoxication in two further German infants mimicking Indian childhood cirrhosis. Path Res Pract 1988;183:39-45.

44. Alt ER, Sternlieb I, Goldfischer S. The cytopathology of metal overload. Int Rev Exp Path 1990;31:165-88.

45. Brewer GJ, Yuzbasiyan-Gurkan V. Wilson's disease: An update, with emphasis on new approaches to treatment. Dig Dis 1989;7:178-93.

46. National Research Council, Food and Nutrition Board, Subcommittee on the 10th Edition of the RDAs. Recommended dietary allowances, 10th ed. Washington DC: National Academy Press, 1989.

47. Health and Welfare Canada, Scientific Review Committee. Nutrition recommendations. Ottawa: Canadian Government Publishing Centre, 1990.

48. Aisen P, Cohen G, Kang JO. Iron toxicosis. Int Rev Exp Path 1990;31:1-46.

49. Lozoff B. Behavioral alterations in iron deficiency. Adv Pediatr 1988;35:331-60.

50. Litovitz TL, Schmitz BF, Holm KC. 1988 Annual report of the American Association of Poison Control Centers national data collection system. Toxicol 1989;7:495-545.

51. Mahoney JR, Hallway PE, Hedlund BE, Eaton JW. Acute iron poisoning; Rescue with macromolecular chelators. J Clin Invest 1989;84:1362-6.

52. Charlton RW, Abrahams C, Bothwell HT. Idiopathic hemochromatosis in young subjects. Arch Path 1967;83:132-140.

53. Blisard K. Neonatal hemochromatosis. Human Pathol 1986;17:376-83.

54. Keusch GT, Farthing MJG. Nutrition and infection. Ann Rev Nutr 1986;6:131-54.

55. Allen JI, Kay NE, McClain CJ. Severe zinc deficiency in humans: Association with a reversible T-lymphocyte dysfunction. Ann Int Med 1981;95:154-7.

56. Kiilerich S, Christiansen C. Distribution of serum zinc between albumin and α-2-macroglobulin in patients with different zinc metabolic disorders. Clin Chim Acta 1986;154:1-6.

57. Baer MT, King JC. Tissue zinc levels and zinc excretion during experimental zinc depletion in young men. Am J Clin Nutr 1984;39:556-71.

58. Patrick J, Dervish C. Leukocyte zinc in the assessment of zinc status. CRC Crit Rev Clin Lab Sci 1984;20:95-114.

59. Shaw JCL. Copper deficiency and non-accidental injury. Arch Dis Child 1988;63:448-55.

60.   Carty H. Brittle or battered. Arch Dis Child 1988;63:350-2.
61.   Levy Y, Zeharia A, Grunebaum M, et al. Copper deficiency in infants fed cows milk. J Pediatr 1985;106:786-8.
62.   Horn N. Menkes' X-linked disease: Prenatal diagnosis and carrier detection. J Inherit Metab Dis 1983;6(suppl 1):59-62.
63.   Spitalny K, Brondum J, Vogt RL, et al. Drinking-water-induced copper intoxication in a Vermont family. Pediatr 1984;74:1103-6.
64.   Pennypacker E, Shrair HR, Lane WT, Schrack WD. Acute copper poisoning. MMWR 1975;29:99.
65.   Walshe JM. Copper: Its role in the pathogenesis of liver disease. Semin Liver Dis 1984;4:252-63.
66.   Goldfischer S, Popper H, Sternlieb I. The significance of variations in the distribution of copper in liver disease. Am J Pathol 1980;99:715-29.
67.   Burk RF. Recent developments in trace element metabolism and function: Newer roles of selenium in nutrition. J Nutr 1989;119:1051-4.
68.   Sunde RA. Molecular biology of selenoproteins. Ann Rev Nutr 1990;10:451-74.
69.   Johnson RA, Baker SS, Fallon JT, et al. An occidental case of cardiomyopathy and selenium deficiency. New Eng J Med 1981;304:1210-2.
70.   Lockitch G, Jacobson BD, Quigley G, et al. Selenium deficiency in low birthweight neonates: An unrecognized problem. J Pediatr 1989;114:865-70.
71.   Smith AM, Picciano MF, Milner JA. Selenium intakes and status of human milk and formula fed infants. Am J Clin Nutr 1982;35:521-6.
72.   Yang G, Ge K, Chen J, Chen X. Selenium-related endemic diseases and the daily selenium requirement of humans. Wld Rev Nutr Diet 1988;55:98-152.
73.   Robinson MF. The New Zealand selenium experience. Am J Clin Nutr 1988;48:521-34.
74.   Jackson ML. Selenium: Geochemical distribution and associations with human heart and cancer death rates and longevity in China and the United States. Biol Tr El Res 1988;15:13-21.
75.   Lockitch G. Selenium: Clinical significance and analytical concepts. CRC Crit Rev Clin Lab Sci 1989;27:483-541.
76.   Lockitch G, Taylor GP, Wong LTK, et al. Cardiomyopathy associated with nonendemic selenium deficiency in a Caucasian adolescent. Am J Clin Nutr 1990;52:572-7.
77.   Volk DM, Cutliff SA. Selenium deficiency and cardiomyopathy in a patient with cystic fibrosis. J Kentucky Med Assoc 1986;84:711-7.
78.   Keen CL, Lonnerdal B, Hurley LS. Manganese. In: Frieden E, ed. Biochemistry of the essential ultratrace elements. New York: Plenum Press, 1984:89-132.
79.   Papavasiliou PS, Kutt H, Millet ST, et al. Seizure disorders and trace metals: Manganese tissue levels in treated epileptics. Neurol 1979;29:1466-73.
80.   Freeland-Graves JH, Behmardi F, Bales CW, et al. Metabolic balance of manganese in young men consuming diets containing five levels of dietary manganese. J Nutr 1988;118:764-73.
81.   Hambidge KM, Sokol RJ, Fidanza SJ, Goodall MA. Plasma manganese concentration in infants and children receiving parenteral nutrition. J Parenter Enteral Nutr 1989;13:168-71.
82.   Dahlstrom KA, Ament ME, Medhin MG, Meurling S. Serum trace elements in children receiving long-term parenteral nutrition. J Pediatr 1986;109:625-630.
83.   Lockitch G. Molybdenum. In: Werner M, ed. CRC handbook of clinical chemistry, Vol. IV. Boca Raton, FL: CRC Press, 1989:255-60.
84.   Bougle D, Voirin J, Bureau F, et al. Molybdenum. Acta Paediatr Scand 1989;78:319-20.
85.   Anderson RA. Chromium metabolism and its role in disease processes in man. Clin Physiol Biochem 1986;4:31-41.
86.   Freund H, Atamian S, Fischer JE. Chromium deficiency during total parenteral nutrition. JAMA 1979;241:496-9.
87.   Brown RO, Forloines-Lynn S, Cross RE, Heizer WD. Chromium deficiency after long-term total parenteral nutrition. Dig Dis Sci 1986;31:661-4.

88. Kien CL, Veillon C, Patterson KY, Farrell PM. Mild peripheral neuropathy but biochemical chromium sufficiency during 16 months of "chromium-free" total parenteral nutrition. J Parenter Enteral Nutr 1986;10:662-4.

89. Carter JP, Kattab A, Abd-El-Hadi K, et al. Chromium (III) in hypoglycemia and in impaired glucose utilisation in kwashiorkor. Am J Clin Nutr 1968;21:195-202.

90. Machlin LJ. Handbook of vitamins: Nutritional, biochemical and clinical aspects. New York: Marcel Dekker, 1984.

91. Weigel B, Zlotkin S. Vitamin supplements: Are they necessary? Contemp Pediatr 1990:8-13.

92. Elsas LJ, McCormick DB. Genetic defects in vitamin utilization. Part I: General aspects and fat-soluble vitamins. Vitam Horm 1986;43:103-44.

93. Sklan D. Vitamin A in human nutrition. Prog Food Nutr Sci 1987;11:39-55.

94. Zachman RD. Retinol (vitamin A) and the neonate: Special problems of the human premature infant. Am J Clin Nutr 1989;50:413-24.

95. Hathcock JN, Hattan DG, Jenkins MY, et al. Evaluation of Vitamin A toxicity. Am J Clin Nutr 1990;52;183-202.

96. Leung A. Carotenemia. Adv Pediatr 1987;34:223-48.

97. Underwood BA. Methods for assessment of vitamin A status. J Nutr 1990;120:1459-63.

98. Gibson RS. Assessment of the status of vitamins A, D, and E. In: Principles of nutritional assessment. New York: Oxford University Press, 1990:377-412.

99. Webb AR, Holick MF. The role of sunlight in the cutaneous production of vitamin D_3. Ann Rev Nutr 1988;8:375-99.

100. Suda T, Shinki T, Takahashi N. The role of vitamin D in bone and intestinal cell differentiation. Ann Rev Nutr 1990;10:195-211.

101. DeLuca HF. The vitamin D story: A collaborative effort of basic science and clinical medicine. FASEB J 1988;2:224-36.

102. Bikle DD, Gee E. Measurement of free vitamin D metabolite levels: Biological and clinical significance. In: Norman AW, Schaefer KL, Grigoleit HG, Herrath DV, eds. Vitamin D: Molecular, cellular and clinical endocrinology. Berlin: Walter de Gruyter, 1988:703-9.

103. Riancho JA, del Arco C, Arteaga R, et al. Influence of solar irradiation on vitamin D levels in children on anticonvulsant drugs. Acta Neurol Scand 1989;79:296-9.

104. Salle BL, Senterre J, Glorieux FH, et al. Vitamin D metabolism in preterm infants. Biol Neonate 1987;52(Suppl 1):119-30.

105. Mehls O, Wolf H, Wille L. Vitamin D requirements and vitamin D intoxication in infancy. Int J Vitam Nutr Res 1989;Suppl 30:87-94.

106. Marx SJ. Vitamin D and other calciferols. In: Scriver CR, Beaudet AL, Sly WS, Valle D, eds. Metabolic basis of inherited disease, 6th ed. New York: McGraw-Hill, 1989:2029-45.

107. Davies M. High-dose vitamin D therapy: Indications, benefits and hazards. Int J Vitam Nutr Res 1989;Suppl 30:81-6.

108. Jones G, DeLuca HF. High-performance liquid chromatography of vitamin D and its application to endocrinology. In: Makin HLJ, Newton R, eds. High-performance liquid chromatography in endocrinology. Berlin: Springer-Verlag, 1988;95-139.

109. Sokol RJ. Vitamin E and neurologic deficits. Adv Pediatr 1990;37:119-48.

110. Ogihara T, Miki M, Kitagawa M, Mino M. Distribution of tocopherol among human plasma lipoproteins. Clin Chim Acta 1988;174:299-306.

111. Traber MG, Sokol RJ, Burton GW, et al. Impaired ability of patients with familial isolated vitamin E deficiency to incorporate alpha-tocopherol into lipoproteins secreted by the liver. J Clin Invest 1990;85:397-407.

112. Bendich A, Machlin LJ. Safety of oral intake of vitamin E. Am J Clin Nutr 1988;48:612-9.

113. Phelps DL. The role of vitamin E therapy in high-risk neonates. Clin Perinatol 1988;15:955-63.

114. Aranda JV, Chemtob S, Laudignon N, Sasyniuk BI. Furosemide and vitamin E. Pediatr Clin N Am 1986;33:583-602.

115. Arrowsmith JB, Faich GA, Tomita DK, et al. Morbidity and mortality among low birth weight infants exposed to an intravenous Vitamin E product, E-Ferol. Pediatr 1989;83:244-9.

116. Farrell PM, Levine SL, Murphy MD, Adams AJ. Plasma tocopherol levels and tocopherol-lipid relationships in a normal population of children as compared to healthy adults. Am J Clin Nutr 1978;31:1720-6.
117. Mino M, Miki M, Miyake M, Ogihara T. Nutritional assessment of vitamin E in oxidative stress. Ann NY Acad Sci 1989;570:296-310.
118. Cynamon HA, Isenberg JN. Characterization of vitamin E status in cholestatic children by conventional laboratory standards and a new functional assay. J Pediatr Gastroenterol Nutr 1987;6:46-50.
119. Lemoyne M, Van Gossum A, Kurian R, et al. Breath pentane analysis as an index of lipid peroxidation: A functional test of vitamin E status. Am J Clin Nutr 1987;46:267-72.
120. Uotila L. The metabolic functions and mechanism of action of vitamin K. Scand J Clin Lab Invest 1990;50:109-17.
121. Olson RE. The function and metabolism of Vitamin K. Ann Rev Nutr 1984;4:281-337.
122. Shearer MJ. Vitamin K and vitamin K-dependent proteins. Br J Haematol 1990;75:156-62.
123. Suttie JW. Recent advances in hepatic vitamin K metabolism and function. Hepatol 1987;7:367-76.
124. Hathaway WE. New insights on vitamin K. Hematol Oncol Clin N Amer 1987;1:367-79.
125. Kries Rv, Shearer MJ, Gobel U. Vitamin K in infancy. Eur J Pediatr 1988;147:106-112.
126. Marks J. The safety of the vitamins: An overview. Int J Vitam Nutr Res 1989;(Suppl 30):12-20.
127. Lee M, Schwartz RN, Sharifi R. Warfarin resistance and vitamin K. Ann Int Med 1981;94:140-1.
128. Sanders MN, Winkelmann RK. Cutaneous reactions to vitamin K. J Am Acad Dermatol 1988;19:699-704.
129. Haas RH. Thiamin and the brain. Ann Rev Nutr 1988;8:483-515.
130. Davis RE, Icke GC. Clinical chemistry of thiamin. Adv Clin Chem 1983;23:93-140.
131. Wyatt DT, Noetzel MJ, Hillman RE. Infantile beriberi presenting as subacute necrotizing encephalomyelopathy. J Pediatr 1987;110:888-91.
132. Handler CE, Perkin GD. Anorexia nervosa and Wernicke's encephalopathy: An underdiagnosed association. Lancet 1982;ii:771-2.
133. Naidoo DP, Singh B, Haffejee A, et al. Acute pernicious beriberi in a patient receiving parenteral nutrition. S Afr Med J 1989;75:546-548.
134. Seear MD, Norman MG. Two cases of Wernicke's Encephalopathy in children: An underdiagnosed complication of poor nutrition. Ann Neurol 1988;24:85-7.
135. Poggi V, Rindi G, Patrini C, et al. Studies on thiamine metabolism in thiamine-responsive megaloblastic anaemia. Eur J Pediatr 1989;148:307-11.
136. Wyatt DT, Erickson MM, Hillman RE, Hillman LS. Elevated thiamine levels in SIDS, non-SIDS, and adults: Postmortem artifact. J Pediatr 1984;104:585-8.
137. Sauberlich HE. Newer laboratory methods for assessing nutriture of selected B-complex vitamins. Ann Rev Nutr 1984;4:377-407.
138. Mount JN, Heduan E, Herd C, et al. Adaptation of coenzyme stimulation assays for the nutritional assessment of vitamins B_1, B_2 and B_6 using the Cobas Bio centrifugal analyser. Ann Clin Biochem 1987;24:41-6.
139. Baines M, Davies G. The evaluation of erythrocyte thiamin diphosphate as an indicator of thiamin status in man, and its comparison with erythrocyte transketolase activity measurements. Ann Clin Biochem 1988;25:698-705.
140. McCormick DB. Two interconnected B vitamins: Riboflavin and pyridoxine. Physiol Rev 1989;69:1170-98.
141. Bates CJ. Human riboflavin requirements and metabolic consequences of deficiency in man and animals. Wld Rev Nutr Diet 1987;50:215-65.
142. Rudolph N, Parekh AJ, Hittelman J, et al. Postnatal decline in pyridoxal phosphate and riboflavin. Am J Dis Child 1985;139:812-5.
143. Gibson RS. Assessment of the status of thiamin, riboflavin, and niacin. In: Principles of nutritional assessment. New York: Oxford University Press, 1990:425-44.
144. Rhead WJ. Inborn errors of fatty acid oxidation in man. Clin Biochem 1991;24:319-29.

145. van Eys J. Nicotinic acid and nicotinamide. In: Machlin LJ. Handbook of vitamins, 2nd ed. New York: Marcel Dekker, 1991:311-40

146. Hankes LV. Nicotinic acid and nicotinamide. In: Machlin LJ. Handbook of vitamins. Nutritional, biochemical and clinical aspects. New York: Marcel Dekker, 1984:199-244.

147. Coronary Drug Project Research Group. Clofibrate and niacin in coronary heart disease. JAMA 1975;231:360-81.

148. Patterson DJ, Dew EW, Gyorkey F, Graham DY. Niacin hepatitis. South Med J 1983;76:239-41.

149. Fu CS, Swendseid ME, Jacob RA, McKee RW. Biochemical markers for assessment of niacin status in young men: Levels of erythrocyte niacin coenzymes and plasma tryptophan. J Nutr 1989;119:949-55.

150. Leklem JE. Vitamin B6. In: Machlin LJ. Handbook of vitamins, 2nd ed. New York: Marcel Dekker, 1991:341-92.

151. Merrill AH, Henderson JM. Diseases associated with defects in Vitamin B6 metabolism or utilization. Ann Rev Nutr 1987;7:137-56.

152. Driskell JA. Vitamin B6. In: Machlin LJ. Handbook of vitamins. Nutritional, biochemical and clinical aspects. New York: Marcel Dekker, 1984:379-401.

153. Minns R. Vitamin B6 deficiency and dependency. Dev Med Child Neurol 1980;22:795-9.

154. Fowler B. Recent advances in the mechanism of pyridoxine responsive disorders. J Inher Metab Dis 1985;8(Suppl 1):76-83

155. Bendich A, Cohen M. Vitamin B6 safety issues. Ann NY Acad Sci 1990;585:189-201.

156. Kroll JS. Pyridoxine for neonatal seizures: An unexpected danger. Dev Med Child Neurol 1985;27:377-9.

157. Ubbink J, Bissbort S, Van den Berg I, et al. Genetic polymorphism of glutamate-pyruvate transaminase (alanine aminotransaminase): Influence on erythrocyte activity as a marker of vitamin B6 nutritional status. Am J Clin Nutr 1989;50:1420-8.

158. Gibson RS. Assessment of vitamin B6 status. In: Principles of Nutritional Assessment. New York: Oxford University Press, 1990;445-60.

159. Davis RE, Nicol DJ. Folic acid. Int J Biochem 1988;20:133-9.

160. Belaiche J, Cattan D. Cobalamin absorption and acquired forms of cobalamin malabsorption. In: Zittoun JA, Cooper BA, eds. Folates and cobalamins. Berlin; Springer-Verlag, 1989:71-84.

161. Botez MI. Neuropsychiatric illness and deficiency of vitamins B12 and folate. In: Zittoun JA, Cooper BA, eds. Folates and cobalamins. Berlin; Springer-Verlag, 1989:145-59.

162. Zittoun J, Marquet J. Inherited disorders of cobalamin metabolism. In: Zittoun JA, Cooper BA, eds. Folates and cobalamins. Berlin; Springer-Verlag, 1989:219-30.

163. Cooper BA. Inherited defects of folate metabolism. In: Zittoun JA, Cooper BA, eds. Folates and cobalamins. Berlin: Springer-Verlag, 1989:199-214.

164. Carmel R. Diagnosis of megaloblastic anemia. In: Zittoun JA, Cooper BA, eds. Folates and cobalamins. Berlin; Springer-Verlag, 1989:20-39.

165. Padh H. Cellular functions of ascorbic acid. Biochem Cell Biol 1990;68:1166-73.

166. Moser U, Bendich A. Vitamin C. In: Machlin LJ. Handbook of vitamins, 2nd ed. New York: Marcel Dekker, 1991:195-232

167. Rivers JM. Safety of high-level vitamin C ingestion. Int J Vitam Nutr Res 1989;Suppl 30:95-102.

168. Jacob RA, Omaye ST, Skala JH, et al. Experimental vitamin C depletion and supplementation in young men. Ann NY Acad Sci 1987;498:333-46.

169. Jacob RA. Assessment of human vitamin C status. J Nutr 1990;120:1480-5.

170. Omaye ST, Schaus EE, Kutnink MA, Hawkes WC. Measurement of vitamin C in blood components by high-performance liquid chromatography: Implication in assessing vitamin C status. Ann NY Acad Sci 1987;498:389-401.

171. Bonjour J-P. Biotin. In: Machlin LJ. Handbook of vitamins, 2nd ed. New York: Marcel Dekker, 1991:393-427.

172. Sweetman L, Surh L, Baker H, et al. Clinical and metabolic abnormalities in a boy with dietary deficiency of biotin. Pediatr 1981;68:553-8.

173. Mock DM, DeLorimer AA, Liebman WM, et al. Biotin deficiency: An unusual complication of parenteral alimentation. N Eng J Med 1981;304:820-3.
174. Nyhan WL. Multiple carboxylase deficiency. Int J Biochem 1988;20:363-70.
175. Fox HM. Pantothenic Acid. In: Machlin LJ. Handbook of vitamins, 2nd ed. New York: Marcel Dekker, 1991:429-51.
176. Eissenstat BR, Wyse BA, Hansen RG. Pantothenic acid status of adolescents. Am J Clin Nutr 1986;44:931-7.
177. Wittwer CT, Schweitzer C, Pearson J, et al. Enzymes for liberation of pantothenic acid in blood: Use of plasma pantetheinase. Am J Clin Nutr 1989;50:1072-8.
178. Heird WC, Winters RW. Total parenteral nutrition: The state of the art. J Pediatr 1975;86:2-16
179. Heyman MB. General and specialized parenteral amino acid formulations for nutrition support. J Am Diet Assoc 1990;90:401-8.
180. Greene HL, Hambidge KM, Schanler R, Tsang RC. Guidelines for the use of vitamins, trace elements, calcium, magnesium, and phosphorus in infants and children receiving total parenteral nutrition. Am J Clin Nutr 1988;48:1324-42.
181. Cochran EB, Phelps SJ, Helms RA. Parenteral nutrition in pediatric patients. Clin Pharm 1988;7:351-67.
182. Rigaud D, Serog P, Legrand A, et al. Quantification of lipoprotein X and its relationship to plasma lipid profile during different types of parenteral nutrition. J Parenter Enteral Nutr 1984;8:529-34.
183. Zlotkin SH. Identification of fat overload during total parenteral nutrition. J Pediatr 1988;115:498.
184. Schmidt-Sommerfeld E, Penn D, Wolf H. Carnitine deficiency in premature infants receiving total parenteral nutrition: Effect of L-carnitine supplementation. J Pediatr 1983;102:931-5.
185. Spear ML, Stahl GE, Hamosh M, et al. Effect of heparin dose and infusion rate on lipid clearance and bilirubin binding in premature infants receiving intravenous fat emulsions. J Pediatr 1988;112:94-8.
186. Paust H, Schroder H, Park W. Intravascular accumulation of lipid in the very-low-birth-weight infant. J Pediatr 1983;103:668-9.
187. Brans YW, Duton EB, Andrew DS, et al. Fat emulsion tolerance in very low birth weight neonates: Effect on diffusion of oxygen in the lungs and on blood pH. Pediatr 1986;78:79-84.
188. Merritt RJ. Cholestasis associated with total parenteral nutrition. J Pediatr Gastroenterol Nutr 1986;5:9-22.
189. Matos C, Avni EF, Van Gansbeke D, Pardou A, Struyven J. Total parenteral nutrition (TPN) and gallbladder diseases in neonates: Sonographic assessment. J Ultrasound Med 1987;6:243-8.
190. Brooke OG, Lucas A. Metabolic bone disease in preterm infants. Arch Dis Child 1985;60:682-5.
191. Sedman AB, Klein GL, Merritt RJ, et al. Evidence of aluminum loading in infants receiving intravenous therapy. N Eng J Med 1985;312:1337-43.
192. McIntosh N. Rickets of prematurity. Bone 1984;1:26-7.
193. MacFarlane K, Bullock L, Fitzgerald JF. A usage evaluation of total parenteral nutrition in pediatric patients. J Parenter Enteral Nutr 1991;15:85-8.

Respiratory Disorders

Michele C. Walsh-Sukys, M.D.   L. Kyle Walker, M.D.
Billie Lou Short, M.D.

INTRODUCTION

This chapter describes the clinical picture of the most common pediatric respiratory disorders seen in the neonatal and pediatric intensive care setting. By far, the most common disorder encountered in the neonatal intensive care unit is respiratory distress syndrome. This single entity is associated with 30% of all neonatal deaths and 50–70% of premature deaths in the United States. This disorder is most commonly found in the preterm infant; disorders such as persistent pulmonary hypertension, pneumonia, and meconium aspiration are diseases of the term infant and are far less common than respiratory distress syndrome. A very common finding in premature infants who have resolved their pulmonary disease is apnea of prematurity, which can be so severe that mechanical ventilation is needed. Infants who require ventilator or oxygen support may sustain lung injury from such therapies, called "bronchopulmonary dysplasia." This disorder is more commonly seen in the very immature infant (< 28 w gestation).

The older child's respiratory diseases are much less homogenous when compared to the newborn, but in general can be grouped into upper and lower airway diseases. Although upper airway diseases can be emergent, life-threatening disorders, they represent only a small number of the admissions to a pediatric intensive care unit as compared to the lower respiratory disorders.

Lower airway disease can be divided into disorders of the bronchi and conducting airways and diseases of the alveoli. Each is discussed in detail in this chapter.

NEONATAL RESPIRATORY DISORDERS

Respiratory Distress Syndrome

Respiratory Distress Syndrome (RDS), formerly called hyaline membrane disease, is due to pulmonary surfactant deficiency. Surfactant deficiency is usually a developmental condition related to immaturity of the neonatal lung, but any number of insults may perturb the complex and delicate enzymatic systems responsible for surfactant synthesis and produce a picture indistinguishable from that seen in the preterm infant. Thus, RDS has been described in term infants and in older children as well as adults.[1] However, prematurity remains the single most important risk factor for RDS. The incidence and severity of RDS decreases with increasing gestational age, with fully 70% of those infants born at 28–30 w gestation manifesting full-blown RDS. In the classical presentation of RDS, a premature infant may appear well initially, but shortly after birth may develop tachypnea, signs of compromised respiration, and use of the accessory muscles of ventilation (grunting, nasal flaring, and intercostal retractions). Hypoxemia is the presenting feature on arterial blood gas analysis, but increases of PCO_2 are seen as the disease progresses. Radiographic study of the chest reveals a hazy ground-glass appearance in mild RDS, while complete opacification of the lung fields may be seen in more severe disease. Clinical symptoms worsen over the first 3–5 d of life and then begin to subside slowly. Clinical improvement is frequently heralded by a urinary diuresis.[2]

Because the primary defect in RDS is surfactant deficiency, much exciting research has focused on the development and administration of natural or synthetic surfactants. Surfactant is a lecithin-phospholipid synthesized by Type II alveolar epithelial cells which decreases surface tension within alveoli so that less pressure is required to hold alveoli open and maintains alveolar expansion by varying surface tension with alveolar size. Numerous controlled trials of exogenous surfactant administration have produced conflicting results (Table 2–1).[1, 3-14] Overall, these studies have shown that the severity of RDS has been reduced, but the impact on chronic lung disease and mortality has been more variable. Symptomatic support of the infant with RDS using supplemental oxygen and mechanical ventilation remains the mainstay of therapy.

TABLE 2–1. Results of Controlled Trials of Exogenous Surfactant Administration in the Treatment of Respiratory Distress Syndrome (RDS)

Investigators	Preparation*	Time of Administration	Number of Doses	Beneficial Effect
Chu et al., 1967	DDPC	After first breath	One	None
Morley et al., 1981	Dry DPPC:PG	At birth	One	Reduced mortality
Fujiwara et al., 1984	Surfactant TA	After ventilation	One	Reduced mortality
Halliday et al., 1984	DPPC	After ventilation	One	None
Wilkinson et al., 1985	Dry DPDC:PG	Trial 1: Before ventilation	One	None
		Trial 2: After ventilation	One	None
Hallman et al., 1985	Human surfactant from amniotic fluid	After ventilation	One	Reduced mortality and severity of RDS
Enhorning et al., 1985	Cow lung surfactant extract	Before ventilation	One	Reduced mortality and severity of RDS
Kwong et al., 1985	Calf lung surfactant extract	Before ventilation	One	Reduced severity of RDS; no change in mortality or BPD**
Shapiro et al., 1985	Calf lung surfactant extract	Before ventilation	One	Reduced severity of RDS; no change in mortality or BPD
Merritt et al., 1986	Human surfactant from amniotic fluid	At birth and later	Multiple	Reduced mortality and bronchopulmonary dysplasia
Gitlin et al., 1987	Surfactant TA	After ventilation	One	Reduced severity of RDS; no change in mortality or BPD
Kendig et al., 1991	Calf lung surfactant extract	At birth vs. later	Multiple	Reduced in those treated at birth
Dunn et al., 1991	Calf lung surfactant extract	At birth vs. later	Multiple	Reduced severity of RDS and BPD

Adapted from: Notler RH, Shapiro DL. Clin Perinatol 1987; 14:433.
*DPPC, Dipalmitoyl phosphatidylcholine; dry DPPC:PG, a dry powder of egg phosphatidylglycerol; surfactant TA, a surfactant extracted from minced cow lungs and enriched with DPPC and other additives.
**BPD, Bronchopulmonary dysplasia

The dawn of the era of surfactant replacement therapy has brought the need for a rapid postnatal test for surfactant deficiency. It is likely that these tests will be derived from those currently in use for *in utero* assessment of fetal lung maturity using amniotic fluid. The large number of tests currently in use suggests that none is entirely satisfactory. Physical measurements of surfactant do not measure individual phospholipids, but instead test non-chemical properties such as optical density, microviscosity, and foam stability. These all have the advantage of simplicity and speed, but have not been well correlated with clinical outcome. Biochemical assays of maturity are more widely used.

Measurement of the ratio of lecithin to sphingomyelin is the most common assay employed. Sphingomyelin content is constant in amniotic fluid during the third trimester, while the concentrations of all phospholipids rise dramatically after 35 w. Thus, sphingomyelin serves as a convenient reference phospholipid against which changes in lecithin can be compared. A second biochemical technique involves direct assay of the major phospholipid components of surfactant, with phosphatidylglycerol the most common component utilized. In the research setting, measurement of surfactant protein-A concentration by either ELISA or RIA techniques has been used successfully.

Persistent Pulmonary Hypertension of the Newborn

Persistent Pulmonary Hypertension of the Newborn (PPHN) is a pathophysiologic state related to sustained postnatal increase of pulmonary vascular resistance. This frequently leads to increased pulmonary artery pressure and a right-to-left shunt at the patent ductus arteriosus and/or the foramen ovale. The shunt is a dynamic event and may improve or worsen in response to therapeutic maneuvers or environmental stimuli. Profound and refractory hypoxemia is the ultimate consequence of PPHN.

PPHN is generally seen in post-mature infants, but also may be seen in near-term and term babies. Many different neonatal and perinatal factors may predispose to the development of PPHN (see Table 2–2), but it is seen most commonly with Meconium Aspiration Syndrome (MAS). Whatever the original insult, asphyxia and hypoxemia combine to promote pulmonary vasoconstriction.[15] If the condition persists over a long period of time, medial hypertrophy can occur, with extension of muscle into the normally nonmuscularized small pulmonary arteries. Once muscular proliferation occurs, the hypertension is usually irreversible and fatal.[16]

TABLE 2–2. Conditions Associated with Persistent Pulmonary Hypertension of the Newborn (PPHN)

Prenatal and Perinatal Conditions	Postnatal Conditions
Prolonged maternal aspirin or indomethacin therapy	Neonatal asphyxia
Maternal pregnancy-induced or chronic hypertension	Meconium aspiration syndrome
Maternal intravenous drug use	Sepsis neonatorum
Oligohydramnios	Pulmonary hypoplasia
Placental insufficiency and intrauterine hypoxia	Congenital diaphragmatic hernia
Postmaturity	Respiratory distress syndrome
Meconium-stained amniotic fluid	Cold stress
Perinatal asphyxia	Hypoglycemia
	Hypocalcemia
	Systemic hypotension
	Myocardial dysfunction
	Polycythemia and hyperviscosity

PPHN should be considered in newborns with or without respiratory compromise and with refractory hypoxemia.[17] Arterial blood gases will confirm hypoxemia. Simultaneous preductal (right radial artery) and postductal (usually umbilical artery) gases are useful to document a right-to-left shunt at the ductal level. It must be remembered that a shunt at the atrial level will equalize the preductal and postductal gases. A hyperoxia test may be both diagnostic and therapeutic. Supplemental oxygen is increased to 100% and a blood gas obtained after 20 min. Hypoxemia will improve if due to pulmonary parenchymal disease, but will remain if related to either PPHN or cyanotic heart disease. If hypoxemia is not relieved by supplemental oxygen, a two-dimensional echocardiogram should be obtained to assess for PPHN and to exclude cyanotic heart disease. Echocardiographic systolic time intervals have been used to assess pulmonary vascular resistance noninvasively. The right pre-ejection period is prolonged in PPHN (> 0.37), presumably due to increased modality, which is very useful in assessing the level and direction of shunts as well as in quantifying tricuspid and pulmonic regurgitation.

Much work has been directed toward identifying the biochemical mediators of PPHN.[18-20] It is clear that vasoconstriction and vasodilation result from a complex interplay of numerous hormonal and intercellular factors, including but not limited to prostacyclins, thromboxane, bradykinin, the leukotrienes, angiotensin II, and calcium. No single mediator has been found to be related to or diagnostic of PPHN.

Although two decades have passed since its first description, the treatment of PPHN remains controversial. Hyperventilation was introduced as a treatment for PPHN in 1980 and has since been widely adopted.[21, 22] However, no large, prospective trial has validated its efficacy, and uncontrolled reports cite mortality ranging from 30–50%. The use of hyperventilation induces alkalosis, which in turn triggers vasodilation, but the cost paid in barotrauma and oxygen toxicity are considerable. In addition, cerebral blood flow is impaired at extremes of alkalosis, which may account for the high rate of neurodevelopmental impairment seen in survivors of this therapy.[23-26] In 1985, Wung and James reported on their experience with a conservative ventilation regime with excellent survival.[27]

Clearly, a well-controlled randomized trial is critically needed to determine the most efficacious therapy for PPHN. Some infants fail to respond to conventional ventilation, regardless of the technique used. In these infants, selective pulmonary vasodilation is attempted.[28-31] Unfortunately, no vasodilator is specific to the pulmonary vascular bed; systemic hypotension is a frequent result of treatment. For infants in whom all other therapies have failed, support with extracorporeal membrane oxygenation (ECMO) may be life saving[32] (see discussion below).

Neonatal Pneumonia

Pneumonia is the most common form of neonatal infection. Pneumonia may be acquired transplacentally *in utero*, by aspiration of infected amniotic fluid at the time of delivery or by hematogenous spread from another focus of infection. Intrauterine pneumonia frequently occurs following prolonged rupture of the amniotic membranes. Some autopsy series have reported findings of intrauterine pneumonia in 5–35% of cases. Pneumonia may follow infection with the same organisms typically responsible for neonatal sepsis. If the diagnosis is considered at or shortly after birth, the primary organisms responsible are *Group B Streptococcus, E. coli, Klebsiella, Listeria,* and non-typable *H. influenzae.* If pneumonia occurs more than one week after birth, the same organisms may be involved but *S. aureus, Pseudomonas, Serratia* and *Candida* must be included in the differential diagnosis. Viral pneumonia may be present at birth or shortly thereafter. Nosocomial viral pneumonia with respiratory syncytial virus, ECHO, and adenovirus have been reported both sporadically and in epidemics.

Diagnosis of pneumonia is made on the basis of clinical findings of cyanosis, tachypnea, labored respirations, apnea, and lethargy. The classic hallmarks of rales, dullness to percussion, cough, and sputum production seen in older patients are usually absent in newborns. A chest radiograph will confirm the diagnosis. It is important to note that pneumonia due to *Group B Streptococcus* is radiographically indistinguishable from respiratory distress syndrome. Therefore, all infants with RDS must be evaluated and treated for infection until the diagnosis is excluded. Tracheal aspirate specimens obtained in intubated patients may not be helpful in the diagnosis due to the high rate of colonization with the same bacteria seen in infection. The presence of large numbers of polymorphonuclear cells with intracellular organisms on a gram stain of a tracheal specimen is more helpful in establishing an etiology for infection. Bacteremia may be present in as many as 30% of infants with pneumonia; blood cultures are therefore helpful in identifying a causative organisms.

Neonatal pneumonia must be treated with intravenous antibiotics directed against the causative organisms. The optimal duration of therapy has not been rigorously evaluated, but generally treatment for 10–14 d is recommended.

Apnea of Prematurity

Apnea of prematurity results from developmental immaturity of the respiratory control centers which improves as the infant matures.[33] Apnea is defined as a cessation of respiration which lasts at least 15 s. It is frequently accompanied by cyanosis, hypotonia, and bradycardia. The incidence and severity of apnea varies inversely with gestational age; the least mature infants are the most affected. Approximately 50% of all infants with birth weights less than 1500 g require intervention for apnea. An understanding of the pathophysiology of apnea may allow rational therapeutic intervention.

Respiratory neurons are located on the ventrolateral surface of the medulla and the pons. Von Euler proposed that the center receives input from both chemoreceptors and mechanoreceptors and then alters rhythmic discharges of the medullary centers responsible for sending efferent impulses to the respiratory musculature.[34] Immaturity appears to adversely influence the rhythmic firing of the brainstem neurons. Peripheral stimuli may influence respirations through chemical receptors that monitor PaO_2, $PaCO_2$, and pH. These chemoreceptors are located both centrally and peripherally. The normal response to hypercarbia in term neonates and in adults is to increase minute ventilation. The response to hypercarbia is blunted in preterm infants. Gerhardt and Bancalari found that apneic infants did not increase minute ventilation as effectively as nonapneic infants.[35] This is believed to reflect a low sensitivity of the respiratory center to hypercarbia and seems again to be a function of immaturity.

Hypoxemia is the other major chemical mediator of respiration. Older children and adults show an immediate increase in ventilation when placed in a hypoxic environment and suppress ventilation when placed in an oxygen-enriched environment. However, when challenged with a low inspired oxygen concentration, both term and preterm newborns briefly increase ventilation and then return to their resting level. Once the infant is 2–3 weeks old, hyperventilation in response to hypoxia is sustained, just as it is in older children. The mechanism responsible for this inappropriate response to hypoxia remains controversial. Traditionally the response is attributed to initial chemoreceptor stimulation, followed by hypoxic depression of the respiratory centers. Other proposed mechanisms include modulation of respiratory center response by endorphins, fatigue of the respiratory muscles, and hypoxia-induced increases in cerebral blood flow, which then lead to cerebral hypocapnia and respiratory depression.

Apnea may occur when the central drive to respiratory muscle fails, leading to a simultaneous cessation of both chest wall movement and airflow. This mechanism is termed "central apnea." In the past, central apnea was believed to be the exclusive mechanism responsible for apnea in the preterm infant. However, by measuring chest wall movements simultaneously with nasal air flow, investigators have demonstrated a cessation of air flow despite continued respiratory muscle activity. This has been termed "obstructive apnea." Although obstruction may be the exclusive mechanism responsible for apnea in a given infant, the most common pattern observed is a central respiratory pause either preceded by or followed by an obstruction. This pattern has been termed "mixed apnea" and represents the predominant form of apnea in 50% of infants. Brief episodes of apnea are more likely to be centrally mediated, whereas episodes longer than 15 s frequently have an obstructive component.

The upper airway of the preterm infant is susceptible to obstruction at the pharyngeal and hypopharyngeal levels. This obstruction may be aggravated by passive flexion of the neck and conversely may be relieved by passive extension.[36, 37] Pharyngeal tone is diminished in preterm infants. During inspiration, negative pressure generated by contraction of the diaphragm may collapse the pharyngeal musculature. For the collapsed airway to open, the infant must generate sufficient pressure by activation of the upper airway muscles such as the genioglossus to overcome surface adhesive forces (Figure 2–1). Infants with apnea fail to activate the genioglossus in response to induced end-expiratory airway occlusion, whereas preterm infants without apnea prolong the activity and the intensity of genioglossus activity.[38, 39] Thus, infants with apnea appear to lack an important mechanism for resolving the apneic episode.

Apnea as the final common response of immature respiratory regulatory centers may be associated with a large number of diverse factors in susceptible preterm infants (Figure 2–2). The diagnosis of apnea of prematurity can only be made after other potentially trigger-

FIGURE 2–1. Obstructive apnea may result when forces which initiate collapse of the upper airway are not adequately balanced by dilating forces of the upper airway muscles.

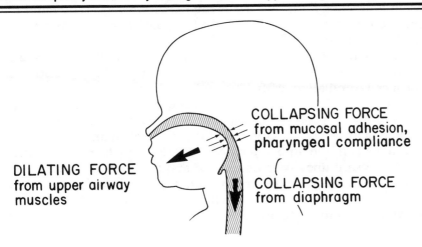

From: Martin RJ, Miller MJ, Carlo WA. Neonatal-perinatal medicine: Diseases of the fetus and newborn. J Pediatr 1986:109;733. Reprinted with permission.

FIGURE 2–2. Apnea may rise in response to a staggering number of insults which perturb the immature respiratory system.

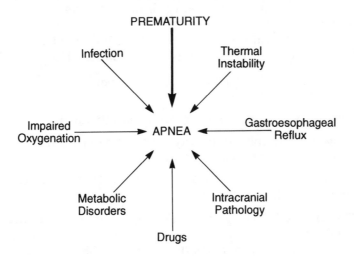

From: Martin RJ, Miller MJ, Carlo WA. Neonatal-perinatal medicine: Diseases of the fetus and newborn. J Pediatr 1986:109;733. Reprinted with permission.

ing events have been evaluated and excluded. All preterm infants less than 34 w gestation should be monitored continuously with a cardio-respiratory monitor until they are greater than 34 w gestation and free of apnea events for at least a week.[40] The goal of immediate management of an apneic episode is to restore adequate ventilation and to relieve hypoxemia. Gentle stimulation is frequently sufficient to arouse the infant and resolve the apneic episode. If stimulation is unsuccessful, artificial ventilation with bag and mask must be initiated. The infant's neck may be gently extended to overcome pharyngeal obstruction. Continuous positive airway pressure (CPAP) administered by nasal prongs at 2–5 cm H_2O may reduce obstructive and mixed apnea by stinting open the upper airway.[37] CPAP is ineffective in central apnea. Methyxanthines such as caffeine and theophylline may be effective in the treatment of refractory apnea regardless of the mechanism.[41] Infants are free of toxicity at plasma concentrations of theophylline of 5–10 mg/L and caffeine of 8–20 mg/L.

Bronchopulmonary Dysplasia

Low-birth-weight infants who have required support with oxygen and mechanical ventilation may have persistent chronic pulmonary dysfunction, which was termed Bronchopulmonary Dysplasia (BPD) by Northway and co-workers.[42] Some authors have labeled BPD as an iatrogenic disease, which implies some degree of therapeutic misadventure. An alternative view is that BPD is the inevitable consequence of exposure of the developing bronchopulmonary tree to oxygen and ventilation, spontaneous or mechanical, many weeks "too soon" in terms of biologic maturity.

There is no universally accepted definition of BPD. One of the most commonly used is that proposed by Bancalari:

1. a requirement for positive-pressure ventilation for greater than three days in the first week of life;

2. respiratory symptoms for greater than 28 days;

3. a need for supplemental oxygen for greater than 28 days to maintain a PaO_2 over 50 mmHg; and

4. a chest roentgenogram showing persistent infiltrates alternating with normal or cystic changes.[43]

The risk of BPD is greatest among the most immature infants. In one study of infants who received mechanical ventilation, 72% of infants weighing less than 1000 g developed BPD, compared to 22% of infants between 1250–1500 g. The incidence of BPD varies dramatically between centers and is influenced not only by the definition used within each center, but also by treatment approaches within each center.[44]

The natural history of BPD is not completely understood. Mortality varies from 11% to 73% in different reports. Most patients who die do so within the first year of life. The incidence of sudden death is increased sevenfold over that seen in normal infants.[45] Infants who survive BPD frequently have residual cardiopulmonary dysfunction.[46] Minor respiratory illnesses may unmask limited cardiopulmonary reserve and require rehospitalization. In one study, infants with BPD were rehospitalized an average of 5 times within the first two years of life. Pulmonary symptoms diminish with time, and most children appear clinically well by 3–4 y of age.[47] Nevertheless, pulmonary function abnormalities can be demonstrated in both school-age and adolescent survivors of BPD who appear to be functioning normally in every other way. Cor pulmonale, a frequent accompaniment to BPD, resolves in parallel with the lung disease.

Developmental delays and neurologic abnormalities are seen frequently in infants with BPD.[48] Several investigators have reported that up to 80% of infants with severe BPD had developmental quotients less than 80 at 2–5 y of age. Infants with less severe disease have a better outcome. Severe hearing loss and blindness related to retinopathy of prematurity are also seen with increased frequency in survivors of BPD. It is likely that outcome is related not only to BPD, but to perinatal events which precipitated the premature birth, and to all the concomitant problems related to severe immaturity, such as intraventricular hemorrhage, delayed growth, and recurrent infection.

Our understanding of the pathophysiology of BPD is still in its infancy. Goetzman has proposed that a susceptible host, with an immature lung, asphyxia, or a genetic predisposition suffers acute pulmonary injury because of surfactant deficiency, oxygen toxicity, and/or barotrauma.[49] The initial injury leads to release of oxidants and proteolytic enzymes which cause further lung injury. The lung then heals in an abnormal manner, perhaps aggravated by inadequate nutrition and vitamin deficiencies.[50] The need for continued therapy with oxygen or mechanical ventilation may generate new injury and inhibit healing of prior injury. Superimposed infection may lead to proliferation of inflammatory mediators and cellular cytokines, which create a chronic inflammatory response and prevent normal healing.

The management of the infant with BPD is controversial and fraught with frustration, since the need for continued life-supporting therapies implies continuation of treatments that contributed to the pathogenesis of the disease. The key to eventual recovery is growth. Infants frequently must consume 120–150 kcal/kg/d to meet the increased caloric requirements of breathing and tissue repair and still allow growth. Supplemental oxygen and/or mechanical ventilation may be needed for prolonged periods, which may exceed one year in severely affected infants. Bronchodilators have been demonstrated in short-term studies to improve compliance and reduce airway resistance. Diuretics may also improve compliance.

The use of corticosteroids early in the course of respiratory illness (14–28 d of age) in an attempt to limit inflammatory injury and therefore prevent BPD has been a recent advance in the care of ventilator dependent low-birth-weight infants. In small, short-term studies, infants treated with steroids demonstrated improved lung compliance and an enhanced ability to wean from mechanical ventilation.[51] Treatment was not without side effects, however; hypertension, hyperglycemia, and sepsis were all seen at increased rates. While therapy with corticosteroids ultimately may prove to be beneficial, many questions remain to be answered, including: the population likely to benefit the most from therapy, the most efficacious preparation and dosing regime, and long-term side effects on hormonal development and growth.

Special Needs of the Newborn Intensive Care Unit:
Laboratory Tests and Blood Gas Monitoring

State-of-the-art care of preterm infants in the 1990s requires a laboratory capable of the collection and rapid processing of samples using microtechniques. It is imperative that phlebotomists are trained thoroughly to obtain specimens by capillary sampling from the heel to ensure both minimal trauma to the infant as well as accurate laboratory results. Laboratories must provide a 24 h service for electrolyte, complete blood count, bilirubin, coagulation, microbiology, and blood gas monitoring. Ideally, blood gas measurements should be done in the NICU. Blood gas values should be available within 10–15 mins. Results of emergent studies should be available within 60 min, and of routine studies within 4–6 h. Consultation with a clinical pathologist or laboratory scientist skilled in the problems of newborn infants must also be available around the clock. The microbiology laboratory must be familiar with the unique problems of premature infants with regard to infection, including the pathogenicity of organisms such as *Staphylococcus epidermidis* which might otherwise be dismissed as contaminants.

Bedside monitoring including pulse oximetry and, to a lesser extent, transcutaneous pO_2 and pO_2 monitoring have allowed the caretaking team to make changes in F_iO_2 without the need for an arterial or capillary blood gas, thus decreasing the workload of blood gas laboratories.

Most critically ill newborns will require arterial blood gases every 1–2 h and complete blood count, electrolytes, and calcium concentrations every 12–24 h. Also of importance to the newborn, and especially the preterm infant, is total, direct, and indirect serum bilirubin, which may be needed every 8 h in the first few days of life, and the serum glucose values which are needed to confirm bedside dextrometer measurements. Drug monitoring is also a needed item in the NICU, including serum aminoglycoside, vancomycin, caffeine, and theophylline concentrations. When starting a new drug, concentrations will need to be monitored daily until therapeutic measurements are achieved. Nutritional monitoring must be undertaken if an infant is on hyperalimentation, including serum phosphorus, magnesium, liver function studies, triglycerides, and the routine tests listed above. If a coagulopathy is suspected, coagulation profiles must be available, include platelet counts, prothrombin time, partial thromboplastin time, fibrinogen, D-dimer, and fibrin degradation products.

PEDIATRIC RESPIRATORY FAILURE

Pediatric respiratory failure can be defined as the failure to maintain adequate respiratory gas exchange. Respiratory failure can occur because of dysfunction at the level of the nares and oropharynx, the larynx, the tracheobronchial tree, or the alveolus. The anatomic level of the lesion is a useful way to analyze the different causes of pediatric respiratory failure, since the symptoms and pathophysiology can be quite different. The most common scheme calls for division into upper and lower airway disease. Upper airway disease includes lesions that affect the nose, oropharynx, larynx, and trachea; lower airway disease involves the bronchi, bronchioles, and alveoli.

Upper Airway Disease

Upper airway disease is more prominent in children than in adults due to anatomical differences in the growing and developing airway. At birth, the larynx and epiglottis are located much higher in the neck. The placement is more anterior and closer to the nasopharynx. This positioning renders the infant an obligate nose-breather until 2–6 m of age.[52] With growth, the larynx descends caudally and posteriorly until it reaches the adult positioning at approximately age 10 y. Other differences in the pediatric airway include increased prominence of the tongue and arytenoids, a softer and more elastic larynx and trachea, and, most importantly, a much smaller diameter. Since resistance to flow is related inversely to the fourth power of the radius, decreased diameter causes enormous increases in resistance.

The causes of upper airway disease can be broken down into two categories: congenital anomalies or acquired lesions. Table 2–3 lists some of the more common causes. The symptoms of upper airway obstruction are more indicative of the anatomic level of the lesion rather than the cause. A common symptom is stridor or "noisy" breathing caused by rapid, turbulent flow through an obstructed or narrowed portion of the airway.[52] Inspiratory stridor is common with lesions above or at the level of the larynx, while expiratory stridor is more often seen with lesions below the level of the vocal cords. Stridor with inspiration and expiration often indicates a fixed lesion, such as subglottic stenosis. Other symptoms include a weak or muffled cry, a "barking cough," feeding difficulties, retractions, tachypnea, and tachycardia. Hypoventilation with a rising CO_2 is seen before cyanosis, but both are late findings and signify a need for rapid action.

The most common presentation of upper airway disease is respiratory distress and noisy breathing. Congenital lesions may not be symptomatic at birth, with the exception of choanal atresia, as the children may compensate until a critical degree of obstruction occurs. This decompensation often occurs with an upper respiratory infection. Stridor at or near birth does require evaluation, as it is often an indicator of a congenital problem, the most common being laryngomalacia.

Most causes of stridor and upper airway obstruction in children are caused by infection. The two most common are acute laryngo-

TABLE 2–3. Causes of Upper Airway Obstruction

Congenital Lesions	Acquired Lesions
Intrinsic lesions	Infections
Subglottic stenosis	Retropharyngeal abscess
Web	Ludwig's angina
Cyst	Laryngotracheobronchitis
Laryngocele	Supraglottitis
Tumor	Fungal infection
Laryngomalacia	Peritonsillar abscess
Laryngotracheoesophageal cleft	Diphtheria
Tracheomalacia	Bacterial tracheitis
Tracheoesophageal fistula	Trauma—internal
Extrinsic lesions	Postextubation croup
Vascular ring	Post-tracheostomy removal
Cystic hygroma	Trauma—external
Birth Trauma	Burns—thermal, chemical
Neurologic lesion	Foreign body aspiration
Craniofacial anomalies	Systemic disorders
Metabolic disorders—Hypocalcemia	Neoplasms—internal, external
	Neurologic lesions
	Chronic upper airway obstruction
	Hypertrophic tonsils, adenoids
	Tight surgical neck dressing

From: Rogers MC, ed. Textbook of pediatric intensive care. Williams and Wilkins, 1987. Reprinted with permission.

tracheobronchitis (croup), usually seen in children 6 m to 3 y of age, and acute supraglottis (epiglottitis), which is most common in children 2–6 y of age. Other causes are retropharyngeal abscess, peritonsillar abscess, and bacterial tracheitis. The differential diagnosis usually revolves around distinguishing croup from epiglottitis. Some of the common differences are shown in Table 2–4. Epiglottitis requires a higher sensitivity to the risks of airway occlusion, and most people recommend securing the airway in a controlled fashion. This is best done with a skilled anesthesiologist or anesthetist, usually under inhalational anesthesia in the operating room. More detailed discussions of this problem are available.[52] Croup is less likely to result in sudden obstruction of the airway. If the child tires and obstructs, with croup, the supraglottic structures are not swollen and distorted as in epiglottitis, and an artificial airway is more easily placed.

A final thought about upper airway lesions is that the risk of acute total obstruction in all of these diseases is real, and inability to establish or maintain an airway can result in death. Establishment of an artificial airway such as an endotracheal or tracheostomy tube can be extremely difficult with abnormal or distorted anatomy. This is particularly true in the emergent situation. Sensitivity to tiring, hypercarbia, increased agitation or other signs of impending respiratory failure must be high. Laboratory evaluations most likely to be of help are arterial blood gases. The CBC can sometimes add information if the cause

TABLE 2–4. Clinical Characteristics Differentiating Laryngotracheobronchitis (LTB) from Supraglottitis

Characteristic	LTB	Supraglottitis
Age	6 m to 3 y	2 to 6 y
Onset	Gradual	Rapid
Etiology	Viral	Bacterial
Swelling site	Subglottic	Supraglottic
Symptoms		
Cough/voice	Hoarse cough	No cough; muffled voice
Posture	Any position	Sitting
Mouth	Closed; nasal flaring	Open—chin forward, drooling
Fever	Absent to high	High
Appearance	Often not acutely ill	Anxious; acutely ill
X-ray	Narrow subglottic area	Swollen epiglottis and supraglottic structures
Palpation larynx	Nontender	Tender
Recurrence	May recur	Rarely recurs
Seasonal incidence	Winter	None

From: Rogers MC, ed. Textbook of pediatric intensive care. Williams and Wilkins, 1987.
Reprinted with permission.

is infectious and cultures of the airway and blood often recover an organism in epiglottitis or bacterial tracheitis.

Lower Airway Disease

Lower airway disease can be divided into disorders of the bronchi and conducting airways and diseases of the alveoli. The two most common diseases of the conducting airways include bronchiolitis and asthma, and there is evidence of overlap between the two processes. Acute respiratory failure after injury to the alveolar capillary unit may occur after a variety of insults.[53] These can include infectious pneumonias, inhalational injuries, sepsis, or shock. A list of common causes is presented in Table 2–5.[53] Injury to the alveolar capillary unit is most often a common group of pathophysiologic findings currently referred to in the literature as adult respiratory distress syndrome (ARDS).

TABLE 2–5. Disorders Associated with (Causing) Adult Respiratory Distress Syndrome (ARDS)

Common	Uncommon
Trauma	Drug overdose (e.g., narcotic—idiosyncratic reaction)
Sepsis	Cardiopulmonary bypass
Near drowning	Hemodialysis
Shock	Fat embolism
Surface burns	High altitude
Smoke inhalation	Strangulation
Infectious pneumonia	Toxic gas inhalation
Gram-negative bacteria	Pancreatitis
Viral	Massive transfusion
Pneumocystis	
Aspiration pneumonia	
Disseminated intravascular coagulopathy	

From: Rogers MC, ed. Textbook of pediatric intensive care. Williams and Wilkins, 1987.
Reprinted with permission.

Bronchiolitis

Bronchiolitis is an acute inflammatory disease of the lower respiratory tract which results in obstruction of the small airways.[54] It is most commonly seen in infants 1–2 y of age. The reported incidence of 11.4 cases per 100 children per year in the first year of life falls to 6 per 100 children per year in the second year of life.[55] Viral agents are the cause and include respiratory syncytial virus (the most common identified cause), parainfluenza, rhinovirus, adenovirus, influenza, and occasionally mumps.[54]

Histopathologically, there is an inflammatory lesion of the respiratory epithelium which leads to small airway obstruction. There is necrosis of the ciliated epithelium with proliferation of non-ciliated cells and edema. In addition to the edema, debris builds up in the bronchioles due to lack of cilia, and they become partially or completely obstructed. A chest radiograph will typically show air trapping and peribronchial thickening, with occasional lobar consolidation or collapse. The alveoli may also be involved in the inflammatory process, with infiltrates of lymphocytes and edema seen in the alveolar lining cells.[54]

Clinically, the infants present with expiratory wheezing, tachypnea, retractions, and irritability. There is often a low-grade fever, cyanosis, and feeding difficulties. Auscultation reveals diffuse wheezing, prolonged expiration, and rales. Younger infants have a significant risk of apnea[56] At one time it was commonly thought that bronchiolitis was the cause of all wheezing in children under age 2 y, and that asthma did not appear until a later age. This is clearly not true. Reversible airway obstruction can occur in infants as well as children, and there are questions about an association between severe bronchiolitis as an infant and an increased incidence of asthma in the childhood years.

Asthma

The hallmark of asthma is a reversible diffuse obstruction to airflow caused by narrowing of hyperreactive airways. This obstruction is intermittent and may reverse with or without treatment. Periods between attacks are usually symptom free, although some abnormalities may be detected with pulmonary function testing.[54] The bronchoconstriction can be precipitated by a variety of stimuli, including allergens, infectious agents, exercise, emotional stress, or the administration of certain drugs (see Table 2–6).

TABLE 2–6. Some Factors that Precipitate Bronchoconstriction in Asthma

Allergy (mediator release)	Infections
Histamine	Viral respiratory tract infection
SRS-A	
Prostaglandins	**Pharmacologic Agents**
Thromboxane	β-adrenergic blockade (propranolol)
Other	Prostaglandin inhibitors (aspirin and
Autonomic Imbalance	nonsteroidal anti-inflammatory drugs)
Excessive cholinergic response	
Reduced β-adrenergic responsiveness	**Exercise Induced**
Nonspecific irritant	Psychogenic

From: Rogers MC, ed. Textbook of pediatric intensive care. Williams and Wilkins, 1987. Reprinted with permission.

Autopsy findings in a patient who dies from status asthmaticus show hypertrophy of smooth muscle in the bronchial wall, associated submucosal and mucosal edema, and mucous plugging of the airways.[55] There are several proposed schemata to explain the pathophysiology of asthma, including:

1. allergens and mast cell/histamine/mediator derangements;[58]

2. derangements of the autonomic nervous system with reduced β-drenergic responsiveness;[59] and

3. aberrant bronchial smooth muscle.[60]

Clinically, patients present with gradual or sudden onset of respiratory distress, which is characterized by diffuse wheezing, a prolonged expiratory phase, tachypnea, tachycardia, and cyanosis. This bronchospasm or acute airway obstruction is often responsive to acute administration of β-adrenergic agonists. Progressive, severe airflow obstruction that is unresponsive to therapy with adrenergic drugs and theophylline is defined as status asthmaticus. Current acute therapy includes administration of β-adrenergic agonists such as epinephrine or terbutaline subcutaneously, or metaproterenol (alupent) or salbutamol (albuterol) by aerosol; intravenous theophylline; intravenous corticosteroids; and aerosolized anti-cholinergic agents such as atropine or ipratropium bromide. Patients should have humidified oxygen administered as needed, and they may be dehydrated because of decreased fluid intake and increased, insensible loss. Ventilatory support with intubation and mechanical ventilation may be necessary in face of progressive tiring and hypoventilation, but carries significant risk of mechanical barotrauma. Chronic therapy includes oral theophylline, inhaled cromolyn sodium, inhaled β-adrenergic agonists, and steroids and oral steroids.

The laboratory values of most interest are arterial blood gases. Serum electrolytes can be useful in guiding hydration therapy. The complete blood count (CBC) usually offers little information that would guide therapy. Therapeutic use of theophylline is guided by frequent serum concentrations.

Adult Respiratory Distress Syndrome (ARDS)

The term ARDS was introduced by Ashbaugh et al.[61] in 1967 and its definition now includes the following points:[62]

1. a catastrophic pulmonary or non-pulmonary event in the patient with previously normal lungs;

2. respiratory distress with hypoxemia, decreased pulmonary compliance, and increased shunt (Qs/Qt) fraction;

3. radiologic evidence of diffuse pulmonary infiltrates; and

4. exclusion of left heart disease and congestive heart failure.

The common microscopic findings include degeneration of alveolar epithelial cells and evidence of injury to the pulmonary capillary endothelium with disruption of the alveolar-capillary membrane.[53] There also may be clots and microemboli that extend from the subendothelial space into the capillary lumen.[63] There is development of proteinaceous hemorrhagic edema in the interstitium, alveolar wall, and alveolus because of the loss of alveolar capillary membrane integrity. This proteinaceous fluid can coalesce and form hyaline membranes. Effort to repair this injury results in proliferation of cuboidal type II pneumocytes, migration of white cells, and formation of fibrous tissue which increases the interstitial volume and destroys acinar architecture. If the destruction is great enough, there is life-threatening loss of surface area available for gas exchange.[53] Functionally, there is loss of compliance and reduced lung volumes with severe arterial hypoxemia and a large venous admixture. The hypoxemia is explained by both right-to-left intrapulmonary shunting and ventilation/perfusion mismatch. There is often an increase in pulmonary vascular resistance.

The clinical presentation is usually characterized by a latent period of minimal symptoms, except that of hyperventilation, and then the gradual onset of respiratory distress. There is profound hypoxemia which is unresponsive to supplemental oxygen by face mask or nasal prongs. The chest X-ray is relatively nonspecific, being normal initially and then showing evidence of pulmonary edema without cardiomegaly and an evolving interstitial pattern.[64] Standard therapy includes tracheal intubation and mechanical ventilation in the face of worsening lung disease when the patient is hypoxemic on > 0.5 F_iO_2.[53] Different mechanical ventilatory maneuvers are used, but the most common involves the use of increased positive end-expiratory pressure (PEEP) to increase and maintain alveolar patency and lung volume. This also improves ventilation and perfusion matching.[53] PEEP itself has many side effects, including barotrauma, increased lung water, and a fall in cardiac output. Therefore, measurements of cardiac output and oxygen delivery obtained with various methods are often used to guide therapy if a PEEP of ≥ 15 cmH_2O is used. Other therapy involves treating inciting disorders if possible, careful fluid balance, inotropic agents, and meticulous monitoring of vital signs, blood pressure, and arterial blood gases. There is no specific therapy available, as the actual mode of injury is multifactorial and is still being investigated.

In spite of careful monitoring and aggressive support, the mortality for ARDS remains quite high. Pediatric mortality in the literature ranges from 28% to 90%, with an average of 52%.[53] Most often, death is not from refractory respiratory failure but secondary to sepsis and failure of other major organs.

Extensive laboratory support is necessary to care for these children. These are often the most critically ill patients in the intensive care unit. Careful monitoring of electrolytes and measures of organ function are needed. Rapid determination of arterial blood gases and hemoglobin saturation measurements is essential. Extensive microbiologic support and measurements of nutritional status are often key. Other monitoring devices that provide minute-to-minute tracking of respiratory function are quite useful. In particular, the end-tidal CO_2 monitor and pulse oximetry may improve monitoring and reduce the need for blood sampling.

NEONATAL EXTRACORPOREAL MEMBRANE OXYGENATION (ECMO)

Extracorporeal membrane oxygenation (ECMO) is the use of extracorporeal circulation and gas exchange to provide temporary life support in patients with cardiac or pulmonary failure.[65] The key component of ECMO is the transport of oxygen into blood across a semi-permeable membrane, which can be achieved with the use of a silicone membrane lung (SciMed Life Sciences, Inc., Minneapolis, MN), and a modified cardiopulmonary bypass system.[66] Long-term (5–21 d) support is possible because the membrane lung separates oxygen and blood components and therefore does not result in hemolysis over time, as did the "bubble oxygenators" which were used in cardiopulmonary bypass surgery. Gas exchange is through a simple diffusion process across a gradient (see Figure 2–3).

Patient Selection

ECMO is the *temporary* use of an artificial lung. Because of the invasive nature and systemic heparinization required, there are many limitations to the use of ECMO in the neonatal population. If a neonate's respiratory disorder can be reversed within a 21 d period, it is feasible for ECMO to safely support the patient. After this time, complications such as bleeding and clot formation in the circuit become more difficult to control. For this reason, it is not practical to use ECMO to treat a disease process such as bronchopulmonary dysplasia, which would require a longer period on the system to reverse the chronic lung damage. The common causes of respiratory failure in neonates are generally reversible within a few days (average time on ECMO is 5 d).

Many very-low-birth-weight infants have severe RDS and would appear to be good ECMO candidates, but the heparinization and/or the alterations in pulsatility of blood flow created by ECMO cause a significant incidence of intracranial hemorrhage and thus a prohibitive mortality in this group of infants.[67] Because of the above concerns, the infant considered for ECMO must be > 34 w gestation, have reversible

FIGURE 2–3. Schematic of the silicone membrane lung used in ECMO. Oxygen and carbon dioxide transfer because of simple diffusion across a concentration gradient. The silicone membrane separates the blood and gas phases, thus decreasing the risk for hemolysis.

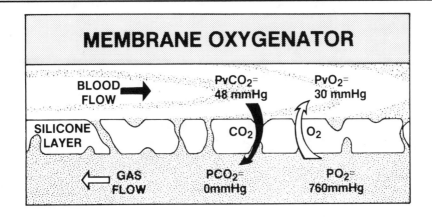

From: Fox W, Polin R (Eds.), Fetal and neonatal physiology. W.B. Saunders, 1991. Reprinted with permission.

lung disease, have less than 10 d of assisted ventilation, and lack an uncontrollable coagulopathy or major intracranial hemorrhage. Institutional criteria predicting an 80% mortality without ECMO[68, 69] should be used to determine when to institute ECMO therapy.

The majority of the pulmonary diseases treated with ECMO are those with underlying persistent pulmonary hypertension resulting in significant right-to-left shunting through the ductus arteriosus and/or foramen ovale, and include meconium aspiration syndrome, severe respiratory distress syndrome, sepsis and/or pneumonia, and congenital diaphragmatic hernia (CDH). Idiopathic, persistent pulmonary hypertension represents almost 20 percent of ECMO cases.[65]

Venoarterial Bypass

In venoarterial (VA) bypass, blood is drained from the right atrium through a catheter placed in the *right internal jugular vein* with the tip of the catheter in the right atrium, deposited into a venous reservoir bag, pumped through a membrane oxygenator where gas exchange occurs, passed through a heat exchanger to warm to body temperature, and returned to the patient through the *right common carotid artery* (see Figure 2–4). This mode of bypass provides excellent support for the heart and lungs. If myocardial ischemia and dysfunction is a major component in the patient's pathology, VA bypass will provide excellent

FIGURE 2–4. Venoarterial ECMO circuit, showing the drainage from the right atrium into the venous reservoir bag, into the membrane lung where oxygenation occurs, warmed to body temperature by the heat exchanger, and returned to the arch of the aorta via the carotid artery catheter.

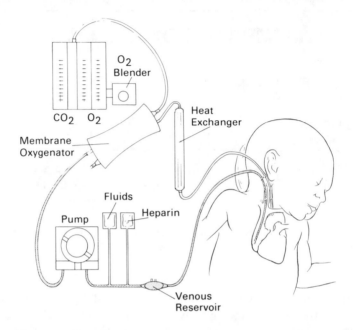

From: Fox W, Polin R (Eds.), Fetal and neonatal physiology. W.B. Saunders Co., 1991. Reprinted with permission.

FIGURE 2–5. Schematic of the venovenous catheter in the right atrium showing the return and outflow portions of the double-lumen single catheter.

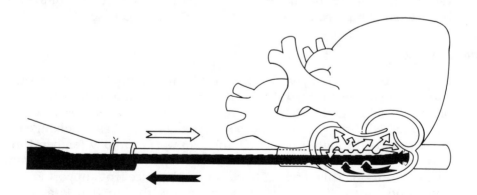

From: Short BL (Ed.), The CNMC ECMO training manual. CNMC, 1991. Reprinted with permission.

cardiac support. Advantages and disadvantages to venoarterial bypass are:

Advantages

- Excellent support of the heart and lungs
- Only one surgical site
- Excellent oxygenation at low flows
- Not dependent on cardiac function

Disadvantages

- Any particles, bubbles, or emboli in the circuit could be infused into the patient's arterial system (i.e., the brain)
- Carotid ligation
- Potential hyperoxia of blood supplying the brain

Venovenous Bypass

Venovenous (VV) bypass is now being used for infants using a single double-lumen venous catheter (The Kendal Co., Mansfield, MA; see Figure 2–5).[70] The inflow and outflow ports of this catheter hook into the circuit as if there were two catheters, and therefore the circuit design is the same as with VA ECMO. Infants treated with VV ECMO must have intact cardiac function, for the heart, not the ECMO pump, must pump the blood. Therefore, this mode of ECMO is limited to less-sick neonates. Those who do not tolerate VV ECMO can easily be converted to VA ECMO by placing an arterial catheter in the carotid artery while using the double-lumen VV catheter as the venous catheter.

Oxygenation During ECMO

ECMO supplies pulmonary support so that the lungs can rest, allowing time for injured lungs to heal. Although VA ECMO can mechanically decrease pulmonary artery pressure by diverting blood flow from the right atrium through the ECMO circuit, the exact mechanism involved in reversal of pulmonary hypertension and/or the underlying pulmonary pathology is unknown. In the first days of ECMO, 60% of the cardiac output (120 mL/kg/min) must flow through the circuit and thus through the membrane lung. As the lungs improve, the arterial blood gases of the infant will improve and the ECMO circuit blood flow rates can be gradually decreased. This period of gradual decrease continues until only 10% of the cardiac output is going through the ECMO circuit. If arterial blood gases remain good, the patient can be successfully taken off ECMO. Infants will require the ventilator for another 24–48 h, but most come off in a 48 h period and off oxygen in 5–7 d.

The CDH infant is the exception, requiring up to 2–3 w to come off the ventilator.

Laboratory Requirements

The infant on ECMO requires a significant amount of laboratory support. The infant may need hourly arterial blood gas measurements from the patient, which can be decreased to 2–4 h if an in-line venous saturation monitor is used. Membrane blood gas measurements should be taken every 8–12 h as a minimum, and more often if clinically indicated. The membrane lung blood gases will have an extremely high PO_2 (350–500 torr) due to the efficiency of the membrane lung. Laboratory tests needed every 8–12 h include hemoglobin, hematocrit, calcium, sodium, potassium, chloride, and CO_2. The membrane lung binds platelets and therefore values will need to be determined every 8 h.[71, 72] Platelet counts are kept between 60,000 and 200,000 mm^3, depending on the bleeding complications of the patient, resulting in 1–2 units of platelets transfused per day. Daily laboratory tests should include phosphorus, magnesium, serum osmolality, BUN, creatinine, and total, direct, and indirect bilirubin. Infants on ECMO require very little sodium replacement (1–2 mEq/kg/d), high potassium replacement (4–5 mEq/kg/d), and relatively high calcium replacement (40–50 mg of elemental calcium/kg/d). Reasons for these requirements are not fully understood.

Prolonged heparinization of the infant requires the use of a bedside test to determine activated clotting times (ACT). Centers use various systems, with the Hemachrone (International Technidyne, Edison, NJ), which uses only 0.25 mL per sample, being the most popular. ACTs are kept between 180–250 s, depending on the bleeding complications in the patient. When disseminated intravascular coagulation is thought to be a problem in an ECMO patient, PT/PTT can be used, but methods to deactivate the heparin effect must be taken. Other clotting tests which should be available are antithrombin III, fibrin degradation products, fibrinogen, and D-dimer. Plasma free hemoglobin concentrations are also needed on a daily basis in the venovenous patients because the high resistance in the VV catheter can cause significant hemolysis.

Laboratory and hematologic support is critical for the patients requiring surgery on ECMO, such as the patient with congenital diaphragmatic hernia. ACT values are kept very low at 180–190 seconds, with platelets > 200,000 mm^3 and fibrinogen concentrations > 150 (mg%). Bleeding can be catastrophic, requiring removal from ECMO and causing death. Blood products, including packed cells, platelets, fresh frozen plasma, and cryoprecipitate, must be available on an emergency basis. Protocols for transfusion of products on ECMO should be developed.

SUMMARY

The respiratory diseases treated in the newborn and pediatric patient are diverse and often life threatening. These cases require an intensive approach to laboratory monitoring, and thus centers caring for these infants must maintain a laboratory capable of microtechniques and very rapid response times to ensure proper care of the patient.

REFERENCES

1. Chu J, Clements JA, Cotton EK et al. Neonatal pulmonary ischemia: Clinical and physiologic studies. Pediatrics 1967;40:709-66.
2. Green TP, Thompson TR, Johnson DE, Lock JE. Diuresis and pulmonary function in premature infants with respiratory distress syndrome. J Pediatr 1983;103:618-23.
3. Morley CJ, Mangham AD, Miller N et al. Dry artificial lung surfactant and its effect on very premature babies. Lancet 1981;i:64-68.
4. Fujiwara T: Surfactant replacement in neonatal RDS. In: Robertson B, van Golde LMG, Batenburg JJ, eds. Pulmonary surfactant. Amsterdam: Elsevier Publishing, 1984:479-504.
5. Halliday HL, McClure G, Reid M et al. Controlled trial of artificial surfactant to prevent respiratory distress syndrome. Lancet 1984;1:476-78.
6. Wilkinson A, Jenkins PA, Jeffrey JA. Two controlled trials of artificial surfactant: Early effects and later outcome in babies with surfactant deficiency. Lancet 1985;ii:287-91.
7. Hallman M, Merritt TA, Jarvenpaa A-L et al. Exogenous human surfactant for treatment of severe respiratory distress syndrome: A randomized, prospective clinical trial. J Pediatr 1985;106:963-69.
8. Enhorning GE, Shennan A, Possmayer F et al. Prevention of neonatal respiratory distress syndrome by tracheal instillation of surfactant: A randomized clinical trial. Pediatrics 1985;76:145-53.
9. Kwong MS, Egan EA, Notter RH et al. A double-blind clinical trial of calf lung lipid for the prevention of hyaline membrane disease in extremely premature infants. Pediatrics 1985;76:585-92.
10. Shapiro DL, Notter RH, Monh FC et al. A double-blind, randomized trial of a calf lung surfactant extract administered at birth to very premature infants for prevention of the respiratory distress syndrome. Pediatrics 1985;76:593-99.
11. Merritt TA, Hallman M, Bloom BT et al. Prophylactic treatment of very premature infants with human surfactant. N Engl J Med 1986;315:785-90.
12. Gitlin JD, Sou CF, Parad RB et al. Randomized controlled trial of exogenous surfactant for the treatment of hyaline membrane disease. Pediatrics 1987;79:31-37.
13. Kendig JW, Notter RH, Cox C et al. A comparison of surfactant as immediate prophylaxis and as rescue therapy in newborns of less than 30 weeks gestation. N Engl J Med 1991;324:865-71.
14. Dunn MS et al. Bovine surfactant replacement therapy in neonates of less than 30 weeks gestation: A randomized controlled trial of prophylaxis versus treatment. Pediatrics 1991;87:377-86.
15. Peckham GJ, Fox WW. Physiologic factors affecting pulmonary artery pressure in infants with persistent pulmonary hypertension. J Pediatr 1978;93:1005-10.
16. Murphy JE, Rabinovitch M, Goldstein JD, Reid LM. The structural basis of persistent pulmonary hypertension of the newborn infant. J Pediatr 1981;98:962-67.
17. Geggel RL, Reid LM. The structural basis of PPHN. Clin Perinatol 1984;11:525-45.
18. Heymann MA, le Biodis J, Soifer SJ, Clyman RI. Leukotriene synthesis inhibition increases pulmonary blood flow in fetal lambs. Chest 1988;93:117S.
19. Murphy JD, Freed MD, Lang P, Epstein M, Frantz I. Prostaglandin-E1 in neonatal persistent pulmonary hypertension. Pediatr Res 1980;14:606-11.

20. Levin DL, Fixler DE, Morriss FC et al. Morphologic analysis of the pulmonary vascular bed in infants exposed *in utero* to prostaglandin synthetase inhibitors. J Pediatr 1978;92:478-83.

21. Drummond WH, Gregory GA, Heymann MA, Phibbs RA. The independent effect of hyperventilation, tolazoline and dopamine on infants with persistent pulmonary hypertension. J Pediatr 1981;98:603-11.

22. Duara S, Gewitz MH, Fox WW. Use of mechanical ventilation for clinical management of persistent pulmonary hypertension of the newborn. Clin Perinatol 1984;11:641-52.

23. Gleason CA, Short BL, Jones MD Jr. Cerebral blood flow and metabolism during and after prolonged hypocapnia in newborn lambs. J Pediatr 1989;115:309-11.

24. Bifano EM, Pfannenstiel N. Duration of hyperventilation and outcome in infants with persistent pulmonary hypertension. Pediatrics 1988;81:657-60.

25. Ferrara B, Johnson DE, Chong P-N, Thompson TR. Efficacy and neurologic outcome of profound hypocapneic alkalosis for the treatment of persistent pulmonary hypertension in infancy. J Pediatr 1984;105:457-61.

26. Hendricks-Munoz KD, Walton JP. Hearing loss in infants with persistent fetal circulation. Pediatrics 1988;81:650-56.

27. Wung J-T, Jones LS, Kilchevsky E, James E. Management of infants with severe respiratory failure and persistence of the fetal circulation, without hyperventilation. Pediatrics 1985;76:488-94.

28. Goetzman BW, Milstein JM. Pulmonary vasodilator action of tolazoline. Pediatr Res 1979;13:942-46.

29. Hageman JR, Farrell EE. Intravenous nitroglycerin (NTG) in the treatment of persistent pulmonary hypertension of the newborn (PPHN). Pediatr Res 1985;19:345A.

30. Klinke WP, Gilbert JAL. Diazoxide in primary pulmonary hypertension. N Engl J Med 1989;302:91-92.

31. Stevenson DK, Kastings DS, Darrall RA Jr et al. Refractory hypoxemia associated with neonatal pulmonary disease: The use and limitations of tolazoline. J Pediatr 1979;95:595-99.

32. Andrews AF, Roloff DW, Bartlett RH. Use of extracorporeal membrane oxygenators in persistent pulmonary hypertension of the newborn. Clin Perinatol 1984;11:729-36.

33. Henderson-Smart DJ, Pettigrew AG, Campbell DJ. Clinical apnea and brain-stem neural function in preterm infants. N Engl J Med 1983;308:353-57.

34. Von Euler C. On the central pattern generator for the basic breathing rhythmicity. J Appl Physiol 1983;55:1647-59.

35. Gerhardt T, Bancalari E. Apnea of prematurity: I. Lung function and regulation of breathing. Pediatrics 1984;74:58-62.

36. Thach BT, Stark AR. Spontaneous neck flexion and airway obstruction during apneic spells in preterm infants. J Pediatr 1979;94:275-81.

37. Miller MJ, Carlo WA, Martin RJ. Continuous positive pressure selectively reduces obstructive apnea in preterm infants. J Pediatr 1985;106:91-94.

38. Carlo WA, Miller MJ, Martin RJ. Differential response of upper airway diaphragmatic activities to airway occlusion in infants. J Appl Physiol 1985;59:847-52.

39. Gauda EB, Miller MJ, Carlo WA et al. Genioglossus response to airway occlusion in apneic vs. nonapneic infants. Pediatr Res 1987;22:683-87.

40. National Institutes of Health Consensus Panel. Development conference of infantile apnea and home monitoring, Sept. 29 to Oct. 1, 1986. Pediatrics 1987;79:292-99.

41. Gerhardt T, McCarthy J, Bancalari E. Effect of aminophylline on respiratory center activity and metabolic rate in premature infants with idiopathic apnea. Pediatrics 1979;63:537-42.

42. Northway NR Jr, Rosan RC, Porter DY. Pulmonary disease following respiratory therapy of hyaline membrane disease. N Engl J Med 1967;276:357-62.

43. Bancalari E, Abdenour GE, Feller R, Gannon J. Bronchopulmonary dysplasia: A clinical presentation. J Pediatr 1979;95:819-23.

44. Avery ME, Todey WA, Keller JB et al. Is chronic lung disease in low birth weight infants preventable? A survey of eight centers. Pediatrics 1987;79:26-30.

45. Werthanner J, Brown ER, Neff EK, Taeusch HW. Sudden infant death syndrome in infants with bronchopulmonary dysplasia. Pediatrics 1982;69:301-4.

46. Smyth JA, Jabachnik E, Duncan WJ et al. Pulmonary function and bronchial hyperreactivity in long-term survivors of bronchopulmonary dysplasia. Pediatrics 1981;68:336-40.

47. Yu VYH, Orgill AA, Lim SB et al. Growth and development of VLBW infants recovering from bronchopulmonary dysplasia. Arch Dis Child 1983;58:791-94.

48. Vohr BR, Bell EF, Oh W. Infants with BPD-growth pattern and neurologic and developmental outcome. Am J Dis Child 1982;136:443-47.

49. Goetzman BW. Understanding bronchopulmonary dysplasia. Am J Dis Child 1986;140:332-34.

50. Frank L, Sosenko IRS. Undernutrition as a major contributing factor in the pathogenesis of bronchopulmonary dysplasia. Am Rev Respir Dis 1988;138:725-29.

51. Avery GB, Fletcher AB, Kaplan M et al. Controlled trial of dexamethasone in respiratory-dependent infants with BPD. Pediatrics 1985;75:106-11.

52. Backofen JE, Rogers MC. Upper airway disease. In: Rogers MC, ed. Textbook of pediatric intensive care. Baltimore, MD, Williams & Wilkins 1987:171-97.

53. Nichols DG, Rogers MC. Adult respiratory distress syndrome. In: Rogers MC, ed. Textbook of pediatric intensive care. Baltimore: Williams & Wilkins 1987:237-71.

54. Chantarojanasiri T, Nichols DG, Rogers MC. Lower airway disease: Bronchiolitis and asthma. In: Rogers MC, ed. Textbook of pediatric intensive care. Baltimore: Williams & Wilkins 1987:199-235.

55. Henderson FW, Clyde WA, Collier AM, et al. The etiologic and epidemiologic spectrum of bronchiolitis in pediatric practice. J Pediatr 1979;95:183-90.

56. Church NR, Anas NG, Hall CB et al. Respiratory syncytial virus related apnea in infants. Am J Dis Child 1984;138:247-51.

57. Dunnill MS. Pathology of asthma. In: Porter R, Birch J, eds. Identification of asthma (Ciba Foundation Symposium Study Group #38). London: Churchill Livingstone 1971:35-50.

58. Kay AB. Basic mechanism in allergic asthma. Eur J Resp Dis (Suppl) 1982;122:9-16.

59. Leff A. Pathogenesis of asthma: Neurophysiology and pharmacology of bronchospasm. Chest 1982;81:224-29.

60. Daniel EE, Davis C, Jones T. Control of airway smooth muscle. In: Hargrave E, ed. Airway hyperactivity, mechanisms and clinical relevance. Proceedings of a symposium. McMaster University. Hamilton, Ontario, Canada: Astra Pharmaceuticals, June 1975.

61. Ashbaugh DG, Bigelow DB, Petty TL, et al. Acute respiratory distress in adults. Lancet 1967;2:319-23.

62. Petty TL. Adult respiratory distress syndrome: Definition and historical perspective. Clin Chest Med 1982;3:3-15.

63. Backofen M, Weible ER. Alterations of the gas exchange apparatus in adult respiratory insufficiency associated with septicemia. Am Rev Respir Dis 1977;116:589-615.

64. Joffe N. The adult respiratory distress syndrome. Am J Roentgen 1974;122:719-32.

65. Stolar CJH, Snedecor SM, Bartlett RH. Extracorporeal membrane oxygenation and neonatal respiratory failure: Experience from the extracorporeal life support organization. J of Pediatr Surg 1991;26:563-71.

66. Short BL, Miller MK, Anderson KD. Extracorporeal membrane oxygenation in the management of respiratory failure in the newborn. Clin Perinatol 1987;14(3):737-48.

67. Cilley RE, Zwischenberger JB, Andrews A et al. Intracranial hemorrhage during extracorporeal membrane oxygenation in neonates. AJDC 1988;142:1320-24.

68. Beck R, Anderson D, Pearson GD et al. Criteria for extracorporeal membrane oxygenation in a population of infants with PPHN. J Pediatr Surg 1986;21(4):297-302.

69. Marsh TD, Wilkerson SA, Cook LN. Extracorporeal membrane oxygenation selection criteria: Partial pressure of arterial oxygen versus alveolar-arterial oxygen gradient. Pediatr 1988;82(2):162-66.

70. Anderson HL, Otsu T, Chapman RA, et al. Venovenous extracorporeal life support in neonates using a double lumen catheter. ASAIO Trans 1989;35:659-63.

71. Anderson JM, Kottke-Marchant K. Platelet interactions with biomaterials and artificial de-
    vices. In: Williams DF, ed. Blood compatibility Vol.I. Boca Raton, FL: CRC Press 1987:103-
    34.
72. Turitto VT, Weiss HJ, Baumgartner HR, et al. Cells and aggregates at surfaces. In: Leonard
    EF, Turitto VT, Vroman L, eds. Blood in contact with natural and artificial surfaces. New
    York: The New York Academy of Sciences 1987:453-67.

Kidney and Urinary Tract Disorders

Elizabeth A. Harvey, M.D., F.R.C.P.(C)

John Williamson Balfe, M.D., F.R.C.P.(C)

INTRODUCTION

The role of the healthy kidney is to maintain the fluid and electrolyte composition of the body within a narrow range of normal despite wide fluctuations in dietary intake of fluid and solute. This is accomplished by a complex process of filtration, reabsorption, and secretion of electrolytes, solutes, and water, mediated by various hormonal systems. Approximately 20% of the cardiac output is delivered to the filtering units of the kidney, the glomeruli, of which there are 1.2 million in each kidney. Passage of water through the glomeruli occurs freely, while passage of electrolytes and solutes is determined by their size and charge. As water and solute travel along the tubular system of the nephron, varying amounts are reabsorbed and secreted to maintain homeostasis. Disruption of this complex process results in clinical disease.

METHODS OF EVALUATION

Evaluation of the child for kidney disease can range from simple screening as part of a routine physical examination to a detailed, specific evaluation based on suggestive clinical features. Children are frightened by hospitals and procedures, especially blood tests.

Therefore, blood tests should be kept to a minimum, and only the smallest specimen necessary taken. Timed urine specimens are particularly difficult to obtain and are often inaccurate, and therefore short timed or spot collections should be done, with results expressed as a concentration ratio to a plasma value or relationship to urinary creatinine. Laboratory results are interpreted in relation to normal children of similar age and size. Functional tests or excretion rates should be related to body weight, surface area, or caloric expenditure. A recent listing of reference laboratory ranges is available.[1]

Electrolytes

Sodium

The reference range for sodium is 135–145 mmol/L. The normal kidney can maintain a normal plasma sodium in spite of a large variation in sodium intake, i.e., 2–1000 mmol/d. The tolerance limits are reduced in renal insufficiency.

Hyponatremia implies a dilution of body solute, either as a result of sodium loss and extracellular fluid (ECF) volume contraction or water retention and ECF volume expansion. Pseudohyponatremia may result from hyperlipidemia, hyperglycemia, or hyperproteinemia, but is rare in children since the aberration must be large. Ion-specific electrodes are free of the effect caused by lipid and protein and are therefore preferred to flame photometry for the measurement of sodium and potassium.

Hypernatremia is usually secondary to a water deficit and is seen in some cases of diarrhea and in infants with diabetes insipidus of pituitary or renal origin. Salt-poisoning is a rare cause of hypernatremia.

Potassium

The reference range for plasma potassium is 3.5–4.5 mmol/L, but is higher in the first few days of life. Maintenance of the ECF potassium concentration is related to hormone control, drugs, disease, and, to a lesser extent, dietary intake.

Hyperkalemia can be the result of excessive potassium intake in patients with renal failure or hypoaldosteronism. Spurious hyperkalemia can occur with thrombocytosis.

Hypokalemia is seen in renal tubular disorders such as Fanconi's syndrome and in hyperaldosteronism, which may occur in hypertension secondary to renal artery stenosis.

Calcium

The reference range for total plasma calcium in a child is 9.0–11.0 mg/dL (2.25–2.74 mmol/L) and for ionized calcium is 4.6–5.2 mg/dL (1.14–1.29 mmol/L) . Much of the plasma calcium is bound to protein (40%) and the remainder exists as free or ionized calcium (50%) or in complex with ions (10%). The ionized calcium is physiologically active. In hypoalbuminemic states, the total calcium is reduced, and if ionized calcium is not available, one can adjust the result by adding 0.09 mg/dL (0.023 mmol/L) for every 0.1 g/dL (1 g/L) that the albumin is < 4.6 g/dL (46 g/L) .

Hypocalcemia may present with tetany and occurs with hypoparathyroidism and vitamin D deficiency rickets. Hypercalcemia occurs with vitamin D toxicity, hyperparathyroidism, and some malignancies.

Hypercalciuria is defined as a urine calcium of > 0.1 mmol/kg/d (4 mg/kg/d) or a calcium/creatinine ratio of > 0.56–0.7 mmol or > 0.2 mg. This disturbance may present as polyuria or hematuria.

Magnesium

The reference range for plasma magnesium is 1.5–2.3 mEq/L (0.75–1.15 mmol/L) for the newborn, 1.4–1.9 mEq/L (0.70–0.95 mmol/L) for children, and 1.3–2.0 mEq/L (0.65–1.00 mmol/L) for adults. Hypomagnesemia is seen in neonatal tetany, diseases with increased gastrointestinal fluid loss, and diuretic therapy. Renal magnesium wasting can occur with Bartter's syndrome and is associated with drugs such as aminoglycosides and cis-platinum.

Urea

The reference range for plasma urea is 5.6–28 mg/dL (2–10 mmol/L) for the newborn, 5–15 mg/dL (1.8–5.4 mmol/L) at 1 to 2 years of age, and 8–20 mg/dL (2.9–7.1 mmol/L) at 2 to 16 years. Urea is the main nitrogen-containing metabolite of protein catabolism. It is synthesized in the liver from ammonia by hepatic enzymes of the urea cycle. Over 90% is excreted by the kidney. Because of tubular reabsorption of urea, especially in the presence of oliguria, urea clearance underestimates glomerular filtration rate (GFR). Although plasma urea does not give a good reflection of GFR, it does give important metabolic data. It is increased in babies who are fed excessive protein or insufficient water, and in states of acute reversible renal failure from dehydration. Assessment of the diet of patients with chronic renal failure is aided by knowing the plasma urea. Each gram of protein leads to the excretion of 0.3 grams of urea.

Creatinine

Creatinine is an endogenous product of muscle metabolism. Its rate of production is proportional to muscle mass and it is excreted predominantly by glomerular filtration (90%), with a small and varying component via renal tubular secretion (10%). Under normal circumstances, the rates of production and excretion are fairly constant. The repeated measurement of plasma creatinine concentration is a useful and simple test of GFR for clinical practice. However, in small children or elderly adults with reduced muscle mass, the plasma creatinine may be in the normal range and not reflect a reduced GFR. It should be noted that the GFR may be reduced as much as 50% without a detectable change in the plasma creatinine concentration. The reference ranges are listed in Table 3–1.

TABLE 3–1. Plasma Creatinine Values for Children

Age in Years	Value in mg/dL (μmol/L)
< 5	< 0.50 (44)
5 – 6	< 0.60 (53)
6 – 7	< 0.70 (62)
7 – 8	< 0.80 (71)
8 – 9	< 0.90 (80)
9 – 10	< 0.99 (88)
10+	< 1.20 (106)

From: American Journal of Clinical Pathology 1978;69:24–31

Glomerular Filtration Rate

The clearance of endogenous creatinine can be used as a measure of GFR, even though it overestimates the result because there is some tubular secretion.

$$Ccr = UcrV/Pcr$$

where:
Ucr = urine creatinine
V = urine volume
Pcr = plasma creatinine

In children of normal body habitus and in a steady state, there are formulae to estimate the Ccr from the plasma creatinine concentration and the patient's height.[2]

$$Ccr = kL/Pcr$$

where:

L = height (cm)

Pcr = plasma creatinine (μmol/L)

k = 29 for pre-term infants,

= 40 for full-term infants,

= 49 for children and adolescent females,

= 62 for adolescent males

There are occasions when the Ccr based on a 24-hour urine is required. However, 24-hour or timed urine collections are difficult. Much work is being done to improve the accuracy and efficiency of measuring GFR. There is considerable experience using a single intravenous bolus injection of isotopic markers, such as ^{125}I iothalamate and 99m Tc diethylenetriamine pentacetic acid (DTPA). The rate of disappearance of the isotope from the plasma estimates the GFR without the need for urine collection. If one assumes a single compartment, fewer blood specimens are required. To improve accuracy, a two-compartment model may be assumed using double rather than single exponential analysis. An even more accurate method can be applied by using the area under the plasma disappearance curve for the GFR agent and dividing this into the quantity of isotope injected.[3] The practical disadvantage is the need for six to nine blood specimens. A constant infusion technique is another accurate method and has pediatric appeal since only one or two blood samples are required.

Tubular Function Tests

The fluid which enters the tubules is a plasma ultrafiltrate devoid of large plasma proteins. The role of the proximal tubule is to reclaim appropriate amounts of filtered glucose, amino acids, electrolytes, phosphate, and bicarbonate. In disease states affecting proximal tubular function, excess amounts of these solutes may be lost in the urine, with subsequent abnormalities of the blood chemistries. Analysis of the urine will assist in diagnosis.[4, 5]

Proximal Tubule

Sodium

The most common test of tubular function is the ability to conserve sodium appropriately to preserve the ECF volume. There is no "normal" value for sodium excretion. In the steady state, the urinary sodium excretion equals dietary intake. In disease states, the urinary sodium concentration should be interpreted in light of the expected normal renal response. With hyponatremic ECF volume contraction, the expected response is excretion of concentrated urine with a sodium concentration < 10 mmol/L. In this situation, high urine sodium (> 20 mmol/L) may be related to proximal tubular defects, diuretics, vomiting, or aldosterone deficiency. Measurement of urinary potassium and chloride concentrations will help clarify the cause. With hyponatremia secondary to water gain (ECF volume expansion), the urine should have a low sodium concentration and be maximally dilute. Failure of this expected response may be seen in the syndrome of inappropriate antidiuretic hormone secretion, or with low effective circulating volume such as occurs with congestive heart failure or hypoalbuminemia. In hypernatremia, usually secondary to water loss with ECF volume contraction, the expected response is excretion of a minimal volume of maximally concentrated urine with a low sodium concentration.

An extremely low urine osmolality will be seen with diabetes insipidus, while a mildly hypertonic urine may occur with an osmotic diuresis or diuretic use.

Potassium

Assessment of potassium excretion is essential in the investigation of hyper- and hypokalemia. Potassium is filtered and completely reabsorbed in the proximal nephron. Urinary potassium excretion is the result of secretion in the late distal convoluted tubule and cortical collecting duct. Since urinary potassium excretion should equal dietary intake, there is no "normal" value. In the face of hypokalemia, a urinary potassium > 20 mmol/L or a daily potassium excretion > 0.5 mmol/kg/d (> 30 mmol/d in adults) suggests a renal cause for the hypokalemia.

The transtubular potassium gradient (TTKG) is an approximation of potassium concentration at the end of the cortical distal nephron, prior to (and corrected for) water reabsorption in the medullary collecting duct. It provides an assessment of aldosterone activity *in vivo* and is calculated as follows:

$$TTKG = \frac{[K]\ urine}{[K]\ plasma} \div \frac{urine\ osmolality}{plasma\ osmolality}$$

where urine/plasma osmolality > 1 and urine sodium > 25 mmol/L.

When the TTKG exceeds 7, mineralocorticoid is present, while a TTKG of less than 4 implies no activity.

Bicarbonate

Normally 80–90% of filtered bicarbonate is reabsorbed in the proximal tubule and normal fractional excretion of bicarbonate is < 10–15%. In proximal renal tubular acidosis (RTA), bicarbonate reabsorption is impaired, resulting in an increased fractional excretion of bicarbonate, above 10–15%. Proximal RTA most often occurs in conjunction with a generalized proximal tubular disorder. The bicarbonate loading test measures bicarbonate excretion and reabsorption at different filtered loads of bicarbonate. During bicarbonate infusion, plasma and urine bicarbonate and creatinine concentrations are measured and plotted against the plasma bicarbonate to determine the bicarbonate threshold.

Glucose

The proximal tubular glucose concentration is the same as that of plasma, as glucose is freely filtered. Ninety percent of filtered glucose is reabsorbed against a concentration gradient in the proximal tubule via a sodium-coupled active transport mechanism. The glucose receptors are "saturable." As blood glucose rises, so does the glucose concentration in the tubular fluid. Proximal glucose reabsorption increases linearly until the receptors are saturated, at which point a maximum value of glucose transport is reached, i.e., the tubular maximum (Tm). The Tm for adults, children, and infants is 300 mg/min/$1.73m^2$ and occurs at a plasma glucose of 180 mg/dL (10 mmol/L). The normal 24 h excretion of glucose should be < 0.5 g/d (2.8 mmol/d). When glucosuria is present, it is important to rule out hyperglycemia. Glucosuria without hyperglycemia may be due to isolated renal glucosuria. It may also be secondary to multiple proximal tubular defects, or may occur in nephrotic syndrome secondary to focal segmental glomerulosclerosis.

Phosphate

Eighty-five to ninety-five percent of filtered phosphate is reabsorbed by the proximal tubule via an active transport system. The 24 h excretion of phosphate is diet dependent, but averages 10–15% of the filtered load. Thus, a normal tubular reabsorption of phosphate (TRP) is greater than 85% and is calculated as follows:

$$TRP\% = 1 - \left(\frac{U_{PO_4}}{P_{PO_4}} \times \frac{P_{Cr}}{U_{Cr}} \right) \times 100$$

where U = urine, P = plasma, PO_4 = phosphate, Cr = creatinine.

An abnormally low TRP results in hypophosphatemia and is associated with generalized disorders of proximal tubular function, tubulointerstitial diseases, hyperparathyroidism, or Vitamin D resistant rickets.

Amino Acids

Normally, 95% of filtered amino acids are reabsorbed in the proximal tubule. Fractional clearances for most amino acids are less than 1%, with the exception of aspartate, serine, glycine, histidine, and taurine, which range from 2–9%. Thus, amounts in excess of 5% of the filtered load are abnormal. Amino aciduria may be generalized and associated with other defects in proximal tubular function. Alternately, it may be due to abnormalities in the transport of neutral amino acids (Hartnup disease), acidic amino acids (benign condition), or cystine and the basic amino acids, which predisposes to urolithiasis. Cystine causes a positive urinary cyanide nitroprusside test.

Chloride

The urinary excretion of chloride is dependent on dietary intake and the state of hydration. With ECF volume contraction, the urinary chloride will be low (< 10 mmol/L) unless the volume contraction is secondary to diarrhea. With acute diuretic use, the chloride will be high in the presence of ECF contraction, as is the case in Bartter's syndrome.

Titratable Acid

The major urine buffer is phosphate. Hydrogen ions buffered with phosphate are referred to as titratable acid. The buffering capacity of phosphate is limited to 20–50 mmol/d, even in severe acidosis. Ammonium provides the extra buffering capacity in sustained acidosis.

Urine pH

The major value of urinary pH measurement is in the detection of bicarbonaturia (pH > 7). It is not a reliable indicator of distal ammonium excretion. However, once a low distal ammonium excretion is suggested by a positive urine net charge (see discussion below), the urine pH will help differentiate low ammonium generation (acid pH) from low distal hydrogen ion secretion (alkaline pH).

Distal Tubule

Urine Net Charge

The urine net charge is an indirect measurement of ammonium production by the distal nephron and is a useful test for assessment of normal anion gap metabolic acidosis. When ammonium is present in the urine, it is usually in the form of ammonium chloride. The urine net charge is calculated as:

Urine net charge = [Cl − (Na + K)] in mmol/L

When urinary chloride concentration exceeds the sum of sodium and potassium (negative net charge), ammonium is present. When chloride is less than the sum of sodium and potassium (positive net charge), little ammonium is present in the urine.

In metabolic acidosis, ammonium is the major route for excretion of hydrogen (see titratable acid). Thus, ammonium excretion should be maximal. When the net charge is positive, the urine pCO_2 should be measured (see discussion below). Excretion of ammonium with an anion other than chloride may mimic a distal renal tubular acidosis (e.g., toluene inhalation). Calculation of the urinary osmolal gap (see discussion below) will reveal an unmeasured anion.

Urine pCO_2

Measurement of the urinary pCO_2 is useful in the assessment of normal anion gap acidosis with a positive urine net charge (low ammonium excretion). It differentiates between failure of distal hydrogen secretion and deficient ammonium production. The pCO_2 must be measured in an alkaline urine (pH > 7). With normal distal hydrogen secretion, the urine pCO_2 will be > 70 mmHg, whereas with defective hydrogen secretion it is < 55 mmHg.

Urine Osmolal Gap

The urine osmolal gap, defined as measured osmolality minus calculated osmolality, is useful for the detection of unmeasured anions. The urine osmolality is calculated as follows:

[2 × (NA + K) + glucose + urea] in mmol/L

When the osmolal gap is > 100 mOsm/L, an unmeasured anion should be suspected.

Renal Tubular Acidosis

Renal tubular acidosis (RTA) is characterized by a normal anion gap, hyperchloremic metabolic acidosis. It may be due to an increased fractional excretion of bicarbonate (Type 2 [proximal] RTA), failure of distal hydrogen excretion or ammonium generation (Type 1 [distal] RTA), or associated with hyperkalemia (Type 4 RTA).

Table 3–2 summarizes the results of the above tests in differentiating the type of renal tubular acidosis.[6] Other tests such as the ammonium chloride loading test or furosemide test may be useful in assessing an acidification defect.

TABLE 3–2. Renal Tubular Acidosis

Test	Proximal	Distal	Hyperkalemic
During Acidosis:			
Urine net charge	negative	positive	positive
Urine pH	< 5.5	> 5.5	< 5.5
Alkali Loading:			
FeHCO3 (%)	> 10–15%	< 5%	> 5–10%
Urine pCO2 (mmHg)	> 70	< 55	≥ 70
Associated defects of tubular function	present	absent	absent
Hypercalciuria/nephrocalcinosis	absent	present	absent

FeHCO3 = fractional excretion of bicarbonate = [(U/P) HCO3 + (U/P) creatinine] x 100

URINARY TRACT INFECTION

Urinary tract infection (UTI) refers in particular to significant numbers of bacteria in the urine. UTI is common, affecting 3% of females and 1% of males in the pediatric age group. The risk of recurrence is 30% following the first UTI and increases to 75% following subsequent infections. The majority of UTIs occur in the absence of an anatomical urinary tract abnormality. However, the occurrence of an infection in the presence of obstruction or vesicoureteric reflux may predispose to renal scarring. Thus, the detection of obstruction, the incidence of which varies from 1–10%, is of paramount importance.

UTIs may be classified on the basis of symptoms, the presence of an underlying anatomic or functional abnormality, or the site of infection. Symptoms of cystitis include dysuria, frequency, and urgency and may be accompanied by foul-smelling or cloudy urine. Pyelonephritis may manifest as flank or abdominal pain, fever, and rigors. In infants, UTI is often accompanied by septicemia and potentially life-threatening metabolic abnormalities.

The approach to UTI in the pediatric age group incorporates diagnosis, localization of infection, treatment, investigation and follow-up.[7-11]

Diagnosis of UTI

The diagnosis of UTI is based on finding significant numbers of microorganisms on urine culture.

Significant Bacteriuria

The term "significant bacteriuria" differentiates true infection from bacterial contamination. Indicators of contamination include low bacterial colony counts, multiple organisms, different organisms on serial culture, or the detection of nonpathogenic organisms. Traditionally, $\geq 10^5$ colony-forming units/mL (CFU/mL) (100×10^6 CFU/L) of a single bacteria is considered diagnostic of infection based on a mid-stream urine collection, as correlated with bladder aspiration and catheterized samples. Colony counts of $\geq 10^3$ CFU/mL (1×10^6 CFU/L) on a catheter specimen or any growth on a suprapubic aspiration specimen is diagnostic of infection. False-negative cultures may occur in dilute urine from a patient with a urinary concentrating defect.

Collection Methods

Collection of urine specimens for culture is difficult in infants and non-toilet-trained toddlers. Thus, various methods of obtaining urine for culture have evolved.

Suprapubic Aspiration

This is considered the "gold standard" for diagnosing significant bacteriuria. The skin is disinfected, the palpable bladder is punctured 1.5 cm above the symphysis pubis, and urine is slowly aspirated. This technique is most suited to infants, in whom the bladder is an intra-abdominal organ. The procedure is time consuming but safe, and contamination of the urine specimen does not occur. Any growth is significant.

Catheter Specimen

Controversy exists over the use of catheterization to obtain urine samples for culture. Introduction of bacteria into the bladder and trauma to the urethra may occur at the time of catheterization. Careful adherence to aseptic technique is essential. Bacterial growth of $\geq 10^3$ CFU/mL (1×10^6 CFU/L) is diagnostic of infection.

Bag Sample

Urine is obtained by cleansing the genitalia with water and affixing a sterile plastic collection bag. The bag is removed promptly once urine is obtained. The sample should then be plated immediately. There is a high incidence of contamination, and a bag sample is most useful when it is negative for significant bacterial growth. A pure growth of the same organism with significant colony counts on two or more occasions suggests infection, especially when associated with pyuria or symptoms.

Mid-Stream Urine (MSU)

To obtain an MSU, the genitalia are washed with a cleansing agent or water two or three times. Voiding is initiated and the mid-portion of the stream is collected. This reduces contamination from urethral or prostatic secretions, though contamination with perineal flora may occur. Significant bacteriuria is $\geq 10^5$ CFU/mL (100×10^6 CFU/L) .

Bacterial Culture

Once obtained, urine for bacterial culture should be plated immediately, using a calibrated loop, onto 5% sheep blood agar and a medium selective for gram-negative bacilli such as MacConkey agar. The culture is incubated for 24 h to obtain a colony count, and a further 12–24 h are necessary for *in vitro* antibiotic sensitivity testing. If immediate plating is not possible, refrigeration at 4° C will maintain stable colony counts for 24 h.

Bacterial culture is expensive and time consuming, and automated, rapid culture methods have been developed. However, they have low sensitivity, especially for low colony counts and slow-growing organisms, making them inappropriate for nosocomial infections and for patients with low-grade bacteriuria.

Ancillary Tests

Tests are available to assist in diagnosis of significant bacteriuria, but are not diagnostic by themselves.

Pyuria

The "gold standard" for pyuria is the WBC excretion rate, with > 400,000 WBC/h correlating significantly with symptomatic UTI, but this method is impractical. Pyuria is defined as > 10×10^6 WBC/L (> 10/mm^3) of uncentrifuged urine, counted with a hemocytometer, or > 10 WBC per high-power field of centrifuged urine. However, direct microscopy suffers from many inaccuracies due to lack of standardization. The presence of pyuria is suggestive of, but not diagnostic for, UTI. In children, pyuria correlates poorly with infection, possibly related to methods of collection or leucocyte excretion rates.

Bacteria

Microscopy for bacteria may assist in the diagnosis of UTI. The presence of ≥ 1 organism per oil immersion field on an uncentrifuged, gram-stained urine correlates with ≥ 10^5 CFU/mL (100 x 10^6 CFU/L) organisms on culture.

Urinary Nitrite

Urinary nitrite is produced by the reduction of dietary nitrate by certain bacteria. It can be detected using an amine-impregnated dipstick, which produces a pink color reaction when positive. False negatives occur in the presence of dilute urine, inadequate dietary nitrates, and non-nitrate reducing bacteria such as *Staphylococcus* and *Enterococcus*. The test is insensitive at colony counts of ≥ 10^5 CFU/mL (100 x 10^6 CFU/L).

Leucocyte Esterase

Leucocyte esterase is an enzyme found in neutrophils, which can be detected by the dipstick method. It correlates best with pyuria rather than UTI. It is as accurate as sediment microscopy in predicting children with insignificant bacteriuria.[12]

Bioluminescence

The bioluminescence assay utilizes the firefly luciferin-luciferase reaction to detect bacterial ATP. False-negatives may occur due to variations in the amount of ATP in different bacterial species and in their metabolic rate. False-positives are associated with antibiotic inhibition of bacteria, slow-growing organisms, and residual leucocyte ATP. Although the bioluminescence assay is more sensitive than nitrite and leucocyte esterase assays,[13] it is expensive.

Localization of Infection

Upper tract infection requires initial treatment with intravenous antibiotics and carries a risk of renal scarring. Thus, early diagnosis and treatment is important. Fever, flank pain, and systemic illness points to a diagnosis of pyelonephritis, but infants may have only non-specific symptoms. Hence, a variety of tests have arisen to aid with localization:

The Stamey Test

The Stamey test is considered the standard in localizing upper tract infection. It involves cystoscopic irrigation of the bladder, selective ureteral catheterization, and culture of urine obtained from both ureters as well as the bladder. It is 100% specific, except in the presence of vesicoureteric reflux. The need for instrumentation of the urinary tract, which in children requires general anesthesia, limits its usefulness.

The Fairley Test

The Fairley test involves washing out the bladder with a mixture of saline, fibrolysin plus deoxyribonuclease, and antibiotic, followed by further rinsing with saline and culture of urine at intervals through an indwelling catheter. While the test has a sensitivity of 90% in adults, it is unreliable in children with vesicoureteric reflux and in patients with neurogenic bladders.

Antibody-Coated Bacteria

This test is based on the premise that invasion of renal tissue by bacteria will elicit an antibody response, whereas mucosal involvement will not. Antibodies coat the offending bacteria and can be detected in the urine using immunofluorescence techniques. However, high false-positive and false-negative rates occur, and the results are unreliable in children.

β_2-Microglobulin

β_2-microglobulin is a small plasma protein synthesized by nucleated cells. It is freely filtered and completely reabsorbed in the proximal tubule. When tubular damage occurs, as in pyelonephritis, increased amounts of β_2-microglobulin are found in the urine. Limitations of the test in children include the need for a 24 h collection of urine, as well as continuous alkalinization of the urine, as the protein is destroyed by an acid pH.

Urinary Lactate Dehydrogenase Isoenzyme Assays

Isoenzymes 4 and 5 of lactate dehydrogenase (LDH) are present in large quantities in the renal medulla and are released into the urine during infection. Total urinary LDH and isoenzyme fractions are measured. Total LDH and isoenzyme 5 correlate best with upper tract disease. Urine must be kept cool during collection as enzyme activity decreases at room temperature, and the patient must not be on nitro-furantoin, as it denatures LDH. This test is not currently in general use.

Miscellaneous Methods

Other non-invasive methods of localization of UTI are available, but they have uncertain diagnostic usefulness and their application to pediatrics is limited. Tests include antibody to Tamm-Horsfall protein, serum C-reactive protein, urinary β-glucuronidase assay, maximal renal concentrating ability, and serum antibody to O antigens. Detailed discussions are given by Pappas and Sheldon.[10, 11]

Treatment, Investigation, and Follow-up

These aspects of urinary tract infection are beyond the scope of this chapter. Recent reviews are available.[7-9, 14]

PROTEINURIA

The presence of an abnormal quantity of protein in the urine is a most reliable marker of renal parenchymal disease. Normal individuals should excrete < 100–150 mg (60 mg/m^2) of protein per day. The new-born may transiently have proteinuria up to 1 g/d.

Low-Grade Proteinuria

Low-grade (< 1 g/d) proteinuria is fairly common and can occur with a number of renal problems:

Asymptomatic Persistent Proteinuria

This is defined as constant proteinuria > 250 mg/d in infants and > 500 mg/d in children. The long-term prognosis for such children is not known, so they should be carefully followed every 3–6 m, measuring the blood pressure and plasma creatinine. A renal biopsy is not necessary as long as the patient is stable. If hematuria is present, the prognosis is guarded

Functional Proteinuria

This occurs with fever, exercise, and congestive heart failure. The urine sediment is normal. The proteinuria should resolve with treatment of the primary problem.

Tubular Proteinuria

This type of proteinuria is found in renal tubular acidosis, Fanconi's syndrome, and Lowe's syndrome. The identifying characteristic of tubular proteinuria is the presence of 25–60% of proteins of low molecular weight. It is generally held that this proteinuria results from failure of tubular reabsorption of plasma proteins.

The dipstick test primarily detects albuminuria. It is based on the tetrabromophenol blue colorimetric test. The turbidimetric test, which uses 10% sulfosalicylic acid, is useful for detecting low-molecular-weight protein. The acid precipitates as little as 0.05–0.1 g/L of low-molecular-weight protein. The precipitate will disappear when brought to a boil and reappear on cooling.

The measurement of β_2-microglobulin (MW = 11,815 daltons) is sometimes used as an index of tubular proteinuria. The ratio of urine albumin to β_2-microglobulin is < 15 in tubular proteinuria, whereas in glomerular proteinuria the ratio is > 1000.

Nephrophthisis

This disease is characterized by polyuria and polydypsia, anemia, and failure to thrive. The proteinuria may be a tubular pattern with a predominance of β_2-microglobulin. There is a tendency to renal salt-wasting. The urine sediment is unremarkable. Renal failure occurs in early adolescence. Tapetoretinal degeneration is the most common association.

Chronic Tubulo-Interstitial Nephritis

This may be secondary to chronic analgesic abuse, toxins such as lead, cadmium, or oxalate, hyperuricemia, hypercalcemia, and hypokalemia. The proteinuria is mild.

Orthostatic Proteinuria

This type of proteinuria is frequent in children, especially adolescents. It is the presence of increased amounts of protein in urine formed when the patient is in the upright position, but not in urine formed when the patient is supine. If the proteinuria is orthostatic and < 1 g/d without sediment abnormalities, serious renal disease is unlikely and a good outcome is predicted, despite reports of abnormal glomerular morphology in a systematic study.

To quantify protein excretion, a split 24 h urine collection is done, one sample at night while the patient is in the supine position and one sample during the day while the patient is ambulatory. An alternative qualitative test is to dipstick the urine for protein on the first void of the day and 2 hours later, which can be done each day for three days.

Heavy Proteinuria (Nephrotic Syndrome)

Nephrotic syndrome is defined as heavy proteinuria (> 3.0 g/1.73 m^2/d or > 50–100 mg/kg/d) with hypoalbuminemia (< 25 g/L; < 2.5 g/dL), edema, and hyperlipidemia. The incidence in children of all forms of the syndrome is 2–4 new cases per 100,000 population per year, with a prevalence of 16 per 100,000, making it the most prevalent glomerular disease in children. There is a male preponderance in early childhood, with 80% of the cases being minimal lesion nephrotic syndrome, compared to only 20% in adults.

Ninety percent of children respond to prednisone, compared to 60% of adults. Cyclophosphamide may produce a permanent remission in frequent relapsers, i.e., patients who experience two relapses in six months or three relapses in one year. Non-responsiveness to prednisone may suggest focal segmental glomerulosclerosis, which may progress to chronic renal failure. A renal biopsy is performed on prednisone-resistant cases.

Rarer causes of nephrotic syndrome are (1) membranoproliferative glomerulonephritis (MPGN), which usually is associated with an active urine sediment and hypocomplementemia, and (2) membranous nephropathy. Children with this type of nephrotic syndrome are generally older than 8 years of age.

Although primary nephrotic syndrome is the most common type, it is necessary to exclude other events or diseases associated with nephrotic syndrome such as:

1. Medications (penicillamine, NSAIDs, gold)

2. Allergens (bee sting, poison ivy)

3. Infections (post-streptococcal glomerulonephritis, infective endocarditis, syphilis, hepatitis B)

4. Neoplasia (carcinoma, lymphoma)

5. Multisystem disease [lupus, Henoch-Schönlein purpura (HSP)]

6. Metabolic (diabetes mellitus, amyloidosis, Fabry's disease)

It is usual to admit new cases to hospital, especially if the edema is significant. Fluids and sodium are restricted and diuretics such as hydrochlorothiazide and spironolactone are prescribed. For severe edema, intravenous albumin (1 g/kg over 4 h) plus furosemide (1 mg/kg) at mid-infusion are given. Prednisone is the main therapy directed towards the proteinuria, giving 2 mg/kg/d in a divided schedule until the urine is protein-free for 5–7 d, at which time the 2 mg/kg is given as a single dose every other morning. In essence, the dose is reduced by a half. The dose of prednisone is reduced by 5–10 mg every two weeks until it is discontinued. Relapses are common, in which case a similar prednisone regimen is reinstituted.

HEMATURIA

Hematuria is defined > 5–10 red blood cells per high-power field in centrifuged urine or dipstick-positive hematuria on qualitative testing. Unlike proteinuria, which usually signifies glomerular disease, hematuria may arise anywhere along the urinary tract. The presence of red blood cell casts is pathognomonic of glomerular bleeding, while brown or smoky urine is highly suggestive. Coexistence of hematuria and proteinuria also implies a glomerular etiology, as does more than 10% dysmorphic RBCs on phase microscopy of the urinary sediment. Blood clots do not occur with glomerular bleeding and suggest a lower urinary tract cause, as does terminal hematuria. Red urine does not always signify blood in the urine; it may be caused by drugs (e.g., pyridium), pigmented foods (e.g., beets), urates, porphyrins, or myoglobin and hemoglobin.

To diagnose true hematuria, a combination of urine dipstick analysis and microscopy is essential. The current dipsticks detect heme pigment, not red cells themselves, and are positive with hemoglobinuria, myoglobinuria, and hematuria. A positive dipstick in the absence of red cells on examination of a fresh sediment suggests hemoglobinuria or myoglobinuria. The former is confirmed by finding pink serum and the latter can be measured directly using radial immunodiffusion.[15-17]

The history is invaluable in determining the cause of hematuria. Dysuria and frequency suggest urinary tract infection; colicky flank pain occurs with renal calculi; a recent upper respiratory tract infection is common in IgA nephropathy; and with postinfectious nephritis, a sore throat occurs 2–3 w previously. Terminal hematuria suggests a lesion in the bladder trigone, initial hematuria occurs with urethral lesions, and blood throughout the stream occurs with bleeding from other sites. A history of trauma, drug ingestion, or bleeding diathesis and a family history of renal disease should be elicited.

Hematuria may be microscopic or macroscopic, and the two may coexist in the same disease entity. Microscopic hematuria occurs with a frequency of 0.5–1.0% in children. The frequency of macroscopic hematuria is 0.13%. Common causes include UTI, trauma, stones, coagulopathy, glomerular diseases, structural abnormalities, and tumors. The causes of hematuria vary with the age of the child. In the newborn, common causes include renal vein thrombosis, birth asphyxia with subsequent acute tubular necrosis, obstruction, and coagulopathies. In infants, hemolytic uremic syndrome, renal vein thrombosis, Wilms tumor and meatal stenosis predominate. In older children, various forms of glomerulonephritis, including HSP, tumors, foreign bodies, trauma, and cystitis are most common.

Investigation

Investigation of hematuria begins with a careful history and physical exam, followed by dipstick examination of the urine, microscopy, and urine culture. Renal imaging studies (e.g., intravenous urogram [IVU] or computerized tomography [CAT] scan) are indicated with a history of trauma or colicky pain suggestive of urolithiasis. Other tests which may be indicated include renal function tests, electrolytes, calcium, phosphorus, hemoglobin, platelets and coagulation parameters, sickle test, serum complements (see discussion below), antinuclear factor, and antistreptolysin titre. Ancillary tests may include audiology and ophthalmology assessments.

Glomerulonephritis (GN)

The acute nephritic syndrome is characterized by hematuria, azotemia, oliguria, edema, and hypertension caused by salt and water retention secondary to a reduced glomerular filtration rate. The presence of red cell casts with or without proteinuria is usual. To diagnose the particular type of GN, the third component of the complement system, C3, used in conjunction with C4 and CH50, is useful. Activation of the classical pathway will result in low concentrations of C3 and C4, whereas with activation of the alternate pathway, only low C3 values occur. Deficiencies of other complement components will give a normal C3 and C4, but a low CH50. The glomerulonephritides commonly associated with low C3 concentrations include systemic lupus erythematosus (SLE), MPGN, GN caused by chronic infections such as bacterial endocarditis or infected ventriculoperitoneal shunts, postinfectious nephritis (usually streptococcal), and inherited abnormalities of the complement system. Diseases usually associated with normal C3 concentrations include HSP, Berger's disease (IgA nephropathy), epidemic hemolytic uremic syndrome, Goodpasture's disease, and hereditary nephritis.[18] Normal values are:

C3:   0–1 y: 60–170 mg/dL (0.6–1.7 g/L)
      > 1 y: 80–180 mg/dL (0.8–1.8 g/L)

C4:   0–6 m: 7–26 mg/dL (0.07–0.26 g/L)
      > 6 m: 10–40 mg/dL (0.1–0.4 g/L)

CH50: ≤ 1:24 (serial dilution bioassay)

A useful approach to classifying a patient into one of the above categories utilizes the serum complement and the clinical assessment of the patient, namely whether the disease process involves multiple organ systems including the kidney, or primarily the kidney, as presented in Table 3–3.

TABLE 3–3. Classification of Glomerulonephritis by Serum C3

C3	Systemic Disease	Renal Disease
Normal	Henoch Schönlein purpura	IgA nephropathy
	Hemolytic uremic syndrome	Hereditary nephritis
	Goodpasture's syndrome	MPGN
Low	SLE	MPGN
	Endocarditis/shunt infection	Postinfectious nephritis
		Complement deficiencies

Other tests are guided by the presumed diagnosis based on the above schema. The most common acute nephritis is post-infectious nephritis, which occurs 1–2 w following a streptococcal pharyngitis or 3–6 w following impetigo. The antistreptolysin O titre is increased in 60–80% of patients with postinfectious nephritis in the absence of early antibiotic treatment (Normal = < 166 Todd units). Other antistreptococcal antibody titers may be increased such as anti-streptokinase and antiDNAase B, and, following impetigo, anti-hyaluronidase. C3 values are initially low and usually return to normal within 4–6 w. Prolonged depression of C3 is more suggestive of MPGN, complement deficiency, or SLE.

The diagnosis of hemolytic uremic syndrome is based on the finding of a microangiopathic hemolytic anemia, thrombocytopenia, and acute renal failure with hematuria and proteinuria. Liver transferases and serum amylase may be increased, along with the usual biochemical abnormalities of acute renal failure. Therapy is supportive with early institution of peritoneal dialysis. The typical presentation of IgA nephropathy is recurrent episodes of gross hematuria immediately following an upper respiratory tract infection, with baseline microscopic hematuria with or without proteinuria. The diagnosis is based on renal biopsy findings of mesangial deposition of IgA. The serum IgA values may be normal, but if increased are suggestive of the diagnosis in the absence of a biopsy. Normal values are:

0–6 m:	8–70 mg/dL	(0.08–0.7 g/L)
6 m – 1 y:	11–90 mg/dL	(0.11–0.9 g/L)
1–2 y:	15–120 mg/dL	(0.15–1.2 g/L)
2–5 y:	22–160 mg/dL	(0.22–1.6 g/L)
5 y – adult:	35–240 mg/dL	(0.35–2.4 g/L)
Adult:	70–310 mg/dL	(0.70–3.1 g/L)

Alport's syndrome or hereditary nephritis is associated with high-frequency nerve deafness and ocular abnormalities and usually has an

X-linked mode of inheritance. Diagnosis is based on multilaminar splitting of the glomerular capillary basement membrane and absence of the Goodpasture antigen on the basement membrane. HSP is a clinical diagnosis based on the presence of a purpuric skin rash, usually of the lower extremities, arthralgias, abdominal pain, and renal involvement, which may range from microscopic hematuria to a mixed nephritic and nephrotic syndrome. Goodpasture's syndrome, which is rare in children, presents with pulmonary hemorrhage and renal disease. The diagnosis is confirmed by finding a circulating antiglomerular basement membrane antibody or by renal biopsy. Complement disorders may be associated with recurrent infections and various forms of renal disease.

Hypercalciuria

Idiopathic hypercalciuria (see earlier section entitled "Methods of Evaluation") without hypercalcemia is a common cause of isolated microscopic hematuria and carries with it an increased risk of future urolithiasis. Hypercalciuria along with hypocitraturia, nephrocalcinosis, and urolithiasis also occurs in distal renal tubular acidosis.[19]

ACUTE RENAL FAILURE

Acute renal failure is defined as a sudden decrease in renal function, accompanied by the accumulation of nitrogenous wastes within the body. It may be accompanied by anuria, oliguria, or polyuria. Six major clinical syndromes are associated with an acute decline in glomerular filtration.

Prerenal Azotemia

Prerenal azotemia is caused by hypotension, hypovolemia, or inadequate renal perfusion such as may occur with hemorrhage or congestive heart failure. Physiological responses result in a reduction in GFR and increased tubular reabsorption of salt and water. Restoration of adequate circulating volume reverses the acute renal failure.

Acute Tubular Necrosis (ATN)

ATN occurs as a result of hypoperfusion, a nephrotoxic injury, or a combination of the two. Removal of the insult does not result in immediate improvement in renal function.

Acute Interstitial Nephritis

Acute interstitial nephritis causes a decrease in GFR because of interstitial inflammation. It is frequently non-oliguric renal failure and is often related to drugs or toxins.

Acute Glomerulonephritis

Acute glomerulonephritis results in a diminished GFR on the basis of vascular inflammation. The most common lesions in children are acute post-streptococcal nephritis and hemolytic uremic syndrome. Recovery of renal function depends on the underlying disease process.

Acute Renovascular Disease

In order for renovascular disease to cause acute renal failure, it must be a bilateral process or occur in a solitary kidney. A common cause in infants is renal vein thrombosis.

Post-renal Azotemia (Obstructive Uropathy)

Post-renal azotemia results from obstruction in the collecting system and may be due to intratubular obstruction (e.g., methotrexate, uric acid) or to extrinsic compression (e.g., tumor). Relief of the obstruction restores a normal GFR.

Examination of the urine sediment is crucial in evaluating the patient with acute renal failure. A sediment with renal tubular epithelial cells, granular casts, and hematuria and proteinuria supports a diagnosis of ATN. RBC casts are found in glomerulonephritis. WBCs and especially eosinophils support a diagnosis of interstitial nephritis. Dipstick hematuria without cellular elements on microscopy is suggestive

TABLE 3–4. Acute Renal Failure

Test	Prerenal	Renal	Postrenal
Urine osmolality (mOsm/kg H_2O)	> 500	250–400	300–400
Urine SG	> 1.020	< 1.010	–
U/P Osm	> 1.3:1	< 1.1:1	–
Urine Na (mmol/L)	< 20	> 40	> 40
FeNA (%)	< 1	> 1	> 3
Renal failure index	< 1	> 1	> 1
U/P Creatinine	> 40	< 20	< 20

SG = specific gravity
U/P Osm = urine to plasma osmolality
FeNa (%) = fractional excretion of sodium = [(U/P) Na + (U/P) creatinine] x 100
Renal Failure Index = U Na + [U/P] creatinine
U/P creatinine = urine to plasma creatinine

of hemoglobinuria or myoglobinuria. In acute renal failure, urinary sodium concentration differentiates between prerenal causes (Na < 10 mmol/L) and intrinsic renal disease (Na > 20 mmol/L). Urine sodium concentration may also be used to assess the adequacy of fluid replacement in the volume contracted patient. Once the ECF space is replete, the urinary sodium will begin to rise. With intrinsic renal disease, the urinary sodium is a guide to the appropriate sodium concentration of replacement fluid.

Various ancillary tests may be necessary for diagnosis. They include urine myoglobin, therapeutic drug monitoring, toxicology screening, creatine kinase, and viral titers.

Management of the patient with acute renal failure involves close monitoring of acid-base and electrolyte status, urea, creatinine, calcium, phosphorus, albumin, magnesium, uric acid, and hematologic and coagulation parameters. Dialysis may be necessary to control the metabolic and fluid disturbances.[20, 21] The laboratory tests useful in assessing patients with acute renal failure are listed in Table 3–4.

CHRONIC RENAL FAILURE

Numerous biochemical abnormalities occur in chronic renal failure (CRF), affecting multiple organ systems. A detailed review is beyond the scope of this chapter, and only salient features are discussed.

Anemia

CRF is characterized by a relative deficiency of erythropoietin, resulting in a progressive normochromic, normocytic anemia. With the advent of recombinant human erythropoietin (EPO), patients with CRF can now maintain satisfactory hemoglobin values without transfusions. Target hemoglobin for patients with CRF on EPO therapy is 9.5–11.5 g/dL (95–115 g/L). Higher hemoglobins can be maintained but may be associated with hypertension and vascular access occlusion. Iron deficiency anemia is common in patients on EPO. Iron supplementation is often necessary, and serial assessment of body iron stores is done. Normal values are:

serum iron = 9–27 µmol/L (50–150 µg/dL)
iron binding capacity = 45–72 µmol/L (251–400 µg/dL)
ferritin = 16–300 µg/L (16–300 ng/mL)

Renal osteodystrophy

CRF is characterized by a decrease in phosphorus excretion, consequent hypocalcemia, and a relative or absolute deficiency of 1,25-

Dihydroxy Vitamin D. This results in secondary hyperparathyroidism and bone disease. Associated factors affecting bone integrity include aluminum toxicity and systemic acidosis. Monitoring of the patient with CRF includes measurement of calcium, phosphorus, alkaline phosphatase, parathyroid hormone level, and occasionally Vitamin D levels. Reference values for phosphate and alkaline phosphatase vary with age.[1] Parathyroid hormone concentrations vary with the laboratory and whether the N-terminal or C-terminal is assayed.

Drug Monitoring

As many drugs or their metabolites are excreted via the kidney, the potential for toxicity, both systemic and renal, exists if drug doses are not adjusted for diminished GFR. The use of therapeutic drug monitoring for patients with CRF taking such drugs as aminoglycosides and vancomycin is essential. Appropriate drug dosing monographs for CRF are available.[22]

Renal Transplantation

The ultimate goal for infants and children with CRF is renal transplantation. As transplantation is still only a treatment and not a cure, children with renal transplants require long-term monitoring and medications. Immediately post-transplantation, electrolyte imbalances are common, including hypocalcemia, hypophosphatemia, and hypomagnesemia. Massive fluid replacement may result in changes in serum osmolality, which should be monitored. Current immunosuppression protocols use a combination of antilymphocyte globulin, cyclosporine, azathioprine, and prednisone. Measurement of cyclosporine values is necessary to achieve concentrations within what is currently regarded as the therapeutic range. Our center aims for concentrations measured by high-pressure liquid chromatography on whole blood of 100–125 µg/L during the first 3 months, 75–100 µg/L from 3–6 months, and 50–75 µg/L after 6 months.

RENIN ANGIOTENSIN SYSTEM

Renin is a proteolytic enzyme (molecular weight 31,000–40,000) predominantly formed and stored in the juxtaglomerular apparatus of the kidney and released into the renal vein and lymph. When released into the circulation, renin acts on its substrate angiotensinogen, an α_2-globulin made mainly in the liver, to give a relatively inactive decapeptide, angiotensin I. Passage through the pulmonary circulation cleaves angiotensin I by a converting enzyme yielding the octapeptide, angiotensin II. A potent vasoconstrictor, angiotensin II also stimulates thirst and secretion of aldosterone, ADH, and catecholamines.

A number of factors control renin release, including renal tubular sodium concentration, renal perfusion pressure, and β-adrenergic tone.

When renal nerves are stimulated, renin release increases. Sympathectomy will decrease baseline renin activity and also decrease renin secretion in response to sodium depletion. Central nervous system stimulation modulates renin release and the renal nerves must be intact for this to occur.

Various factors influencing renin release are listed in Table 3–5.

TABLE 3-5. Factors Influencing Renin Release

Increase in Renin Release	Decrease in Renin Release
DRUGS	DRUGS
Vasodilators	β-Adrenergic blockers
Diuretics	Mineralocorticoids
β-Adrenergic stimulators	α-Adrenergic stimulators
EDTA (vis calcium efflux)	Lanthanum
HORMONES	HORMONES
Glucagon	Mineralocorticoids
Prostaglandins	Vasopressin
Norepinephrine and other catecholamines	Angiotensin
	Atrial natriuretic fator (ANF)
DIET	DIET
Sodium deprivation or loss	Salt load

From: Ingelfinger JR. Hypertension. Philadelphia: WB Saunders, 1982:48.

Hypertension

The causes of hypertension are distinctly different for children as compared to adults. Most infants and children with hypertension have a secondary cause. Hypertension in the neonatal period is not rare. It may be secondary to a renal artery thrombosis from an improperly placed umbilical artery catheter. In a number of hypertensive infants, the cause is unknown; however, they outgrow the problem by age 1 y (transient neonatal hypertension). The older adolescent is more like the adult in that the most common cause is essential or primary hypertension. A child who is age 10 or less and definitely has hypertension will most likely have a secondary cause. Renal disorders are by far the most common cause; however, a number of other causes must be excluded (see Table 3–6).

Investigation

The initial assessment is a thorough physical examination, looking for signs associated with the causal disease, such as upper-limb hypertension in coarctation of the aorta, abdominal bruit in renal artery stenosis, a café au lait skin lesion in neurofibromatosis, or a cushingoid appearance in cases of adrenal corticosteroid excess. The urinalysis and renal function tests are important. Plasma electrolytes and acid base measurements demonstrating a hypokalemic metabolic alkalosis suggest activation of the renin angiotensin system. Pheochromocytoma should be excluded in all patients by obtaining a 24 h urine for vanillylmandelic acid (VMA) and catecholamines. If the screen is positive, a CAT scan of the abdomen or ^{131}I metaiodobenzylguanidine (MIBG) scintigraphy should be requested.

TABLE 3–6. Causes of Hypertension in Children

RENAL:	Parenchymal causes:
	Chronic Pyelonephritis
	Acute or chronic glomerulonephritis
	Congenital defects:
	Polycystic kidney disease
	Segmental hypoplasia
	Ask-Upmark kidney
	Hemolytic uremic syndrome
	Renal transplant
	Renovascular:
	Intrinsic renal artery disease
	Fibromuscular lesions: intimal, medial, perimedial
	Neurofibromatosis
	Arteritis
	Extrinsic renal artery diseases
	Para-aortic tumors
	Para-aortic lymph nodes
	Para-aortic neurofibromata
ENDOCRINE:	Pheochromocytoma
	Congenital adrenal hyperplasia
	Hyperthyroidism
	Primary aldosteronism
VASCULAR SYSTEM:	Coarctation of the aorta
	Takayasu's arteritis
DRUG-RELATED:	Corticosteroids
	Amphetamine overdose
	Licorice
	Oral contraceptives
MISCELLANEOUS:	Essential hypertension
	Wilms tumor
	Neuroblastoma
	Burns

Most of the secondary causes of hypertension are easily excluded, with the exception of renal artery stenosis. The definitive test for renal artery stenosis is a renal arteriogram. However, noninvasive evaluation should be done first. The renin system can be assessed by obtaining a peripheral vein renin and a 24 h urine for sodium excretion. Laragh et al.[23] have developed a nomogram for adults. Administration of the oral angiotensin converting enzyme inhibitor, captopril, has been shown to be useful in a number of adult studies. However, only preliminary results are available for children.

With the patient at rest, a baseline renin is obtained, then captopril is given (0.35–0.7 mg/kg) orally and 60 or 90 minutes later a repeat renin is obtained. A positive test is a plasma renin activity value of ≥ 3.3 ng/L/s (12 ng/mL/h) with an increase of ≥ 2.8 ng/L/s (10 ng/mL/h), or a relative increase of 150%, provided the initial renin value is ≥ 0.8 ng/L/s (3 ng/mL/h). A radionuclide renal scan may be useful as a screening test for renal artery stenosis and as an adjunct to the study, a single dose of captopril, as above, is given 1 h prior to the scan. Captopril will decrease the GFR of the affected kidney, which will manifest as decreased isotopic uptake by the kidney.

Antihypertensive Therapy

The monitoring of the effectiveness of antihypertensive drug therapy is by measuring the patient's blood pressure and looking for side effects. Laboratory tests are not necessary.

Diuretics

Hydrochlorothiazide is the most frequently used diuretic. It is necessary to monitor the patient for hypokalemia. The potassium sparing diuretics such as amiloride can cause hyperkalemia, especially if there is renal failure. Potent loop diuretics such as furosemide can cause serious electrolyte disturbances.

β-Adrenergic Blocking Agents

This group of drugs includes the most commonly used antihypertensives. It is possible to measure blood concentrations of drugs such as propranolol; however, the usual clinical approach is to gradually increase the drug dose to a reasonable concentration while monitoring the heart rate and blood pressure.

Angiotensin Converting Enzyme (ACE) Inhibitors

Captopril and enalapril are the two most commonly used ACE inhibitors. There is a danger of hyperkalemia, especially if combined with a potassium-sparing diuretic.

Sodium Nitroprusside

This is the preferred antihypertensive for the management of hypertensive crises. Prolonged use of this drug can cause cyanide poisoning. Thiocyanate blood concentrations should be monitored in cases of prolonged or high-dose therapy or in patients with renal failure.

Normotensive Hyper-reninemic Conditions

Diseases associated with salt and water loss, such as vomiting and diarrhea, lead to an increased plasma renin concentration. There are pediatric conditions in which the plasma renin can be very high (50–100 fold increase) and can even be diagnostic. Bartter's syndrome is a form of renal sodium and potassium wasting. Such infants and children present with a hypokalemic metabolic alkalosis; in some, hyponatremia and hypomagnesemia are observed. The plasma renin activity is very high, but the blood pressure is normal. The urine has excessive sodium, potassium, and chloride, in spite of low plasma values. Infants with cystic fibrosis, a common genetic disease, can present with identical plasma electrolyte and renin values; however, the urine has very low sodium and chloride values. The salt wasting in these infants is via the sweat. Finally, infants provided with a formula that is low in chloride can mimic Bartter's syndrome; however, their urine will be nearly free of sodium and chloride.

DISTURBANCES OF ELECTROLYTES AND WATER

Pathophysiology

A large fraction of the body mass is water. The total body water is divided into two main compartments, intracellular fluid (ICF) and extracellular fluid (ECF). The ECF space has two major subdivisions, plasma and interstitial fluid. Using the volume of distribution of various markers, it is possible to measure total body water (e.g., using heavy water) and the ECF space (e.g., using bromide) and by subtracting the two, derive the ICF volume. These measurements are not routinely used in clinical medicine. The electrolyte composition of the ECF compared to ICF is quite different. Sodium is the major ECF cation and potassium is the major ICF cation. In the plasma, by subtracting anions from cations, an undetermined anion fraction or anion gap is obtained. It can be grossly calculated by the formula: $Na - (Cl + HCO_3)$ and is normally 10–15 mmol/L. An increased anion gap can be observed in lactic or ketoacidosis. The electrolyte concentration in the ICF is similar to plasma, but differs slightly because of the absence of negatively charged proteins in the ICF (e.g., Gibbs-Donnan equilibrium).

Because in children the body is composed of an even larger proportion of water, the incidence of acute disturbances of salt and water is commonplace. Dehydration or ECF volume contraction can be the result of a reduced intake of salt and water, or increased losses such as from the gastrointestinal tract in diarrhea, in the urine from an osmotic diuresis or adrenal insufficiency, from skin, or from the respiratory tract. Types of dehydration can be classified according to the plasma sodium concentration: isotonic dehydration (sodium 130–150 mmol/L), hypertonic dehydration (sodium > 150 mmol/L), and hypotonic dehydration (sodium < 130 mmol/L).

Frequently, dehydrated patients will also have an acid base and potassium disturbance. In addition, there may be a component of renal failure. Urinalysis for protein, hemoglobin, sediment, specific gravity or osmolality, and sodium concentration will help separate prerenal versus renal failure.

Clinical Management

Acute ECF Volume Contraction

The management of such patients is based on physiological principles. The clinician must determine the following:

1. Type of dehydration (plasma sodium)
2. Magnitude of the dehydration (acute weight loss)
3. Presence of deficit of body potassium (plasma potassium)
4. Nature of the acid-base disturbance (measure blood acid-base status and anion gap)

The patient's electrolyte and water deficits are calculated and then added to the maintenance electrolyte and water requirements. In moderately and severely dehydrated patients, the early phase of management (first 2 h) is directed towards the restoration of circulatory integrity. The remainder of the first day is aimed at partial restoration of ECF sodium and water deficits and partial correction of acid-base disturbances. The final phase (days 1–4) is devoted to replacing potassium deficits, plus any remaining ECF volume and acid-base disturbances. There are comprehensive reviews of the topic.[24, 25]

Renal Tubular Disorders

Bartter's Syndrome

Bartter's syndrome was originally described in children with growth failure associated with a hypokalemic metabolic alkalosis, hyperreninemia, hyperplasia of the juxtaglomerular apparatus, and normal blood pressure.[26] It has since been described in all age groups. It is the result of failure of chloride and consequently potassium and sodium reabsorption in the distal nephron segments. Younger patients can have renal sodium wasting and more severe electrolyte and acid-base disturbances. Hypomagnesemia is present is some patients. The cause is unknown and the diagnosis is one of exclusion of other causes of a similar electrolyte disturbance such as cystic fibrosis, low chloride diet, surreptitious vomiting (as in bulimia), and diuretic or laxative abuse. The main focus of therapy is potassium chloride supplementation. Drugs such as indomethacin, ibuprofen, and amiloride have been used to reduce urinary potassium and water loss. Monitoring the progress of these patients requires serial measurement of plasma electrolytes and acid-base values.

Cystinosis

Fanconi's syndrome is characterized by a number of renal tubular defects involving excessive urinary losses of amino acids, glucose, uric acid, and phosphate. It is frequently associated with urinary sodium and potassium wasting, proximal renal tubular acidosis, tubular proteinuria, and hyposthenuria. There are numerous causes of Fanconi's syndrome, but in children, cystinosis is the most common.

Cystinosis, an autosomal recessive disorder, typically presents in infancy as failure to thrive, polyuria, muscle weakness, photophobia, and rickets.[27] The diagnosis is suggested by the clinical picture, combined with Fanconi's syndrome and a hypokalemic metabolic acidosis. The presence of cystine crystals in the cornea is diagnostic. The diagnosis can also be confirmed by measuring the leucocyte cystine content. The patients are managed by alkali and potassium supplementation and vitamin D if rickets is present. With time, cystine damages the thyroid gland and thyroxine is required. Eventually, renal failure develops and renal transplantation is necessary. Experimental use of cysteamine to slow the progression of the disease is encouraging.

Nephrogenic Diabetes Insipidus

Nephrogenic diabetes insipidus is an inherited X-linked recessive disorder characterized by renal tubular unresponsiveness to antidiuretic hormone.[28] Affected boys present in infancy with hypernatremia associated with polyuria, polydypsia, unexplained fever, and growth failure. The mother who carries the gene may have a urinary concentrating defect. There are many causes of acquired nephrogenic diabetes insipidus which must be excluded, such as medullary cystic disease, hypokalemia, drugs such as lithium, sickle cell disease, and excessive water intake. There may be a positive family history, and with the demonstration of hypernatremia and dilute urine the diagnosis is straightforward. Central diabetes insipidus is excluded by demonstrating unresponsiveness to vasopressin or deamino-8-D-arginine vasopressin (dDAVP). Management of such infants is focused on providing adequate water intake to maintain normonatremia. A low-solute diet is provided and hydrochlorothiazide will decrease free water clearance. Non-steroidal anti-inflammatory drugs such as indomethacin will reduce the polyuria. During the first two years of life, the child is at risk for dehydration with consequent brain injury, and therefore night-time nasogastric tube feeding may be required.

SUMMARY

Although urinary tract and kidney disorders are not extremely common in children, many different disorders occur as has been described in this chapter. An understanding of their physiology and etiology is important in deciding the most appropriate laboratory tests to order.

REFERENCES

1. Barakat AY, Ichikawa I. Laboratory Data. In: Ichikawa I, ed. Pediatric textbook of fluid and electrolytes. Baltimore: Williams and Wilkins, 1990:478-500.
2. Schwartz GJ, Brion LP, Spitzer A. The use of plasma creatinine concentration for estimating glomerular filtration rate in infants, children and adolescents. Pediatric Clinics of North America 1987;34:571-90.
3. Hall JE, Guyton AC, Farr BM. A single-injection method for measuring glomerular filtration rate. American Journal of Physiology 1977;232:F72-F76.
4. Halperin ML, Goldstein MB. Fluid, Electrolyte and acid-base emergencies. Philadelphia: W.B. Saunders, 1988.
5. Morris RCJ, Ives HE. Inherited disorders of the renal tubule. In: Brenner B, Rector FCJ, ed. The kidney, 4th ed. Philadelphia: W.B. Saunders, 1991:1596-1656.
6. Rodriguez-Soriano J, Vallo A. Renal tubular acidosis. Pediatric Nephrology 1990;4:268-75.
7. Stull TL, LiPuma JJ. Epidemiology and natural history of urinary tract infections in children. Medical Clinics of North America 1991;75:287-97.
8. Sherbotie JR, Cornfield D. Management of urinary tract infections in children. Medical Clinics of North America 1991;75:327-38.
9. Kallenius G, Mollby R, Svenson SB. Microbiological aspects of urinary tract infection. In: Halliday MA, Barratt TM, Vernier R, eds. Pediatric nephrology, 2d ed. Baltimore: Williams and Wilkins, 1987:210-17.
10. Pappas PG. Laboratory in the diagnosis of urinary tract infections. Medical Clinics of North America 1991;75:313-25.
11. Sheldon CA, Gonzalez R. Differentiation of upper and lower urinary tract infections: How and when? Medical Clinics of North America 1984;68(2):321-33.
12. Goldsmith BM, Campos JM. Comparison of urine dipstsick, microscopy and culture for the detection of bacteriuria in children. Clin Pediatr 1990;29:214-8.
13. Males BM, Bartholomew WR, Amsterdam D. Leucocyte esteras: Nitrate and bioluminescence assays as urine screens. J Clin Microbiol 1985;22:531-4

14.   Winberg J. Clinical aspects of urinary tract infection. In: Holliday MA, Barratt TM, Vernier RL, eds. Pediatric nephrology, 2nd ed. Baltimore: Williams and Wilkins, 1987:626-63.

15.   Kaplan MR. Hematuria in childhood. Pediatrics in Review 1983;5:99-105.

16.   Norman ME. An office approach to hematuria. Pediatric Clinics of North America 1987;34:545-60.

17.   Stapleton FB. Morphology of urinary red blood cells: A simple guide in localizing the site of hematuria. Pediatric Clinics of North America 1987;34:561-9.

18.   Hebert LA, Cosio FG, Neff JC. Diagnostic significance of hypocomplementemia. Kidney International 1991;39:811-21.

19.   Barratt TM. Urolithiasis and nephrocalcinosis. In: Holliday MA, Barratt TM, Vernier RL, eds. Pediatric nephrology, 2nd ed. Baltimore: Williams and Wilkins, 1987:700-8.

20.   Brezis M, Rosen S, Epstein FH. Acute renal failure. In: Brenner BM, Rector FCJ, eds. The kidney, 4th ed. Philadelphia: W.B. Saunders, 1991:993-1061.

21.   Paul MD. Three stages of acute renal failure. Diagnosis 1986:November:105-11.

22.   Bennett WM. Guide to drug dosage in renal failure. In: Cliical Pharmacokinetics drug data handbook. New Zealand: ADIS Press, 1990:31-84.

23.   Laragh JH, Baer L, Brunner HR, et al. Renin, angiotensin and aldosterone system in pathogenesis and management of hypertensive vascular disease. American Journal of Medicine 1972;52:633-52.

24.   Winters RW, ed. The body fluids in pediatrics. Boston: Little, Brown and Co., 1973.

25.   Ichikawa I, ed. Pediatric textbook of fluid and electrolytes. Baltimore: Williams and Wilkins, 1990.

26.   Stein JH. The pathogenetic spectrum of Bartter's syndrome. Kidney International 1985;28:85-93.

27.   Schneider JA, Schulman Jd. Cystinosis. In: Stanbury JB, Wyngaarden JB, Frederickson DS, Goldstein JL, Brown MS, eds. The metabolic basis of inherited disease, 5th ed. New York: McGraw-Hill, 1983:1844-66.

28.   Niadet P, Dechaux M. Trivin C, et al. Nephrogenic diabetes insipidus: Clinical and pathological aspects. Advances in Nephrology 1984;13:247-60.

Cardiovascular Disorders

*Robert M. Gow, M.B., B.S.   John Dyck, M.D.   Ivan M. Rebeyka, M.D.
Vera Rose, M.D.   Robert M. Freedom, M.D.*

INTRODUCTION

This chapter examines disorders of the cardiovascular system that either have a primary biochemical basis or cause secondary biochemical changes in the body. Abnormalities of specific enzymatic pathways have been shown to cause myocardial pathology, and heart failure often leads to changes in water and electrolyte homeostasis. The patency of the ductus arteriosus is determined by metabolites within the arachidonic acid pathway, and elucidation of this mechanism has allowed the successful pharmacologic manipulation of the ductus. The relationship of the resting membrane potential, action potential, arrhythmias, and electrolyte abnormalities are discussed, as are abnormalities produced by cardiopulmonary bypass. Finally, disorders of lipid metabolism are receiving increased attention, as are the causes of myocardial ischemia in childhood.

CARDIOMYOPATHY

Cardiomyopathy refers to disease of the heart muscle and excludes structural or functional abnormalities which may be due to valvular disease, coronary artery disease, and systemic or pulmonary vascular disease. Diseases of unknown etiology can be called *primary cardiomyopathies*, and diseases of known cause or associated with disorders of other systems are referred to as *secondary cardiomyopathies* or *specific heart muscle diseases.*[1]

Of the many cardiomyopathies presenting in infancy and childhood, those of unknown etiology are most frequent. These diseases remain enigmatic from the biochemical viewpoint, but are generally divided on the basis of their pathophysiology into *dilated, hypertrophic,* and *restrictive* forms. A brief discussion of these entities follows. Perhaps more intriguing to the biochemist and geneticist are the specific heart muscle diseases; a discussion of several of these entities is also included.

Dilated Cardiomyopathy

Idiopathic Dilated Cardiomyopathy (IDC) in childhood is a relatively unique entity. The majority of patients who present with cardiac failure are under 2 years of age.[2] Many conditions have been implicated in the etiology of idiopathic dilated cardiomyopathy, including genetic predisposition, infective processes, immunologic abnormalities, catecholamine excess, and thyroid hormone disorders. To date, no single agent has been identified, and it is likely that the disorder is heterogeneous in etiology.

The major morphologic feature of IDC is dilatation of both ventricles with an overall increase in the myocardial muscle mass. Interstitial myocardial fibrosis accompanied by hypertrophy and atrophy of myocardial cells is seen microscopically. The clinical picture is one of congestive heart failure with tachypnea, tachycardia, diaphoresis, a gallop rhythm, and hepatomegaly. The congestive heart failure is treated and prognosis is guarded, with mortality as high as 63%.

Laboratory studies are rarely rewarding. Red and white blood cell counts are usually normal, and the erythrocyte sedimentation rate (ESR) is often high. Serum albumin and globulins may be abnormally reduced as a result of hepatic insufficiency. Cardiac enzymes are occasionally mildly increased.

Endocardial Fibroelastosis (EFE) is predominantly characterized by focal thickening of the left-sided endocardium. EFE may be primary, or secondary to other structural heart disease such as aortic stenosis. A large number of possible etiologic factors have been suggested. Many cases of EFE are familial, and systemic carnitine deficiency presenting as EFE has been recently described.[3] More than 75% of cases will present in the first year of life. Diagnosis may be suggested by echocardiography and is confirmed by endomyocardial biopsy. Treatment is non-specific and prognosis remains guarded. It is possible that endocardial fibroelastosis is the result of a non-specific response of the heart to a variety of insults.

Hypertrophic Cardiomyopathy

Hypertrophic Cardiomyopathy (HCM) is the current terminology for a condition previously called Idiopathic Hypertrophic Subaortic Stenosis (IHSS) and Hypertrophic Obstructive Cardiomyopathy (HOCM). Many cases are familial and appear to follow an autosomal dominant pattern of inheritance. However, expressivity of the gene is so variable that many familial cases may escape detection.

HCM is characterized histologically by myocyte hypertrophy and myofibril disarray. The basis for both of these pathologic abnormalities remains to be explained. Considerable evidence supports the theory that a genetically determined abnormality of catecholamine function in the heart may play a significant causal role in hypertrophic cardiomyopathy.[4] A greater thickening of the ventricular septum than of the free wall of the left ventricle occurs in the majority of patients and is generally related to disorganization of septal myocardial fibers. Ventricular systolic function is usually normal or supranormal, while diastolic dysfunction predominates. Gradients across the right ventricular outflow tract are common in early infancy, but left ventricular outflow tract gradients predominate in the older age group. The causes of ventricular outflow tract obstruction are multifactorial.

The natural history of hypertrophic cardiomyopathy is extremely variable and is not particularly related to outflow obstruction. Clinical symptoms are those of angina, presyncope, and (only rarely) congestive heart failure; mortality is primarily due to sudden death (arrhythmic or hemodynamic). The management of hypertrophic cardiomyopathy involves improving diastolic dysfunction, relieving left ventricular outflow tract obstruction, and control of arrhythmias.

Restrictive Cardiomyopathy

Restrictive cardiomyopathies are unusual in childhood and are characterized by a significant limitation to ventricular filling. Ventricular systolic function is generally well preserved, but overall ventricular volume may be reduced. The limitation to ventricular filling is usually associated with significant dilation of the atria.

Restrictive cardiomyopathies are most often idiopathic in origin, although some are characterized by an associated eosinophilia. So-called endomyocardial fibrosis and Loeffler's disease would fit into this category. Amyloidosis and hemochromatosis are other examples of restrictive cardiomyopathies. The medical therapy is directed primarily at symptomatic relief; however, corticosteroids and immunosuppressive drugs have been used with some success in those patients with eosinophilic syndromes.

Specific Heart Muscle Diseases

A variety of systemic diseases are associated with morphologic and functional abnormalities of the myocardium. In many conditions, cardiac involvement is a relatively minor problem, while in others it may predominate. Only a few selected conditions are discussed.

Metabolic Disorders Involving the Heart (Table 4–1)

Lysosomal Storage Diseases

This group of inborn errors of metabolism are generally the result of specific enzyme deficiencies resulting in the storage of the enzyme substrate within lysosomes.

Mucopolysaccharidoses. The mucopolysaccharidoses are a clinically diverse group of disorders.[5] They are due to deficiencies of specific degradative, lysosomal enzymes and lead to the accumulation of heparin sulfate, dermatin sulfate, or keratin sulfate. Phenotypic expressions of these defects are characterized by dwarfism, coarse facies, and corneal clouding and are variously referred to as Hurler's, Hunter's, or Scheie's syndromes. Cardiac involvement may take the form of mitral and aortic valve deterioration, leading to regurgitation, coronary artery narrowing, or a dilated or hypertrophic cardiomyopathy. Laboratory diagnosis is made by screening urine for mucopolysaccharides, and by analysis of cultured cells to identify specific enzyme defects.

TABLE 4–1. Primary Cardiomyopathies

Lysosomal Disorders
  Mucopolysaccharidoses (Types 1, 2, 4, 6, 7)
  Mucolipidoses (Types 2, 3)
  Gangliosidoses (G_{M1}, G_{M2})
  Lipidoses (Niemann-Pick, Gaucher's)

Mitochondrial Disorders
  Fatty acid oxidation (Acyl CoA dehydrogenase deficiency)
  Pyruvate metabolism (Leigh's)
  Oxidative phosphorylation (Cytochrome C oxidase deficiency)

Fatty Acid Transport Disorders
  Primary carnitine deficiency
  Secondary carnitine disorders

Glucose Utilization Disorders
  Glycogen storage disease (Types 2, 3, 4)

Alpha-L-iduronidase is deficient in Hurler's and Scheie's syndromes and in the Hurler-Scheie compound. Hunter's syndrome is caused by a deficiency of iduronate sulfatase, while Morquio's syndrome results from a deficiency of galactose-6-sulfatase. Fetal diagnosis from cells obtained at amniocentesis is possible, and plasmapheresis or liver transplantation may ultimately be shown to provide some relief for this difficult group of disorders.

Mucolipidoses. These abnormalities are characterized biochemically by a modest deficiency of lysosomal acid hydrolases and were initially confused with the Hurler/Hunter syndromes. Cardiac involvement is common and takes the form of a hypertrophic cardiomyopathy and valvular degeneration. Diagnosis is made by tissue (liver) biopsy, followed by specific enzyme assay in tissue culture.

Gangliosidoses. Characterized biochemically by a deficiency of beta-galactosidase (G_{M1}), hexosaminidase A, or hexosaminidase B (G_{M2}) the gangliosidoses result in progressive neurologic deterioration and early death. So-called Tay-Sachs disease is the best known of these disorders. Cardiac involvement is common and takes the form of electrocardiographic abnormalities, a hypertrophic cardiomyopathy, occasional coronary artery involvement, and valvular degeneration.

Glycogen Storage Disease Type II. Glycogen storage disease type II is the best known to pediatric cardiologists and is mentioned here because it is a lysosomal disorder unlike the others, which results from a deficiency of a cytoplasmic enzyme. There are two disorders—a severe and mild form—due to deficiency of the enzyme acid maltase. Pompe's disease, the severe infantile form, is universally fatal. Hypotonia, hepatomegaly, and cardiac involvement dominate the clinical picture. Very specific EKG changes and a severe progressive hypertrophic cardiomyopathy constitute the unique cardiac involvement. The milder form presents as a progressive skeletal myopathy and variable cardiomyopathy in the older child and adult.[6]

Lipidoses. The lipidoses (acid lipase deficiency, Farber's syndrome, Niemann-Pick disease, Gaucher's disease, Fabry's disease) are phenotypically distinct disorders in which the clinical picture is dominated by neurologic deterioration. Variable cardiac involvement, often including constrictive pericardial involvement, valve degeneration, and ventricular hypertrophy, may occur.

Cytoplasmic Disorders

Type IV Glycogen Storage Disease is a deficiency of the branching enzyme in glycogen metabolism and may occur with two separate clinical pictures: a severe infantile form and a later-onset form characterized by muscle weakness, hepatomegaly, and the development of a dilated cardiomyopathy.

Cardiac Phosphorylase Kinase Deficiency is a very rare condition and has been described in association with severe, early-onset congestive heart failure secondary to a dilated cardiomyopathy and characteristic EKG findings. Early death has occurred.

Mitochondrial Myopathies

The mitochondrial myopathies are characterized by a "ragged red" appearance of cardiac or skeletal muscle on light microscopy using trichrome stain. The appearance is due to increased numbers of mitochondria and lipid deposits. The cardiomyopathy is usually hypertrophic.[7]

Acyl-CoA Dehydrogenase and Carnitine Deficiencies

Fatty acids are an important substrate for cardiac energy metabolism. They undergo beta-oxidation within the mitochondria, and long-chain fatty acids are transported across the mitochondrial membrane by carnitine. There are separate carnitine transferases which transfer long-, medium-, and short-chain fatty acids to carnitine. Once within the mitochondria, the first step in beta-oxidation is a dehydrogenation catalyzed by acyl-CoA dehydrogenase.

Primary Carnitine Deficiency

Primary carnitine deficiency has been associated with two or three specific clinical presentations and enzyme deficiencies.[8] A syndrome of skeletal myopathy with subclinical cardiac involvement and onset in late childhood or early adolescence has been associated with acyl-CoA dehydrogenase deficiency. A diet rich in short- and medium-chain triglycerides as well as prednisone therapy may be helpful in this condition.

A second syndrome of recurrent hypoglycemia, with or without cardiomyopathy, has been associated with acyl-CoA dehydrogenase deficiency. Treatment with oral carnitine has been suggested. A third clinical syndrome of familial endocardial fibroelastosis with some response to oral carnitine therapy has also been described. 3-methylglutaconic aciduria may also present with short stature, neutropenia, and endocardial fibroelastosis.

Secondary carnitine deficiency is seen in a number of disorders associated with excessive utilization and inadequate dietary intake.

These states can occasionally be associated with a dilated cardiomyopathy.

Kearns-Sayre Syndrome

This clinical syndrome consists of external ophthalmoplegia, retinopathy, and atrioventricular heart block and may represent a common expression of several different metabolic disorders, including cytochrome C oxidase deficiency.

Neuromuscular Disorders

This diverse group of conditions has not been attributable to specific etiologies, yet, on the basis of genetic transmission and biochemical evidence, specific metabolic derangements would seem likely.

Duchenne's Muscular Dystrophy (DMD) is an X-linked myopathy with early onset and progression to death by age 30. Cardiac involvement is inevitable though often not dominant. Abnormalities of the cardiac conduction system as well as the occurrence of arrhythmias are also of note.

Nemaline Myopathy derives its name from the small rod-like structures seen on light microscopy of skeletal muscle. Conduction abnormalities and a dilated cardiomyopathy have been described.

Friedreich's Ataxia is dominated by neurologic findings, with the most common cardiac abnormalities being characteristic EKG findings, particularly widespread T wave inversion, arrhythmias, and a form of hypertrophic cardiomyopathy. Cardiac involvement is the cause of death in the majority of patients. Recently, a mitochondrial malic enzyme deficiency has been described.

Heart Failure

Heart failure is defined as the inability of the heart to deliver oxygen to the tissues at a rate adequate to provide for the metabolic requirements of the body, and can be due to *mechanical/anatomical abnormalities, myocardial abnormalities,* and *abnormalities of cardiac rhythm*.[9] Alternatively, one can view the circulatory system in terms of myocardial mechanics and classify the abnormalities as those of *preload, myocardial contractility,* or *afterload*.

The causes of heart failure vary with age, and in the fetus may be caused by rhythm disturbances, premature closure of the foramen ovale, large arteriovenous fistulae, atrioventricular valve regurgitation, anemia, and myocarditis. Premature birth is often complicated by the presence of a patent ductus arteriosus, which may cause high-output heart failure. In the term infant, heart failure during the first 24 hours of life usually results from myocardial dysfunction secondary to birth asphyxia or metabolic derangements such as hypoglycemia, hypocalcemia, and acidosis. Obstructive lesions of the left side, such as the hypoplastic left heart syndrome, are the usual cause during the first week, while shunt lesions (for example, ventricular septal defect) predominate for the remainder of the first year. After 1 year of age, acquired forms of heart disease, including cardiomyopathies, endocarditis, cardiac arrhythmias, and rheumatic heart disease, assume the leading roles as causes of heart failure.[10]

Pathophysiology of Heart Failure

The circulatory system utilizes many compensatory mechanisms in an effort to supply adequate amounts of oxygen for the metabolic needs of the body. These primarily involve the autonomic nervous system, atrial natriuretic factor, renal mechanisms, and mechanical adaptations.

Autonomic Nervous System

A falling cardiac output will result in reflex autonomic-sympathetic excitation to the heart and peripheral vascular bed and increased circulating concentrations of epinephrine and norepinephrine as a result of increased release by the adrenal glands. There is a concomitant decrease in cardiac parasympathetic activity. Stimulation of beta-1 adrenergic receptors results in increased heart rate and myocardial contractility, while alpha-1 receptor stimulation results in constriction of arteriolar and venous smooth muscle. These combine to maintain blood pressure and cardiac output. Over time, there is a tendency toward down-regulation of the beta receptors in the heart and increased peripheral arteriolar and venous constriction leading to a mismatch between contractility, preload, and afterload. There is evidence that the improved contractility resulting from endogenous or exogenous catecholamines is limited in the developing myocardium.

As a result of changes in the autonomic nervous system and in local metabolic demands, heart failure is associated with a redistribution of the cardiac output away from the skeletal muscle and splanchnic bed and toward the heart, brain, and adrenals.[11] In the early phases of falling cardiac output, increased systemic oxygen extraction compensates for the reduced overall delivery of oxygen to the tissues. Therefore, monitoring of mixed venous oxygen content is a reasonable means of monitoring cardiac output during congestive heart failure.

Renal Mechanisms

Reduced renal blood flow results from renal vasoconstriction which is mediated by both the sympathetic nervous system and renin-angiotensin system and is exacerbated by redistribution of renal blood flow within the kidney. Increased distal tubular reabsorption of sodium results in marked sodium and water retention and expansion of both intravascular and extravascular volume, leading to hyponatremia and edema. Increased tubular reabsorption of sodium tends to occur principally in the ascending limb of the loop of Henle, but is also seen in the distal convoluted tubule. Urine concentrations of sodium are low despite the hyponatremia, unless there is concomitant use of diuretics. Changes in function of the distal tubule are in a large part controlled by the action of aldosterone. The stimulus for the secondary hyperaldosteronism seen in the congestive heart failure appears to be arterial hypovolemia or hypotension. It causes enhanced excretion of both hydrogen and potassium ions, with resultant hypokalemia and alkalosis.[9] The features of secondary hyperaldosteronism may be exaggerated by diuretic induced hypovolemia.

Heart failure leads to increased secretion of renin by the renal nerves, adrenal medulla, and posterior pituitary. Renin then acts upon angiotensinogens to produce angiotensin 1, which is converted to angiotensin 2 by a converting enzyme present largely in the pulmonary circulation. Angiotensin 2 is a potent arterial vasoconstrictor and also stimulates the secretion of aldosterone by the adrenal gland. Antidiuretic hormone concentrations are increased in heart failure and contribute to the water retention and vasoconstriction.[12]

Atrial Natriuretic Factor

Atrial natriuretic factor is one or more peptides released by the cardiac atria in response to atrial distension. They have both a sodium-losing and a diuretic effect and are known to relax vascular smooth muscle. A role for atrial natriuretic factor as a homeostatic mechanism in the control of excessive sodium and water retention seen during heart failure is supposed but remains unclear at the present time.[13]

Mechanical Factors

The Starling mechanism refers to the ability of the cardiac muscle to increase its contractile force in response to increased resting fiber length. Failure of the ventricle to empty itself completely results in an increased end-diastolic volume for the next cycle. The increased contractility of the next ejection phase will produce increased stroke work and stroke volume. Similarly, patients with chronic congestive heart failure retain both sodium and water and show increased filling pressures and end-diastolic volumes of the ventricles.

The Starling mechanism is operative in the developing heart; however, the response of the myocardium appears to be more limited and the newborn myocardium is also less compliant.[14] The combination of these factors may make the neonate more likely to develop congestive heart failure during periods of hemodynamic stress.

Increased ventricular volume (dilatation) with little or no change in pressure causes a significant increase in myocardial wall stress in the failing heart, which is a stimulus for myocardial hypertrophy in the mature heart and myocardial hyperplasia in the neonate.[15] The end result is an increased ventricular muscle mass index and a reduction of wall stress. However, the deleterious effects of such hypertrophy and hyperplasia can be a reduced diastolic function of the ventricle and a reduced perfusion of the subendocardial myocardium.

Patent Ductus Arteriosus

The ductus arteriosus is a normal fetal structure which connects the main or left pulmonary artery and descending aorta, allowing oxygenated blood returning to the heart from the placenta to pass through the right heart and to be shunted away from the lungs, which have a high vascular resistance. In the normal full-term newborn, functional closure of the ductus arteriosus occurs by 48 h of age.[16] Anatomic obliteration of the ductus occurs over several weeks following birth. In the premature infant, it is remarkably common for the ductus arteriosus to remain patent after 48 h of age, and there is an inverse relationship between the patency of the ductus and gestational age. Persistent patency is defined as patency of the ductus arteriosus beyond 3 m of age.

Evidence has accumulated which suggests that normal closure of the ductus results from oxygen-induced contraction and from the withdrawal of vasodilator substances, particularly prostaglandin E_2 and locally produced prostaglandin I_2. The sensitivity of isolated ductal tissue to elevated partial pressures of oxygen has been clearly demonstrated.[17] Arachidonic acid is liberated from cellular membrane glycerophospholipids by the action of phospholipases. There are subsequently two major pathways in the metabolic cascade: the cyclooxygenase pathway, which produces thromboxane and prostaglandin E_2 (PGE_2), I_2 (PGI_2), and F_{2a} (PGF_{2a}), and the lipoxygenase pathway, which produces the leukotrienes. PGE_2, PGF_{2a}, and PGI_2 (prostacyclin) have all been shown to be synthesized and released by ductal tissue. Many different activities have been attributed to these various substances, although few have a clear role in the perinatal period.

Metabolites of arachidonic acid, including thromboxane and the leukotrienes, have not been shown to exert major affects on the ductus arteriosus; however, this remains an area of active research. A contractile response to agents which inhibit the cyclooxygenase enzyme, and thus inhibit the pathway leading to PGE_2 production, has been shown and serves as the basis for pharmacologic manipulation of the ductus arteriosus.[18]

Pharmacologic Manipulation
of the Ductus Arteriosus

Indomethacin is an inhibitor of cyclooxygenase (prostaglandin synthetase) and has been shown to promote ductus closure in up to 90% of infants.[19] Because of highly variable gastrointestinal absorption, intravenous administration is probably preferable. A single dose of indomethacin is effective in about 50% of infants, while closure is achieved after two doses in 75%. The contraindications to indomethacin usage are hyperbilirubinemia, abnormal renal function, intracranial hemorrhage, necrotizing enterocolitis, and thrombocytopenia.[20]

Renal function may be altered by indomethacin. In particular, glomerular filtration may be decreased, as well as free water clearance. These factors may result in hyponatremia and oliguria. At high doses, hyperkalemia may also occur, as may increased creatinine. Most of the renal effects of indomethacin may be explained on the basis of inhibition of prostaglandin E_2 action on the kidney and can be reversed or prevented by furosemide. Indomethacin interferes with platelet function; however, clinical studies have not demonstrated an increase in hemorrhagic complication associated with its use. Indomethacin may displace bilirubin from protein binding sites.

The indications for the use of PGE_1 or PGE_2 to dilate the ductus arteriosus in the setting of congenital heart disease are reasonably well accepted. The conditions for which this therapy are of use include the cyanotic conditions, including tetralogy of Fallot and other conditions involving an obstruction to pulmonary blood flow, and left-sided obstructions, where maintaining patency of the ductus arteriosus allows a free flow of blood from the pulmonary circulation to the descending aorta. PGE_1 is most frequently given as a continuous intravenous infusion at a dose of 0.005–0.1 µg/kg/min. Higher dosages may occasionally improve efficacy and should be considered dependent upon the clinical situation.

A large multi-center trial has examined the side effects of therapy with prostaglandin E_1 in infants with critical congenital heart disease and found at least one side effect in 43% of patients.[20] Cardiovascular complications, including vasodilatation, arrhythmias and hypotension, were reported most frequently, particularly in infants with cyanotic defects. Central nervous system complications, including temperature elevation, "jitters," or seizures, were also quite frequent. Respiratory depression and apnea was the third most common complication, especially in the low-birth-weight infant. Other rare side effects reported include hematologic abnormalities, metabolic derangements, and cortical hyperostosis.

Electrolytes, the Action Potential, and Arrhythmias

The ability to generate action potentials is the distinguishing feature of excitable membranes. The cardiac action potential (AP) is caused by the transmembrane movement of ions in response to an electrical stimulus which depolarizes the membrane to a threshold value and is divided into "phases" which show qualitative and quantitative differences in various cardiac tissues.[21] These phases and their major ionic components are:

> *Phase 0*: the rapid influx of sodium (Na^+) ions, which depolarizes the membrane.
> *Phase 1*: early repolarization, which is carried by potassium (K^+) ions and makes the membrane potential less positive.
> *Phase 2*: the plateau phase, which is characterized by the slow inward calcium (Ca^{++}) current. The degree of plateau current varies in different tissues.
> *Phase 3:* the repolarization phase, which is carried by K^+ ions and returns the membrane potential toward the negative resting value.
> *Phase 4*: the interval when the membrane has returned to its resting value.

Resting Membrane Potential

It is now well established that the resting membrane potential (RMP) depends predominantly on the permeability to K^+ ions.[22] The K^+ ions move across the membrane until a balance is reached between the concentration gradient, which forces the K^+ ions outward, and the electrical gradient, which attempts to draw the K^+ ions inward. When these forces are balanced, the potential is stabilized and can be described by the Nernst equation

$$E_k = RT / F \ln [K]_o / [K]_i$$

where:
R is the gas constant
T is the absolute temperature
F is the Faraday number

ln is the logarithm to base e
$[K]_0$ and $[K]_i$ are the extracellular and intracellular
potassium concentrations, respectively.

The RMP is negative with respect to the outside of the membrane
and is usually constant in atrial and ventricular myocardium at values
between –80 mV and –95 mV. The Nernst equation is a reasonable approximation of the events responsible for the RMP; however, the Goldman constant-field equation takes the observed small inward Na^+
current into account and is probably more accurate. The membrane
potential varies with external K^+ concentration, with increases in the
extracellular K^+ causing the RMP to become less negative. Decreases in
the external K^+ concentration cause hyperpolarization of the membrane. However, within the physiologic range of K^+ concentrations, de-
viations from the Nernst relationship are seen due to a depolarizing
Na^+ current.

Phase 0: The Rapid Inward Current

In atrial muscle, ventricular muscle, and Purkinje fibers, depolarization is produced by an increase in membrane conductance for Na^+ ions
which move along their electrochemical gradient. dV/dT describes the
rate of change of the potential (V) with respect to time, and its peak
value is indicated by V_{max}, which is dependent on instantaneous membrane potential. The rate of Na^+ entry into the cells is dependent on the
number of available channels and the magnitude of the electrochemical gradient. V_{max} is also one of the determinants of conduction velocity. Consequently, any perturbations which alter the RMP (K^+
concentration, ischemia) may alter the V_{max} and conduction velocity.
The activation of the Na^+ current is brief (< 1 msec), and the inactivation process starts almost immediately. Inactivation is voltage-dependent and can be modified by altering the membrane potential. As the
membrane repolarizes, the portion of channels in the resting state increases. Inactivation has been removed in nearly all the Na^+ channels
at a resting potential of –90 mV.

Phase 1: Transient Outward Current

At the same time that the Na^+ current is inactivating, a transient outward current is responsible for the early, rapid repolarization which
precedes the plateau. It would appear that this current is carried by K^+
ions, although depolarization opens a chloride channel which allows
the inward movement of chloride down its electrochemical gradient
(outward current).

Phase 2: Plateau

The plateau is a balance between a number of currents which show different time- and voltage-dependent characteristics. As the membrane potential starts to repolarize, a slow inward current is activated. This current is carried predominantly by Ca^{++}, although a residual Na^+ current is thought to play some role. Unopposed, the slow inward current would again depolarize the membrane. The plateau phase terminates both by inactivation of calcium channels, and activation of repolarizing K^+ currents.

Phase 3: Rapid Repolarization

The delayed rectifier is a time- and voltage-dependent K^+ current which is activated toward the end of the plateau. A large outward current is generated, which returns the membrane potential toward the resting level. At the same time, the slow inward current is inactivated, allowing the delayed rectifier to proceed unopposed.

Potassium

Hypokalemia

Hypokalemia may be seen in situations of abnormal fluid loss (such as vomiting, diarrhea and early ileostomy drainage), as well as with diuretic therapy. Endocrine causes are well recognized, particularly Cushing's syndrome, hyperaldosteronism, and diabetic ketoacidosis.

Electrophysiologic Effects: A low serum K^+ value can affect the cardiac action potential at several sites.[22] Initially, hyperpolarization of the RMP occurs in all fibers exposed to moderate hypokalemia, as predicted by the Nernst equation. At very low values of external K^+, the membrane potential deviates from that predicted and may depolarize. The repolarization phase is prolonged in Purkinje fibers and myocardium, causing a prolongation of the action potential. Spontaneous diastolic depolarization is increased in cardiac tissues, which may give rise to automatic rhythms. Conduction may be slowed if impulses arrive at incompletely repolarized tissue.

Electrocardiographic Effects: As can be expected from the cellular effects of hypokalemia, the electrocardiogram shows changes in repolarization and conduction.[23] These are evidenced by ST segment depression, large U waves with prolongation of the QU interval, and QRS widening. Nearly 80% of patients with plasma K^+ below 2.7 mmol/L show electrocardiographic abnormalities, compared with 10% with 3.0–3.5 mmol/L.

Arrhythmias: The increased diastolic depolarization seen in isolated tissues has its clinical counterpart in the presence of ectopic rhythms. Plasma K^+ concentrations below 3.2 mmol/L are associated with ventricular ectopy in 28% of patients, while supraventricular ectopic complexes are seen in 22%.[24] Hypokalemia may also cause reversible atrioventricular block. Delayed conduction in atrial and ventricular myocardium due to hypokalemia may be the substrate for a reentry circuit. Severe arrhythmias, such as ventricular fibrillation and *torsade de pointes*, have been described in K^+-deficient states. Digitalis toxicity is enhanced by hypokalemia, and infusions of K^+ can be effective in suppressing the abnormal ectopic activity seen with elevated digoxin levels.

Hyperkalemia

Elevated K^+ concentrations can occur with renal failure, hypoaldosteronism (congenital or acquired), renal tubular defects (sickle cell disease, post-renal transplantation), and cell damage (crush injuries, acidosis).

Electrophysiologic effects: At a cellular level, increasing the external K^+ concentration causes depolarization of the RMP, as predicted by the Nernst equation. Potassium conductance increases and the repolarization process (phase 3) becomes more rapid, with a consequent shortening of the action potential.[25] Spontaneous diastolic depolarization decreases in Purkinje fibers, which should lead to a decrease in automaticity. However, the "gap" between threshold potential and RMP decreases, causing an increase in excitability. Further decrease in the RMP will slow conduction and decrease tissue excitability.

Electrocardiographic effects: The earliest electrocardiographic sign of hyperkalemia is the appearance of tall, peaked T waves. This change is followed by a decrease in amplitude and widening of the P wave and eventual QRS widening. The plasma level at which these changes occur is variable, with QRS widening being reported at levels less than 7 mmol/L, or not until 9–11 mmol/L. Acidosis, hyponatremia, and hypocalcemia potentiate the cardio-toxic effects of hyperkalemia.

Arrhythmias: A wide range of rhythm disturbances may be seen with increased plasma K^+ concentrations.[25] Ventricular arrhythmias are more common than supraventricular arrhythmias. The slowing of conduction due to hyperkalemia may predispose to reentry beats, which can be either single or repetitive. The concomitant shortening of the action potential may allow a premature beat to induce an arrhythmia such as ventricular fibrillation. AV node conduction is either enhanced (minimal increase in plasma K^+) or slowed (higher concentrations).

Magnesium

Magnesium (Mg^{++}) deficiency has been associated with cardiac effects, and the importance of Mg^{++} in both the generation and treatment of cardiac arrhythmias is being increasingly recognized.[26] The major causes of hypomagnesemia are malnutrition states, chronic diarrhea and malabsorption, renal tubular acidosis, exchange transfusions, and diuretic therapy.

Electrophysiologic effects: The exact effects of Mg^{++} on the cardiac action potential are poorly defined. Mg^{++} has a modulating effect on the mechanisms which promote homeostasis of the major intracardiac ions K^+, Na^+, and calcium (Ca^{++}). The action potential does not appear to be altered if K^+ and Ca^{++} concentrations remain normal. Hypomagnesemia leads to loss of intracellular K^+, and an increase in intracellular Na^+ which may lead to increased excitability.[26]

Electrocardiographic effects: The electrocardiogram in isolated hypomagnesemia may show slight T wave changes, although concomitant electrolyte abnormalities may dominate the electrocardiogram. Severe Mg^{++} deficiency will produce QRS changes similar to hypokalemia, while elevated concentrations may cause slowing of conduction in the AV node and specialized conduction tissue.[26]

Arrhythmias: Mg^{++} deficiency appears to exacerbate the pro-arrhythmic nature of other electrolyte abnormalities. In particular, ventricular extrasystoles in hypokalemic patients may not disappear until both K^+ and Mg^{++} are corrected. The arrhythmias from digoxin toxicity may be worse in the presence of hypomagnesemia. Atrial and ventricular arrhythmias may occur in hypomagnesemic states, and Mg^{++} infusion has an antiarrhythmic effect in certain circumstances. The severe drug-induced ventricular arrhythmia *torsade de pointes* may be successfully treated by rapid infusion of Mg^{++}, regardless of the serum Mg^{++} concentration.[26] Mg^{++} infusion has had limited success in other (particularly atrial) arrhythmias.

Hypocalcemia

The major causes of hypocalcemia are hypoparathyroidism, malabsorption syndromes, Vitamin D deficiency, renal tubular acidosis, prematurity in infants, birth asphyxia, and diabetes in mothers of infants.

Electrophysiologic and electrocardiographic effects: Hypocalcemia causes a widening of the action potential which is due to prolongation of the plateau (phase 2), with a decrease in the amplitude. Consequently, the electrocardiogram shows a lengthening of the repolarization process, which is evidenced by an increase in the duration of the ST segment and the overall QT interval.[27]

Arrhythmias: The long QT interval in hypocalcemia does not appear to be pro-arrhythmic, and moderate hypocalcemia has been shown to suppress ventricular and supraventricular ectopic beats. AV block may occur.

Hypercalcemia

Causes of hypercalcemia include hyperparathyroidism, Vitamin D intoxication, chronic renal failure, thyroid disorders and malignancy.

Electrophysiologic and electrocardiographic effects: The plateau of the action potential (phase 2) is shortened and the amplitude increased by hypercalcemia.[28] Although spontaneous diastolic depolarization of Purkinje fibers may be increased, there does not appear to be a concomitant increase in automatic rhythms. The electrocardiogram shows parallel shortening of the ST segment and QT interval. Delayed conduction may be indicated by a widening of the QRS complex.

Arrhythmias: Hypercalcemia has not been shown to predispose to increased automaticity and ectopic rhythms. Sudden deaths have occurred in patients with hyperthyroid crisis, which might be attributed to a ventricular arrhythmia.

THE DYSLIPIDEMIAS

Lipid disorders in children are a major concern because of their key role in the development of arterial lesions, and there is good evidence supporting the concept that the prevention of atherosclerosis should be considered for children at increased risk because of the presence of dyslipidemia.[29] (For further discussion on lipoprotein composition and metabolism, refer to Chapter 15).

Most studies relating diet and plasma cholesterol to vascular disease show increased concentrations of low density lipoprotein cholesterol (LDL-C) and diminished levels of high density lipoprotein cholesterol (HDL-C). Increased concentrations of triglyceride (TG) are also predictive, but this relationship may be due to some extent to a tendency of persons with high TG concentrations to be overweight and to have low levels of HDL-C. Obese children tend to have increased TG and low HDL-C concentrations, a situation which can usually reversed by weight control. In children, the patterning of body fat also appears to be related to lipid and lipoprotein concentrations, and it has been shown that a truncal distribution of adipose tissue in early life is associated with development of adverse concentrations of lipids, lipoproteins, and apolipoproteins.

Morphologic studies have described the early changes of atherosclerosis in childhood and demonstrated myo-intimal arterial thickening in infants, which can progress or regress. Oxidative changes have been shown to trigger uptake of LDL in the arterial wall. Lipid is demonstrated intracellularly within the foamy macrophages in early arterial lesions and extracellularly when plaque formation progresses. Immunologic injury of the coronary endothelium is the primary mechanism of transplant atherosclerosis, and the process is aggravated by hyperlipidemia, which probably results from treatment with immunosuppressives such as prednisone. Experimental studies in animal models have related dietary saturated fat concentration to the development as well as regression of atherosclerotic lesions. In the primate model, new and early lesions are the most responsive to dietary lipids, particularly in the adolescent animals, while lesions in advanced stages could not be changed.

Epidemiologic studies which connect diet and plasma lipid levels to heart disease have been extended to large numbers of free living populations of children and adolescents, as in the Bogalusa Heart study in Louisiana[30] and the Muscatine study in Iowa.[31] Cross-cultural studies have examined the distribution of serum lipids in children from populations with low rates of coronary disease in comparison with children from high-risk populations. There is no population difference of lipid profiles at birth, indicating that environmental factors are the cause of these cross-cultural differences. The child's genetic makeup can also have an effect on lipid levels within a given population and could determine the intensity of the environmental impact.

Genetic conditions which cause hypercholesterolemia through inherited biochemical defects usually are expressed in early childhood. This is best demonstrated in familial hypercholesterolemia (FH), a Mendelian dominant disorder which is the result of a genetic alteration or deletion of the gene for the LDL receptor on the surface of body cells.[32] FH is the most commonly recognized genetic disorder of lipoprotein metabolism in childhood and is fully expressed at birth and in infancy, leading to the development of premature atherosclerotic disease in the third or fourth decade (1 : 500 population incidence). If a child inherits one abnormal gene from each parent, there is complete absence of receptors which results in a fourfold elevation of blood cholesterol and LDL-C, leading to premature death from disease, usually in the first or second decade. Fortunately, this condition is rare (1 : 1,000,000 population). It should be noted that some children with hypercholesterolemia and a positive family history of premature vascular disease could have other as yet poorly defined heritable factors affecting the LDL receptor pathway. The pediatric implications of heterozygous FH have been recently reviewed.[33] Secondary causes of hyperlipidemia may also be seen in childhood. In particular, glycogen storage disease and biliary atresia may be associated with elevated lipids in the first year of life, while endocrine disorders (e.g., hypothyroidism and diabetes mellitus) and renal disease may be responsible later in childhood.

Chapter 15 discusses the biochemistry and clinical aspects of the dyslipidemias in more detail.

MYOCARDIAL ISCHEMIA

Although myocardial ischemia and infarction are considered rare in children, there are a number of congenital and acquired causes.[34] The most common congenital cause is anomalous origin of the left coronary artery from the pulmonary artery. Early studies suggested that this lesion alone may account for 25% of all the cases of myocardial infarction in childhood.[35]

Kawasaki disease is a vasculitis of unknown etiology which has its most significant effects when it involves the coronary arteries. Aneurysmal dilatation of the coronary arteries occurs in 15% to 25% of cases; however, the incidence has been significantly reduced since the initiation of immunoglobulin therapy in the early stages of the disease. Myocardial infarction occurs in a small proportion of the cases.

Ischemia results from an imbalance between oxygen supply and demand. This situation may be seen when myocardial hypertrophy is present, particularly if there is associated hypoxemia. The ischemia may be localized to the subendocardial region or the papillary muscles, and can be seen in such conditions as aortic stenosis, severe pulmonary stenosis, and in the hypoplastic ventricles of pulmonary atresia with intact ventricular septum. Hypoxia may also contribute to the transient myocardial ischemia seen with perinatal asphyxia.

Under normal conditions, myocardial energy production is predominantly an aerobic process which produces acetyl CoA via the metabolism of glucose and glycogen.[36] Certain enzymes within the glycolytic pathway (for example, phosphofructokinase, pyruvate dehydrogenase, glycogen phosphorylase) act as regulatory sites which are affected by hormonal and non-hormonal factors. Under adverse conditions, glyceraldehyde-3-phosphate dehydrogenase is inhibited by the intermediate metabolites which accumulate during ischemia, with the end result being a block of glycolysis. Fatty acid oxidization is the other major source of energy in cardiac muscle. After uptake into the cell, fatty acyl CoA is formed, which serves as a substrate for acyl transfer and beta oxidation.

Ischemia has a profound effect on myocardial energetics. ATP production is decreased and NADH accumulates within the cell. The increased levels of NADH inhibit glycolysis and fatty acid oxidation.[36] Alterations in the metabolism of ATP lead to increased concentrations of dephosphorylated metabolites of the nucleotides and subsequent loss from the cell. Increases in hydrogen ion concentration occur, resulting in cell damage. Ionic exchange mechanisms may be inhibited, causing calcium overload.

Elevation of circulating concentrations of cardiac enzymes has been used as a marker of myocardial damage from ischemia. Serum glutamic oxaloacetic transaminase (AST), lactate dehydrogenase (LDH) and creatine kinase (CK) are the principal enzymes in clinical use. It is believed that the enzymes are released after irreversible tissue injury, and there are many determinants of the plasma concentrations attained.[37] Because these enzymes are present in many tissues, the specificity is reduced; however, the sensitivity is excellent.

Measurement of isoenzymes of LDH and CK has improved the specificity. The isoenzymes of LDH are composed of four subunits which are different combinations of a heart (H) or muscle (M) type and show different electrophoretic mobilities. LDH_1 is present in heart muscle and is the component released after myocardial infarction. Similarly, CK isoenzymes are dimers of either muscle (M) or brain (B) subunits. CK-MB is found almost exclusively in heart muscle and increased concentrations are very specific for myocardial injury. Time-activity curves have been used successfully to estimate infarct size in adults.

In adults, the first enzyme released after acute myocardial infarction is CK, which is elevated by 4–6 hours, peaks by 24 hours, and declines over 3–4 days. The peak level is two- to tenfold above normal. AST activity is increased by 6–12 hours, peaks at 18–36 hours, and is also normal by 3–4 days. LDH, on the other hand, has the slowest rise, with initial increase being present by 24–48 hours, peaks occurring within 3–6 days, and levels returning to normal by 14 days. It appears that increase of the LDH_1 fraction precedes increases in the total LDH and may be present by 8–24 hours. There is some evidence that the enzyme changes in children with myocardial infarction are qualitatively similar to adults, but the peak concentrations (especially of CK) may be reduced.[34]

BIOCHEMICAL CHANGES ASSOCIATED WITH CARDIOPULMONARY BYPASS

The central purpose of cardiopulmonary bypass is to permit surgery within the heart by artificially maintaining the function of both the heart and lungs. Cardiopulmonary bypass, however, does not reproduce normal cardiorespiratory function and represents an abnormal physiological state whereby arterial blood flow to the body is temporarily provided by means of extracorporeal circulation using a pump oxygenator. Accordingly, the use of cardiopulmonary bypass for intracardiac repair of congenital heart malformations results in numerous biochemical and physiologic changes that persist into the postoperative period. At present, the mechanisms responsible for many of these physiologic changes remain incompletely understood but probably relate to suboptimal organ perfusion secondary to arteriovenous shunting, as well as the damaging effects of cardiopulmonary bypass on blood components as a consequence of their contact with foreign surfaces within the extracorporeal circuit.

The successful recovery of the patient following cardiac surgery involving cardiopulmonary bypass is dependent upon the careful monitoring of organ system function to detect early deviation from the pattern of normal postoperative convalescence.

Serum Electrolyte Changes

Postoperative fluid and electrolyte changes in patients subjected to cardiopulmonary bypass differ considerably from that of other patients undergoing major surgical procedures without cardiopulmonary bypass. Patients in congestive cardiac failure usually have an increased total body water content preoperatively, which is increased by the interstitial fluid accumulation that occurs when hemodilution perfusion is used during bypass. Furthermore, marked postoperative Na^+ and water retention leads to further expansion of the extracellular fluid space.[38] In general, intravascular volume tends to fall, with an associated increase in extracellular fluid space. These changes in total body fluid distribution occur maximally during the second postoperative day and persist for more than one week.[39]

Sodium

Postoperative hyponatremia is almost always dilutional in nature, secondary to excess water retention, and can be managed in most patients by fluid restriction. Hyponatremia does not require aggressive treatment unless the serum Na^+ falls below 125 mmol/L. However, infants are unable to conserve sodium as efficiently as older patients because of renal immaturity, and may require the careful administration of Na^+.

Hypernatremia is often seen in critically ill infants when large amounts of sodium bicarbonate have been required to correct a metabolic acidosis associated with low cardiac output.

Potassium

Hypokalemia commonly occurs postoperatively and is related to the loss of K^+ during the phase of early postoperative diuresis. Depleted total body K^+ secondary to preoperative diuretic therapy also predisposes the cardiac surgical patient to hypokalemia. Although infants appear less prone to ventricular arrhythmias with hypokalemia, the risk of digitalis toxicity is increased in the presence of low serum K^+ concentrations.

Hyperkalemia may occur during the immediate postoperative phase when large volumes of high K^+ cardioplegic solution are administered to arrest or stop the heart during intracardiac repair. This initial hyperkalemic phase typically resolves within several hours following cardiopulmonary bypass. Persistent or delayed hyperkalemia suggests that low cardiac output or renal failure has complicated the postoperative recovery period and will be exacerbated by the presence of metabolic acidosis. Frequent serum K^+ determinations are warranted during the initial postoperative period as the classic progression of T wave changes on the electrocardiogram are not reliable.

Calcium

Cardiopulmonary bypass is frequently associated with alterations in ionized serum Ca^{++} concentrations, both intraoperatively as well as during the postoperative period. Changes in ionized Ca^{++} concentrations are usually due to the chelating effects of citrate in blood products used in the cardiopulmonary bypass circuit or administered peri-operatively.

Significant hypocalcemia may occur in newborn infants during the early postoperative phase. Several factors likely predispose the neonate to hypocalcemia: (1) prematurity, with inadequate Ca^{++} stores and parathyroid function; (2) stress leading to endogenous steroid production; (3) administration of sodium bicarbonate; and (4) increased serum citrate concentrations secondary to administration of stored blood products.

Magnesium

Alterations in Mg^{++} metabolism following cardiopulmonary bypass may be associated with clinically significant hypomagnesemia and can predispose the patient to serious cardiac arrhythmias. Cardiac surgical patients frequently have depleted intracellular Mg^{++} stores because of preoperative diuretic therapy. The decrease in serum Mg^{++} may be exacerbated by its binding to the citrate present in stored blood products used in bypass prime solutions or administered postoperatively.

Serum Glucose

Serum glucose values following cardiopulmonary bypass are typically increased due to the high glucose content of priming solutions as well as endogenous catecholamine release. The hyperglycemia rarely reaches dangerous concentrations and is useful in promoting a postoperative diuresis. However, postoperative glucose values vary markedly and hypoglycemia is occasionally seen in newborn infants who have poorly developed mechanisms for glucose regulation. Serum glucose concentrations should be monitored every 4–6 hours during the first postoperative day, as the changes in glucose concentrations occur unpredictably. Marked changes in serum glucose values appear more commonly when hypothermic total circulatory arrest is employed.

Renal Function

Acute renal failure is an uncommon event following intracardiac surgery but does occur more frequently in infants than in older children and adults.[40] Renal dysfunction usually is encountered in association with low cardiac output, but other factors that contribute to postoperative renal failure include preoperative renal dysfunction, nephrotoxic drugs, sepsis and massive hemoglobinuria related to red blood cell trauma from the pump oxygenator, and excessive transfusions or blood transfusion reactions. Furthermore, patients with congenital heart disease commonly have associated abnormalities of renal structure and function. The appropriate management of peri-operative renal dysfunction is dependent upon early detection of renal failure. As oliguria is frequently present in the early postoperative period, blood urea nitrogen and creatinine concentrations should be monitored at least daily for 2–3 days and more often if renal failure is present or suspected. In the presence of renal failure, more frequent monitoring of serum K^+, Na^+, chloride, Ca^{++}, and pH is indicated.

Postbypass Liver Function

Jaundice in the early postoperative period is infrequent following cardiac surgery, but may result from (1) increased bilirubin production secondary to multiple transfusions of stored blood preparations with red blood cells having a shortened life span, or excessive hemolysis with prolonged bypass durations; or (2) hepatocellular dysfunction due to either decreased perfusion of the liver or increased venous pressure with passive liver congestion. Jaundice appearing later in the postoperative course should alert one to the possibility of systemic infection from a viral (hepatitis) or bacterial (generalized sepsis) source.

Amylase

Acute pancreatitis is unusual following operations involving cardiopulmonary bypass, especially in pediatric cardiac surgical patients. However, postoperative pancreatitis is associated with a high mortality rate, as it is usually encountered in the presence of severely low cardiac output. Despite the rarity of clinical pancreatitis, significant increases of both serum and urinary amylase occur following cardiopulmonary bypass, with concentrations frequently rising more than tenfold.[41]

Endocrine Alterations

The systemic response cardiopulmonary bypass is associated with significant alterations in endocrine homeostasis. Numerous studies have documented a substantial release of endogenous catecholamines in association with cardiopulmonary bypass. The use of hypothermia during bypass contributes to the abnormal catecholamine release. Plasma epinephrine concentrations increase at the onset of bypass, reaching levels ten times normal, and the increase persists for a number of hours postoperatively. Plasma norepinephrine concentrations appear to rise to a lesser extent. Cardiopulmonary bypass produces a massive release of vasopressin or antidiuretic hormone (ADH), with increases up to 20 times basal levels that persist postoperatively.

The effect of cardiopulmonary bypass on metabolic function is characterized by a state of catabolism. Lipid metabolism becomes dominant as free fatty acid concentrations rise secondary to catecholamine release, while carbohydrate metabolism is deranged with impaired insulin release and glucose utilization. Increased plasma cortisol concentrations are universally seen in response to the metabolic stress of surgery and persist for more than 48 hours following cardiopulmonary bypass.[42]

The effects of bypass on thyroid metabolism are poorly understood. Recent studies have suggested that cardiopulmonary bypass simulates the "euthyroid sick syndrome," with significant depression of free triiodothyronine concentrations while thyroxine concentrations remain with the normal range.

CONCLUSIONS

The clinical biochemist plays an integral role in the management and diagnosis of many cardiac diseases in children. At an investigative level, the discovery of abnormal metabolic pathways in previously uncharacterized cardiomyopathies has resulted from a multidisciplinary approach. It is likely that the number of "idiopathic" cardiomyopathies will decrease in number as more sophisticated biochemical analysis identifies specific metabolic abnormalities in many of these patients.

The delineation of the arachidonic acid pathway and its role in ductal patency lead to the successful pharmacologic manipulation of the ductus arteriosus, which has had far-reaching benefits in clinical cardiology.

The biochemical laboratory has a critical role to play in the day-to-day management of many children with heart disease. As has been demonstrated, derangements of the serum electrolytes have far-reaching consequences for the myocardium. Similarly, the treatment of heart failure, and cardiopulmonary bypass, may be complicated by fluid and electrolyte disturbances.

Finally, myocardial ischemia needs to be managed appropriately in the pediatric age group, and there is evidence that significant ischemia and infarction is frequently unrecognized.[35] It appears that "standard" clinical and electrocardiographic signs may be inadequate to detect ischemia in children. Consequently, diagnostic cardiac enzymology will assume an increasing importance, and valid questions about its sensitivity and specificity in the pediatric age group need to be answered.

REFERENCES

1. Report of The WHO/ISFC Task Force on the Definition and Classification of Cardiomyopathies. B Heart J 1980;44:672-73.
2. Pacquet M, Hanna BD. Cardiomyopathy. In: Garson A Jr, Bricker JT, McNamara DG, eds. The science and practice of pediatric cardiology. New York: Lea & Febiger, 1990: 1617-46.
3. Tripp ME, Katcher ML, Peters HA, et al. Systemic carnitine deficiency presenting as familial endocardial fibroelastosis. New Engl J Med 1981;305:385-90.
4. Wenger NK, Abelmann WH, Roberts WC. Cardiomyopathy and specific heart muscle disease. In: Hurst JW, Schlant RC, Rackley CE, Sonnenblick EH, Wenger NK, eds. The Heart, 7th ed. New York: McGraw Hill, 1990:1278-1347.
5. McKusick VA, Neufeld EF. The mucopolysaccharide storage diseases. In: Stanbury JE, Wyngaarden JB, Frederickson DS, Goldstein JL, Brown HS et al., eds. The metabolic basis of inherited disease, 5th ed. New York: McGraw Hill, 1983:751-77.
6. Caddell JL. Metabolic and nutritional diseases. In: Adams FH, Emmanoulides GC, Riemenschneider TA, eds. Heart disease in infants, children, and adolescents, 4th ed. Baltimore: Williams and Wilkins, 1989:750-77.
7. Mackay EH, Brown RS, Pickering D.. Cardiac biopsy in skeletal myopathy: Report of a case with mitochondrial abnormalities. J Pathol 1976;120:35-42.
8. Gelb BD. Metabolic heart disease. In: Garson A, Bricker JT, McNamara DG, eds. The science and practice of pediatric cardiology. New York: Lea & Febiger. 1990:1656-83.
9. Rackley CE, Sonnenblick EH. Pathophysiology of heart failure. In: Hurst JW, Schlant RC, Rackley CE, Sonnenblick EH, Wenger NK, eds. The heart, 7th ed. New York: McGraw Hill, 1990:387-418.
10. Talner NS. Heart Failure. In: Adams FH, Emmanoulides GC, Riemenschneider TA, eds. Heart disease in infants, children, and adolescents, 4th ed. Baltimore: Williams and Wilkins, 1989:890-911.
11. Fischer DJ. Mechanisms of congestive heart failure. In: Garson A, Bricker JT, McNamara DG, eds. The science and practice of pediatric cardiology. New York: Lea & Febiger, 1990:244-49.
12. Share L. The role of vasopressin in cardiovascular regulation. Physiol Rev 1988;68:1248-84.

13. Raine AEG, Erne P, Burgess E, et al. Atrial natriuretic peptide and atrial pressure in patients with congestive heart failure. N Engl J Med 1986;315:533-37.

14. Romero TE, Freidman WF. Limited left ventricular response to volume overload in the neonatal period. Ped Res 1979;13:910-15.

15. Berman W, Christensen D. Effects of acute preload and afterload stress on myocardial function in newborn and adult sheep. Biol Neonate 1983;43:61-66.

16. Allen HD, Goldberg SJ, Valdes-Cruz LM, Sahn DJ. Use of echocardiography in newborns with patent ductus arteriosus: A review. Pediatr Cardiol 1982;3:65-70.

17. Oberbonsli-Weiss I, Heymann MA, Rudolph AM, Mehner KL: The pattern and mechanisms of response to oxygen by the ductus arteriosus and umbilical artery. Pediatr Res 1972;6:693-700.

18. Coceani F, White E, Badach E, Olley PM. Age dependent changes in the response of the lamb ductus arteriosus to oxygen and ibuprofen. Can J Physiol Parmacol 1979;57:825-31.

19. Corbet AJ. Medical manipulation of the ductus arteriosus. In: Garson A, Bricker JT, McNamara DG, eds. The science and practice of pediatric cardiology. New York: Lea & Febiger, 1990:2108-25.

20. Lewis AB, Freud MD, Heymann MA et al: Side effects of therapy with prostaglandin E, in infants with critical congenital heart disease. Circulation 1981;64:893-98.

21. Fozzard HA, Arnsdorf MF: Cardiac electrophysiology. In: Fozzard HA, Haber E, Jennings RB, et al., eds. The heart and cardiovascular system. New York: Raven Press, 1986:1-30.

22. Hecht H, Heath J, Maier ES, et al. The cellular basis of the electrocardiographic changes associated with alterations in serum potassium. J Clin Invest 1957;36:897.

23. Surawicz B, Braun AH, Crum WB, et al. Quantitative analysis of the electrocardiographic pattern of hypopotassemia. Circulation 1957;16:750-63.

24. Davidson S, Surawicz B: Ectopic beats and atrioventricular conduction disturbances in patients with hypopotassemia. Arch Intern Med 1967;120:280-85.

25. Ettinger PO, Regan TJ, Oldewurtel HA, et al. Hyperkalemia, cardiac conduction and the electrocardiogram: A review. Am Heart J 1974;88:360-71.

26. Keller PK, Aronson RS. The role of magnesium and cardiac arrhythmias. Prog Cardiovasc Dis 1990;32:433-48.

27. Rardon DP, Fisch C: Electrolytes and the heart. In: Hurst JW, Schlant RC, Rackley CE, et al., eds. The heart, 7th ed. New York: McGraw Hill, 1990:1557-70.

28. Surawicz B: The interrelationship of electrolyte abnormalities and arrhythmias. In: Mandel WJ, ed. Cardiac arrhythmias: Their mechanisms, diagnosis and management, 2nd ed. Philadelphia: JB Lippincott, 1987:81-100.

29. Lauer RM, Lee J, Clarke WR, et al. Cholesterol screening in childhood. In: Roche AF, ed. Prevention of adult atherosclerosis during childhood. Columbus, OH, Ross Laboratories, 1988:97-102.

30. Freedman DS, Shear CL, Srinivisan SR, et al. Tracking of serum lipids and lipoproteins in children over an 8-year period: The Bogalusa Heart Study. Prev Med 1985;14:203-16.

31. Clarke WR, Schrott HG, Leaverton PE, et al. Tracking of blood lipids and blood pressures in school age children: The Muscatine Study. Circulation 1978;58:626-34.

32. Brown MS, Goldstein JL. A receptor-mediated pathway for cholesterol homeostasis. Science 1986;232:34-47.

33. Cortner JA, Coates PM, Gallagher PR. Prevalence and expression of familial combined hyperlipidemia in childhood. J Pediatr 1990;116:514-19.

34. Towbin JA. Myocardial infarction in childhood. In: Garson A Jr, Bricker JT, McNamara DG, eds. The science and practice of pediatric cardiology. New York: Lea & Febiger, 1990:1684-1722.

35. Franciosi RA, Blanc WA. Myocardial infarcts in infants and children. 1. A necropsy study in congenital heart disease. J Pediatr 1968;73:309-19.

36. Morgan HE, Neely JR. Metabolic regulation and myocardial function. In: Hurst JW, Schlant RC, Rackley CE, et al., eds. The heart, 7th ed. New York: McGraw Hill, 1990:91-105.

37. Sobel BE. Cardiac enzymes and other macromolecular markers of myocardial injury. In: Hurst JW, Schlant RC, Rackley CE, et al., eds. The heart, 7th ed. New York: McGraw Hill, 1990:972-74.

38. Breckenridge IM, Digerness SB, Kirklin JW. Increased extracellular fluid after open intracardiac operation. Surg Gynecol Obstet 1970;131:53-56.

39. Beattie HW, Evans G, Garnett ES, et al. Albumin and water fluxes during cardiopulmonary bypass. J Thorac Cardiovasc Surg 1974;67:926-31.

40. Chesney RW, Kaplan BS, Freedom RM, Haller JA. Acute renal failure: An important complication of cardiac surgery in infants. J Pediatr 1975;87:381-88.

41. Hennings B, Jacobson G. Postoperative amylase secretion. A study following thoracic surgery with and without extracorporeal circulation. Ann Clin Res 1974;6:215-22.

42. Hirvonen J, Huttunen P, Nuutinen L, Pekkarinen A. Catecholamines and free fatty acids in plasma of patients undergoing cardiac operations with hypothermia and bypass. J Clin Pathol 1978;31:949-55.

Growth Disorders

Raphaël Rappaport, M.D.   Jean-Claude Souberbielle, Ph.D.

INTRODUCTION

Growth from birth to adolescence is closely related to health, so any deviation from the normal growth rate may be the presenting symptom or the complication of an intercurrent disease, or lead to the diagnosis of a defect in skeletal development or its endocrine control. A number of biochemical tools contribute to the diagnosis. Their use is initially guided by the clinical analysis. The majority of problems related to growth that occur in the childhood period are due to growth retardation rather than to increases in growth.

PHYSIOLOGY OF GROWTH

Growth from birth until adulthood is determined by genetic and environmental factors. Among these is nutrition, which is essential to allow the optimal effect of hormones and growth factors. Therefore, a long-lasting, chronic disease can impair growth by interfering with nutrient intake and utilization, as well as by impairing specific organ functions and imposing a condition of chronic stress.

The endocrine control of skeletal growth is primarily dependent on growth hormone (GH) secretion and bioactivity as is demonstrated by pituitary dwarfism. It has been shown that GH does not stimulate bone growth or cartilage activity *in vitro* by direct action, but needs the presence of a growth factor initially called somatomedin and now known as insulin-like growth factor I, or IGF I. This somatomedin hypothesis has been verified by the finding that IGF I is produced by the liver and most cells of the body and that it stimulates target cells, in particular cartilage growth plates, thereby controlling endochondral ossification. More recently, this classical view has been challenged by the evidence of a direct effect of GH on cartilage. It is now appreciated that locally produced IGF I, stimulated by GH, acts by an autocrine/paracrine mechanism. The cell-to-cell interaction is superimposed on the endocrine circulating IGF effect. GH and IGF I are necessary for other hormones, such as thyroid hormones and sex steroids, to fully express a complete and appropriate stimulation of skeletal growth.

Growth Hormone and Growth Factors

The GH/IGF I axis is presently viewed as central to the control of growth (see Figure 5–1). Schematically, the growth response depends on (1) the availability of both GH and IGF I, which are assessed by measurement of their circulating concentrations; and (2) on their biological activity, which may depend on the molecular form of GH, on the presence of specific binding proteins, on their receptors, and on as yet poorly defined cartilage and bone factors involved in the tissue responsiveness to endocrine control.

Growth Hormone

Human GH (hGH) is a protein secreted by the pituitary gland, with a molecular weight of 22 kD consisting of a single peptide chain of 191 amino acid residues. The hGH genes reside within a cluster of five loci: normal GH, or GH 1; two human chorionic somatomammotropin, or hCS A and B; one hCS pseudogene; and a variant GH, or GH 2, only expressed in the placenta. Expression of the GH gene GH1 utilizes two different splicing sequences. This alternative splicing forms the basis of the 20 kD variant of hGH. The two 22 kD and 20 kD forms are cosecreted and circulate in the plasma in percentages of 80 and 20, respectively, independently of age and sex.[1]

Neuro-endocrine Control

The pituitary receives information from the central nervous system through the hypothalamus, which receives and modulates a large number of neurotransmitters as well as hormonal and metabolic signals.[2] The final common pathway for integration of these signals involves two hypothalamic neuropeptides which are hypophysiotropic hormones: somatostatin (somatotropin release inhibiting factor, or

FIGURE 5–1. The Endocrine and Paracrine Control of Skeletal Growth

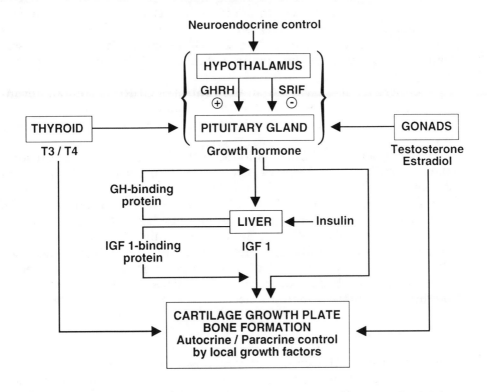

From: Rappaport R. A touch of growth. Horm Res, in press. Reprinted with permission.

SRIF), which has an inhibitory influence, and growth hormone releasing hormone, or GHRH, which exerts a stimulatory effect. Many of the studies demonstrating neuro-endocrine control come from experiments on rodents, such as those designed to selectively exclude the effect of one of the hormones using specific antibodies.[3] Although it is known that there are definite species differences, it is likely that in the human most of the other hypothalamic neuropeptides or monoamines also act via the SRIF/GHRH pathway.

The GHRH neurones are mainly located in the arcuate nucleus. GHRH (secreted as GHRH 1-44) selectively stimulates *in vitro* and *in vivo* growth hormone secretion. Analogs have been synthesized such as the GHRH 1-29, which has an activity identical to that of the natural peptide. A partial loss of responsiveness, also considered as partial receptor desensitization with depletion of GH stores, has been observed in normal human subjects receiving several boluses of GHRH. This effect is much less striking than the severe desensitization observed in the effect of gonadotropin releasing hormone analogs and seems to have no clinical relevance. In contrast, the GH response to a supramaximal dose of GHRH was preserved during 14 days' continuous GHRH infusion with increased serum IGF I concentrations. This observation established the therapeutic potential of GHRH in children with hypopituitarism.

Other signals play a role in the control of GHRH secretion. For instance, the *in vitro* secretion of GHRH is inhibited by IGF I. This control may involve hypothalamic GHRH production at a post-transcriptional level.[4]

Somatostatin, or SRIF, is found in the hypothalamus but also in the pancreas. It is a family of peptides including somatostatin-14 and somatostatin-28, which is the most potent. Newly synthesized molecules have a longer half-life. SRIF exerts its activity through specific pituitary membrane receptors, inhibiting both GH and thyroid stimulating hormone (TSH) secretion. SRIF inhibits or modulates GH secretion by blocking the stimulatory effect of GHRH. It also mediates the GH and IGF I negative-feedback effect on growth hormone secretion which stimulates SRIF release. SRIF does not interfere with GRF binding to pituitary somatotrophs.[5]

GH Secretion Patterns

The patterns of GH secretion vary among species. Generally, bursts or pulses of secretion occur at variable intervals, separated by periods during which GH sometimes fails to reach detectable concentrations. In the human, GH is episodically secreted in intermittent bursts, the majority of which occur during the night. During the day, GH secretion may be related to exercise, stress, and nutrient intake. A new method for calculating the secretory rate, deconvolution analysis, provides information of clinical relevance.[6]

Rat experiments indicate that SRIF is important for maintaining low basal concentrations, whereas pulsatile GH secretion is dependent on GHRH activity. In addition, variations in SRIF secretion contribute to the pattern of pulsatile secretion. Hence, the control of GH secretion depends on asynchronous periodic release of GHRH and SRIF; pulses of GH secretion would be expected to occur at times of maximal GHRH and minimal SRIF activity. It has been stated that the variability in the response of GH to a supramaximal dose of GHRH in normal subjects reflects varying hypothalamic SRIF secretion at time of GHRH stimulation.

Resting concentrations of GH in plasma taken at random vary with age. At birth, the mean concentration is 33 ng/mL. It declines within a few months to the prepubertal concentration of 3–5 ng/mL until the pubertal rise. These changes go along with parallel changes in secretion rates as estimated from spontaneous profiles. GH secretion rises during abrupt hypoglycemia and is suppressed by acute hyperglycemia. A high-protein meal or intravenous infusion of amino acids induces release of GH, probably by hypothalamic control. During fasting or in protein-deprived, malnourished children, growth hormone secretion is stimulated. This effect is possibly due to the suppression of the normal feedback control of plasma IGF I. It is of interest that obesity induces a blunted GH response to pharmacological stimulation to GHRH, and to exercise. Stress is a potent stimulus of GH release. A characteristic feature is the sleep-associated rise of GH; this nocturnal rise is mainly related to sleep onset and is correlated with EEG changes of slow-wave sleep, although the phenomena are not directly interdependent.

GH Binding Protein and GH Receptor

Fifty percent of the circulating GH is estimated to be in a complexed form in association with a specific high-affinity and low-capacity binding protein. This protein has more affinity for the 22 kD than the 20 kD form of GH. It represents the extracellular portion of the monomeric GH receptor.[7] It is hypothesized that the binding protein may have an effect on the *in vivo* kinetics of GH, prolonging its biological activity. It may dampen the pulsatile variations in the pituitary secretion of GH. Another possibility is provided by the correlation between plasma binding activity and the number of receptors present, essentially in the liver. Although regulation of that binding activity by hormones has been demonstrated, this view remains questionable, since the mechanism of production of the binding protein, probably by proteolytic cleavage, in humans remains unknown.

Lack of plasma binding activity has only been observed in the Laron syndrome, wherein there is complete GH insensitivity due to genetic defects of the GH receptor.[8, 9] A possible consequence of GH heterogeneity in human circulation and binding to carrier proteins may be the well-known discrepancy between immunoassayable and bioassayable GH in plasma. This may also represent a limitation of our current understanding of the control of skeletal growth by GH.

Insulin-like Growth Factors

Growth hormone exerts its growth-promoting effect on somatic tissues by inducing peptide growth factors, termed insulin-like growth factors (formerly somatomedins). Specific peptides of this kind are IGF I and IGF II. These factors were isolated on the basis of their insulin-like effects on fat and muscle, their GH-dependent effect on cartilage, and their mitogenic effect on cultured fibroblasts. They regulate functional cell differentiation. Their biological role is determined primarily by the receptors expressed in the target cells and the tissue expression of their genes.[10, 11]

Both IGF I and IGF II structures are very similar to proinsulin, and it is thought that both IGFs and insulin have evolved from a common ancestor. The gene structures of the IGFs have been well investigated. The IGF I gene is localized on the long arm of chromosome 12; the IGF II gene is on chromosome 11, downstream from the insulin gene. The expression of IGFs' genes varies between organs and during development in the fetus. It is generally considered that IGF II is dominant in embryonic fetal life. In contrast, IGF I is present in the fetal circulation at low concentrations and increases from birth to adulthood. As the expression of IGF I in liver appears to parallel its serum concentration, it is likely that in the postnatal life the liver is the major source of IGF I in circulation.

GH has a key role in regulating IGF production, and the production of IGF I (more than IGF II) is dependent on the presence of mature growth hormone receptors. IGF I increases gradually in serum until puberty. At puberty, its dramatic increase is GH-mediated under the control of sex steroids.[12, 13] IGF I production is also dependent on other hormones. Thyroid hormones may modulate the GH effect on liver production of IGF I. Insulin may participate in the control of IGF I release, as has been shown in experimental animals. The role of glucocorticoids is not elucidated, although high doses may suppress circulating IGF I concentrations.

There are two specific IGF receptors. The type 1 IGF receptor has a structure similar to that of the insulin receptor. It cross-reacts weakly with insulin. The type 2 receptor essentially binds IGF II. Its structure is very different from that of the type 1 receptor and its function is unknown. Growth effect would therefore depend mostly on the IGF type 1 receptor.

IGF Binding Proteins

IGFs circulate in bound forms with specific binding proteins localized in two main fractions in serum: the 150 kD complex, which contains most of the IGFs, and the 40 kD complex. Several binding proteins have been isolated, and some are produced by recombinant technique.[14, 15] The major binding protein is IGF BP-3, incorporated in the 150 kD complex together with an 80 kD acid-labile subunit. It has also been shown that IGF BP-3 is induced by IGF I itself. It is glycosylated and consists of a 54 kD and a 47 kD component. As for IGF I, IGF BP-3 concentration shows little change over 24 h. In contrast, the 40 kD complex shows an inverse relationship with growth hormone. It contains two other IGF binding proteins, IGF BP-1 and IGF BP-2. Both are influenced by nutrition and insulin secretion. Their function may be minimal in respect to postnatal growth.

The binding proteins lengthen the half-life of the IGF peptides and change their clearance. They also control biological activity by modulating their binding to cell surface receptors. They have been shown to have both inhibitory and stimulatory effects. This is a critical issue currently under investigation.

Endocrine and Paracrine Control of Growth

The concept of IGF I as principal GH-dependent agent of postnatal growth is consistent with the extreme situation of Laron dwarfism, wherein serum IGF I is barely detectable but concentrations of GH are normal to high. Recombinant human IGF I stimulates growth of hypophysectomized mice and of Snell dwarf mice and is able to mimic the effects of GH on epiphyseal plate width and trabecular bone formation, confirming that it is acting as a potent endocrine factor. In addition, IGF I produces both positive nitrogen balance and hypercalcuria in patients with GH insensitivity.[16]

It is now recognized that GH, in addition to controlling IGF I production, has a direct effect on growth of tissues. According to the Green hypothesis, GH would induce differentiation of precursors of prechondrocytes with clone formation, whereby these cells acquire the capacity to produce IGF I and to respond to it.[17] It was suggested that this activation of the IGF I gene is independent of the effect of GH on the liver and results from a direct interaction between GH and cartilage. Furthermore, pulsatile treatment with physiological doses of GH induces a 3–5 fold increase in concentrations of IGF I mRNA in rat growth plates, whereas continuous infusion is less effective. Thus, the local paracrine and autocrine action plays a major role in skeletal growth: IGFs act primarily as local regulators of cell growth and differentiation. However, it is still difficult to determine the respective role of systemic and locally produced IGF I. This dual mechanism may explain the poor correlation between circulating IGF I concentrations and growth rates. The highest growth rates observed in infancy, accompanied by the lowest blood IGF I concentrations, may reflect a predominant paracrine/autocrine control at that age.

Isaksson et al. have proposed a sequence of events leading to bone growth, as a dual effector theory for GH action: the effect of GH is limited to a precursor cell population which differentiates and thereby produces local IGF I and IGF binding proteins leading to chondrocyte proliferation and differentiation.[18]

Thyroid Hormones

Thyroid hormones play a central role in skeletal maturation. They stimulate GH secretion and control the effect of GH on IGF I production. In addition, thyroid hormones require the presence of GH to exert a full effect, since GH accelerates the conversion of thyroxine into its active metabolite, triiodothyronine. However, it is likely that thyroid hormones also have a direct effect on the skeleton, as thyroid treatment accelerates bone maturation in pituitary dwarfs not treated with hGH.

Sex Steroids and Pubertal Growth

Growth at puberty is dependent on the interaction of GH, IGF I, and sex steroids. Height increase accelerates and skeletal maturation results in fusion of the epiphyseal cartilages when the final height is reached. Secretion of GH is increased by sex steroids through augmented amplitude of GH secretion episodes, although frequency of pulses is not affected. The threshold concentration of GH secretion required to obtain a pubertal growth is not known. There is some evidence that it may be low.

Estrogen, in low doses, stimulates growth without an increase in IGF I concentrations, and similar findings have been reported in boys receiving oxandrolone, an anabolic steroid. These findings correspond to *in vitro* evidence that chondrocytes respond to estradiol and dihydrotestosterone with an increased synthesis of proteoglycans. In addition, the presence of estrogen receptors has been demonstrated in these cells, with a higher affinity for estrogen at puberty than before puberty. These findings provide a rationale for the therapeutic use of low doses of sex steroids at initiation of puberty in hypogonadotrophic patients.

Glucocorticoids

There is no evidence that cortisol at physiological concentrations regulates growth. However, glucocorticoids at pharmacological doses do inhibit cartilage activity and decrease GH secretion.

Growth and Nutrition

Growth retardation occurs during chronic malnutrition or voluntary reduction of caloric intake as in anorexia nervosa. The characteristic sequence of events includes increased GH secretion, low IGF I concentrations reflecting a state of cellular resistance to GH. Fasting induces a decrease in membrane GH-binding capacity and/or a post-receptor defect resulting in decreased ability to generate IGF I. IGF I circulating concentrations therefore appear to be a sensitive index of nutritional status.[19] Insulin is essentially acting indirectly by allowing normal final utilization, as neither cartilage nor bone tissue in culture show a response to that peptide.

Catch-up Growth

Catch-up growth with a return to the child's own growth curve occurs after any temporary growth disturbance such as malnutrition, corticotherapy, renal acidosis, or chronic dehydration. Catch-up growth may be incomplete if the disease is not fully cured or if it has caused permanent cellular lesions. Its mechanism is not well understood; factors such as nutrition and GH secretion may play a role.

DIAGNOSTIC BASIS FOR BIOCHEMICAL INVESTIGATION

Short Stature

Failure to grow and/or short stature may be the presenting symptom of endocrine disorders or chronic diseases.[20] A number of causes must therefore be ruled out before the diagnosis of genetic or constitutional short stature is considered. Most of these causes are presented in Table 5–1. This is the framework for radiological and biochemical investigation. The most frequently encountered chronic diseases are malnutrition, chronic disorders of digestive absorption, chronic renal failure, emotional deprivation, and primary skeletal disorders. Endocrine causes include late-onset hypothyroidism, growth hormone deficiency, and delayed puberty.

At first, a critical analysis of the child's growth should be performed, focusing on his or her perinatal history, growth curve, weight-to-height ratio, and growth rate for chronological age and for bone age using appropriate reference data. Causes of growth retardation vary with age (Table 5–2). Specific problems arise with abnormal timing of puberty (Table 5–3). In most cases, the clinical features generally provide a valuable guideline for the choice of biochemical and hormonal evaluation (Table 5–4).

One should focus on treatable causes of short stature. Therefore, it may be advisable to perform a laboratory screening for diseases such as renal failure and coeliac disease and to consider the possibility of thyroid or GH deficiency. The latter is a crucial issue (Table 5–5). Another approach relates to known chronic diseases, during which growth failure may be severe and long lasting.

TABLE 5–1. Causes of Growth Failure and Short Stature

Clinical Diagnosis	Biochemical Findings
Genetic short stature	Normal
Constitutional delay in growth	Normal
Constitutional delay in puberty	Transient GH deficiency; Delayed sex steroid secretion
Intra-uterine growth retardation	Possible GH deficiency
Psychosocial dwarfism	Low or normal GH, low IGF I
Malnutrition, protein-calorie deficiency or chronic disease	Normal or high GH, low IGF I
Genetic bone disease	Normal
Turner syndrome in girls	46,XO karyotype
Hormonal abnormalities GH deficiency	
Isolated deficiency	Low GH, low IGFI
Multiple pituitary deficiency	+ low T4, low cortisol and absence of puberty
Genetic hypopituitarism	Low GH, low IGF I
Genetic GH insensitivity	Lack of GH binding; low IGFI; Normal or high GH
Other hormones Hypothyroidism (primary)	Low T4, high TSH
Cortisol excess	High urinary cortisol
Diabetes mellitus (not controlled)	High HbA1C
Diabetes insipidus (not controlled)	Chronic dehydration

TABLE 5–2. Etiology of Growth Retardation According to Age

Infancy	Intrauterine growth retardation Calorie deficiency (malnutrition, coeliac disease) Metabolic diseases, renal failure Hypothyroidism Hypopituitarism
Childhood	Genetic short stature Calorie deficiency (psychosocial dwarfism, coeliac disease) GH deficiency Hypothyroidism Genetic bone disease Turner syndrome (girls) Cushing syndrome
Puberty	Constitutional delay Turner syndrome (girls) Hypopituitarism Anorexia nervosa Chronic diseases

TABLE 5–3. Typical Investigation for Growth Disturbance in Relation to Abnormal Puberty

Clinical Presentation	Estradiol* Testosterone DHEAS	LH/FSH*	Diagnosis
Delayed Puberty (retarded growth	low	low	delayed puberty hypogonadotropinism
and bone maturation)	low	high	primary gonadal failure
Precocious puberty	high	pubertal level	central precocious puberty
(accelerated growth and bone maturation)	high	low	primary gonadal hyperfunction
	DHEAS high	normal	premature pubarche
	17 OHP high	normal	congenital virilizing adrenal hyperplasia

*indication of concentration by comparison with normal for chronological age
DHEAS = Dehydroepiandrosterone Sulfate
17 OHP = 17-hydroxyprogesterone
LH = Luteinizing Hormone
FSH = Follicle Stimulating Hormone

It may be relevant to consider the various mechanisms of growth retardation in such affected children before deciding therapy. These mechanisms may be quite variable, such as primary metabolic disturbances, treatment-related iatrogenic negative effects on growth, secondary skeletal lesions, and/or resistance to endogenous GH, caloric and protein deprivation, or psychosocial disturbance. The laboratory investigation will help in assessing some of these hypotheses in a given case. In growth retardation, it may be useful to consider the information provided by the combined evaluation of GH and IGF I secretion, as described in Table 5–6.

Tall Stature

In the case of short stature, the diagnosis is largely based on the clinical assessment. Children presenting with tall stature generally have no disease but are extremes of normal variation. However, accelerated growth with advanced bone maturation in a child who was initially of normal stature suggests primary endocrine disorders such as hyperthyroidism, hyperandrogeny, or precocious puberty. Hormonal evaluation is required with various approaches, depending on age, sex, and pubertal status of the child.

TABLE 5–4. Growth Retardation: Guidelines for Clinical and Biochemical Evaluation

Cause	Clinical Signs	Plasma Biochemical/ Hormonal Signs	Possible Diagnosis
Familial and neonatal history	Parental short stature and/or pubertal delay	Normal	Genetic/constitutional growth retardation
	Poor economic status	Normal GH, low IGF I	Calorie/protein deficiency
	Disturbed family, child abuse	Normal GH, low IGF I	Psychosocial dwarfism
	Small for date and/or dysmorphic features	Normal	Intrauterine growth retardation
		Normal	Chromosomal, skeletal disorders
Endocrine causes	GH deficiency features, hypoglycemia or growth retardation associated with midline defects or perinatal asphyxia secondary to cranial irradiation or brain tumor	Low GH, low IFG I	Isolated GH deficiency or multiple pituitary deficiencies
	isolated (sporadic or familial)	Low GH, low IGFI	Isolated GH deficiency (GRF deficiency); GH gene deletion
		High GH, low IFGI	GH receptor mutation: GH insensitivity
	Hypothyroidism	Low T4/T3, high TSH	Primary hypothyroidism
	Obesity, osteoporosis	High plasma/urinary cortisol	Cushing syndrome
	Corticoid therapy	Low DHEA sulfate	Iatrogenic
	Delayed puberty	Lack of sex steroid secretion	Delayed puberty (transient or organic)
	Polyuria, polydipsia	Failure to concentrate urines	Diabetes insipidus with vasopressin deficiency
	Diabetes mellitus	Normal GH, low IGF I	Poor control
Non-endocrine causes	Anemia, rickets	Low 25OHD3, anemia, low iron	Vitamin D deficiency and iron deficiency
	Turner features (girl)	46, XO karyotype	Turner syndrome
	Low weight for height	Normal GH, low IGF I	Malnutrition, anorexia nervosa
	Chronic diarrhea	Antigliadin antibodies, low folate	Coeliac disease
	Abdominal pain, fever	Accelerated sedimentation rate	Crohn's ileitis
	Anemia, edema	Increased creatinine, urea	Chronic renal failure
	Polyuria, polydipsia	Failure to respond to vasopressin	Diabetes insipidus with vasopressin resistance

TABLE 5–5. Elements of Routine Evaluation of a Child with Short Stature and/or Decreased Growth Rate

History and physical examination

Skull X-ray, bone age on left hand

CBC, folate, carotene, antigliadin antibodies, ESR

Plasma electrolytes, creatinine, BUN

Karyotype in females

Thyroid function: T4, TSH

Growth hormone response to pharamacological stimulation and/or spontaneous profiles on nightime or 24 hr.

IGF I and IGF BP 3

TABLE 5–6. Growth Retardation due to Abnormalities of the Growth Hormon/IGF I Axis Classified According to Plasma Concentrations

LOW GH, LOW IGF I

Primary GH Deficiency
Genetic:	Autosomal dominant or recessive, X-linked recessive GH gene mutation
Idiopathic:	Isolated GH deficiency (probable GHRH deficiency)

Primary Multiple Pituitary Hormone Deficiency
Genetic:	Autosomal or X-linked, recessive Pituitary differentiation factor gene mutation
Developmental:	Midline defects (cleft lip and palate) Pituitary aplasia Optic-septo dysplasia
Organic:	Cranial irradiation Hypothalamic-pituitary tumors Trauma
Idiopathic:	Perinatal trauma and asphyxia Pituitary stalk interruption (on MRI)

Secondary GH Deficiency
  Chronic malnutrition
  Hemochromatosis, psychosocial dwarfism, thalassemia

HIGH GH, LOW IGF I

Primary GH Insensitivity
  Laron-type dwarfism (GH receptor gene mutation and absent plasma GH binding protein)
  Genetic dwarfism with low GH receptor activity (pygmy)

Secondary GH Insensitivity
  Acute fasting
  Chronic malnutrition, protein-calorie deficiency

Bioinactive but Immunoreactive GH
  No definitely proven case of abnormal endogenous GH with normal response to exogenous hGH

HIGH GH, NORMAL TO HIGH IGF I

Chronic renal failure with excess in IGF BP-3 (supposed resistance to GH/IGF I)
Primary IGF I receptor defect (not demonstrated)

HORMONAL AND BIOCHEMICAL INVESTIGATION: CLINICAL SIGNIFICANCE

Growth Hormone Secretion

GH Assays

Growth hormone in plasma consists of various molecular forms which may not be equally recognized in different assays.[1] Until recently, polyclonal competitive radioimmunoassays were used in routine evaluation, with fairly satisfactory agreement between most assay systems. Technical improvements have led to new assays such as immunoradiometric assay (IRMA) with monoclonal or polyclonal antibodies, immunoenzymometric assay (IEMA or ELISA), immunofluorometric assay (IFMA), and oligoclonal assay (OCA). However, each assay may provide different results, as a number of factors can be the source of variability.

Standards used for the assay may be natural extractive pituitary GH, containing several forms of GH, as provided by the National Institute for Biological Standards, United Kingdom, or highly purified forms of GH, and eventually recombinant GH. The use of monoclonal antibodies has been the main cause of discrepancy.[21, 22] For instance, one antibody does not recognize the 20 kD form; others have variable affinity for dimeric forms.[23] Hence, polyclonal antisera may be more universal reagents for routine assays. It is also useful to have complete information for each assay with respect to the recognition of the main GH circulating forms. In a given assay, a matrix effect may induce additional variation when horse serum, free GH plasma,[24] or veronal buffer (personal data) is used. It has been suggested that the high-affinity protein binding GH might interfere in the serum assay, but a survey of different assays has shown that such a binding protein effect is not frequent and most often is quite negligible.

For clinical use, it is important to have full information on the characteristics of the assay to determine reference values in physiological conditions and to have a comparison with other current assays when growth hormone deficiency is to be diagnosed. Distinct discriminant values may be needed for various assays. A high degree of relative correlation has been found between assays, but absolute potency estimates have differed.[21] It would be preferable to have them compared to a reference assay, for which the best choice would be a polyclonal antibody. In addition, some studies should take into account time-related changes of molecular forms of circulating GH after stimulated or spontaneous pulse secretion.

The radioreceptor assay has some limitations and is no longer routinely used. Among the *in vitro* bioassays, the most interesting and promising is the NB2 mode lymphoma cell proliferation assay. It is based on the human GH lactogenic property, which stimulates cell proliferation in a dose-dependent fashion.[25]

Measurement of GH Secretion

The diagnosis of growth hormone deficiency is based on the evidence of low circulating growth hormone concentrations and inferred low secretion. The use of random basal values has failed to be diagnostic because of spontaneous pulsatility. Therefore, the most widely used procedure is pharmacological stimulation of GH secretion. Quite a large number of stimuli, acting through still poorly identified mechanisms, are used in clinical practice. It is not known which is most closely related to physiological growth hormone secretion. The commonly used stimuli include clonidine, L-Dopa, ornithine, insulin-induced hypoglycemia, and glucagon-propranolol. The arginine stimulation test is less potent and has more false-negative results. By convention, failure to achieve a maximum stimulated GH concentration of 7 or 10 ng/mL using conventional RIAs defines classical GH deficiency. This cut-off value should be lower when using some of the monoclonal assays.

Because of the variability of the peak GH response, use of two different stimuli is recommended. It is generally accepted that concordant decreased responses to two consecutive tests are sufficient for a diagnosis of GH deficiency. This is most frequently observed in patients with severe GH deficiency, decreased growth rate, and typical features of hypopituitarism, or in children with organic pituitary deficiency. Difficulties in the assessment of GH secretion arise when children with isolated short stature are investigated in view of hGH therapy. A great many studies have been performed to determine the best diagnostic procedure. The pharmacological stimulation tests often provide discrepant results when two consecutive tests are performed.[26] Furthermore, the level of response may vary according to the stimulus used for testing.

Therefore, assessment of spontaneous GH secretion by sampling at frequent intervals or by continuous withdrawal during 12–24 h periods has been proposed, with results expressed as spontaneous peak values or integrated concentrations of GH (IC-GH). This method also allows the calculation of secretion rates and metabolic clearance using complex mathematical models with deconvolution analysis.[6] The measurement of spontaneous secretion concentrations was found to be highly reproducible when continuous withdrawal was used.[26] It is generally accepted that some children with low stimulated GH concentrations have spontaneous GH profiles and IC-GH in the normal range,[27] but the contrary can also occur.[28]

To interpret the individual data, one must also take into account the large range of IC-GH values obtained in normal children.[27, 29] The occurrence of such a discrepancy has led to the concept of neurosecretory dysfunction. This is an ill-defined condition which may only reflect inevitable discrepancies between various methods for which diagnostic cut-off values remain arbitrary and rely on limited information in the child with normal stature. Other techniques may provide additional information, such as measurement of urinary excretion of GH and plasma IGF I concentrations (see discussion below). Whatever the technique used, thyroid function should be normal or adequately replaced at time of testing. In boys with delayed puberty, transient low GH secretion may be corrected by short administration of testosterone, such as 100 mg/M^2 every two weeks for two months. Therefore, it may be useful to evaluate these boys only after short-term testosterone administration.

In conclusion, the most widely recognized procedure is the use of two consecutive stimulation tests. An overnight spontaneous GH profile is probably more reliable but less practical and more costly. It is largely agreed that it is essentially a clinical investigation tool. Basal IGF I concentration measurement may be a convenient screening procedure. Urinary GH measurement has not yet proved to be a reproducible and reliable diagnostic tool. Finally, because of the difficulty in classifying borderline cases, it remains necessary to consider the results in light of the clinical assessment and eventually to repeat testing during follow-up.

Urinary GH

GH is excreted in the urine with natural 22 kD GH. A very small fraction of injected GH is recovered in the urine. The GH excretion in hypopituitary children is significantly diminished; however, in idiopathic growth failure, as assessed by current plasma GH measurements, some children have values in the range of classical GH deficiency.[30] Urinary GH measurement has some pitfalls and difficulties: quality, duration of urine collection, poor reproducibility over several days, and cumbersome assays unless a direct measurement can be performed with a highly sensitive antibody. Similarly, quantitation of urinary IGF I should be performed. At present, urinary GH assays have not proved to be more reliable than the conventional diagnostic approach. They remain to be validated as screening procedures in the future.

Markers of GH Action

As described above, the circulating concentrations of IGF I and eventually IGF BP-3 reflect the secretion of growth hormone and at present should be considered to be the best markers of GH activity in relation to growth. The only important limitation is their close dependence on the nutritional status. Other markers more specifically related to skeletal growth have been studied. The serum concentrations of protein constituents of the connective tissues have been shown to be correlated with the rate of growth and to increase after GH administration. Therefore, radioimmunoassays have been performed for the measurement of serum type I procollagen,[31] type III procollagen,[32] or osteocalcin, also called bone gal protein.[33] The latter is specifically secreted by the osteoblasts. However, none of these marker measurements may contribute to the etiology of a diagnosis of short stature.

GH Binding Protein

At present, in plasma the high-affinity protein can be measured as a GH binding activity, using various separation techniques.[34, 35] Simpler assay techniques should allow a more thorough evaluation of its physiological and clinical significance. Its concentration is very low at birth, rises during childhood, and reaches adult values by age 20–30 years. Its measurement provides useful clinical information for rare but specific conditions of GH insensitivity; it is undetectable in Laron dwarfism because of mutations in extracellular binding domains of the GH receptor. In certain short populations, such as the African pygmies and New Guinea people, a decreased concentration of GH binding protein was found, possibly indicating a partial end organ resistance.[36] It remains to be seen if this approach can be extended to patients with constitutional short stature.

Insulin-like Growth Factors

IGF Assays

The initial radioimmunoassay, until recently the most widely used, was a direct measurement of IGF I (Somatomedin-C) in serum and plasma samples. It was a preincubation with antiserum before adding the tracer, a so-called nonequilibrium technique, and thereby avoided the interference from binding proteins. This technique is affected by many variables, such as the sample type—serum, heparin, or EDTA plasma—and handling conditions—acidification, freeze thawing, or age of sample.[37] This easy and inexpensive technique is useful, since the affinity of the anti-IGF I antibodies most widely used, such as that provided by the National Institutes of Health, have a higher affinity than binding proteins for IGF I. In this assay, normal male adult plasma is used as a standard to which an arbitrary concentration of 1 unit/mL is attributed. However, it is now necessary to remove the binding proteins in order to measure the total amount of circulating IGF I.

Acid gel filtration represents the reference technique, but it is difficult to apply to routine measurements. Alternative techniques to remove binding proteins are currently used: microcolumns C18 or acid ethanol extraction.[10] The latter technique has been improved by a cryoprecipitation step which reduces residual IGF BPs to a level that does not interfere with the immunoassay.[38] In any case, high-affinity antisera are needed for the radioimmunoassay. As a reference standard, recombinant IGF I use now allows expression of concentrations in ng/mL and comparison between laboratories. Whatever the extraction technique used, the possibility of significant interferences of binding proteins needs to be considered when dealing with pathological states.

For IGF II measurement, variable antibodies have been used: polyclonal antibody with minimal cross-reactivity with IGF I, specific antibody prepared against a synthetic peptide derived from the C domain of IGF II, or a competitive protein binding assay.[10]

IGF I Significance

The concentrations of IGF I in serum have been studied from birth until adolescence, and quite a number of reference values are available.[39] They show differences in absolute values but a substantial agreement in age-related changes, with a progressive increase in concentration during childhood and a marked increase at puberty. IGF I secretion is essentially growth hormone dependent, provided there is no malnutrition or chronic disease, since the latter may be accompanied by low plasma IGF I values. Because IGF I concentrations show little diurnal variation, it was supposed that its measurement would contribute to the diagnosis of GH deficiency. In most cases of short stature, GH secretion and plasma IGF I are now measured in combination.

Several studies investigated the diagnostic value of IGF I measurement. It was found that most but not all children with a low GH response to provocative stimulation had plasma IGF I values below the normal range for age. Although GH-sufficient children with short stature may have low IGF I concentrations, the conclusion of a recent study indicated that IGF I values may have clinical use in predicting GH response to stimulation.[40] Whatever technique is used, there is an overlap between normal short and GH-deficient children which is even more likely to occur in children below age 6 years when physiological values are in the low range.

Because of their age dependence, the data preferably should be expressed as age- and sex-related Z score values, taking into account age and the pubertal status, for better interpretation of individual data and group comparison.[39] Such a procedure requires appropriate normative data. Because of the strong influence of nutrition, plasma IGF I concentration may also be used to monitor therapy for malnutrition. Recovery from deprivation correlates with increasing plasma IGF I. This a more sensitive measure of recovery than assays for plasma pre-albumin, retinol binding protein, or transferrin.

IGF Binding Proteins

According to the present nomenclature, IGF BP-1 and IGF BP-3 are two serum-binding proteins which may have clinical importance. IGF BP-3 secretion is greatly GH-dependent, with low concentrations in patients with GH deficiency or genetic insensitivity. Its concentrations measured by RIA[41] increase soon after birth and remain constant thereafter until puberty. Changes during puberty are not well documented. There is no circadian variation.

IGF BP-3 is bound to the large 150 kD complex and does not cross the capillary barrier. Large variability in concentrations of IGF BP-3 were found in hypopituitary patients, and its contribution to the diagnosis of GH deficiency is still controversial. The development of new RIAs may rapidly contribute to its evaluation. It may be expected that IGF BP-3 is a reliable marker of GH activity in early childhood because of its high plasma concentration at that age. A characteristic feature of chronic renal failure is an increase in IGF BP-3, as well as in other IGF binding proteins. IGF BP-3 is decreased in chronic malnutrition and during prolonged fasting.[15]

IGF BP-1 circulating concentrations decline from birth to puberty. They are low in normal children. There are considerable diurnal variations with a nocturnal peak. IGF BP-1 is found in amniotic fluid and maternal serum during gestation. It is increased during fasting, chronic malnutrition, and noncontrolled diabetes. In GH-deficient children, there is an inverse correlation between IGF BP-1 and GH concentrations. It has been shown that IGF BP-1 concentrations are inversely correlated to plasma insulin, and low IGF BP-1 values also have been reported in states of insulin resistance.[36] Only preliminary results have been reported on IGF binding proteins in the urine.[36] The availability of recombinant IGF BPs in the near future may lead to a better evaluation of metabolic and endocrine abnormalities.

Reference Values

Because of difficulty in investigating children with normal stature, only a few studies provide reference data for GH response to pharmacological stimulation, GH secretion as calculated from spontaneous profiles, and IGF I concentration in plasma. Furthermore, these reference data depend on the type of assay used by the authors, as noted the accompanying figure and tables. The following data were selected:

1.   Peak GH responses to pharmacological stimulation (Table 5–8)
2.   Spontaneous GH during nighttime (Figure 5–2)
3.   Plasma IGF I and IGF II concentrations (Table 5–7)

FIGURE 5–2. The Mean Nighttime GH Concentration in Normal Children According to Bone Age (top panel) and Pubertal Stage (bottom panel). Individual values (points) and 95% confidence limits are presented. GH assay: polyclonal antibody at Hazeltone Biotechnologies.

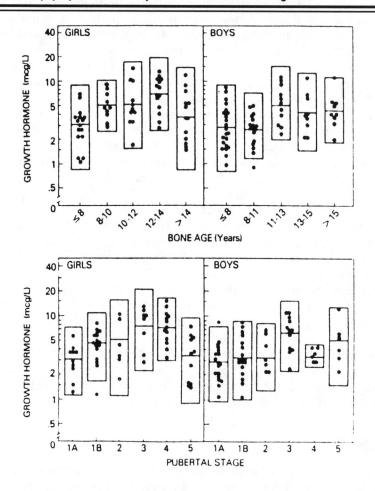

From: Rose SR, Municchi G, Barnes KM et al. Spontaneous growth hormone secretion increases during puberty in normal girls and boys. J Clin Endocrinol Metab 1991:73;428-35. Reprinted with permission.

TABLE 5–7. Plasma IGF I and IGF II Concentrations by Age and Sex (values obtained by RIA after acid gel filtration)

Age (yr)	NORMAL			NORMAL SHORT STATURE			GH DEFICIENCY		
	n	IGF-I	IGF-II	n	IGF-I	IGF-II	n	IGF-I	IGF-II
Boys									
<3	10	77 ± 33	480 ± 85	3	38 ± 39	477 ± 640	0		
3–5	9	157 ± 103	573 ± 259	5	80 ± 75	244 ± 100*	9	28 ± 17*	288 ± 227*
6–8	15	211 ± 112	607 ± 185	9	99 ± 41*	339 ± 139*	9	38 ± 20*	271 ± 137*
9–11	10	301 ± 173	505 ± 189	8	148 ± 109	580 ± 380	11	101 ± 94*	409 ± 380
12–14	38	466 ± 188	500 ± 114	5	207 ± 94	490 ± 171	5	92 ± 76*	352 ± 164
>15	14	516 ± 139	531 ± 107	1	252	384	4	73 ± 75*	603 ± 201
Girls									
<3	10	134 ± 53	419 ± 145	0			0		
3–5	15	247 ± 175	526 ± 201	3	103 ± 52	300 ± 129	7	31 ± 35*	273 ± 145*
6–8	20	298 ± 151	601 ± 228	4	198 ± 42	704 ± 119	8	47 ± 67*	452 ± 444
9–11	16	366 ± 109	522 ± 135	4	196 ± 126*	412 ± 220	7	60 ± 59*	286 ± 138*
12–14	26	521 ± 164	498 ± 116	1	90	231	7	54 ± 23*	509 ± 361
>15	14	464 ± 141	466 ± 145	1	122	824	1	25*	669

Values expressed as mean ± SD nanograms per milliliter. Means were compared by repeated analysis of variance for each age group.

*Significantly different from normal patients (P <0.05). IGF-I and IGF-II concentrations in normal short and GH-deficient children were not significantly different form each other in any other group.

From: Rosenfeld RG, Wilson DM, Lee DK. Insulin-like growth factors I and II in evaluaiton of growth retardation. J Pediatr 1986; 109:428–433. Reprinted by permission.

TABLE 5–8. Peak GH Responses to Clonidine Stimulation Before and During Puberty

	PUBERTAL STAGE		
	I	II – III	IV – V
Male	16.9 ± 6.7	17.8 ± 7.7	26.5 ± 12.0
Female	12.8 ± 5.1	18.3 ± 9.0	35.5 ± 5.1

GH assay = NHPP polyclonal antibody, expressed in ng/ml
95% of normal children have peak GH responses to paired clonidine and arginine or insulin stimulation > 10 ng/mL before puberty and > 14 ng/mL in late puberty. The mean peak GH response varies according to simulation: 21.0 ± 10.7 (SD) with clonidine, 13.1 ± 6.1 with arginine, and 14.2 ± 4.3 ng/mL with insulin.
From: Zadik Z, Chalew SA, Kowarski A. Assessment of growth hormone secretion in normal stature children using 24-hour integrated concentration of GH and pharmacological stimulaton. J Clin Endocrinol Metab 1990; 71:932–936. Reprinted by permission.

REFERENCES

1. Baumann G. Growth hormone binding proteins and various forms of growth hormone: Implications for measurements. Acta Paediatr Scand 1990;370:72-80.
2. Martin JB. Neural regulation of growth hormone secretion. N Engl J Med 1973;288:1384-93.
3. Tannenbaum GS, Painson JC, Lapointe M, Gurd W, McCarthy GF. Pituitary hypothalamic somatostatin. Interplay of somatostatin and growth hormone-releasing hormone in genesis of episodic growth hormone secretion. Metabolism 1990;39:35-9.
4. Thorner MO, Vance ML, Evans WS et al. Physiological and clinical studies of GRF and GH. Recent Prog Horm Res 1986;42:589-640.
5. Frohman LA, Downs TR, Kelijman M, Clarke IJ, Thomas G. Somatostatin secretion and action in the regulation of growth hormone secretion. Metabolism 1990;39:43-5.
6. Veldhuis JD, Carlson ML, Johnson ML. The pituitary gland secretes in bursts: Appraising the nature of glandular secretory impulses by simultaneous multiple-parameter deconvolution of plasma hormone concentrations. Proc Natl Acad Sci USA 1987;84:7686-90.
7. Kelly PA, Djiane J, Postel-Vinay MC, Edery M. The prolactin/growth hormone receptor family. Endocr Rev 991;12:235-51.
8. Amselem S, Duquesnoy BS, Attree O et al. Laron dwarfism and mutations of the growth hormone-receptor gene. N Eng J Med 1989;321:989-95.
9. Rosenbloom AL, Guevara-Aguirre J, Rosenfeld RG, Fielder PJ. The little women of Loja: Growth hormone-receptor deficiency in an inbred population of southern Ecuador. N Engl J Med 1990;323:1367-74.
10. Daughaday WH, Rotwein P. Insulin-like growth factors I and II. Peptide, messenger ribonucleic acid and gene structures, serum, and tissue concentrations. Endocr Rev 1989;10:68-91.
11. Hintz RL. Peptide growth factors, oncogenies, and growth. Curr Opin Pediatr 1990;2:786-93.
12. Martha PM, Rogol AD, Veldhuis JD, Kerrigan JR, Goodman DW, Blizzard RM. Alterations in the pulsatile properties of circulating growth hormone concentrations during puberty in boys. J Clin Endocrinol Metab 1989;69:563-70.
13. Rose SE, Municchi G, Barnes KM et al. Spontaneous growth hormone secretion increases during puberty in normal girls and boys. J Clin Endocrinol Metab 1991;73:428-35.
14. Binoux M, Roghani M, Hossenlop P, Hardouin S, Gourmelen M. Molecular forms of human IGF binding protein: Physiological implications. Acta Endocrinol 1991;124:41-7.

15.   Baxter RC. Insulin-like growth factor (IGF) binding proteins: The role of serum IGF BPs in regulating IGF availability. Acta Paediatr Scand 1991;372:107-14.

16.   Walker JL, Malinowska MG, Romer TE, Pucilowska JB, Underwood LE. Effects of the infusion of insulin-like growth factor I in a child with growth hormone insensitivity syndrome (Laron dwarfism). N Engl J Med 1991;324:1483-88.

17.   Green H, Morikawa M, Nixon L. A dual effector theory of growth hormone action. Differenciation 1985;29:195-8.

18.   Lindhal A, Isgaard J, Isaksson O. Growth and differentiation. Clin Endocrinol Metab 1991;5:671-87.

19.   Isley WL, Underwood LE, Clemmons DR. Dietary components that regulate serum somatomedin-C concentrations in humans. J Clin Invest 1983;71:175-82.

20.   Van den Brande L, Rappaport R. Normal and abnormal growth. In: Bertrand J, Rappaport R, Sizonenko PC, eds, Pediatric endocrinology. Baltimore: Williams & Wilkins, in press.

21.   Reiter EO, Morris AH, McGillivray MH, Weber D. Variable estimates of serum growth hormone concentrations by different radioassay systems. J Clin Endocrinol Metab 1988;66:68-71.

22.   Celniker AC, Chen AB, Wert RM, Sherman B. Variability in the quantitation of circulating growth hormone using commercial immunoassays. J Clin Endocrinol Metab 1989;68:469-76.

23.   Bowsher RR, Apathy JM, Ferguson Al, Riggin RM, Henry DP. Cross reactivity of monomeric and dimeric biosynthetic human growth hormone in commercial immunoassays. Clin Chem 1990;63:362-66.

24.   Felder RA, Hall RW, Martha P et al. Influence of matrix on concentrations of somatotropin measured in serum with commercial immunoradiometric assays. Clin Chem 1989;35/7:1423-26.

25.   Friesen HG. Receptor assays for growth hormone. Acta Paediatr Scand 1990;370:87-91.

26.   Zadik Z, Chalew SA, Kowarski A. Assessment of growth hormone secretion in normal stature children using 24-hour integrated concentration of GH and pharmacological stimulation. J Clin Endocrinol Metab 1990; 71:932-6.

27.   Rose SR, Ross JL, Uriarte M, Barnes KM, Cassorla FG, Cutler GB. The advantage of measuring stimulated as compared with spontaneous growth hormone levels in the diagnosis of growth hormone deficiency. N Engl J Med 1988;319:201-7.

28.   Donaldson DL, Pan F, Hollowell JG, Stevenson JL, Gifford RA, Moore WV. Reliability of stimulated and spontaneous growth hormone (GH) levels for identifying the child with low GH secretion. J Clin Endocrinol Metab 1991;72:647-52.

29.   Rose SR, Municchi G, Barnes KM et al. Spontaneous growth hormone secretion increases during puberty in normal girls and boys. J Clin Endocrinol Metab 1991;73:428-35.

30.   Albini CH, Sotos J, Sherman B, Johanson A et al. Diagnostic significance of urinary growth hormone measurements in children with growth failure: Correlation between serum and urine growth hormone. Pediatr Res 1991;29:619-22.

31.   Carey DE, Goldberg B, Ratzan SK, Rubin KR, Rowe DW. Radioimmunoassay for type I procollagen in growth hormone-deficient children before and during treatment with growth hormone. Pediatr Res 1984;19:8-11.

32.   Danne T, Grüters A, Schuppan D, Quantas N, Enders I, Weber B. Relationship of procollagen type III propeptide-related antigens in serum to somatic growth in healthy children and patients with growth disorders. J Pediatr 1989;114:257-60.

33.   Johansen JS, Jensen SB, Ris BJ, Rasmussen L, Zachmann M, Christiansen C. Serum bone Gla protein: A potential marker of growth hormone (GH) deficiency and the response to GH therapy. J Clin Endocrinol Metab 1990;71:122-26.

34.   Baumann G. Growth hormone binding proteins: Biochemical characterization and assays. Acta Endocrinol 1991;124:21-6.

35.   Fontoura M, Hocquette JF, Clot JP et al. Regulation of the growth hormone binding proteins in human plasma. Acta Endocrinol 1991;124:10-3.

36.   Cohen P, Fielder PJ, Hasegawa Y, Frisch H, Giudice LC, Rosenfeld RG. Clinical aspects of insulin-like growth factor binding proteins. Acta Endocrinol 1991;124:74-85.

37.   Furlanetto RW. Pitfalls in the somatomedin C radioimmunoassays. J Clin Endocrinol Metab 1982;54:1084-6.

38.   Breier BH, Gallagher BW, Gluckman PD. Radioimmunoassay for insulin-like growth factor I: Solutions to some potential problems and pitfalls. J Endocrinol 1991;128:347-57.

39.   Rosenfeld RG, Wilson DM, Lee PDK. Insulin-like growth factors I and II in evaluation of growth retardation. J Pediatr 1986;109:428-33.

40.   Lee PDK, Wilson DM, Rountree L, Hintz RL, Rosenfeld RG. Efficacy of insulin-like growth factor I levels in predicting the response to provocative growth hormone testing. Pediatr Res 1990;27:45-51.

41.   Rutanen EM, Pekonen F. Assays for IGF binding proteins. Acta Endocrinol 1991;124:70-3.

42.   Rappaport R. A touch of growth. Horm Res, in press.

The Diagnosis of Pediatric Reproductive Disorders

Claude J. Migeon, M.D.   *Gary D. Berkovitz, M.D.*
Patricia Y. Fechner, M.D.

INTRODUCTION

Human reproduction is necessary for the conservation of the species and is based on well established patterns of sexual dimorphism that are determined at sex differentiation. Reproductive function covers nearly the whole life span of human subjects. The first major stage is the *sex differentiation*, which takes place during fetal life and which includes the fertilization of the egg by a sperm, followed by establishment of chromosomal sex and the development of the fetus along male or female lines. Infancy and childhood are not considered as important periods for reproduction, although there is a process of learning and rehearsal of future sex life during that time. The next major stage is *puberty*, during which the gonads and sex organs mature. This is followed by the stage of *male-female bonding, pregnancy,* and *child rearing*. Post-menopausal age in women and old age in men are considered to have little relevance to the life cycle of reproduction, although grandparents may play an important role in inculcating the societal values of the family to the youth.

This chapter focuses specifically on *reproductive disorders* as related to *sexual differentiation* and *pubertal development*.

SEXUAL DIFFERENTIATION

Biochemistry and Physiology

The sexual differentiation of the human fetus is a complicated process which involves various types of cell differentiation and cell multiplication. In a simplified manner, one can describe four major steps:

1. Fertilization and determination of genetic sex
2. Formation of organs common to both sexes
3. Gonadal differentiation
4. Differentiation of the internal ducts and external genitalia

Fertilization

Without doubt, the first step in sex differentiation takes place at fertilization. An egg with a complement of 23 chromosomes, including an X chromosome, will be conjugated with a sperm which includes either a 23,X chromosome complement or a 23,Y complement. Hence, at conception the first diploid cell has either a 46,XX or 46,XY complement, which establishes the *genetic sex*.

Formation of Organs Common to Both Sexes

Following the rapid cell multiplication of the fertilized egg, there is cell differentiation with formation of various sex organs similar in both sexes, specifically the *gonadal ridges*, the *internal ducts*, and the *external genitalia*.[1] The genital ridges can be easily recognized by 5 w of gestation. At that time, they already have been invaded by the germ cells which have migrated from the wall of the yolk sac and have entered the fetus by way of its caudal part. The eventual differentiation of the germ cells into ova or spermatogonia will occur later and will be based on whether the gonad has become an ovary or a testis.

By 6 w of fetal life, fetuses of both sexes have two sets of internal ducts, the *Müllerian ducts* and the *Wolffian ducts*. The external genitalia at 6 w gestation appear female and include a genital tubercule, the genital folds, urethral folds and a urogenital sinus.

Gonadal Differentiation

This important event is the commitment of the gonadal ridge to become either an ovary or a testis. In males, the commitment to testicular determination is triggered by the product of a gene located on the Y chromosome (Figure 6–1). This product has been termed "testis determining factor" (TDF). As shown in Figure 6–1, the locus of this gene recently has been mapped to the area near the pseudoautosomal region of the short arm of the Y chromosome.[2] A gene from the TDF locus was isolated and named "sex determining region Y chromosome" (SRY). It is now well established that the product of the SRY gene is necessary for testis determination[2] and that SRY is identical with TDF. However, it is also clear that a number of other genes located both on the X chromosome and on autosomes are necessary for the formation of normal male gonads. At this time, it is not clear whether SRY triggers all these other genes simultaneously, or whether there is an orderly cascade in which SRY triggers a second gene, the product of which triggers a third, and so on.

FIGURE 6–1. Map of the Short Arm of the Y Chromosome (Yp)

The upper part of the figure shows the loci of SRY and ZFY genes in relation to the pseudoautosomal region of the Y chromosome. The lower part of the figure shows the locus of the testis-determining factor (TDF) and the map of the various probes used for mapping studies, including pY53.3, a 2.1kb fragment of genomic DNA which contains the sex determining region of the Y (SRY).

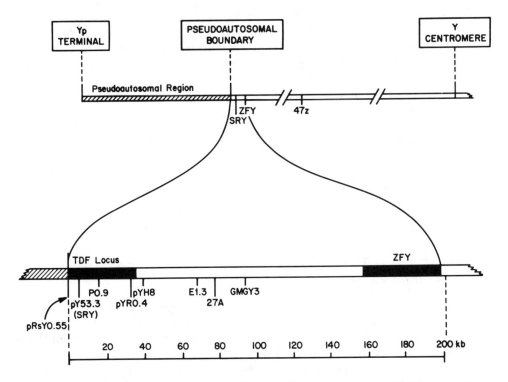

From: Migeon CJ, Berkovitz GD. Congenital defects of the external genitalia in the newborn and prepubertal child. In Carpenter SE, Rock J, eds. Pediatric and adolescent gynecology. New York: Raven Press, 1992:79.

Histologically speaking, the first sign of testicular determination is the appearance of *Sertoli cells*, which rapidly agglutinate to each other to form the seminiferous tubules.[3] In this process, the Sertoli cells surround the germ cells and isolate them from the rest of the testis. About 2 w after the appearance of the Sertoli cells, *Leydig cells* can be detected in the interstitial spaces and steroid secretion starts shortly thereafter.

It is important to note that the Sertoli cells will secrete the Müllerian inhibiting substance (MIS) shortly after their differentiation. Although the granulosa cells also secrete MIS, its production occurs much later in relation to the start of its production by the Sertoli cells.

Shortly after their appearance, the Leydig cells begin producing the male hormone, testosterone.[4] Testosterone arises from the transformation of cholesterol by a series of biosynthetic steps, as shown in Figure 6–2. Most of these steps involve a hydroxylation requiring electron transfer and a specific cytochrome P450 for each step. Cytochrome P450scc is needed for hydroxylation of carbons 20 and 22, as well as for the removal of the cholesterol side chain.

As to cytochrome P450c17, it permits 17α-hydroxylation as well as removal of the two carbon side chain, resulting in formation of C19 steroids or *androgens*. The enzyme 3β-hydroxysteroid dehydrogenase (3β-HSD) transforms the inactive Δ^5-steroids to active Δ^4-compounds, whereas 17-ketoreductase converts androstenedione to testosterone and 5-α reductase converts testosterone to dihydrotestosterone.

In the absence of SRY, such as in 46,XX subjects or 46,XY individuals who have a deleted or mutant SRY gene, the bipotential gonadal ridge becomes an ovary. At present, it is not clear whether one (or several) gene product(s) is(are) required for ovarian determination. The cells which give rise to the Sertoli cells in the male gonad differentiate as granulosa cells in the ovary. These cells eventually surround the germ cells to form primordial follicles. As to the cells which give rise to Leydig cells in the testis, they also occur in the ovary but in much smaller number and are located near the hilus and form the hilar cells.

Differentiation of the Internal Ducts
and External Genitalia

The mechanisms by which the ducts and genitalia differentiate have been established by the pioneering work of Jost and Josso.[5]

In the male, the testicular secretion of testosterone permits the development of the Wolffian ducts, whereas the secretion of MIS by the Sertoli cells inhibits the Müllerian ducts, which eventually disappear. Both testosterone and MIS express their effects locally. For example,

FIGURE 6–2. Biosynthetic Pathway of Testosterone from Cholesterol

It requires two cytochromes P450 (P450scc and P450c17) as well as a 3β-ol-dehydrogenase (3β-SDH) and a 17-ketosteroid reductase. The figure also shows the pathway from cholesterol to the adrenal steroids, cortisol and aldosterone.

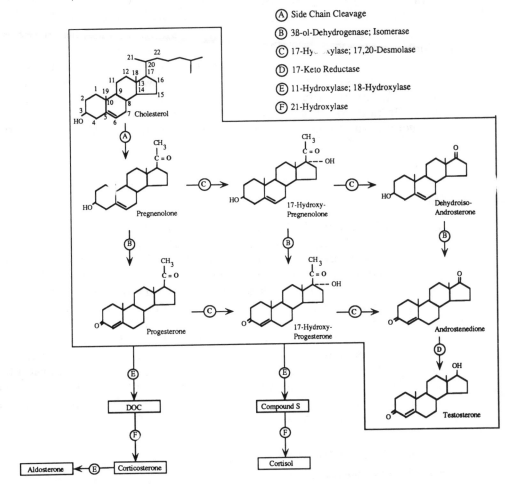

the absence of a testis on one side results in the development of a female duct with absence of a male duct on that side, whereas the presence of a normal testis on the other side results in normal formation of a Wolffian duct and normal inhibition of the Müllerian duct on that side.

The masculinization of the external genitalia by the high concentrations of testosterone in the male starts around 8 w of gestation. The growth of the genita. tubercule and of the urethral folds results in the formation of the penis and of a penile urethra. As to the labio-scrotal folds, they enlarge and fuse, starting from the posterior part to form the scrotum. The full masculinization of the external genitalia of the male requires the local metabolism of testosterone to dihydrotestosterone, a more potent androgen.[6]

It must be added that the process of masculinization of the male fetus requires the presence of a normal androgen receptor, a protein which is coded by a gene located on chromosome Xq12.[7]

In the female, the absence of ovarian secretion of testosterone results in the disappearance of the male ducts whereas the lack of secretion of MIS at the appropriate time results in development of the female ducts. In addition, the absence of androgen results in growth arrest of the genital tubercule forming the clitoris, while the folds become the labia majora and minora.

Abnormal Sexual Differentiation

In view of the complexity of normal sexual differentiation described above, it is not surprising that abnormalities of sexual differentiation can have many causes. The disorders which can occur after the gonads have been committed to becoming ovaries or testes are now well understood. They are either an abnormal masculinization of a female fetus (female pseudohermaphroditism) or an insufficient masculinization of the male fetus (male pseudohermaphroditism). As to the disorders associated with the early part of gonadal differentiation, they are not well characterized or understood. The model for the genetic control of gonadal differentiation indicates that testis determination occurs in the presence of SRY or a mutation that permits testis determination even in the absence of SRY. If SRY is absent or SRY action fails to occur, ovarian determination takes place.

Disorders Related to Abnormal
Gonadal Differentiation

On the basis of our present knowledge, one could make a classification on the basis of the presence or absence of normal testis-determining genes. As shown in Table 6–1, *conditions lacking testis determination* include normal 46,XX females, the "47,XXX superfemales," the 45,X Turner syndrome and its variants, and the 46,XY females (complete or pure gonadal dysgenesis or Swyer's syndrome). *The conditions with normal or partial testis determination* (Table 6–2) include normal 46,XY males, the 47,XXY Klinefelter syndrome, "45,X males," "46,XX males," 46,XX true hermaphrodites, the mosaic 45,X/46,XY, 46XY true hermaphrodites, and the 46,XY partial gonadal dysgenesis.[8]

TABLE 6–1. Conditions with Absent SRY Gene Product

	Normal Female 46,XX	"Super-Female" 47,XXX	Turner 45,X 45,X/46,XX (Variants)	"46,XY Female" 46,XY [-]
External Genitalia	F	F	F	F
Internal Ducts	F	F	F	F
Gonads				
In utero	Ovaries	Ovaries	Ovaries	Ovaries
Adults	Ovaries	Ovaries	Streaks (ovaries rarely)	Streaks
Fertility	Yes	Yes (limited)	No (yes rarely)	No

[-] Deleted or Mutant SRY. Mutation of another gene needed for SRY action.

TABLE 6–2. Conditions with Normal or Partial Testis-Determining Function

	46,XY Normal	47,XXY Klinefelter	45,X Male	46,XX Male	46,XX True H	45,X/ 46,XY	46,XY True H	46,XY Partial Gonadal Dysgenesis
External Genitalia	M	M	M	M	Amb	M/Amb/F	Amb	Amb
Internal Ducts	M	M	M	M	Variable	Variable	Variable	Variable
Gonads								
In utero	Testes	Testes	Testes	Testes	Ovo-testes	Variable	Ovo-testes	Ovo-testes (?)
Adults	Testes	Testes* (no sperm)	Testes* (no sperm)	Testes*	Ovo-testes	Variable	Ovo-testes	Dysgenetic gonads
Fertility	Yes	No	No	No	Variable	Variable	Variable	No

*Hyalinized Tubules

Disorders Related to Abnormalities
Other than Gonadal Differentiation

The causes of *female pseudohermaphroditism* are listed in Table 6–3. As can be seen, abnormal amounts of androgens can arise from the fetus (congenital adrenal hyperplasia) or from the mother.[9]

In 46,XY *male pseudohermaphroditism* (Figure 6–3), the concentrations of testosterone in the newborn may be low (*steroid enzyme defect, partial gonadal dysgenesis, true hermaphroditism*). If the concentrations of testosterone are normal, the possibilities are *5-reductase deficiency, androgen insensitivity,* or *"timing defect."*[10]

TABLE 6–3. Classification of Female Pseudo-Hermaphroditism In Subjects with 46,XX Karyotype

Excess fetal androgen
  21-Hydroxylase deficiency
    Partial (simple virilizing form)
    More Complete (salt-losing form)
  11-Hydroxylase deficiency (hypertensive form)
  3β-Hydroxysteroid dehydrogenase deficiency
Excess maternal androgen
  Iatrogenic
  Virilizing tumor of ovary or adrenal
Congenital abnormalities
  Structural or teratogenic factors

FIGURE 6–3. Diagram of the Causes of Ambiguous Genitalia in 46,XY Infants

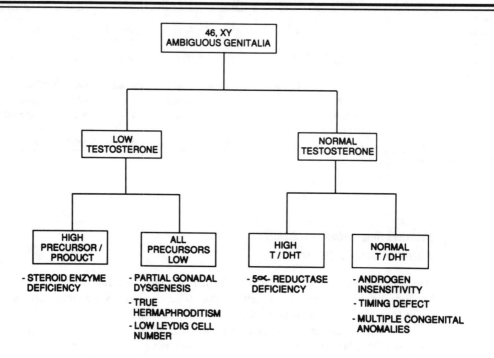

From: Migeon CJ, Berkovitz GD. Congenital defects of the external genitalia in the newborn and prepubertal child. In Carpenter SE, Rock J, eds. Pediatric and adolescent gynecology. New York: Raven Press, 1922:84.

Clinical and Laboratory Evaluation of Ambiguous Genitalia in the Newborn Period

It is of interest that the diagnosis of sex at birth is made rather superficially by visual evaluation of the appearance of the external genitalia. Clearly, this is sufficient in the large majority of cases.

The fact the genitalia appear appropriately formed does not rule out the possibility of abnormalities. For example, a normal-appearing female may have an abnormal karyotype such as 47,XXX super female, 45,X (Turner syndrome) or, rarely, 46,XY pure gonadal dysgenesis. Similarly, a normal-appearing male may have an abnormal karyotype such as 47,XXY (Klinefelter syndrome) or, rarely, 46,XX (46,XX male). Complete deficiency of one of the enzymes needed for cortisol biosynthesis can result in full masculinization of the genitalia of a female fetus. However, in such cases, no gonads are palpated in the scrotum.

Ambiguous external genitalia in newborns usually are related to partial rather than complete forms of the various disorders described above. This complicates further the diagnosis of the etiology of the problem. The evaluation of the infant must be carried out as an emergency, first because life-threatening symptoms such as salt loss can develop, and second because a decision must be made as rapidly as possible about whether the infant will be reared as male or female.

The work-up needed for this situation has been discussed previously.[11] The measurement of the various precursors of androgens as well as testosterone and dihydrotestosterone should be done. A karyotype should also be obtained, and the genital structures should be evaluated by sonogram and genitogram. Following is a recommended schedule for tests which takes in consideration the physiology of steroid secretion in the newborn and the turnover times of some of the tests.

Day 1 or 2: Karyotype, including study of fluorescent Y chromosome and of possible mosaicism. Concentrations of testosterone and dihydrotestosterone in single blood sample in order to compare the values of these two steroids.

Day 3 or 4: Concentrations of 17α-hydroxyprogesterone, 17α-hydroxypregnenolone, and androstenedione, also in a single blood sample.

Day 5 or 6: Sonogram of the gonads and internal ducts followed by genitogram (retrograde injection of contrast substance through the uro-genital sinus).

Day 10 to 12: Repeat concentrations of 17α-hydroxyprogesterone, 17α-hydroxy-pregnenolone, androstenedione, testosterone, and dihydrotestosterone.

In addition, throughout the period of evaluation it is important to check concentrations of serum electrolytes and blood glucose at least once a day. This is necessary in order to detect the possibility of the development of an adrenal crisis with salt loss and hypoglycemia.

Although sex chromosomes do not always reflect the genetic endowment of a subject, the karyotype remains capital in the diagnosis of the cause of ambiguous genitalia. As shown in Figure 6–4, a 46,XX karyotype will orient toward the possibility of female pseudo-hermaphroditism and true hermaphroditism. With a 46,XY karyotype, the possibility of male pseudo-hermaphroditism, true hermaphroditism, and partial gonadal dysgenesis will be considered.

The study of the concentrations of androgens and their precursors will be helpful in further delineating the causes of the ambiguous genitalia. In 46,XY subjects with low testosterone concentrations, increased androgen precursor values will permit determination of the enzyme deficiency involved (Table 6–4), whereas low precursor values will suggest partial gonadal dysgenesis or true hermaphroditism. In 46,XY subjects with normal male concentrations of testosterone a high testosterone/dihydrotestosterone (T/DHT) ratio (> 12 in newborns) will make the diagnosis of 5α-reductase deficiency, whereas a normal T/DHT ratio will suggest either androgen insensitivity (i.e., androgen receptor abnormality) or a "timing defect."

Reference Ranges

Cytogenetic Laboratory

We have already emphasized the importance of careful karyotype studies. It must be emphasized that a search for mosaicism should be carried out, since the presence of a Y chromosome in 5% of cells or even less can result in gonadal differentiation along male lines. For this reason, a search for fluorescent Y can be helpful, even though the fluorescence arises from the long arm of the chromosome whereas the short arm bears the SRY gene, near the junction with the pseudo-autosomal region.

Molecular Biology Laboratory

Molecular genetic techniques are not yet routine, but they may become more so in the future. Specifically, studies of the SRY gene can be done using polymerase chain reaction (PCR) amplification and sequencing of this gene. This permits the detection of the presence of this gene, as in 46,XX males, or of its deletion or mutation, as in 46,XY females.[12]

FIGURE 6–4. Diagram of the Causes of Ambiguous Genitalia in Infants, Depending upon the Sex Chromosome Complement (46,XY, 46,XX, or Other Karyotypes)

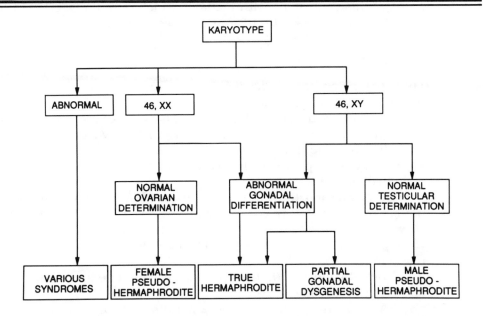

From: Migeon CJ, Berkovitz GD. Congenital defects of the external genitalia in the newborn and prepubertal child. In Carpenter SE, Rock J, eds. Pediatric and adolescent gynecology. New York: Raven Press, 1922:83.

TABLE 6–4. Enzymes Involved In the Biosynthesis of Testosterone from Cholesterol and Clinical Results of Their Deficiency

Enzyme Deficiency	Genitalia in Males	Genitalia in Females	Other Symptoms	Congenital Adrenal Hyperplasia
P450scc				
Complete	Female	Female	Salt Loss	+
Partial	Ambiguous	Female	–	+
3β-HSD				
Complete	Female	Female	Salt Loss	+
Partial	Ambiguous	Ambiguous	–	+
P450c17				
Complete	Female	Female	Hypertension	+
Partial	Ambiguous	Female	Hypertension	+
17-ketoreductase	Ambiguous	Female	–	0
5α-reductase	Ambiguous	Female	–	0

Another application of this technique is being investigated for the study of the androgen receptor gene. PCR amplification of each of the 8 exons of this gene along with methods which permit detection of point mutations can be used to rule out androgen insensitivity.[13]

Hormonal Assays

Study of the concentrations of androgens and their precursors are particularly important. In a normal male infant, the concentrations of testosterone are about half of the values of adult males at age 1–3 d; then they tend to decrease somewhat until age 6–7 d, when they go back to 150–300 ng/dL (5.2–10.4 nmol/L) for the next 8–12 w of life. This is followed by a drop to very low concentrations for the rest of infancy and childhood until puberty.[14]

By comparing the ratio of androstenedione to testosterone (in a normal male at 1–2 w of age, usually < 1) and of testosterone to dihydrotestosterone (range = 2.5–7.5), it is possible to determine whether there is a deficiency of 17-ketoreductase and 5α-reductase, respectively.

Normal concentrations of plasma testosterone and androstenedione are shown in Figure 6–5.

The placenta secretes large amounts of progesterone and 17α-hydroxyprogesterone; these steroids cross to the fetus, and their concentrations at birth in cord blood and in the infant are extremely high. However, their half-life is quite short, and by the third day of life values are representative of the infant's secretion of these steroids (a similar comment applies to androstenedione). If the results of the progesterone and 17α-hydroxyprogesterone concentrations obtained at 3 d are inconclusive, it might be necessary to repeat these assays at 6-7 d of life.

The concentrations of plasma 17α-hydroxyprogesterone are particularly important to the diagnosis of congenital adrenal hyperplasia due to 21-hydroxylase deficiency. However, there can be a major cause of error if this steroid is measured directly on plasma by routine RIA. Normal newborns have huge concentrations of Δ^5-steroids conjugated as sulfates, which have a markedly prolonged half-life and which interfere with the assay of 17α-hydroxyprogesterone. The concentrations of Δ^5-steroid-sulfates decrease slowly with age, so that their interference becomes minimal by 2-4 m of age. For this reason, most laboratories use a purification procedure for the determination of this steroid in infants up to 4–6 m of age. In our laboratory, we use a Sephadex-LH20 column chromatography of the plasma extract; it has the advantage of purifying and separating progesterone and 17α-hydroxyprogesterone.

Normal concentrations of plasma 17α-hydroxyprogesterone are shown in Figure 6–6.

FIGURE 6–5. Concentrations of Plasma Testosterone and Androstenedione in Normal Male and Female Infants, Children, and Adults. (To convert testosterone and androstenedione to S.I. units [nmol/L], multiply by 0.0347 and 0.0349)

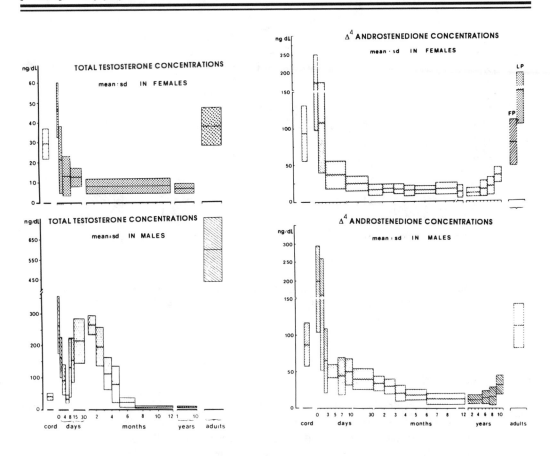

From: Migeon CJ, Forest MG. Androgens in biological fluids. In: Rothfeld B, ed.. Nuclear medicine in vitro, 2d ed. Philadelphia: J.B. Lippincott, 1983:156-57.

ABNORMALITIES OF PUBERTY

Puberty is the series of events which permit a child to become a young adult. These events occur in an orderly fashion, resulting in adult secretion of gonadal hormones and in attainment of reproductive capacity. Puberty involves the maturation of the gonads or *gonadarche* and the secretion of adrenal androgens or *adrenarche*.

FIGURE 6–6. Concentrations of Plasma 17α-hydroxyprogesterone in Normal Male and Female Infants

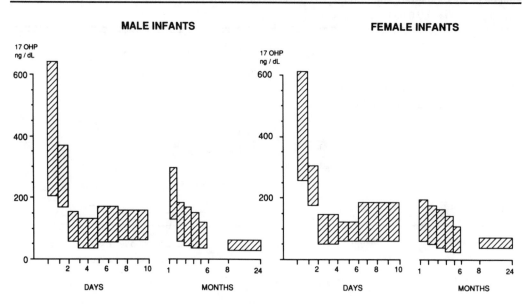

Adapted from: Forest MG, Cathiard AM. Ontogenic study of plasma 17α-hydroxyprogresterone in the human. Pediatric Research 1979;12:6-11.

Biochemistry and Physiology

During childhood, hypothalamic gonadotropin releasing hormone (GnRH) is suppressed, leading to low concentrations of pituitary gonadotropins, luteinizing hormone (LH), and follicle stimulating hormone (FSH). The first indication of puberty is the release of the inhibition of the GnRH secretion. The pulsatile secretion of GnRH every 60–90 min leads to a pulsatile pattern of LH and FSH. This occurs initially during sleep. As puberty progresses, the pulsatile pattern also occurs during the day, until there is no longer a diurnal pattern of secretion.

A gradual rise in the adrenal androgens—dehydroepiandrosterone (DHEA), dehydroepiandrosterone sulfate (DHEA-S), and androstenedione—starts 1–2 y prior to the physical changes of puberty (age 6–7 y in girls and 7–8 y in boys). The cause of the increase in androgen production has been postulated to be the secretion of a pituitary peptide hormone, probably related to but different from ACTH. This presumed hormone is called Adrenal Androgen Stimulation Hormone (AASH).

Females

The normal age of onset of puberty in females is 8–13 y. The first signs of puberty are usually the growth spurt and the development of breast buds. However, in 15% of girls, the first sign of puberty is the development of pubic hair. Tanner and Marshall have devised a scale for staging breast and pubic hair development in females (Table 6–5), where stage I is prepubertal and stage V is adult.[15] Pubertal development is usually completed in 2–6 y, and menarche usually occurs at Tanner stage IV, i.e., 2.3 ± 1.0 y after the onset of breast bud development. In girls, the pubertal growth spurt begins with breast budding but is maximal in mid-puberty. The current average age of menarche is 12.8 y (range 10–16 y). In many girls, the early menstrual cycles are anovulatory until the mechanism for LH surge has matured.

Males

Tanner developmental stages of external genitalia and pubic hair are also used to describe the progression through puberty (Table 6–5), with Tanner stage I being prepubertal and Tanner stage V being adult.[16]

The average age for the onset of puberty in boys is 9–14 y. Most boys complete puberty in 3–4.5 y. In contrast to girls, the pubertal

TABLE 6–5. Stages of Adolescent Sexual Development

Stage*	Mean Age (yrs) ± SD	Male	Mean Age (yrs) ± SD	Female
B2		—	11.1 ± 1.1	Breast "bud" areolar diameter increases
G2	11.6 ± 1.1	Testes 2.5–3.2 cm; thinning of scrotum		—
P2	13.4 ± 1.1	Sparse, long		On labia majora
B3		—	12.1 ± 1.1	Further enlargement; glandular tissue present
G3	12.8 ± 1.1	Testes 3.3–4.0 cm; pigmentation of scrotum; penis enlarged		—
P3	13.9 ± 1.5	Darker, curlier, coarser		Extend to mons
B4		—	13.1 ± 1.1	Areola forms secondary mound
G4	13.7 ± 1.1	Testes ≥ 4.1 cm; further penile enlargement		—
P4	14.3 ± 1.1	Extend to pubis		Extend to pubis
B5		—	15.3 ± 1.7	Adult
G5	14.9 ± 1.6	Testes ≥ 4.5 cm; adult penis		—
P5	15.1 ± 1.1	Adult		Adult

*B = breast stage, G = gonadal stage, P = pubic hair stage

growth spurt in boys occurs later in pubertal development (Tanner stages III-IV for genitalia). This growth spurt results from increased testosterone and growth hormone production. IGF-I concentrations rise through puberty and peak at Tanner stage IV. The onset of spermatogenesis occurs at about Tanner stage IV for genitalia.

The earliest sign of puberty in a boy is the enlargement of testes. Testes greater than 2.5 cm in length (or 3 cc in volume) are consistent with the onset of puberty. The increase in testicular size is predominantly secondary to an increase in seminiferous tubule size. But there is also an increase in the Leydig cell size. The further increase in genitalia and pubic hair development are primarily due to increasing testosterone production through puberty.

Precocious Puberty

Precocious puberty is the onset of puberty in girls prior to age 8 y or in boys prior to age 9 y.[17] These children present with tall stature for their age and secondary sex characteristics. *Central precocious puberty* is a premature activation of the hypothalamic GnRH pulse generator, whereas *peripheral precocious puberty* is independent of GnRH function.[18] In addition, one distinguishes *contrasexual precocity*, in which there is excessive production of estrogens in males or excessive production of androgens in females.

The incidence of precocious puberty is much greater in girls than in boys.

Central Precocious Puberty

In this type of precocity, there is early activation of the hypothalamic GnRH pulse generator, resulting in pubertal LH/FSH pulse patterns. The etiologies of central precocious puberty are listed in Table 6-6. The idiopathic forms are much more frequent in girls than in boys, accounting for the markedly greater incidence of all types of sexual precocity in girls. The incidence of precocious puberty due to an identifiable CNS lesion is approximately the same in both sexes.

TABLE 6–6. Etiologies of Central Precocious Puberty

1. Idiopathic
2. Central Nervous System Involvement
   a) Tumor: Hamartoma, Astrocytoma, Glioma
   b) Neurofibromatosis
   c) Injuries: Hydrocephalus, Meningitis, Encephalitis, Head Trauma
3. Severe Primary Hypothyroidism

Peripheral Precocious Puberty

Children with peripheral precocious puberty do not have a mature hypothalamic-pituitary-gonadal axis. Rather, the stimulus for the sex steroid production is independent of the GnRH pulse generator. In girls the sexual precocity is due to estrogen exposure, whereas in boys the sexual precocity is due to androgen exposure. The etiologies of peripheral precocious puberty are summarized in Table 6–7.

Both gonadal and adrenal tumors are extremely rare in both sexes. McCune-Albright syndrome is thought to be due to an abnormality of a G-protein subunit associated with the LH-receptor that results in the secretion of gonadal steroids despite the absence of LH stimulation.

Contra-sexual Precocious Puberty

Gynecomastia appearing before the onset of puberty in a male is extremely rare and may be caused by an estrogen secreting adrenal tumor. Virilization and hirsutism in prepubertal girls are also rare and may be due to congenital adrenal hyperplasia or an androgen secreting adrenal or ovarian tumor.

Incomplete Precocious Puberty

Premature thelarche is the isolated development of breasts in girls before age 8 y. It usually occurs in the first 4 years of life, and often it regresses completely. A transient increase in LH/FSH and estradiol concentrations can be observed on occasion. However, gonadotropin and steroids are usually low and there is no activation of the GnRH pulse generator. In addition, there is no estrogenization of the vaginal mucosa and no significant advance in bone age. In some of the patients, one small ovarian cyst can be found by pelvic sonogram. In such cases, the cyst is the source of estrogens. Rupture and disappearance of the cyst result in breast regression.

TABLE 6–7. Etiologies of Peripheral Precocious Puberty

GIRLS	BOYS
McCune-Albright Syndrome (café au lait spots, precocious puberty and fibrous dysplasia)	McCune-Albright Syndrome
	Testicular Tumors
	Masculinizing Tumors
Ovarian Tumors (Cysts)	Congenital Adrenal Hyperplasia
Feminizing Adrenal Tumors	Ectopic hCG Tumors
Ectopic hCG Tumors	Premature Leydig Cell Maturation

Premature adrenarche occurs between age 4–8 y. There is predominantly pubic hair development, often only on the labia in girls. In addition, there may be apocrine odor and axillary hair. There may be a mild to moderate acceleration of growth velocity with a slight advancement of bone age. Estrogen and testosterone concentrations are prepubertal, but there is an increased concentration of adrenal androgens, particularly DHEA and DHEA-S, which may rise to pubertal values. Gonadotropins remain prepubertal. Puberty occurs at a normal time in these individuals.

Evaluation of Precocious Puberty

The evaluation of children with precocious puberty should begin with a complete history with particular attention to:

- the age at onset of pubertal signs
- the rapidity of progression of symptoms
- history of CNS insult
- family history of puberty
- medications (contraceptive pills, androgens, etc.) accessible to the child
- the growth curve, to assess an acceleration of growth velocity.

On physical examination, a careful neurologic work-up should be obtained and pubertal staging should be made. In males, the testes should be palpated for the presence of a mass. Virilization with no testicular enlargement in boys implies an extra-testicular source of androgens. The skin should also be examined for café au lait spots, which could indicate McCune-Albright syndrome, or for lesions of neurofibromatosis; both conditions are associated with precocious puberty.

Initial laboratory evaluation to determine whether the precocious puberty is of central or peripheral origin should include the determination of the concentration of *gonadotropins* (LH/FSH), *gonadal steroids* (testosterone, estradiol) and *adrenal steroids* (17-hydroxyprogesterone [17-OHP], androstenedione [Δ], DHA and DHA-sulfate). In addition, a *bone age* and a set of *thyroid function tests* (T_4 RIA, T_3 resin uptake, T_{index}, and TSH) should be obtained. In order to minimize the effect of episodic LH/FSH secretion, it is recommended that 4 serial blood samples be obtained at 20 min intervals. Assays can be obtained using a blood pool of the 4 samples, or preferably on each sample. Depending on the results of basal values, work-up will be performed as shown in Figure 6–7.

If pubertal values of gonadotropins and gonadal hormones are found, then *central precocious puberty* must be considered and a differential diagnosis of its various causes must be done as shown in Table

FIGURE 6–7. Diagram of the Work-up of Children with Signs of Precocious Puberty

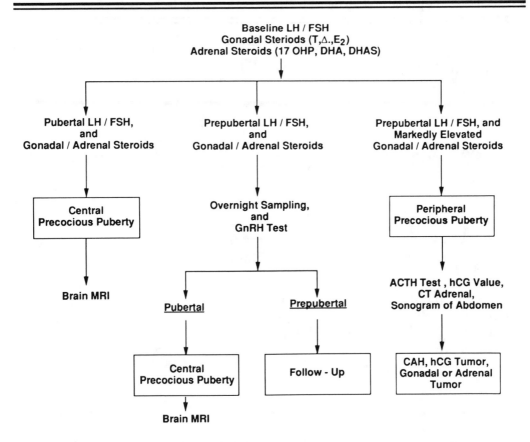

6–6. A brain MRI is important in order to study the possibility of tumors.

If prepubertal values of LH/FSH and steroids are reported, it will be necessary to perform an overnight blood sampling (every 20 min from 2 AM to 6 AM for LH/FSH, and every hour for gonadal steroids) and a GnRH test (at 8 AM, an IV slow push of 100 micrograms of GnRH is given, followed by blood sampling every 20 min for 2 h). Because LH/FSH are secreted only at night in the early stages of puberty (Figure 6–8), a daytime sampling may give misleading information. As to the GnRH test, it will result in LH/FSH concentrations in the adult range if the subject is in early puberty (stage II). When the results of the overnight sampling and GnRH tests are indicative of a prepubertal status, close follow-up is in order.

The presence of markedly increased gonadal and/or adrenal steroids along with prepubertal LH/FSH will suggest a peripheral cause for the sexual precocity (see Table 6–7). An ACTH test (0.25 milligrams of

FIGURE 6–8. Pattern of LH Concentrations in Pre-puberty, Early-to-mid Puberty, Mid-to-late Puberty and Adulthood. The pattern of sleep stages is also shown for each pubertal stage.

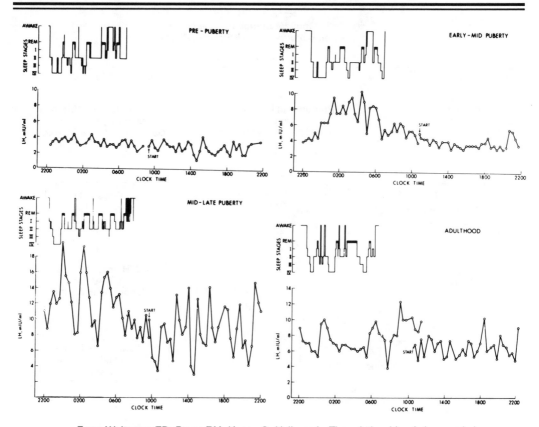

From: Weitzman ED, Boyar RM, Kapen S, Hellman L. The relationship of sleep and sleep stages to neuroendocrine secretion and biological rhythm in man. Rec Prog Horm Res 1975;31:399.

1–24 ACTH, IV slow push, is given followed by blood sampling at 0, 30, and 60 min for 17-hydroxyprogesterone and progesterone) will help determine whether congenital adrenal hyperplasia is the cause of precocity. An increased hCG concentration will suggest an hCG producing tumor. CT of adrenal glands and sonogram of abdomen/pelvis may also be indicated.

Patients with McCune-Albright syndrome present the triad precocious puberty, fibrous dysplasia, and café au lait spots, although they may have only two signs of the triad. A bone scan is necessary to look for the changes of fibrous dysplasia.

Delayed Puberty

Definition and Classification

We usually consider that puberty is delayed in a male in whom there is no noticeable testicular enlargement by the age of 14 y and in females if there is no breast development by the age of 13 y. In girls, the definition of primary amenorrhea is the lack of menstrual period by age 16 y or by the failure to menstruate within about 3 y of the onset of breast development.[19]

In many cases the delayed puberty will eventually resolve and result in normal maturation. However, in other cases the delayed puberty will be associated with a hypogonadism that will remain for a life time.

The classification of the causes of delayed puberty is based on whether the problem is central, i.e., related to the hypothalamus-pituitary, or is due to primary gonadal deficiency (Table 6–8). This permits us to distinguish *hypogonadotropic hypogonadism* from *hypergonadotropic hypogonadism*. In the first condition there is an inability to produce LH/FSH, whereas in the second condition a defect in gonadal function results in a compensatory increase of the secretion of GnRH by the hypothalamus and LH/FSH by the pituitary. A GnRH test showing little or no increase of gonadotropin concentration is typical of the prepubertal state due to central disorders, whereas the GnRH test will show an accentuated response of LH and FSH in primary gonadal disorders.

TABLE 6–8. Classification of the Causes of Delayed Puberty

	Site of Defect	Gonadotropin	LH/FSH Response to GnRH	Gonadal Steroids
Constitutional delay, Reversible hypogonadotropism	Delayed maturation of hypothalamus	Low	Prepubertal	Low
Permanent hypogonadotropism	Hypothalamus or pituitary	Low	Prepubertal or absent	Low
Hypogonadotropism related to increased androgens	Adrenal or gonadal androgens	Low	Prepubertal	Elevated
Hypergonadotropic hypogonadism	Gonads	Elevated	Accentuated	Low

Constitutional Delay and Reversible Hypogonadotropism

The term *constitutional delay* applies to subjects whose pubertal maturation occurs after the normal average age but is eventually established and is normal from there on. This is the most common cause of pubertal delay, particularly in boys.

Certain conditions result in a *delayed secretion of gonadotropins* that is reversible following the correction of the original condition. Such conditions include malnutrition, as in starvation or anorexia nervosa, the latter problem arising more often in girls than in boys. Another delaying factor is strenuous exercise. It has been observed in children involved in competitive sports such as gymnastics, swimming, running. A number of systemic diseases (severe cardiovascular or respiratory disorders, inflammatory bowel disease, renal tubular acidosis, poorly controlled diabetes mellitus) can also result in delay of gonadotropin secretion. There have also been cases of delayed puberty reported to be related to psychopathological problems. As already mentioned, an improvement in all those conditions will eventually result in the development of puberty.

Permanent Hypogonadotropic Hypogonadism

As seen in Table 6–9, tumors as well as other destructive disorders of the pituitary hypothalamic area can result in an inability to secrete GnRH and/or LH/FSH. Similarly, various congenital anomalies of the central nervous system can result in hypogonadotropism. Some of them are associated with various syndromes such as septo-optic dysplasia, Kallmann's syndrome, and some cases of Prader-Willi syndrome. In some patients, the anatomical anomaly cannot be determined and the etiology is termed "idiopathic hypopituitarism."

TABLE 6–9. Permanent Hypogonadotropic Hypogonadism as Cause of Delayed Puberty

1. Tumors of Pituitary, Hypothalamus, Optic Chiasma, Third Ventricle
   Adenoma, Craniopharyngioma
   Glioma, Dysgerminoma
2. Destructive Disorders
   Histiocytosis, Sarcoidosis, Lupus
3. Head Trauma
   Hemorrhage
4. Congenital Anomalies
   Pituitary Aplasia
   Deficient LH/FSH or GnRH secretion related to various syndromes
   Idiopathic Hypopituitarism

Hypogonadotropism Related to Increased Androgen Secretion

In some cases, the androgens arise from the adrenals (virilizing adrenal tumor or congenital adrenal hyperplasia due to 21-hydroxylase deficiency or to 11-hydroxylase deficiency). In other cases, the androgens are gonadal in origin. In girls, it can be related to polycystic ovaries or ovarian tumors (adrenal rest tumor, hilar cell tumor, arrhenoblastoma). In boys, this might be related to a Leydig cell tumor.

The clinical picture in such cases is that of androgen effects including virilism without estrogenic effect in girls and without testicular development in boys. Clearly, the treatment of such conditions is to remove or suppress the origin of androgen hypersecretion. This will permit the establishment of puberty.

Hypergonadotropic Hypogonadism

In these patients it is necessary to correlate the appearance of the external genitalia with the karyotype. When the karyotype is requested, instructions should be given to look for mosaicism and search for fluorescent Y chromosome. In most instances it will also be important to obtain a sonogram of the abdomen in order to obtain information about the ovaries and Müllerian ducts in girls and of the testes in males whose gonads are not palpable in the scrotum. A careful physical examination as well as a complete recording of the medical history will also be important in establishing the cause of the hypergonadotropic hypogonadism.

Hypergonadotropic Hypogonadism with Normal Appearing Female External Genitalia (Table 6-10)

If a normal 46,XX karyotype is obtained, one must consider a number of conditions. The *46,XX gonadal dysgenesis* might be recognized on the basis of the abdominal sonogram, which would show the presence of streak gonads. The *steroid enzyme deficiencies* are characterized by an inability to synthesize androgens and estrogens. In the P450c17-deficiency there is a concomitant hypertension, whereas the deficiency of either 3β-HSD or P450scc is usually associated with a salt-losing syndrome. As to the other ovarian disorders, they will have a history of *autoimmune abnormality*, *chemotherapy* and/or *radiation*, or of *surgical operation* for bilateral ovarian torsion or tumor. The syndrome of *resistant ovaries* is usually diagnosed by exclusion of all other possible abnormalities.

TABLE 6–10. Hypergonadotropic Hypogonadism with Normal Female External Genitalia

---

1. Karyotype 46,XX

    a) 46,XX Gonadal Dysgenesis

    b) Steroid Enzyme Deficiency
        P450c17, 3βD-HSD, P450scc

    c) Resistant Ovaries

    d) Other Ovarian Disorders
        Oophoritis (auto-immune)
        Radiation, Chemotherapy
        Bilateral Torsion or Tumor

2. Karyotype 46,XY
    a) 46,XY "Pure Gonadal Dysgenesis"
    b) Steroid Enzyme Deficiency
        P450c17, 3β-HSD, P450scc
    c) Androgen Insensitivity Syndrome

3. Karyotype 45,X and Variants
    Turner Syndrome

4. Karyotype 47,XXX

If a 46,XY karyotype is reported, then one should consider the *46,XY pure gonadal dysgenesis.* In this condition, the gonadal tissue disappears fairly early in fetal life, resulting in completely normal female phenotype and streak gonads which can be detected by sonogram. As to the *steroid enzyme deficiencies* in subjects with 46,XY karyotype, they must be complete in order to result in a female phenotype, this being rather rare. Finally, there is the possibility of *androgen insensitivity syndrome* characterized by the presence of testes in the abdomen or the labial folds with normal male testosterone secretion. In these subjects, the lack of androgen receptor function results in an inability to express androgen effects. Although there is a short vagina, there are no Müllerian structures and little or no Wolffian structures. The LH concentrations are always elevated, but much less than in other conditions of hypergonadotropic hypogonadism. At puberty, the subjects develop breasts, but usually no pubic or axillary hair, and of course no menstruation. The locus of the androgen receptor gene is on the X chromosome, and androgen insensitivity is an X-linked disorder.

If the karyotype is 45,X (or one of its variants), one is dealing with *Turner syndrome.* This condition is characterized by streak gonads and short stature, as well as many other congenital malformations. The patients have an increased incidence of cardiovascular malformations, particularly coarctation of the aorta. There is also an increased incidence of thyroid antibodies and of hypothyroidism, and frequently congenital kidney malformations. The latter might be observed at the time of the abdominal sonogram.

Finally, the karyotype can on occasion be 47,XXX, sometimes termed "super female." Some of these patients tend to have a delayed puberty, and many of them have premature menopause.

Hypergonadotropic Hypogonadism with Normal
Male External Genitalia (Table 6–11)

If the karyotype is 46,XY, the diagnosis of *"vanishing testes"* will be made if gonads cannot be localized. This syndrome is thought to be due to a destruction of the testes taking place after gonadal differentiation, since the normal male external genitalia is evidence of previous androgenic masculinization. In *Noonan's syndrome* or *"male Turner syndrome,"* one can observe a number of the congenital malformations found in 45,X Turner syndrome, including the short stature. However, the testicular function may be fairly normal as far as Leydig cell function is concerned, but most of patients are azoospermic. One could also be dealing with *partial testicular dysgenesis*, a poorly understood syndrome characterized by partial but variable malformation of the testes usually with a variably decreased Leydig cell function.

One must also consider the possibility of an *autoimmune disorder* involving the testes. As to a *trauma* or *tumor* of the gonads, it must be bilateral in order to result in hypogonadism. In other cases, there is a previous history of *radiation* or *chemotherapy*, as in the treatment of a leukemic disorder in childhood.

TABLE 6–11.
Hypergonadotropic-Hypogonadism with
Normal Male External Genitalia

1. Karyotype 46,XY
   a) Anorchia ("Vanishing Testes")
   b) Noonan's Syndrome (Male Turner)
   c) Partial Testicular Dysgenesis
   d) Other Testicular Disorders
      Inflammation (auto-immune)
      Bilateral Trauma or Tumor
      Radiation-Chemotherapy

2. Karyotype 46,XX
   "46,XX Males"

3. Other Karyotypes
   a) 47,XXY (Klinefelter) and Variants
   b) Some 47,XYY
   c) Some 45,X/46,XY

In "46,XX males," it is thought that a part of the Y chromosome has been translocated to one of the two X's. For all purposes, such a patient is somewhat similar to a subject with 47,XXY Klinefelter syndrome. Some of these patients, as well as some with a 47,XYY complement and those with a mosaicism 45,X/46,XY, present with delayed puberty.

Evaluation of Delayed Puberty

Based on the classification described above, the first step is to determine the gonadotropin function by measuring LH/FSH concentration in serum as well as the response to the administration of GnRH. The methods used are similar to those described for sexual precocity.

If there is *hypogonadotropism*, it is usually easy to determine whether the etiology is a hypersecretion of androgens. The androgens to be measured include the adrenal androgens (DHA, its sulfate, and androstenedione) as well as testosterone. If *21-hydroxylase deficiency* is considered, then plasma 17-hydroxyprogesterone concentration should also be determined, whereas if *11-hydroxylase deficiency* is possible, plasma 11-deoxycortisol concentration must be measured. In some patients it might be necessary to use a dexamethasone suppression test: complete androgen suppression will be obtained in congenital adrenal hyperplasia, but no such suppression will be observed in cases of *virilizing adrenal or ovarian tumors.*

As to the *reversible forms* of hypogonadotropism, they can usually be suspected by appropriate history. However, this might not always be possible, in which case the work-up of suspected *permanent hypogonadotropism* must be carried out. This usually includes an MRI of the head as well as the full work-up of the other pituitary hormones, specifically growth hormone, TSH, and ACTH. The brain MRI will usually detect tumors as well as other destructive processes. It will also detect *pituitary aplasia* as well as *septo-optic dysplasia*. However, in some cases no abnormality of the pituitary hypothalamic area will be found, in which case one can entertain the diagnosis of *idiopathic hypopituitarism*.

If *hypergonadotropism* has been demonstrated, then a karyotype must be obtained. If there is an abnormality of sex chromosomes (such as 45,X or 47,XXY), or if the sex chromosome complement of the karyotype is normal but incongruous with the phenotype of the external genitalia of the patient (46,XX male, 46,XY female), then the diagnosis can readily be made. On the other hand, if the karyotype is that expected for the phenotype of the external genitalia, then the diagnosis may be slightly more complicated. In those patients, a sonogram of the abdomen can be helpful in determining the status of the gonads. In some male patients with scrotal testes, gonadal biopsy may be necessary to determine the type of lesion present.

REFERENCES

1. Langman J. Medical embryology, 2nd ed. Baltimore: Williams and Wilkins, 1969.
2. Koopman P, Gubbay J, Vivian N, Goodfellow P, Lovell-Badge R. Male development of chromosomally female mice transgenic for Sry. Nature 1991;351:117-21.
3. Magre S, Jost A. The initial phases of testicular organogenesis in the rat: An electron microscopy study. Arch Anat Microsc Morphol Exp 1980;69:297-318.
4. Ewing L, Brown BL. Testicular steroidogenesis. In: Johnson AD, Gomes WR, eds. The testis, Vol 4. New York: Academic Press, 1977:239-87.
5. Josso N, Picard JY. Antimüllerian hormone. Physiol Rev 1986;66:1038-90.
6. Siiteri PK, Wilson JD. Testosterone formation and metabolism during male sexual differentiation in the human embryo. J Clin Endocrinol Metab 1974;38:113-25.
7. Migeon BR, Brown TR, Axelman J, Migeon CJ. Studies of the locus for androgen receptor: Localization on the human X chromosome and evidence for homology with Tfm locus in the mouse. Proc Natl Acad Sci USA 1981;78:6339-43.
8. Grumbach MM, Conte FA. Disorders of sexual differentiation. In: Wilson JD, Foster DW, eds. Williams textbook of endocrinology, 8th ed. Philadelphia: WB Saunders, 1992:853-951.
9. Donohoue PA, Berkovitz GD. Female pseudohermaphroditism In: Rock JA, ed. Seminars in reproductive endocrinology, Vol. 5, No. 3. New York: Thieme-Stratton Medical Publishers, 1987:233-41.
10. Migeon CJ. Male pseudohermaphroditism. Annales d'Endocrinologie (Paris) 1980;41:311-43.
11. Migeon CJ, Berkovitz GD. Congenital defects of the external genitalia in the newborn and prepubertal child. In: Carpenter SE, Rock J, eds. Pediatric and adolescent gynecology. New York: Raven Press, 1992:77-94.
12. Berkovitz GD, Fechner PY, Marcantonio SM, Bland G, Stetten G, Goodfellow PN, Smith KD, Migeon CJ. The role of the sex-determining region of the Y chromosome (SRY) in the etiology of 46,XX true hermaphroditism. Hum Genet 1992;88:411-16.
13. Brown TR, Lubahn DB, Wilson EM, French FS, Migeon CJ, Corden JL. Naturally occurring mutant androgen receptors from subjects with complete androgen insensitivity are defective in transcriptional activation. Molecular Endocr 1990;4:1759-72.
14. Forest MG, Sizonenko PC, Cathiard AM, Bertrand J. Hypophyso-gonadal function in humans during the first year of life. I. Evidence for testicular activity in early infancy. J Clin Invest 1974;53:818-28.
15. Marshal WA, Tanner JM. Variations in pattern of pubertal changes in girls. Arch Dis Child 1969;44:291-303.
16. Marshal WA, Tanner JM. Variations in pattern of pubertal changes in boys. Arch Dis Child 1970;45:13-23.
17. Grumbach MM, Styne DM. Puberty: Ontogeny, neuroendocrinology, physiology, and disorders. In: Wilson JD, Foster DW, eds. Williams textbook of endocrinology, 8th ed. Philadelphia: WB Saunders, 1992:1139-221.
18. Kaplan SL, Grumbach MM. Pathogenesis of sexual precocity. In: Grumbach MM, Sizonenko PC, Aubert ML, eds. Control of the onset of puberty. Baltimore: Williams and Wilkins, 1990:620-68.
19. Job J-C, Chaussain J-L, Toublanc J-E. Delayed puberty. In: Grumbach MM, Sizonenko PC, Aubert ML, eds. Control of the onset of puberty. Baltimore: Williams and Wilkins, 1990:588-619.

Disorders of the Thyroid Gland

Wellington Hung, M.D., Ph.D., F.A.A.P., F.A.C.P.

INTRODUCTION

Thyroid hormones are essential for the general growth and development of the infant and child, particularly in the differentiation and function of the central nervous system. They are necessary elements in the maturational events involved in the transition of the newborn to the adult.

The thyroid gland is bi-lobed and the lobes are connected by an isthmus. The isthmus usually overlies the region of the second to fourth tracheal cartilages. In normal children, the right lobe is often the larger of the two lobes. The thyroid gland produces the thyroid hormones $3,5,3',5'$-thyroxine (T_4), and $3,5,3'$-triiodothyronine (T_3).

Thyroid hormone homeostasis is controlled by the hypothalamus and pituitary gland. Thyrotropin-releasing hormone (TRH) is produced by several hypothalamic nuclei and is secreted into the hypophyseal portal system and carried to the anterior pituitary to bind to cell membrane receptors on thyrotrophic cells. The structure of TRH has been shown to be pyroglutamyl-histyl-prolinamide, and this tripeptide has been synthesized. TRH stimulates the thyroid cells to increase the synthesis and release of T_4 and T_3. These hormones, in turn, feed back on the pituitary thyrotroph to suppress synthesis of TSH.

In the human fetus, pituitary TSH is detectable at 8–10 w of gestation.[1] Pituitary TSH concentrations are low until 16 w of gestation and are increased significantly at 28 w. Serum TSH is detectable at 10 w of gestation.[2]

The secretion of TSH is pulsatile; the pulse frequency being about 8–12 pulses per 24 h and the pulse amplitude about 0.5 mU/L. In children and adolescents, serum TSH concentrations exhibit a circadian rhythm.[3] The serum TSH concentrations reach a nadir in the late afternoon, rise to a peak around midnight, remain on a plateau for several hours, and then decrease. The nocturnal rise is sleep-independent.

Feedback control of TSH secretion occurs at both the pituitary and hypothalamic levels. At the pituitary, low concentrations of circulating thyroid hormones result in increased TSH secretion, while increased concentrations of thyroid hormones suppress TSH secretion. Feedback inhibition by thyroid hormones on the thyroid gland itself has been described.

THYROID HORMONE SYNTHESIS

Iodine and amino acids are essential substrates for the formation of T_4 and T_3. After iodide is absorbed from the gastrointestinal tract, it enters the iodine pool of the body. From the pool, iodide is removed by trapping in the follicular cells of the thyroid gland or is excreted in the urine.

Immediately after entrance of iodide into the thyroid, iodination of organic compounds occurs and is dependent upon oxidation of iodide to iodine. Thyroid hormones are first synthesized as a prohormone, thyroglobulin (Tg). Thyroglobulin is a glycoprotein consisting of amino acids connected in peptide linkage. Tg is a normal secretory product of the thyroid gland and can be measured by radioimmunoassay (RIA) in the serum. Interlaboratory variations for serum values exist because an international standard has not been established.

T_4 and T_3 are secreted by the thyroid gland in a T_4:T_3 ratio of 10:1. Twenty percent of T_3 is directly secreted by the thyroid, while 80% is converted from T_4 by peripheral deiodination, catalyzed by T_4-5'-deiodinase.

In pathologic states, a greater proportion of T_3 comes from direct thyroidal secretion. T_3 is three to four times more potent than T_4.

Although T_4 and T_3 secretion is primarily regulated by TSH, it may also be regulated by iodide and various growth factors. Extrathyroidal T_3 production is also regulated; it is decreased by starvation and virtually all illnesses, increased by overfeeding, decreased in hypothyroidism, and increased in hyperthyroidism.

Most, if not all, thyroid hormone actions are mediated by regulation of gene expression, through binding of T_3 receptor complexes to specific response elements of different genes. The T_3 nuclear receptors are structurally similar to many steroid hormone receptors. The affinity of the receptor for T_3 is approximately tenfold higher than the affinity for T_4.

3,3',5'-triiodothyronine, or reverse T_3 (RT_3), is formed primarily from peripheral monodeiodination of T_4. The inner ring deiodination of T_4 by 5'-deiodinase forms RT_3. The distinction between formation of T_3 and RT_3 does not appear to be a random event and may be one of the host defense mechanisms against protein deficiency. The metabolic activity of RT_3 is almost nil.

TRANSPORT OF THYROID HORMONES

Transport of T_4 and T_3 in plasma involves binding to protein carriers. Approximately 75% of serum T_4 is bound to an inter-alpha globulin (T_4-binding globulin of TBG); 20% is bound to albumin and 5% to a prealbumin, thyroxine-binding prealbumin (TBPA). T_4 binds with approximately 10 times the affinity of T_3 to these protein carriers, and this accounts for the much greater concentration of T_4 and T_3 found in normal plasma. A small amount of T_4 is loosely attached to erythrocytes. It is estimated that although free and bound T_4 are in equilibrium, at any given time only 0.016% to 0.064% of the total circulating T_4 is not bound. This minute fraction is referred to as free thyroxine (FT_4). Although quantitatively insignificant, the free hormone concentrations indicate more accurately the metabolic status of an individual, since only in this form can it traverse the cellular membranes and exert its function.

PHYSIOLOGIC CHANGES OF THYROID FUNCTION TESTS DURING THE PEDIATRIC AGE

The proper interpretation of serum TSH, T_4, T_3, RT_3, thyroid hormone binding ratio (THBR), and Tg concentrations in pediatric patients requires a knowledge of the age-dependency of these hormones. Importantly, pre-term and small-for-gestational-age (SGA) newborns have serum thyroid hormone values different from those of full-term newborns.

THYROID-STIMULATING HORMONE

Serum TSH can be measured by RIA, and conventional RIA can easily detect patients with primary hypothyroidism; however, because of assay insensitivity, RIA cannot differentiate low-normal from abnormally low values. In the early 1980s, immunometric assays (IMA) for serum TSH became available that are referred to as "sensitive" TSH (sTSH) or second-generation TSH assays. The sTSH-IMA are approximately 10 to 100 times as sensitive as TSH-RIA and are capable of discriminating very low TSH values found in hyperthyroidism from those found in healthy euthyroid patients.[4] These assays have a sensitivity of 0.1 mU/L. These second-generation sTSH assays are currently used in clinical practice. Efforts to develop still more sensitive assays have led to a third generation of assays utilizing immunochemiluminescence assay[5] that are becoming available to the clinician. The third-generation assay has an approximately tenfold greater sensitivity of 0.01 mU/L. This assay will allow differentiation of patients with nonthyroidal illnesses and low serum TSH values from hyperthyroidism. This assay also will allow more precise adjustment of exogenous thyroxine dosage prescribed to hypothyroid patients. Suppression of the serum TSH concentration measured by sensitive assays has been shown to be highly predictive of a suppressed response to TRH stimulation, thus obviating the need in most situations for performing a TRH test (see discussion below).

In the newborn infant, there is a great increase in serum TSH concentrations at the time of birth. An acute increase in values occurs within the first few minutes of life, and peak values are observed approximately 30 min following delivery.[1] Values decrease rapidly thereafter, falling to 50% of the peak values by 2 h of life. Serum TSH concentrations decrease further, so that by 48 h of age they are only slightly higher than cord blood values. The complete explanation for this striking increase in TSH concentrations is not known. There is evidence that the increase may be due, at least in part, to the drop in body temperature experienced by the newborn after delivery. Serum TSH values from birth to age 20 y are presented in Table 7–1.

TABLE 7–1. Serum TSH Values (mIU/L) by Age Determined by sTSH (Immunoradiometric Assay) or Third-Generation Assay (Chemiluminescence Assay)

Age	Serum TSH
Birth – 4 d	1.0–38.9
2 w – 20 w	1.7–9.1
21 w – 24 m	0.8–8.2
25 m – 20 y	0.7–5.7

From: Nichols Institute Reference Laboratories, San Juan Capistrano, CA. Reproduced with permission.

THYROTROPIN-RELEASING HORMONE (TRH) STIMULATION TEST

Synthetic TRH causes release of TSH from the anterior pituitary glands of normal children. Serum TSH values increase in normal children and adolescents within 10 min after intravenous administration of TRH, peak at 20–45 min, and then decline to baseline values by 2 h. The TRH test allows us to (1) distinguish hypothalamic TRH deficiency from pituitary TSH deficiency as the cause of hypothyroidism; (2) evaluate pituitary TSH reserve; and (3) offer a confirmatory test for hyperthyroidism. As previously mentioned, the availability of sTSH assays obviates the need to perform TRH testing in most instances.

THYROXINE-BINDING GLOBULIN

The TBG concentration is high in cord blood and decreases to adult values by 20 years of age (see discusion below). Serum TBG values at term are higher in healthy, full-term newborns than in SGA newborns. A positive correlation is present between serum TBG and thyroid hormone concentrations.

Serum concentrations of TBPA are higher in the full-term newborn than in the SGA newborn; however, the serum concentration of TBPA is *lower* in the SGA newborn than in the premature newborn. Serum TBG values from birth to age 19 y are presented in Table 7–2.

TABLE 7–2. Thyroxine-Binding Globulin by RIA
[values expressed in mg/dL (mg/L)]

Age	Males	Females
Cord Blood (full-term)	1.9–3.9 (19–39)	1.9–3.9 (19–39)
1–5 d	2.2–4.2 (22–42)	2.2–4.2 (22–42)
1–11 m	1.6–3.6 (16–36)	1.7–3.7 (17–37)
10–19 y	1.4–2.6 (14–26)	1.4–3.0 (14–30)

From: Nichols Institute Reference Laboratories, San Juan Capistrano, CA. Reproduced with permission.

The serum concentrations and binding of the thyroxine-binding proteins vary with physiologic and pathologic states (Table 7-3) and affect serum T_4 and T_3 concentrations.[7] Alterations in TBG concentration or binding usually do not affect the FT_4, and it is therefore useful to measure this if one suspects an abnormality in the serum values of T_4-binding proteins.

TABLE 7–3. Causes of Abnormal Serum Concentration and/or Binding of Thyroxine-Binding Proteins

	TBG	TBPA
Hypothyroidism	inc	
Genetic	inc or dec	N
Estrogens	inc	dec
Pregnancy	inc	dec
Hepatic Disease	inc or dec or N	dec
Androgens	dec	dec
Anabolic Steroids	dec	
Nephrosis	dec	
Severe Hypoproteinemia	dec	
Phenytoin (Dilantin)	dec	
Glucocorticoids (High Dosage)	dec	dec
Salicylate (Aspirin)	N	dec
Heroin	inc	
Methadone	inc	
Acute Stress		dec
Chronic Illness		dec
Thyrotoxicosis		dec

inc = increased; dec = decreased; N = normal

FAMILIAL DYSALBUMINEMIA

This is an autosomal disorder in which affected patients synthesize albumin with increased affinity and/or capacity to bind T_4 but not T_3. These patients have increased serum T_4 and free T_4 (FT_4-I) indices, but their serum T_3 and TSH values are normal and they are clinically euthyroid. The FT_4I values are high because the abnormal binding involves only T_4 and is not recognized by the THBR study (see discussion below). A similar abnormality in TBPA has been reported.

TABLE 7–4. Age-Related Values for Serum T$_4$ and T$_3$
[values expressed in μg/dL (nmol/L)]

Age	T$_4$	T3
Cord		
30 w	5.7–15.6 (73.5–201.2)	
25 w	6.1–16.8 (78.7–216.7)	
40 w	6.6–18.1 (85.1–233.5)	
45 w	7.1–19.4 (91.6–250.3)	
Term	6.6–17.5 (85.1–225.8)	14–86 (0.22–1.32)
1–3 d	11.0–21.5 (141.9–277.4)	100–740 (1.54–11.40)
1–4 w	8.2–16.6 (105.8–214.1)	100–300 (1.54–4.62)
1–12 m	7.2–15.6 (92.9–201.2)	100–260 (1.54–4.00)
1–5 y	7.0–15.0 (90.3–193.5)	95–250 (1.46–3.85)
6–10 y	6.5–13.5 (83.9–174.2)	95–240 (1.46–3.70)
11–15 y	5.0–11.7 (64.5–151.0)	80–215 (1.23–3.31)
16–20 y	4.5–11.8 (58.1–152.2)	80–210 (1.23–3.23)

From: Fisher DA. The thyroid gland. In: Brook CGD, ed. Clinical paediatric endocrinology, 2d ed. Oxford: Blackwell Scientific Publications 1989:313.

THYROXINE

Peak serum concentrations of T$_4$ in the newborn are reached 24 h after birth (see Table 7–4) and then slowly decrease over the first weeks of life.[9] Healthy premature and SGA newborns have qualitatively similar but quantitatively decreased changes in T$_4$ when compared to full-term newborns. During the first 7 weeks of life, serum T$_4$ values are significantly lower in SGA than in full-term infants, and even lower values are present in premature infants. After approximately 50 days of age, comparable serum T_4 concentrations are present in all three maturity groups of infants. Between 1 and 15 years of age, there is a gradual decrease in concentration of T_4 with increasing age. Causes of hyperthyroxinemia are listed in Table 7–5, some of which have been presented in Table 7–3. It is important to remember that hyperthyroxinemia does not equal hyperthyroidism.

Causes of decreased serum thyroid hormone binding or hypothyroxinemia are listed in Table 7–6. Inherited TBG disorders are X-linked and may be complete or partial. Salicylates and furosemide in high doses may cause decreased T_4 and T_3 binding because they are competitive physicochemical inhibitors of T_4 and T_3 binding to TBG. Patients with severe non-thyroidal illnesses may have low albumin and TBPA values, and therefore T_4 and T_3 binding are decreased.

TABLE 7–5. Causes of Hyperthyroxinemia in Pediatrics

I.	Hyperthyroidism
II.	Increased Serum Binding of Thyroid Hormones
	A. TBG
	B. Thyroxine-binding albumin
	1. Familial dysalbuminemic hyperthyroxinemia
	C. TBPA
	1. Inherited abnormal TBPA
	D. Anti-T_4 antibodies
III.	Non-Thyroidal Illnesses
	A. Medical illnesses
	B. Psychiatric illnesses
IV.	Drug-Induced Hyperthyroxinemia
V.	Generalized thyroid hormone resistance

FREE THYROXINE (FT₄)

The principal methods for measuring FT_4 are as follows:

1.   indirect tracer equilibrium dialysis (ED)

2.   direct immunoassays

3.   free T_4 index (FT_4-I).

The concentration of cord FT_4 is higher than the mean maternal value, but the difference is not statistically significant. Serum FT_4 concentrations peak at 24 h of life and then decrease slowly over the first weeks of life. Similar to T_4, serum FT_4 concentrations correlate positively with increasing gestational age and birth weight. FT_4 concentrations decrease progressively with age during childhood. Age-related values of free T_4 are presented in Table 7–7.

TABLE 7–6. Causes of Decreased Serum Thyroid Binding or Hypothyroxinemia in Pediatrics

I.	Hypothyroidism
II.	Decreased Thyroxine-Binding Proteins
	A. Thyroxine-binding globulin
	1. Androgens
	2. Anabolic steriod hormones
	3. Inherited complete or partial TBG deficiency
	4. Non-thyroidal illnesses
	5. Glucocorticoids
	B. Thyroxine-binding pre-albumin
	1. Non-thyroidal illnesses
	2. Glucocorticoids
	C. Thyroxine-binding albumin
	1. Non-thyroidal illnesses
III.	Drug-Related Inhibition of Binding
	A. Salicylates in high doses
	B. Furosemide in high doses
IV.	Illness-Related Inhibition of Binding
	A. Protein inhibitors
	B. Fatty acid inhibitor

TABLE 7–7. Age-Related Values of Free T_4 by Equilibrium Dialysis [values expressed in ng/dL (pmol/L)]

Age	Free T_4
Birth – 4 d	2.2–5.3 (28.4–68.4)
2 w – 20 w	0.9–2.2 (11.6–28.4)
21 w – 24 m	0.7–1.9 (9.0–24.5)
25 m – 20 y	0.8–2.3 (10.3–29.7)
8 y – 20 y	0.6–2.0 (7.7–25.8)

From: Nichols Institute Reference Laboratories, San Juan Capistrano, CA. Reproduced with permission.

The conventional free T_4 index (FT_4-I) is an estimate for serum FT_4. It is calculated from two test results: the total T_4-RIA and the thyroid hormone binding ratio (THBR). The THBR is a new term for the T_3 uptake test, emphasizing its distinction from T_3-RIA. The THBR provides information about the available binding sites of TBG. Normal values for age vary with the test procedure and the *individual laboratory*. THBR varies shortly after birth, but does not change significantly between 1 year of age and adulthood (see Table 7–8).

FT_4-I values at various ages calculated from total T_4 and THBR are presented in Table 7–9.

TABLE 7–8. Thyroid Hormone Binding Ratio (THBR) by Age

Age	THBR
Cord Blood (full-term)	0.70–1.11
1–3 d	0.83–1.17
1 w	0.70–1.05
1–12 m	0.70–1.05
1–3 y	0.78–1.14
3–10 y	0.75–1.18
Pubertal	0.85–1.15

From: Pediatric Endocrine Syllabus, Endocrine Sciences, Calabasas, CA. Reproduced with permission.

TABLE 7–9. Free T_4 Index (arbitrary units) Calculated from T_4 and THBR

Age	Free T_4 Index
Cord Blood (full-term)	6.0–13.2
1-3 d	9.9–17.5
1 w	7.5–15.1
1-12 m	5.0–13.0
1-3 y	5.4–12.5
3-10 y	5.7–12.8
Pubertal Children & Adults	4.2–13.0

From: Pediatric Endocrine Syllabus, Endocrine Sciences, Calabasas, CA. Reproduced with permission.

THYROGLOBULIN

Under physiological conditions, Tg can be found in low concentrations in the blood and values in cord blood are higher than the maternal values. Age-related values are presented in Table 7–10.

TABLE 7–10. Thyroglobulin (ng/mL or μg/L)

Age	Thyroglobulin
TERM INFANT	
Cord Blood	5–65
1 d	6–93
3 d	9–148
PREMATURE INFANT (27–31 w)	
1 d	107–395
10 d	49–163
30 d	17–63
PREMATURE INFANT (31–34 w)	
1 d	147–277
10 d	32–112
30 d	19–51
7–12 y	20–52
13–18 y	9–27

From: Fisher DA. The thyroid gand. In: Brook CGD, ed. Clinical paediatric endocrinology, 2nd ed. Oxford: Blackwell Scientific Publications, 1989:312.

MISCELLANEOUS THYROID TESTS

Antibodies to T_4 and T_3

On very rare occasions, patients, particularly those with Graves' disease, CLT, and non-thyroidal illnesses, may have serum antibodies to T_4 or T_3.[11] Depending on the method used, the value for T_4 may be spuriously high or low. RIA methods based on double antibody techniques will give higher values than methods using talc or charcoal to separate bound and free hormones.

Circulating antithyroid hormone autoantibodies can cause artifactual effects on RIAs for total and FT_4 and T_3 and give the clinician confusing information about a patient's thyroid status; i.e., discrepancies between physical findings and laboratory thyroid hormone tests results.[12] In this situation, the presence of autoantibodies to T_4 or T_3 should be considered. Radiobinding assays for detection of anti-T_3 and anti-T_4 autoantibodies are available from commercial laboratories.

Thyroid Antibodies

A variety of antibodies have been associated with thyroid autoimmune diseases.[13] The classic thyroid autoantibodies are directed against thyroglobulin and against thyroid cell membrane antigens. These auto-antibodies include anti-thyroglobulin (ATG) and antimicrosomal antibodies (AMA). Recent evidence indicates that AMA are directed predominantly against the membrane-bound thyroid peroxidase enzyme.[14] Antithyroid peroxidase antibodies (Anti-TPO) can be measured, and this assay is more specific than the AMA test for diagnosis of autoimmune thyroid disease.

Other antibodies of clinical importance are directed against the TSH receptor. There are a number of methods for measuring TSH receptor antibodies (TRAb). Assays for TSH receptor stimulating immunoglobulin (TSI) have been developed, and TSI is now believed to produce the hyperthyroid state in Graves' disease.[15]

In patients with Graves' disease who are to be treated with antithyroid drugs, the finding of very high serum concentrations of TSI prior to starting therapy indicates the high probability of failure of therapy. The assay is also useful in predicting those patients who will relapse at the end of the drug treatment period.

Radioactive Thyroidal Uptake and Scintiscanning

Normal values for 24 h thyroidal ^{123}I uptake vary geographically because of regional variations in dietary iodine content and therefore must be determined locally for each part of the country. This test is being used less frequently in pediatric patients because of several factors:

1. The increased intake of stable iodides through food preservatives, antiseptics, and drugs has lowered the normal range of uptake, so it may not discriminate between normal subjects and patients with hypothyroidism.

2. Although ^{123}I reduces the dose of radiation to the thyroid gland as compared with ^{125}I or ^{131}I, some tissue radiation is still present.

3. The test is time-consuming and moderately expensive.

Thyroid scintiscanning may be useful in determining the etiology of congenital hypothyroidism—i.e., ectopia or aplasia of the thyroid gland—and in the evaluation of nodules of the thyroid gland and goiters.

Ultrasonography is useful for determining thyroid size in pediatric patients and in determining the cause of diffuse goiters.[16] Data on thyroid volume in normal controls have been published. There is no significant difference in thyroid volume between boys and girls, and there is a gradual increase in volume with age.

APPLICATION OF THYROID FUNCTION TESTS TO THE MORE COMMON THYROID PROBLEMS IN PEDIATRIC PATIENTS

Hyperthyroidism

In over 90% of pediatric patients, hyperthyroidism is due to Graves' disease. Graves' disease is an autoimmune disease in which TSI bind to and stimulate the thyroid gland to secrete excessive amounts of T_4 and T_3, resulting in the clinical manifestations of thyrotoxicosis. Given a patient in whom there is clinical reason to suspect hyperthyroidism, the initial tests should include serum total T_4, total T_3, and sTSH. In almost all pediatric patients with Graves' disease, both serum T_4 and T_3 are increased and sTSH is abnormally suppressed. However, a few patients will have hyperthyroidism due to isolated increases in serum T_3 (T_3-toxicosis), and the serum T_4 is normal or even low. Measurement of T_4 and FT_3 can be used in place of total T_4 and T_3 if the clinician suspects that increased serum concentrations of thyroid hormones may be abnormally affected by the patient's serum thyroxine-binding proteins. An extremely rare cause of hyperthyroidism in pediatric patients is excessive secretion of TSH from a pituitary tumor (see causes of hyperthyroxinemia listed in Table 7–5). Radioactive iodine uptake studies and TRH testing are rarely necessary to establish a diagnosis of hyperthyroidism. TSI assay is not indicated for diagnostic purposes.

Comparison of serum test results in hyperthyroxinemic and hypothyroxinemic states is shown in Table 7–11. Hyperthyroxinemia is not synonymous with hyperthyroidism.

Very rarely, an euthyroid pediatric patient may have increased serum T_4 and/or a normal FT_4-I but normal values of sTSH. Possible causes of this combination of findings include familial dysalbuminemic hyperthyroxinemia or the presence of anti-T_4 and/or anti-T_3 antibodies. If thyrotoxicosis factita is suspected, it can be ruled out by determination of serum hTg. Since hTg is produced by the thyroid gland, its serum concentration will be decreased in thyrotoxicosis factita.

Hypothyroidism

In pediatric patients with suspected hypothyroidism, the most specific and sensitive screening test is the serum total T_4 concentration. Specificity is increased by determining the serum FT_4 or FT_4-I, thereby eliminating those patients with low serum TBG. Accuracy is improved by measuring serum sTSH. Patients with mild hypothyroidism due to *primary* hypothyroidism have increased sTSH even when the serum T_4 and FT_4 concentrations are only borderline low. However, in the presence of hypothalamic or pituitary disease causing hypothyroidism, the sTSH concentrations are low or in the normal range.

TRH testing might allow distinguishing patients with hypothalamic hypothyroidism from those with pituitary hypothyroidism. The
classic response to TRH in patients with hypothalamic hypothyroidism
is a delayed increase in serum TSH following TRH administration. In
pituitary hypothyroidism, TSH should not increase after TRH administration. However, there have been exceptions in both categories.

TABLE 7–11. Comparison of Serum Thyroid Function Tests in Hyperthyroxinemic and Hypothyroxinemic States

	T_4	Free T_4 Index	Free T4	T3	sTSH
HYPERTHYROXINEMIC STATES					
Euthyroid					
Hyperthyroxinemia					
Non-thyroidal illnesses (Euthyroid sick syndrome)	inc	inc	inc	N, dec	N
Drug-induced	inc	inc	inc	N, dec	N, inc
High TBG states	inc	N	N	inc	N
Dysalbuminemia	inc	inc	N	N	N
Generalized thyroid hormone resistance	inc	inc	inc	inc	N, inc
Hyperthyroidism	inc	inc	inc	inc	dec
HYPOTHYROXINEMIC STATES					
Non-thyroidal illnesses (Euthyroid sick syndrome)	dec	dec	N	dec	inc, N, dec
Low TBG states	dec	dec	N	N, dec	N
Primary hypothyroidism	dec	dec	dec	dec	inc
Secondary hypothyroidism	dec	dec	dec	dec	dec

inc = increased, dec = decreased, N = normal

Neonatal Screening for Hypothyroidism

The incidence of congenital hypothyroidism in non-endemic areas of
the world is approximately 1 in 4,000 live births.[17] Congenital hypothyroidism is the most common endocrine cause of infant mental retardation that is preventable with early therapy. Recent experience
indicates that large-scale, routine screening of newborns for congenital
hypothyroidism is practical and cost-effective. Filter-paper disc blood
spots are collected in the neonatal period and eluates utilized for measurement of TSH and T_4. In most screening programs in the United
States, the primary screening test is the T_4, and in those samples with
T_4 values in the lower 10%, a follow-up measurement of TSH in the

same sample is performed. All neonates with suspected hypothyroidism by screening tests require follow-up measurement of serum TSH and T_4 before a definitive diagnosis of hypothyroidism is made.

False-positive and false-negative results occur with filter-paper thyroid screening and must be followed with serum testing if indicated.[18]

NON-THYROIDAL ILLNESSES

A variety of non-thyroidal illnesses (NTI) produce alterations in thyroid function in non-hospitalized, but more frequently in hospitalized, pediatric patients in whom no intrinsic thyroid disease exists.[19] The pathologic states producing these alterations include any acute or chronic medical illness, trauma, major surgery, caloric restriction and fasting, and acute psychiatric disorders. The precise mechanism(s) responsible for the changes in thyroid hormone indices with NTI has not been elucidated.

The most common thyroid hormone abnormality in NTI is a depression in serum total T_3 and FT_3 concentrations producing the "low T_3 state." In this condition, the serum FT_4 and sTSH concentrations are normal.

A subgroup of patients with the low T_3 state may also have a low serum T_4 concentration producing the "low T_3–low T_4 state." The serum sTSH is low in this situation.

EVALUATION OF THYROID STATUS IN PATIENTS RECEIVING LEVO-THYROXINE THERAPY

Treatment of Hypothyroidism

In the patient treated for primary hypothyroidism, the correct dose of levo-thyroxine is that dose that normalizes the clinical symptoms and the serum T_4 and sTSH concentrations. Monitoring the serum sTSH concentration to be sure that it remains in the normal range will prevent over-treatment with levo-thyroxine, which is especially important in pediatric patients.[4] In patients with hypothyroidism due to hypothalamic or pituitary failure, restoration of serum T_4 to the normal range is the only laboratory blood test available for determining the appropriate replacement dose of levo-thyroxine. If a patient has a normal T_4 or FT_4 but increased sTSH, the most likely explanation is poor compliance. The patient probably ingested enough levo-thyroxine just prior to the office visit to raise the T_4 and FT_4, whereas sTSH concentrations reflect more the long-term average hormonal status.

Unsubstantiated Hypothyroidism

Pediatricians are occasionally presented with patients receiving thyroid hormone therapy for unsubstantiated hypothyroidism, in which case the question of whether the correct diagnosis was made needs to be answered. If the original diagnosis is in question, the answer can be obtained by discontinuing the hormone abruptly and measuring serum T_4 or FT_4 and sTSH 6 weeks later. Nearly all patients with primary hypothyroidism will have a low serum T_4 and increased sTSH at that time, whereas euthyroid patients will have a normal serum T_4 after a transient drop below normal. Failure to find an increased sTSH value combined with a low T_4 raises the possibility of pituitary hypothyroidism which can be investigated by a TRH test.

A variation of the above thyroid hormone withdrawal test has been devised in situations where there is a reluctance to discontinue thyroid hormone therapy completely.[20] In this test, the patient is given Liothyronine (L-triiodothyronine sodium salt) in replacement doses for 28 days. Serum T_4 is measured at the end of this time, while the patient is still receiving Liothyronine. In patients with primary or secondary hypothyroidism, serum T_4 concentrations are below 1.0 µg/dL (12.9 nmol/L). Euthyroid patients have serum T_4 concentrations above 1.2 µg/dL (15.5 nmol/L).

GOITERS

The incidence of goiters in school-age children and adolescents is approximately 4–6%. The most common cause is autoimmune chronic lymphocytic thyroiditis (CLT), or Hashimoto's thyroiditis. CLT is the single most frequent thyroid disease seen in pediatrics and is the most common cause of acquired hypothyroidism. Colloid or simple goiter is the second most common cause of euthyroid goiters in pediatric patients. The patient with CLT is usually clinically euthyroid and the goiter is completely asymptomatic.

The presence of ATG and particularly anti-TPO autoantibodies is consistent with the diagnosis of CLT. However, antithyroid antibodies may not be detected even in histologically proven cases. Serum values of T_4 and T_3 may be normal, low, or even high. Serum TSH concentrations are usually normal, but may be increased despite normal serum T_4 concentrations. Thyroid scintiscanning may show thyromegaly with asymmetrical or patchy areas of radioisotope uptake. A definite diagnosis of CLT may require fine-needle biopsy.

Almost all pediatric patients with colloid goiters are asymptomatic and euthyroid. These patients have normal thyroid function studies and no detectable serum antithyroid antibodies.

THYROID CANCER

Carcinoma of the thyroid gland is rare in pediatrics. Almost all patients are clinically euthyroid. Serum T_4, T_3, and TSH determinations are helpful in determining the functional status of the thyroid gland but are not useful in establishing a diagnosis. Serum Tg lacks specificity as a marker of thyroid cancer when used preoperatively, but is useful in detecting postoperative recurrence of differentiated thyroid carcinoma. The measurement of serum calcitonin is essential if one suspects medullary thyroid carcinoma. Patients with this tumor may have normal or elevated basal values of serum calcitonin that increase after intravenous infusion of calcium or pentagastrin.

Thyroid scintiscanning is not particularly helpful in distinguishing between benign and malignant thyroid lesions. A definitive diagnosis of malignancy can be made only by histopathologic examination.

EFFECTS OF DRUGS ON THYROID HORMONE MEASUREMENTS

Pediatricians are occasionally required to determine whether patients may have hypothyroidism or hyperthyroidism at a time when they are taking medications that alter thyroid function tests. The effects of commonly prescribed drugs on thyroid function are presented in Tables 7–3 and 7–6.

Phenytoin (Dilantin) therapy in euthyroid pediatric patients results in a decrease in serum T_4 and FT_4 values to subnormal values and either normal or slightly decreased values of serum T_3 and FT_3.[21] Serum TSH is in the normal range. Treatment of patients with carbamazepine (Tegretol)[21] and rifampin results in subnormal concentrations of FT_4.

Some drugs act predominantly by decreasing the rate of peripheral conversions of T_4 and T_3. These drugs include glucocorticoids in "stress" doses and propranolol hydrochloride in high doses. This results in decreased concentrations of serum T_3 and FT_3, normal or increased concentrations of serum T_4 and FT_4, and usually normal serum TSH concentrations. Large doses of glucocorticoids, however, may cause serum sTSH values to be suppressed and may also depress TBG and TBPA values, resulting in decreased serum concentrations of T_4 and sTSH.

Dopamine infusions in the large doses used in intensive-care units can cause decreased serum concentration of sTSH.

CLINICAL SYNDROMES OF THYROID HORMONE RESISTANCE

Several forms of incomplete resistance of thyroid hormones have been described.[22] In one variety of thyroid hormone resistance, the resistance is thought to affect only the pituitary cells. These patients have goiters and increased serum total and free T_4 and T_3. Serum TSH is secreted in supranormal quantities, and the normal negative feedback control of TSH secretion appears to be insensitive to thyroid hormones. Since the peripheral tissues respond in the normal manner, clinical hyperthyroidism is present. In these patients, the presence of a TSH-secreting pituitary adenoma should be ruled out. The serum alpha-subunit of TSH is almost always increased in the presence of a thyrotroph adenoma.

Patients with the generalized resistance form—that is, pituitary and peripheral resistance to T_4 and T_3—will present with goiters, increased serum total and free T_4 and T_3, and TSH. However, these patients are *euthyroid* or *mildly hypothyroid*.

Thyroid hormone resistance syndromes must be excluded in patients with increased serum T_4 and T_3 concentrations in order that inappropriate therapeutic measures not be initiated in an attempt to decrease the serum thyroid hormone concentrations.[23]

REFERENCES

1. Fisher DA, Polk DH. Development of the thyroid. Bailliere's Clin Endocrinol Metab 1989;3:627-57.
2. Thorpe-Beeston JG, Nicolaides KH, Felton CV et al. Maturation of the secretion of thyroid hormone and thyroid-stimulating hormone in the fetus. New Engl J Med 1991;324:532-6.
3. Rose SR, Nisula BC. Circadian variation of thyrotropin in childhood. J Clin Endocrinol Metab 1989;68:1086-90.
4. Nicoloff JT, Spencer CA. The use and misuse of the sensitive thyrotropin assay. J Clin Endocrinol Metab 1990;71:553-8.
5. Spencer CA, LoPresti JS, Patel A et al. Applications of a new chemiluminometric TSH assay to subnormal assessment. J Clin Endocrinol Metab 1990;70:453-60.
6. Nichols Institute Reference Laboratories, San Juan Capistrano, CA.
7. Cavalier RR, Pitts-River R. The effect of drugs on the distribution metabolism of thyroid hormones. Pharmacol Reviews 1981;33:55-80.
8. Pediatric Endocrine Diagnostic Syllabus, Endocrine Sciences, Calabasas, CA.
9. Fisher DA. The thyroid gland. In: Brook CGD, ed., Clinical paediatric endocrinology, 2nd ed. Oxford: Blackwell Scientific Publications 1989:313.
10. Fisher DA. The thyroid gland. In: Brook CGD, ed., Clinical paediatric endocrinology, 2nd ed. Oxford: Blackwell Scientific Publications 1989:312.
11. Sakata S, Nakamura S, Miura K. Autoantibodies against thyroid hormones or iodothyronine. Ann Int Med 1985;103:579-89.
12. Pryds O, Hadberg A, Kastrup KW. Circulating autoantibodies to thyroid hormones: A diagnostic pitfall. Acta Pediatr Scand 1987;76:685-7.
13. Bottazzo GF, Doniach D. Autoimmune thyroid disease. Ann Rev Med 1986;37:353-9.
14. Portman L, Hamada N, Heinrich G et al. Antithyroid peroxidase antibody in patients with autoimmune thyroid diseases: Possible identity with antimicrosomal antibody. J Clin Endocrinol Metab 1985;61:1001-3.
15. Zakarija M, McKenzie JM, Hoffman WH. Prediction and therapy of intrauterine and late-onset neonatal hyperthyroidism. J Clin Endocrinol Metab 1986;62:386-71.
16. Chanoine JP, Toppet V, Lagasse R, Spehl M et al. Determination of thyroid volume by ultrasound from the neonatal period to late adolescence. Eur J Pediatr 1991;150:395-9.

17. Fisher DA, Dussault JH, Foley TP et al. Screening for congenital hypothyroidism: Results of screening one million North American infants. J Pediatr 1979;94:700-5.
18. Willi SM, Moshang Jr T. Diagnostic dilemmas: Results of screening tests for congenital hypothyroidism. Pediatr Clinics N Am 1991;38:555-66.
19. Zucker AR, Chernow B, Fields AI et al. Thyroid function in critically ill children. J Pediatr 1985;107:552-4.
20. Harney BP, Stein RB, Nicoloff JT. Triiodothyronine withdrawal test. Clin Res 1974;22:117A.
21. Larkin JG, MacPhee GJS, Beastall GH et al. Thyroid hormone concentrations in epileptic patients. Eur J Clin Pharmacol 1989;36:212-16.
22. Refetoff S, Salazard A, Smith TJ et al. The consequences of inappropriate treatment due to failure to recognize the syndrome of pituitary and peripheral tissue resistance to thyroid hormone. Metabolism 1983;32:822-34.
23. Hopwood NJ, Sauder SE, Shapiro B et al. Familial partial peripheral and pituitary resistance to thyroid hormone: A frequently missed diagnosis? Pediatrics 1986;78:1114-22.

CHAPTER

8

Disorders of the Adrenal Gland

G. Michael Addison, M.A., M.B., B.Chir., M.Sc., Ph.D.

ADRENAL CORTEX

Steroid Structure and Nomenclature

The naturally occurring steroids are based on a four ring structure, the cyclopentanoperhydrophenanthrene nucleus (Figure 8–1). The nucleus is modified by the introduction of hydroxyl and carbonyl groups, aliphatic side chains, and the production of unsaturated double bonds to produce the steroid hormones. Orientation of the substituted groups is either toward the reader, α, or away, β, with the plane of the steroid nucleus in the plane of the page. A systematic nomenclature has been described for steroids by the International Union of Pure and Applied Chemistry (IUPAC),[1] but in order to facilitate usage the important steroids and metabolites have been given shorter common names (Table 8–1). It is the author's opinion that the older nomenclature wherein steroid hormones were identified by single letters should be abandoned.

Biosynthesis of Adrenal Steroids

The adrenal cortex synthesizes three classes of steroid hormones; glucocorticoids, mineralocorticoids, and androgens. Classical pathways for the synthesis of these steroids (Figure 8–2) have been established

FIGURE 8–1. Steroid Structure

The identification of the four carbon rings and the numbering of the individual carbons is shown for the basic steroid nucleus and cholestane, the nucleus of cholesterol.

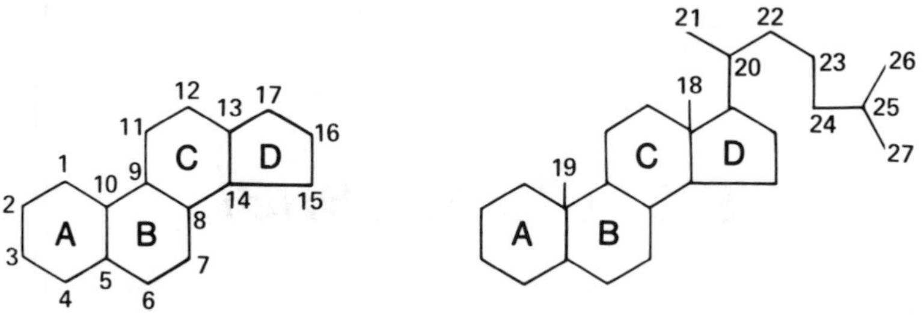

Cyclopentanoperhydrophenanthrene

Cholestane

for many years, but with the advent of the newer techniques of molecular biology there has been considerable increase in our knowledge of the enzymes involved in steroidogenesis. A brief outline is given below. Further details are available elsewhere.[2, 3]

Adrenal steroids are derived from cholesterol, which either enters the cell in the form of LDL or is possibly synthesized *in situ* from acetate. Cholesterol is converted to the C21 steroid pregnenolone with the loss of a 6-carbon side chain. This is believed to involve three steps: 20α-hydroxylation, 22-hydroxylation, and the oxidative cleavage of the C20–C22 bond. Alternative routes for the metabolism of pregnenolone exist. In the synthesis of glucocorticoids, the first step is the 17-hydroxylation to 17α-hydroxypregnenolone, which is then converted by oxidation at C3 and isomerization to 17α-progesterone (17OHP). This is

TABLE 8–1. Adrenal Steroid Nomenclature

Common Name	IUPAC Nomenclature
Cholesterol	cholest-5-en-3β-ol
Pregnenolone	3β-hydroxypregn-5-en-20-one
Progesterone	pregn-4-ene-3, 20-dione
17α-hydroxypregnenolone	3β, 17α-dihydroxypregn-5-en-20-one
17α-progesterone	17α-hydroxypregn-4-ene-3, 20-dione
11-deoxycortisol	17α, 21-dihydroxypregn-4-ene-3, 20-dione
11-deoxycorticosterone	21-hydroxypregn-4-ene-3, 20-dione
Cortisol	11β, 17, 21-trihydroxypregn-4-ene-3, 20-dione
Corticosterone	11β, 21-dihydroxypregn-4-ene-3, 20-dione
18-hydroxycorticosterone	11β, 18, 21-trihydroxypregn-4-ene-3, 20-dione
Aldosterone	11β, 21-dihydroxy-18-al-pregn-4-ene-3, 20-dione
Dehydroepiandrosterone	3β-hydroxyandrost-5-en-17-one
Androstenedione	androst-4-ene-3,17-dione

FIGURE 8–2. Pathways of Adrenal Steroid Biosynthesis

The enzymes catalyzing each step are:

1. P450scc (20,22-desmolase)
2. 3β-hydroxysteroid dehydrogenase
3. P450c17 (17α-hydroxylase)
4. P450c21 (21-hydroxylase)

5. P450c11β (11-hydroxylase)
6. P450c11β (corticosterone methyloxidase I and II)
7. P450c17 (17,20 desmolase)
8. Steroid sulphotransferase

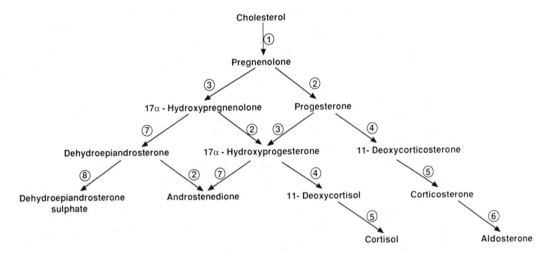

termed the Δ^5 pathway. 17OHP is further metabolized to cortisol by hydroxylations at C21 and C11.

Adrenal androgens are also derived from 17α-pregnenolone, but there is loss of the 2-carbon side chain to yield the C19 steroid dehydroepiandrosterone (DHA) before oxidation at C3 and isomerization to androstenedione. Testosterone is probably not produced in the normal adrenal gland, but adrenal androgens can be converted to testosterone by peripheral metabolism.

The mineralocorticoids do not have a hydroxyl group at C17, and synthesis proceeds via the Δ^4 pathway from pregnenolone to progesterone. Hydroxylations at C21 and C11 produce corticosterone, which is converted to aldosterone in a two-step procedure involving hydroxylation at C18 and subsequent dehydrogenation. An alternative pathway involving a second C18 hydroxylation followed by loss of a water molecule has been proposed.

Six enzymes are involved in the above pathways, four of these are cytochrome P450 oxidases (Table 8–2). The fifth, 3β-hydroxysteroid dehydrogenase:Δ^{5-4} oxosteroid isomerase (3βHSD), is a non-P450 oxidase enzyme. It is of interest that four of the enzymes—P450scc, P450c17,

P450c11β, and 3βHSD—catalyze more than one reaction. However, there appears to be only one active gene for each of the four steroidogenic cytochrome P450s which have been assigned to different chromosomes (Table 8–2). A single gene for 3βHSD has been assigned to chromosome 1, but there is some evidence for the existence of tissue-specific isoenzymes which could result from post-transcriptional or post-transactional modification. Other tissues which produce steroid hormones, including the ovary and testis, lack P450c11β and P450c21 activity and cannot produce glucocorticoids or mineralocorticoids.

The sixth enzyme is steroid sulphotransferase, which converts DHA to DHA sulphate (DHAS), which is the major adrenal androgen.

The adrenal cortex is divided into three zones, a subcapsular zona glomerulosa; the zona reticularis, next to the adrenal medulla; and separating these two, the zona fasciculata.

Functionally, the glomerulosa acts as a separate gland, producing only mineralocorticoids and in particular aldosterone. Cells of the glomerulosa lack P450c17 activity and possess the 18-dehydrogenase activity of P450c11β. Cells of the fasciculata and reticularis do not possess the 18-dehydrogenase activity of P450c11β and therefore cannot synthesize aldosterone. In the human, the function of the fasciculata and reticularis is to produce glucocorticoids and adrenal androgens respectively, although the separation of this function is not absolute.

The recent development in our knowledge of the molecular genetics of steroidogenesis, and in particular the multifunctional nature of P450c11β and P450c17, have complicated rather than simplified the understanding of steroid hormone biosynthesis.[4] It is easy to under-

TABLE 8–2. Adrenal Steroid Biosynthetic Enzymes

Enzyme	Previous Name	Cellular Localization	Chromosome	Gene	EC Number
P450scc	20,22-desmolase	Mitochondria	15q23-q24	CYP11A	1.14.15.6
3β-hydroxsteroid dehydrogenase, Δ^{5,4}-oxo-steroid isomerase	unchanged	Microsome	1p13	HSDB3	1.1.1.51 5.3.3.1
P450c17	17-hydroxylase	Microsome	10q24–q25	CYP17	1.14.99.9
P450c17	17,20-desmolase	Microsome	10q24–q25		—
P450c11β	11β-hydroxylase	Mitochondria	8q21–q22	CYP11B	1.14.15.4
P450c11β	18-hydroxylase (corticosterone methyl oxidase I)	Mitochondria	8q21–q22	CYP11B	1.14.15.5
P450c11β	18-dehydrogenase (corticosterone methyl oxidase II)	Mitochondria	8q21–q22	CYP11B	—
P450c21	21-hydroxylase	Microsome	6p21.3	CYP21	1.14.99.10
Steroid sulphotransferase	unchanged	—	—	—	2.8.2.15

stand that the gene for P450c17 is not expressed in some adrenocortical cells (glomerulosa), but as yet there is no explanation as to why all three activities of P450c11β are expressed in glomerulosa cells but only two, the 11 and 18 hydroxylase, are found in the remainder of the cortex. These questions and others have caused some scientists to question the classical pathways of steroidogenesis[5, 6] and to propose that many of the properties of the steroid biosynthetic pathways are a consequence of the physical organization of the enzymes as multifunctional units.

Control of Adrenal Steroid Biosynthesis[4, 7]

The chief regulator of adrenal glucocorticoid and androgen biosynthesis is the pituitary polypeptide ACTH. The available evidence does not support the hypothesis of an alternative androgen-stimulating hormone. ACTH has both acute and chronic effects which are the consequence of the binding of ACTH to a specific receptor on the cell surface and the resultant stimulation of the production of cyclic adenosine monophosphate (AMP). The primary acute effect is to increase binding of cholesterol to P450scc; other effects include the stimulation of the hydrolysis of cholesterol esters and enhanced transport of cholesterol into the mitochondria, probably involving the steroid carrier protein 2. The result of these effects is a rapid increase in hormone production.

The chronic effect of ACTH is to increase the synthesis of not only the steroidogenic cytochrome P450s but also associated proteins and enzymes involved in electron transfer—adrenodoxin, adrenodoxin reductase, and NADPH-cytochrome P450 reductase.

ACTH is also involved in the maintenance of adrenal cortical mass. Stimulation of the adrenal with ACTH leads to hypertrophy of cells. This action appears to be mediated by other factors, e.g., insulin-like growth factor 2 (IGF2) through a paracrine effect. Other mitogenic factors are involved with ACTH to cause hyperplasia.

ACTH release from the anterior pituitary is in turn controlled by another peptide hormone corticotrophin releasing factor (CRF). A circadian rhythm of ACTH secretion with a peak in the morning and a nadir in the late evening is paralleled by changes in plasma cortisol concentration. Superimposed on this basic rhythm, CRF and hence ACTH release can be stimulated by a large number of "stress" factors. The release of ACTH is also controlled through a negative feedback loop by plasma cortisol (glucocorticoid) concentration. Reduction of cortisol concentration for whatever reason will result in an increased release of ACTH, producing in turn the acute and chronic effects of ACTH on the adrenal and resulting in restoration of appropriate plasma cortisol concentration. If the adrenal cortex is unable to synthesize cortisol as a result of an inherited disorder of steroid biosynthesis, then the negative feedback loop will be interrupted. Prolonged effects of ACTH result in the increase of adrenocortical mass and overproduction of steroid precursors, which is termed congenital adrenal hyperplasia (CAH). If the cortex is damaged by a disease process, it may be unable to respond to increased plasma ACTH concentrations.

Aldosterone biosynthesis is controlled directly by the extracellular concentrations of sodium and potassium and also by the renin-angiotensin system. There is a feedback control loop between aldosterone and renin synthesis mediated by extracellular sodium. A decrease in ECF sodium stimulates renin release and production of angiotensin II, which in turn stimulates aldosterone synthesis and sodium retention by the renal tubules. ACTH does not appear to have a major effect on mineralocorticoid biosynthesis, at least in normals, but may be important in patients in salt-losing states.[8]

There is histological evidence that the adrenal cell is pluripotential[9] and it is possible that the life of a single adrenal cell involves migration as it ages through the glomerulosa via the fasciculata to the reticularis, where it eventually dies. In turn, it will synthesize mineralocorticoid, glucocorticoid, and adrenal androgens. It has been suggested that the vascular system of the adrenal gland can support a metabolic gradient of steroids between the various zones which can influence the cell to produce different steroid hormone, depending on its position in the cortex.

Catabolism and Excretion of Steroids[10]

Steroids are excreted principally in the urine after undergoing one or more enzymic modifications to render them more water soluble. These may include reduction, oxidation, hydroxylation, side chain cleavage, and conjugation, usually as glucuronides or sulphates. The liver is the main organ of steroid catabolism, but other tissues, including the adrenal itself, are also involved. Analysis of the products of steroid catabolism may sometimes cause diagnostic difficulties if it is not appreciated that the liver can convert Δ^5 to Δ^4 steroids, i.e., pregnenolone derivatives to progesterone derivatives.

Urine contains large numbers of steroid metabolites which used to be determined mainly based on the chemical reactions of substituted groups, e.g., 17-hydroxysteroids, oxosteroids, and oxogenic steroids, but these have largely been displaced by specific plasma assays (usually radioimmunoassays) or gas chromatographic techniques for specific metabolites. The major urinary metabolites of cortisol are given in Table 8–3.

TABLE 8–3. Urinary Steroid Metabolites of Cortisol

Metabolite	Mean Excretion (%)
Free C21 Steroids	
Cortisol	1.7
Cortisone	1.7
Conjugated C21 Steroids	
Tetrahydrocortisol	17.8
Allotetrahydrocortisol	9.5
Tetrahydrocortisone	24.1
20α-cortol	1.9
20β-cortol	4.5
20α-cortolone	11.4
20β-cortolone	8.2
Conjugated C19 Steroids	
11-oxoetiocholanolone	3.1
11β-hydroxyetiocholanolone	3.9
11β-hydroxyandrosterone	1.0
Other Neutral Steroids	11.4

Investigation of Adrenal Function

Tests of adrenal function are of two types. In the first, basal secretion of the steroids is measured using a single plasma or urine sample. Dynamic tests, on the other hand, require two or more samples and are used to test the integrity of the control mechanisms of the hypothalamic-pituitary-adrenal (HPA) axis. The use of computer-assisted imaging technology has enhanced the investigation of adrenal disorders considerably and allows a more selective use of biochemical tests in individual patients.

Several adrenal steroids, including cortisol, 17OHP, androstenedione, testosterone, and aldosterone, can be assayed in saliva. The salivary concentration of unconjugated steroids closely correlates with the plasma free steroid concentration. Saliva has been used as an alternative test in clinical situations such as the diagnosis of Cushing syndrome or adrenal hypofunction or in monitoring therapy of 21-hydroxylase deficiency CAH.[11, 12] Steroid concentration in saliva is 1–5% of plasma concentration and separate pediatric reference ranges should be established.

Basal Tests

Glucocorticoids

It should be noted that reference ranges quoted below for plasma cortisol determinations both in basal and dynamic tests usually have been derived from the now abandoned fluorometric methods. Modern radio-immunoassay methods are much more specific and give values 85–90% of those given by fluorimetry.

Plasma Cortisol. A random cortisol estimation is difficult to interpret due to the variability of cortisol excretion during the day and should be avoided if possible. Age-related quantitative data for plasma cortisol concentration in the first few weeks of life is contradictory, but there is a much wider range of cortisol concentration, particularly in neonates, and a nadir at 7 days. Diurnal rhythm and adult values are achieved by 3 months.

Urine Free Cortisol. This is a useful screening test for excess cortisol production (Cushing syndrome). An excretion of < 200 nmol/2 h in urine is found in normal children.

Mineralocorticoids

In order to test the adrenal end of the renin-aldosterone feedback loop, it is necessary to measure both aldosterone and renin. It is essential to know the plasma and urinary electrolytes and hence the patient's sodium balance in order to interpret the results. Thus, there is no simple test of mineralocorticoid production. It is, however, useful to measure renin alone in the control of the therapy of 21-hydroxylase deficiency CAH to monitor mineralocorticoid replacement.

Because renin measurements are highly method dependent, it is inappropriate to publish reference ranges which should be established in each laboratory. Both plasma renin and aldosterone fall throughout childhood, but there is insignificant correlation between them when population-based reference ranges are established.[13] Reference ranges are best constructed by measuring both hormones in the same blood sample and plotting the results on a graph. Results from patients can be assessed by plotting on the graph of normal results and assessing any disturbance of the relationship between renin and aldosterone.

Adrenal Androgens

Age-related reference ranges for the adrenal androgens androstenedione DHA and DHAS are given in Table 8–4. Unlike the glucocorticoids, concentrations of adrenal DHA and DHAS are relatively stable in blood and timing of samples is less critical. Androstenedione, on the other hand, shows considerable circadian variation.

Steroid Hormone Precursors

In certain adrenal disorders, especially steroid biosynthetic defects and adrenal tumors, large quantities of steroid precursors may be secreted

TABLE 8–4. Reference Ranges for Adrenal Steroids in Infancy, Childhood and Puberty*

Age	17α-Hydroxyprogesterone ng/100ml (nmol/L)	Dehydroepiandrosterone ng/100ml (nmol/L)		Dehydroepiandrosterone Sulphate µg/100ml (µmol/L)	Androstenedione ng/100ml (nmol/L)		Aldosterone ng/100ml (nmol/L)
	M + F	M	F	M + F	M	F	M + F
0–1 d	170–2500 (5–75)	320–1100 (11–39)	460–1200 (16–42)	15–370 (0.4–10)	15–145 (0.5–5.0)	15–175 (0.5–6.0)	
1–7 d	30–350 (1–10)	90–870 (3.0–30)	120–930 (4–32)	4–110 (0.1–3.0)	20–110 (0.7–3.8)	25–95 (0.9–3.3)	
7–28 d	0–250 (0–8.0)	45–580 (1.5–20)	90–580 (3–20)	4–33 (0.1–1.2)	25–160 (0.9–5.5)	9–90 (0.3–3.0)	
1–12 m	0–170 (0–5.0)	9.0–290 (0.3–10)	17–170 (0.6–6.0)	0.4–11 (0.01–0.3)	6–90 (0.2–3.0)	6–145 (0.2–5.0)	5.8–110 (0.16–3.0)
1–4 y	0–100 (0–3.0)	12–90 (0.4–3.0)	20–45 (0.7–1.6)	7.0–75 (0.2–2.0)	6–35 (0.2–1.2)	6–45 (0.2–1.5)	2.5–36 (0.07–1.0)
4–10 y (P1)	0–100 (0–3.0)	25–300 (0.9–10)	12–200 (0.4–7.0)	4–180 (0.1–4.8)	25–190 (0.8–3.0)	3–60 (0.1–2.0)	1–22 (0.03–0.6)
P2	0–130 (0–4.0)	50–580 (1.8–20)	60–1700 (2.0–60)	40–260 (1.0–7.0)	15–120 (0.5–4.0)	30–145 (1.0–5.0)	1.5–2.2 (0.04–0.06)
P3	30–200 (1.0–6.0)	130–640 (4.5–22)	125–1900 (4.4–65)	75–280 (2.0–7.5)	18–145 (0.6–5.0)	30–200 (1.0–7.0)	1.5–2.2 (0.04–0.06)
P4	30–230 (1.0–7.0)	190–730 (6.5–25)	170–1700 (6.0–60)	90–330 (2.5–9.0)	15–220 (0.5–7.5)	18–260 (0.6–9.0)	1.5–2.2 (0.04–0.06)
P5	30–250 (1.0–8.0)	230–730 (8.0–25)	220–810 (7.5–28)	110–440 (3.0–12.0)	40–260 (1.3–9.0)	18–260 (0.6–9.0)	1.5–2.2 (0.04–0.06)

*Note: These reference ranges are for guidance only. They have been derived from published and unpublished sources using different methodologies and varying numbers of subjects. In addition, parametric statistics frequently have been used when the data clearly are not normally distributed. Readers are advised to consult the local laboratory for more relevant reference ranges or to develop their own.

by the gland. These may be detected in blood or urine. In the latter
case, analysis by gas-liquid chromatography,[14, 15] with or without mass
spectroscopy, is required, and this is the province of specialized and
experienced laboratories.

17α-hydroxyprogesterone (17OHP)

As with cortisol, 17OHP has a marked circadian rhythm. Timing
of samples is important in infants and children but not crucial in neonates if specimens are being used for the diagnosis of 21-hydroxylase
deficiency CAH, since circadian rhythm is not yet established. Age-
related reference ranges are given in Table 8–4.

11-Deoxycortisol

The immediate precursor of cortisol, 11-deoxycortisol is increased
in 11-hydroxylase deficiency CAH. This metabolite has not been studied in depth to provide an age-related reference range. Normal concentrations in childhood are < 60 nmol/L.

Dynamic Tests

Hypothalamic-Pituitary-Adrenal (HPA) Axis

Circadian Rhythm

ACTH and cortisol secretion has a pronounced diurnal rhythm,
with a peak between 0800 and 1000 h and a nadir between 1800 and
0200 h. The circadian rhythm can be assessed by means of paired
blood specimens taken at the appropriate times. This test is not reliable immediately after hospitalization, when stress temporarily
abolishes the rhythm. Its main use is in screening patients for Cushing
syndrome, in which the circadian rhythm is lost. The relationship
between the two hormones can be assessed by measuring ACTH in the
same samples.

Dexamethasone Suppression Tests

Overnight Single Dose. This is a screening test for hypercortisolism
and is performed by giving a dose of 1 mg dexamethasone at 2400 h
and taking a blood specimen for the determination of plasma cortisol
at 0800 h. In the normal child, the morning plasma cortisol is markedly suppressed.

Low-Dose Dexamethasone. Following a basal 24 h urine collection
for urine free cortisol determination, the patient is given 5 μg/kg dexamethasone every 6 h for 48 h. A second 24 h urine collection is then

made. Diurnal plasma cortisol determinations also can be made on days 1 and 4. Failure to suppress either the urine free cortisol or the plasma cortisol establishes the diagnosis but not the etiology of Cushing syndrome.

High-Dose Dexamethasone. This test, which is rarely required in pediatric practice, is similar to the low-dose test, the difference being that the dose of dexamethasone is increased to 2 mg every 6 h. The test is used to help distinguish pituitary Cushing disease from hypercortisolism due to adrenal tumors. This distinction is more easily made by imaging.

Metyrapone Test

Metyrapone (2-methyl-1,2-bis-(3′-pyridyl)-propan-1-one) inhibits steroid 11β-hydroxylase, resulting in a decrease in the synthesis of cortisol. If the HPA axis is normal, the consequence is a reduction in the negative feedback control on ACTH synthesis and release. As a result of the increased plasma ACTH, the adrenal cortex is stimulated and there is increased secretion of the cortisol precursor 11-deoxycortisol (compound S), which can be measured in the plasma.

Standard Metyrapone Test. Oral metyrapone, 3.0 mg/m^2, is given every 4 h for 6 doses. Blood is collected 4 h after the last dose for the estimation of cortisol, 11-deoxycortisol, and ACTH. Alternatively, three 24 h urine collections for the determination of 17-oxogenic steroids should be made to include a basal day, the treatment day, and post-treatment day. A failure to respond to metyrapone could be due to a failure of pituitary reserve or adrenal response. The urinary 17-oxogenic steroid measurements will not distinguish these two, while the plasma determinations will.

Short Metyrapone Test. 30 mg/kg metyrapone is given at 2400 h and a blood specimen taken for measurement of cortisol, 11-deoxycortisol, and ACTH at 0800 h.

Insulin Hypoglycemia (Stress) Test

Hypoglycemia produced as a response to intravenous insulin is a potent stress stimulus for the release of ACTH. It is often used to test the secretion of growth hormone simultaneously. The normal dose of soluble insulin, 0.1–0.15 U/kg, should be reduced to 0.05 U/kg if ACTH deficiency is strongly suspected. *Precautions must be taken to ensure immediate treatment is available should a severe response to insulin occur.* For HPA axis assessment, samples are taken at 0 (fasting), 15, 30, 60, and 120 min for glucose and cortisol. ACTH can also be measured at these times. For an adequate test, the blood glucose should fall to < 2.2 mmol/L. Plasma cortisol should rise at least 250 nmol/L and a peak should exceed 550 nmol/L in a normal response.

ACTH Stimulation Tests

These tests are used to examine the ability of the adrenal cortex to respond to stimuli, or occasionally to help differentiate steroid biosynthetic defects by increasing the total or exaggerating the relative production of steroid precursors.

Short ACTH Test. A basal blood specimen is followed by administration of 250 µg/m^2 Synacthen® (1-24 ACTH), either intramuscularly or intravenously. Further blood specimens are taken at 30 and 60 min for the measurement of cortisol. A rise of plasma cortisol by at least 250 nmol/L and a peak value of > 550 nmol/L indicates a normal response. An insufficient response may be due to either primary adrenal disease or prolonged absence of endogenous ACTH stimulation of the gland.

17OHP can be measured using this test in the evaluation of 21-hydroxylase deficiency. This is especially useful if the patient has been started on therapy as a consequence of a clinical diagnosis or in the evaluation of heterozygotes or patients with late-onset CAH.

Long ACTH Test. Following a baseline cortisol estimation, an oral dose of 1 mg Synacthen® is given daily for 3 days. A second blood specimen is taken 6 h after the third dose. In normals and patients with secondary adrenal deficiency, there will be a rise of at least three times the basal value to a peak of > 800 nmol/L. In primary adrenal disease, the response to the prolonged administration of Synacthen® is suppressed.

Mineralocorticoids

As mentioned above, the close interrelationship between aldosterone and renin requires that both be measured simultaneously in the investigation of disorders of mineralocorticoid production. In addition, testing requires knowledge and manipulation of the electrolyte status of the patient.

Salt (Sodium) Restriction

DAY 1: Measure baseline plasma electrolytes, aldosterone, and renin. Collect 24 h urine for electrolytes and creatinine.

DAYS 2-6: Administer a low-sodium diet, 10–20 mmol/d; collect 24 h urines on days 5 and 6 for electrolytes and creatinine.

DAY 6: Collect plasma for electrolytes, aldosterone, and renin after the patient has been erect for 1 h.

In normal subjects, the urine sodium excretion will fall to < 20 mmol/l and the plasma renin and aldosterone will rise by a factor of three.

Diseases of the Adrenal Cortex

Classification of adrenocortical disorders is complex. In Tables 8–5 and 8–6, an initial separation into primary and secondary disorders has been made, with subsequent divisions based on whether the disease produces under- or over-function of the gland. The steroid hormones can be looked at individually under each of the headings, but it should

TABLE 8–5. Classification of Pediatric Primary Adrenocortical Disorders

Adrenocortical Hyperfunction	Adrenocortical Hypofunction
Glucocorticoid excess	Glucocorticoid deficiency
Adrenal adenoma	Steroid biosynthetic defects:
Adrenal carcinoma (iatrogenic)	21-hydroxylase deficiency
Mineralocorticoid excess	17α-hydroxylase deficiency
Adrenal glomerulosa adenoma (Conn syndrome)	11β-hydroxylase deficiency
Adrenocortical nodular hyperplasia	Congenital unreponsiveness to ACTH
Steroid biosynthetic defects:	Mineralocorticoid deficiency
17α-hydroxylase deficiency	Steroid biosynthetic defects
11β-hydroxylase deficiency	Corticosterone methyl oxidase deficiency
Adrenal tumors secreting deoxycorticosterone	(CMOD) type I and II
or corticosterone	Adrenal androgen deficiency
Dexamethasone suppressible hyperaldosteronism	Steroid biosynthetic defect
Adrenal androgen excess	17, 20-desmolase deficiency
Adrenal adenoma	Delayed adrenarche
Adrenal carcinoma	Mixed adrenal steroid deficiency
Steroid biosynthetic defects	Steroid biosynthetic defects
21-hydroxylase deficiency	20, 22 desmolase deficiency
11β-hydroxylase deficiency	3β-hydroxysteroid dehydrogenase
Mixed adrenal hormone excess	deficiency
Adrenal tumors	21-hydroxylase deficiency
	Combined 17α-hydroxylase and
	17, 20-desmolase deficiency
	Congenital adrenal hypoplasia
	Adrenoleukodystrophy
	Wolman disease
	Adrenal crisis of acute infection
	(Waterhouse-Friderichsen syndrome)
	Autoimmune adrenal disease

TABLE 8–6. Classification of Pediatric Secondary Adrenocortical Disorders

Adrenocortical Hypofunction	Adrenocortical Hyperfunction
Hypopituitarism	Pituitary tumors
Isolated ACTH deficiency	Ectopic ACTH secreting tumors
Hypothalamic defect	Hyperaldosteronism secondary to renal disease
Intracranial tumors, craniopharyngioma	Pseudohyperaldosteronism
Adrenal suppression as a consequence of glucocorticoid therapy	
Following removal of unilateral adrenal tumor	
Steroid therapy in mothers during pregnancy	

be emphasized that, particularly with inborn errors of steroid biosynthesis, deficiency of one steroid hormone is not infrequently associated with deficiency or excess of another.

Many of the conditions listed in Tables 8–5 and 8–6 are extremely rare. The most common primary disorders are 21-hydroxylase deficiency CAH and adrenal tumors, while the most common secondary disorders are adrenal hypofunction resulting from steroid therapy and hypopituitarism. Adrenocortical disease should be suspected in any child with unexplained disturbances of electrolyte metabolism and in abnormalities of sexual maturation.

21-Hydroxylase Deficiency CAH

CAH due to a deficiency of 21-hydroxylase is the most common inborn error of adrenal steroid biosynthesis. It manifests itself in four clinical forms: salt loss, prenatal virilization of females, precocious sexual development in late infancy and childhood, and a late-onset or nonclassical form. The first three are usually diagnosed in infancy or childhood, but rare cases are found among adults. Approximately two-thirds are salt wasting. Non-classical CAH usually presents in females in adolescence or adulthood with signs of androgen excess. The prevalence of the infantile forms is approximately 1:7000 to 1:12,000 births. Rarely, a very high prevalence occurs in closed ethnic groups, e.g., 1:500 found in Yupik Inuits in Alaska. On the other hand, the prevalence of non-classical CAH is much higher, at 1:100 in Caucasian populations and 1:30 in Ashkenazi Jews.

All types of 21-hydroxylase deficiency are due to defects of the CYP21 gene (previously called CYP21B) on chromosome 6. This is one of a pair of reduplicated genes. The second, CYP21P (previously known as CYP21A), is a highly homologous but nonfunctional pseudogene. The two genes are situated in the class III region of the HLA complex, and each is closely linked to two complement genes, C4A and C4B respectively (Figure 8–3). The reduplication facilitates unequal cross-over at meiosis, with the possibility of total loss of the functional CYP21 gene or its conversion by a combination of variable quantities of DNA from CYP21 and CYP21P to a gene which is not capable of producing native enzyme. Point mutations can also occur.

The complex molecular pathology of 21-hydroxylase deficiency[16] has helped in part to explain the different clinical manifestations of the disease. Patients who are homozygous for CYP21 gene deletions or large-scale gene conversions or compound heterozygotes for both major gene defects usually are found to have salt wasting. On the other hand, point mutations on one chromosome associated with mild or severe alleles on the other chromosome also have been associated with classical salt wasting CAH. Simple virilizing 21-hydroxylase deficient patients with both CYP21 alleles severely affected have not been described so far, and the mutations associated with this variety of 21-hydroxylase deficiency have not been identified. Non-classical CAH has been associated with a G to T (val to leu) mutation.

While it is interesting to try to link the different clinical presentations of 21-hydroxylase deficiency to specific genetic abnormalities, it should be noted that families with affected siblings, presumably with

FIGURE 8–3. Map of Human Chromosome 6

The 21-hydroxylase gene is shown within the class III HLA cluster. The active gene 21 and pseudogene 21P are shown in relationship to the two reduplicated complement genes, C4B and C4A.

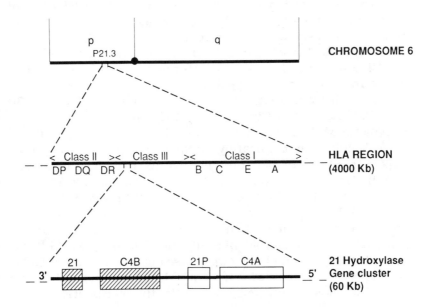

the same genetic defects, can have different clinical phenotypes. It is therefore probable that the phenotypic variability of 21-hydroxylase deficiency is due in part to other factors. There is some evidence that 21-hydroxylase (P450c21) exists in heterogeneous forms with different substrate specificities, at least in the bovine adrenal.[17] This heterogeneity may result from post-transitional modification, e.g., differential gene splicing or alteration in sialic acid content or phosphorylation. Thus, the question of relating genotype to phenotype in 21-hydroxylase deficient CAH remains to be resolved.

Of great interest is the recent observation of aldosterone production in patients homozygous for CYP21 deletion or with one allele being deleted and the other coding for a nonfunctional protein. Although extra adrenal 21-hydroxylation cannot be ruled out entirely, evidence points to another enzyme in the adrenal gland with 21-hydroxylase activity, possibly induced by high levels of precursors.[18]

Diagnosis

21-hydroxylase deficiency should be suspected in patients with any of the clinical presentations described above. In salt-losing states or in patients with ambiguous genitalia, diagnosis is urgent. The use of urinary pregnanetriol estimation has been abandoned in favor or the measurement of plasma 17OHP concentrations by immunoassay. In infantile forms, the concentration of 17OHP is normally greatly increased, but patients with non-classical CAH may have basal plasma 17OHP within the normal range. Heterozygotes for severe forms of 21-hydroxylase deficiency may have elevated basal 17OHP concentrations. Differentiation of these groups can be aided by using a short ACTH stimulation test, with measurement of 17OHP, cortisol, and 11-deoxycortisol. Non-classical CAH patients will have an increase of 17OHP > 40 nmol/L (normals < 15 nmol/L) at 30 min. Differentiation of heterozygotes is accomplished by the use of 17OHP : deoxycortisol ratios which are increased above the normal value of < 12 at 30 min.

The finding of an increased 17OHP concentration is not confined to patients with 21-hydroxylase deficiency. They are frequently found in sick full-term or healthy premature infants who may also be hyponatremic, and therefore give rise to diagnostic confusion.[19, 20] It may be necessary to do several 17OHP estimations and also a short ACTH test to help diagnosis. Patients with 21-hydroxylase deficiency may have basal plasma cortisol within the normal range and some increase on ACTH stimulation. In addition, increased 17OHP has been reported in other steroid biosynthetic defects, e.g., 11β–hydroxylase and 3β-hydroxysteroid dehydrogenase defects. The findings have led to the reports of combined 11β- and 21-hydroxylase deficiencies. However, the most likely explanation is the peripheral metabolism of steroid precursors, e.g., 17-hydroxypregnenolone to 17OHP ($\Delta^5 \rightarrow \Delta^4$). GLC of urine steroid metabolites may help resolve these problems.

Screening[21]

Following the development of 17OHP assays from dried blood spots,[22] neonatal screening programs for the early detection of 21-hydroxylase deficiency have been established successfully in North America, Europe, and Japan. Since salt-wasting infants usually present with life-threatening salt-losing crises in the second week of life, the timing of screening is critical and must be early enough to allow detection before onset of symptoms. There are problems with cross-reacting steroids in neonatal blood which may give a false-positive test, and also increased concentrations of 17OHP are found in premature and low-birth-weight infants. Screening for 21-hydroxylase deficiency, although practical, remains an area of controversy and has not been universally adopted.[23, 24]

Prenatal Diagnosis and Treatment

Since the masculinization of female fetuses occurs in the latter part of the first trimester of intrauterine life, early identification of fetuses at risk and treatment with dexamethasone has been attempted in order to prevent these changes.[25, 26] Infants are identified as female by chromosome analysis and as affected by the use of a combination of amniotic fluid 17OHP concentrations and HLA typing of amniotic cells, or by DNA analysis using chorionic villus sampling.

The results of this approach in infants at risk have been the absence of virilization in a third, minor or partial virilization in a further third, and severe virilization in the remaining third. It has been suggested that the results could be improved by starting treatment as early as possible in pregnancy, even pre-conception, and stopping treatment if the fetus is found to be male or unaffected. The effectiveness of dexamethasone in suppressing the fetal adrenal can be assessed by measuring maternal urinary estriol, which is derived from fetal dehydroepiandrosterone by placental metabolism.

11β-Hydroxylase Deficiency

11β-hydroxylase deficiency is the second most common inborn error of steroid biosynthesis but accounts for only 5–15% of cases.[27] Presentation is similar to 21-hydroxylase deficiency, but hypertension is also present in the majority of cases. Patients may have hypoglycemia and alkalosis. Biochemical diagnosis is established by finding an increased plasma deoxycortisol concentration or a raised urinary excretion of tetrahydro-deoxycortisol.

Clinical variants of 11β-hydroxylase deficiency have been described.[28] In the severe form, it appears that 11β-hydroxylation of both 17-hydroxy and 17-deoxysteroids is affected, while in milder forms only 11β-hydroxylation of 17-hydroxysteroids is reduced.

The cause of the hypertension in these patients is unclear. The suggestion that it is caused by the increased plasma concentration of deoxycorticosterone does not fit clinical findings of normotensive patients with high concentrations or severe hypertension in patients with only mild increases of plasma deoxycorticosterone. An alternative suggestion is that the steroid causing hypertension could be 18-hydroxy,11-deoxycorticosterone because of the multiple activities of cytochrome P45011β.

3β-Hydroxysteroid Dehydrogenase, Δ⁵⁻⁴ Oxosteroid Isomerase Deficiency

3β-hydroxysteroid dehydrogenase, $\Delta^{5\text{-}4}$ oxosteroid isomerase (3βHSD) is found also in ovary, testis, liver, and brain. Deficiencies of all groups of steroids are found in patients with 3βHSD deficiency, but because the enzyme is present in the gonads and is required for androgen biosynthesis, ambiguous genitalia can be found in both males and females.

The classical form of 3βHSD deficiency is associated with salt loss which is usually severe, but mild and non-salt-losers have been described. The condition does not always present with the same severity in families. A non-classical form of 3βHSD has been described which presents in females with premature adrenarche, oligomenorrhea, and/or hirsutism; it is reported to be present in 15% of hirsute women.

Diagnosis is made by measuring the Δ^5 steroids 17α-hydroxy-pregnenolone and pregnenolone in plasma, or by estimating the $\Delta^{5:}\Delta^4$ ratio of steroid metabolites in urine.

Inborn Errors of Aldosterone Biosynthesis

Two types of aldosterone biosynthetic defect have been described, corticosterone methyloxidase deficiency types I and II (CMOD I and II). Almost all patients described have had CMOD II. Presentation is usually with failure to thrive, dehydration, hyponatremia, and hypokalemia. Older children may have failure to grow and/or postural hypotension, and affected siblings have been described without symptoms.

Diagnosis depends on elimination of other causes of hyponatremia associated with salt wasting. Biochemical diagnosis requires the measurement of plasma aldosterone and renin; aldosterone is normal or low in the presence of a high renin concentration. Measurement of urinary aldosterone, metabolites of aldosterone and its precursors, deoxycorticosterone and corticosterone, and their 18-hydroxyl derivatives help differentiate the condition from pseudohypoaldosteronism.[29]

Steroid-Producing Adrenal Tumors

Adrenal tumors producing steroids are very rare. Approximately 5% of all pediatric adrenal tumors arise in the cortex, and the incidence is between 0.1 and $0.4/10^6$/year. There is an increased incidence in early childhood, and female-to-male ratios between 2 : 1 and 5 : 1 have been reported. Adrenocortical carcinomas are said to be more common than carcinoma,[30] but this has been disputed.[31]

The clinical presentation of adrenal tumors in children is predominantly one of precocious puberty and/or virilization. This may be associated with signs of hypercortisolism (Cushing syndrome), or even occasionally feminization. Aldosterone secreting tumors and asymptomatic (non-hormone producing) tumors are very rare but form a higher proportion of adrenal tumors in adults.

The role of the biochemistry laboratory in establishing the diagnosis of adrenal tumor has been modified considerably by modern computerized imaging techniques. However, there remains the problem of differentiating benign adenomata from malignant carcinomas, which is sometimes difficult even with histology. Measurement of plasma and urinary steroids and responses to trophic hormones and suppression tests have all been used. Because of the rarity of the tumors, large series take many years to collect, during which testing procedures and methodologies change; hence, it becomes difficult to evaluate the most useful biochemical markers. In addition, certain techniques such as GLC involve hydrolysis of conjugates before analysis, complicating comparisons with RIA techniques which measure conjugates such as dehydroepiandrosterone sulphate (DHAS).

Serum hormone measurements are claimed to have advantages over urine, but the difficulties of obtaining suitable urine collections from children are overemphasized and it is a non-invasive technique. In addition, GLC of urinary steroid metabolites allows the detection of unusual steroids which may be useful markers both in diagnosis and in monitoring treatment.

Two major patterns of steroid secretion have been observed in pediatric virilizing adrenal tumors.[32] In the first of these, urinary ketosteroid excretion is high (> 50 μmol/24h), serum testosterone is markedly raised for age, and the principal steroid produced is dehydroepiandrosterone (DHA). In the second major pattern, urinary ketosteroid excretion is lower (< 20 μmol/24h), serum testosterone is moderately raised, and the major steroid produced is 11βhydroxyandrosterone. Both patterns can be associated with either adenoma or carcinoma, although carcinoma is more frequent and the prognosis worse in the group producing DHA. However, the overall prognosis of adrenal tumors in children is relatively good following surgery.

Tumors detected in early infancy are sometimes associated with increased excretion of 16-oxygenated-3β-hydroxyl-5-ene steroids, which are produced normally in the neonatal period. These tumors lack 3βHSD activity.

Cushing Syndrome in Children

Accurate figures on the incidence of Cushing syndrome in children are not available, but it is of the same order as that for adrenal tumors. It should be noted that many patients diagnosed as having Cushing syndrome in adult life have symptoms that began in childhood. The differential diagnosis of Cushing syndrome from simple obesity and iatrogenic Cushing syndrome from the therapeutic use of exogenous steroids are common pediatric problems.

Cushing syndrome may result from overproduction of ACTH as a consequence of hypothalamic-pituitary disease (Cushing disease) or from ectopic ACTH secretion from non-adrenal tumors. As a consequence of the increased circulating ACTH, the patients have bilateral adrenal hyperplasia. Approximately 50% of all pediatric cases of Cushing syndrome are ACTH dependent, the majority of these being in the older age group. The remaining cases are ACTH independent and are caused by adrenal adenomas or carcinomas. Rare syndromes causing ACTH independent disease are primary adrenal micronodular dysplasia (PAND) and McCune-Albright syndrome.

The biochemical diagnosis of Cushing syndrome is relatively simple. The most useful initial screening tests are the 24 h urine free cortisol excretion[33] or the overnight dexamethasone test. Urine free cortisol can be raised in the very obese. If these tests give borderline or increased values, a low-dose dexamethasone test will separate patients whose cortisol is raised for reasons of stress, in whom the plasma or urinary cortisol will be normalized.

The differential diagnosis of the various etiologies of Cushing syndrome requires the measurement of plasma ACTH concentration, performance of the high-dose dexamethasone suppression test, and the results of imaging procedures of the pituitary and adrenal areas. Unmeasurable plasma ACTH is diagnostic of primary adrenal disease, usually a tumor. However, ACTH within the "normal range" may be caused by Cushing disease or ectopic ACTH. It should be remembered that ACTH is normally suppressed by increased cortisol production; therefore, even though the ACTH concentration falls within the normal range, it is, in fact, inappropriately increased. Imaging may resolve the problem, but selective venous sampling and the establishment of the presence of an ACTH gradient may be required. High plasma ACTH concentration is usually associated with ectopic ACTH. The high-dose dexamethasone suppression test can give both positive and negative results in either pituitary or adrenal Cushing syndrome.

The other tests previously used in the diagnosis of Cushing syndrome—diurnal rhythm of plasma cortisol, insulin tolerance test, and metyrapone test—are almost certainly no longer of value.

Adrenocortical Hypofunction

Decreased production of one or more of the adrenal steroid hormones may be caused by one of a large heterogeneous group of conditions.[34] (See Tables 8-5 and 8-6.) These may be primary disease of the adrenal glands or be secondary resulting from either decreased stimulation by ACTH or renin as a consequence of hypothalamic-pituitary disease or renal disease, respectively.

The predominant etiologies of the adrenal hypofunction vary according to age. In the neonate and in early infancy, steroid biosynthetic defects, sporadic or familial congenital adrenal hypoplasia, panhypopituitarism, and maternal steroid therapy are the major causes. In later infancy and childhood, iatrogenic adrenal suppression as a result of glucocorticoid therapy is by far the major cause, with inborn errors of steroid biosynthesis, autoimmune adrenal disease, adrenoleukodystrophy (peroxisomal disease), and hypopituitarism also contributing to cases of adrenal hypofunction. Acute destruction of the adrenal gland in fulminating infection (Waterhouse-Friderichsen syndrome) is found at any age.

The biochemical diagnosis of adrenocortical hypofunction is established by use of tests of basal steroid hormone excretion, of the intactness of the HPA axis, and by the response of the adrenal to the stimulus of exogenous ACTH. The measurement of plasma ACTH is extremely helpful in distinguishing primary from secondary adrenal failure. Diurnal rhythm of ACTH and cortisol secretion is often maintained in primary or secondary disease and is not a useful test. The insulin stress test should be used with great caution in the diagnosis of adrenal failure if there is a danger of severe hypoglycemia, and in most cases of severe hypoadrenalism the short ACTH test can be adequately substituted.[35]

One of the most common but difficult biochemical problems associated with the assessment of adrenal hypofunction is the testing of the status of the HPA axis prior to or after withdrawal of glucocorticoid therapy. The question being asked is whether or not the HPA axis can respond to natural stress conditions—e.g., infection or trauma—to produce appropriate quantities of cortisol. A normal response to pharmacological tests such as insulin hypoglycemia or ACTH stimulation tests may not accurately reflect the true status of the HPA axis and the ability of the patient to respond to stress with an adequate secretion of cortisol. The metyrapone test may be more useful in these circumstances, but 11-deoxycortisol assays are not readily available. Recently, a new low-dose ACTH test using 1 μg 1–24 ACTH has been described which is claimed to be useful in assessing responsiveness in patients currently taking steroids.[36] It may be that the use of adrenal responses to different amounts of ACTH will be the most suitable test of adrenal hypofunction, but this has not yet been validated in children.

ADRENAL MEDULLA

The adrenal medulla has a different embryological derivation from the adrenal cortex and is normally considered as separate in terms of biochemistry, physiology, and pathology. However, there exist strong interrelationships between the adrenal cortex and medulla.[37] This is most obvious when considering response to stress: both cortisol and epinephrine (adrenaline) are released in response to stressful stimuli, and there is well recognized modulation of tissue sensitivity to epinephrine by cortisol. There is also some evidence for reciprocal cooperation between steroid and catecholamine synthesis.

The pathology of the adrenal medulla consists essentially of two disorders, both tumors: neuroblastoma and pheochromocytoma. The diagnosis of these conditions depends heavily on the measurement of catecholamines and their metabolites.

Catecholamine Biosynthesis

The adrenal medulla produces two principal catecholamines, norepinephrine (noradrenaline) and its methylated derivative, epinephrine, in the ratio 1:9. These are produced from the amino acid tyrosine by a series of enzymatic steps (Figure 8–4). Tyrosine hydroxylase converts tyrosine to dihydroxyphenylalanine (DOPA), which is then metabolized to the physiologically active metabolite dopamine through the action of DOPA-decarboxylase. Norepinephrine and epinephrine are produced from dopamine by the sequential action of dopamine β-hydroxylase and phenylalanine N-methyl transferase (PMNT), respectively.

The formation of DOPA takes place in the mitochondria, where activity of the rate-limiting enzyme tyrosine hydroxylase is regulated by ACTH and by feedback inhibition from epinephrine and norepinephrine. Synthesis of dopamine and epinephrine occurs in the cytoplasm, but dopamine β-hydroxylase activity is found in chromaffin

FIGURE 8–4. Biosynthesis of Catecholamines

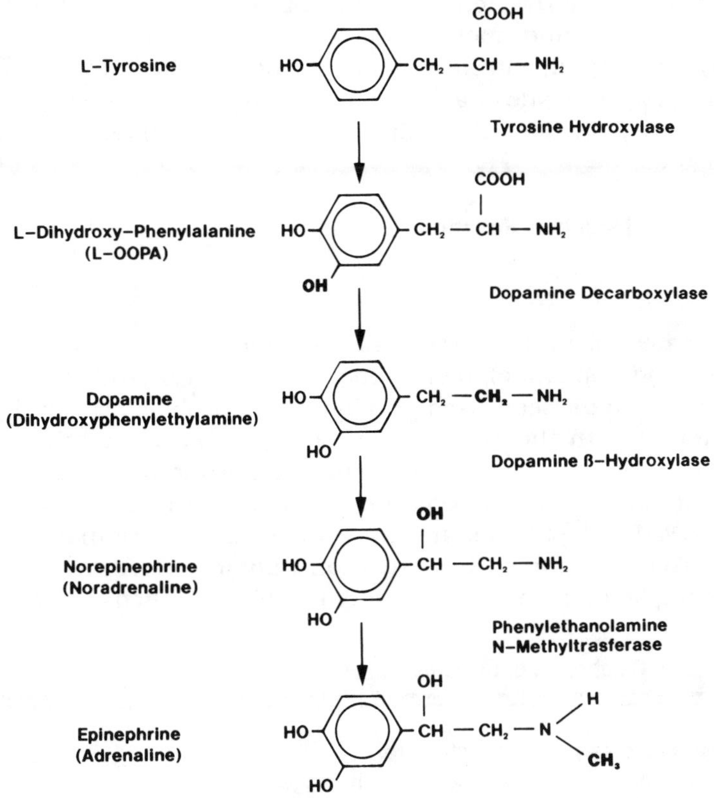

L–Tyrosine — $HO-\bigcirc-CH_2-\underset{|}{\overset{COOH}{CH}}-NH_2$

Tyrosine Hydroxylase

L–Dihydroxy–Phenylalanine (L–OOPA) — $HO-\bigcirc-CH_2-\underset{|}{\overset{COOH}{CH}}-NH_2$ (OH)

Dopamine Decarboxylase

Dopamine (Dihydroxyphenylethylamine) — $HO-\bigcirc-CH_2-CH_2-NH_2$ (HO)

Dopamine ß–Hydroxylase

Norepinephrine (Noradrenaline) — $HO-\bigcirc-\underset{|}{\overset{OH}{CH}}-CH_2-NH_2$ (HO)

Phenylethanolamine N–Methyltrasferase

Epinephrine (Adrenaline) — $HO-\bigcirc-\underset{|}{\overset{OH}{CH}}-CH_2-N\underset{CH_3}{\overset{H}{<}}$ (HO)

storage granules. Conversion of norepinephrine to epinephrine is sensitive to local corticosteroid concentrations. Catecholamine synthesis also occurs in the autonomic nervous system and in the brain, although the balance of the different bioactive catecholamines synthesized differs in these tissues.

Catecholamine Metabolism

In catecholamine catabolism (Figure 8–5), a considerable number of closely related metabolites are produced from DOPA, dopamine, norepinephrine, and epinephrine.[38] The important ones from the clinical laboratory diagnostic point of view are the metanephrines, normetanephrine and metanephrine, produced from norepinephrine and epinephrine respectively and usually measured as total metanephrines; homovanillic acid (HVA, 4-hydroxy-3-methoxy-phenylacetic acid), produced from dopamine; and 4-hydroxy-3-methoxy-mandelic acid (HMMA), also known as vanillylmandelic acid (VMA), produced from dopamine, norepinephrine, and epinephrine. These metabolites are produced by the action of two enzymes, catechol-O-methyl transferase (COMT) and monoamine oxidase (MAO). Both enzymes are widely distributed, with high concentrations in liver, brain, and sympathetic nervous tissue. Catecholamines and their O-methylated derivatives are excreted in the urine, partly as sulphate and glucuronide conjugates.

Investigation of Adrenal Medullary Function

Urine

Total catecholamines, free catecholamines (norepinephrine, epinephrine, and dopamine), metadrenalines, and HVA and HMMA excretion in urine have all been used to diagnose neuroblastoma and pheochromocytoma. With the development of HPLC and electrochemical detectors, the group assays (total catecholamines and metadrenalines) are of reduced usefulness in pediatric practice; with very rare exceptions, HVA, HMMA, dopamine, and norepinephrine determinations are sufficient. Total metadrenaline excretion remains useful as a preliminary screening test for pheochromocytoma. HPLC methods, as well as allow-

FIGURE 8–5. Catabolism of Catecholamines

The enzymes catalyzing each step are:
1. Monoamine oxidase and aldehyde dehydrogenase
2. Catechol-O-methyl transferase

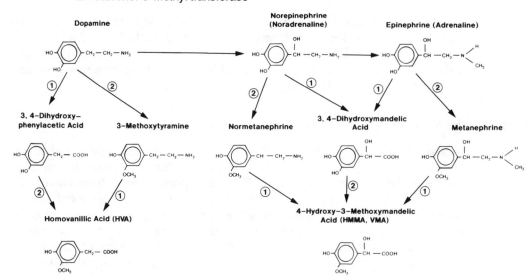

ing more specific differentiation of the individual catecholamines, overcome almost all the problems of interferences from drugs and dietary substances which caused serious problems with the older chemical methods.

For a long time, diagnosis has rested on the use of 24 h urine collections, with results expressed either as absolute quantity excreted per day or as a ratio to the amount of creatinine excreted. Because of the real but overemphasized problems of collecting 24 h urine specimens, particularly from very young children, a number of groups have used random urine collections[39] and expressed results as creatinine ratios. Available information on sensitivity and specificity of random urine collections is sparse. However, there is some indication that this technique could miss smaller tumors unless several specimens are analyzed.[40] Both adrenal catecholamine secretion and renal creatinine excretion have circadian rhythms, and to be more useful there is a need to standardize the time of the random urine collection.

Because of the instability of some of the catecholamines and metabolites at neutral pH, urines must be acidified to pH 1 immediately after voiding. HVA and VMA appear to be stable in unacidified urine when collected onto filter paper for population screening (see discussion below). Additional precautions to be taken before urine collection include the avoidance of stressful procedures such as surgery, which will give rise to a physiological increase in catecholamine excretion.

The urine excretion of catecholamines and metabolites is age related even when corrected for creatinine, and reference ranges quoted in the literature for the same or different methods vary widely. It is therefore important, as for the adrenal steroids, for each laboratory to establish and use its own reference range relevant to the techniques used. Selection of the control group should be done with care; healthy children may not be the most appropriate, and the use of hospitalized or ill patients should be considered.[41] Seasonal variation in catecholamine excretion has been reported, but this has not proven to be a practical problem.

Reference ranges derived in our laboratory using HPLC and electrochemical detection from 24 h collections from hospitalized patients are given in Table 8–7.

The measurement of total HVA—i.e., free plus conjugated HVA—has been proposed as a useful alternative investigation when the free urinary HVA is borderline.[42] However, the alternative measurement of dopamine and/or noradrenaline was not considered in these patients.

Plasma

As an alternative to urine collections, the measurement of epinephrine, norepinephrine, dopamine, and metabolites, both free and conjugated, has been used. The advantages are that there is no requirement for

TABLE 8–7. Reference Ranges for Catecholamines and Their Metabolites*

AGE	UPPER LIMIT** OF NORMAL EXCRETION mmol/mol creatinine (μg/mg creatinine)			
	Norepinephrine	Dopamine	HMMA (VMA)	HVA
<1 year	0.25 (0.37)	1.8 (2.4)	15.0 (26.3)	22.0 (35.5)
1–2 years	0.20 (0.30)	1.5 (2.0)	12.0 (21.1)	17.0 (27.4)
3–4 years	0.15 (0.22)	0.9 (1.22)	8.0 (14.0)	15.0 (24.2)
5–9 years	0.14 (0.21)	0.8 (1.08)	7.0 (12.3)	10.0 (16.1)
10–15 years	0.11 (0.16)	0.7 (0.95)	7.0 (12.3)	7.0 (11.3)

*NOTE: These reference ranges were derived from urines collected over 18–24 hours into sufficient acid to reduce pH to below 3.0. The reference population consisted of patients in whom an adrenal medullary tumor was suspected, but whose final diagnosis excluded neuroblastoma or pheochromocytoma. Analysis was by HPLC with electrochemical detection.
**The upper limit of normal is defined as the 0.95 fractile, determined using non-parametric methods.

24 h collections; that interferences from drugs are reduced; that the measurements are suitable for monitoring catecholamine secretion in response to stimuli, i.e., in dynamic tests; and that plasma can be used in anuric patients. Against these, however, are several major disadvantages: lack of stability of catecholamines in plasma, requiring special handling procedures; lower concentrations, requiring more sensitive assays; and single-point estimations of fluctuating concentrations are obtained, rather than the integrated values obtained using timed urines. In addition, plasma catecholamine concentration is affected by a number of physiological variables, including age, circadian rhythms, exercise, posture, temperature, feeding, stress, and electrolyte balance, as well as pathological conditions such as heart disease, diabetes, hypertension, etc.[43] This means that plasma catecholamine determinations should be performed under carefully controlled and standardized conditions.

Information on age-related pediatric reference ranges for plasma catecholamines is very limited, and only very small numbers of subjects have been studied.[44] What information is available suggests that plasma free epinephrine and norepinephrine are raised in infants under 2 years of age. In studies using mass fragmentography of much larger numbers of subjects, an exponential decline of plasma HMMA and HVA concentrations was shown throughout childhood, with changes in concentration of 40X and 5X for HVA and HMMA respectively between the first day of life the late teens.[45]

Pheochromocytoma

Pheochromocytomas are very rare catecholamine-secreting tumors arising from the adrenal medulla or less commonly from extra-adrenal chromaffin tissue. Patients frequently present with headache, and on examination are found to be hypertensive; alternative presenting symptoms include profuse sweating and diarrhea. Some patients are asymptomatic but are found to be hypertensive on routine health examinations. Approximately 1% of children with hypertension have pheochromocytoma,[46] although it is probable, as with adrenocortical tumors, that a number of patients who present with pheochromocytoma in adulthood have had symptoms beginning in childhood.

Tumors are found more frequently in boys (M:F ratio 1.8 : 1), and 35–40% are single tumors of the adrenal medulla. Twenty percent of children have bilateral adrenal tumors, while the remainder have single extra-adrenal tumors or multiple tumors. Early studies reported low prevalence (10%) of malignancy, similar to that in adults, but more recent studies have given prevalence rates for malignancy as high as 60%.

Familial pheochromocytomas are well recognized either as a separate entity or in association with disorders such as multiple endocrine neoplasia, neurofibromatosis, and von Hippel-Lindau syndrome.

The biochemical diagnosis of pheochromocytoma has been the subject of much study and controversy. These arguments concern not only whether plasma or urine is the optimum specimen, but which analyte or combination of analytes give the best sensitivity and specificity. These arguments relate more to the needs of adult patients, in whom the differentiation from benign essential hypertension is a major logistical problem. In the pediatric population, the measurement of 24 h urinary total metadrenalines and free catecholamine excretion will detect almost all cases. Occasional false positives due to stress or exogenous catecholamine administration may be found. If the index of suspicion is high and urine results persistently normal when the patient is hypertensive, then plasma catecholamine determinations may help, but these have not proved necessary in our series.

Neuroblastoma

Neuroblastoma accounts for 7–10% of all pediatric malignancies, with an annual incidence of 1 : 100,000 children. However, the overall incidence figure disguises the fact that neuroblastoma is predominantly a disease of infancy, being the most common non-hemopoietic tumor in the first two years of life.

The role of the laboratory in the diagnosis, prognostic evaluation, and monitoring of treatment of children with neuroblastoma has been studied extensively. Interpretation of the data is confusing and is complicated by the fact that there is still considerable debate as to exactly which tumors should be included under the heading of neuroblastoma. A number of other neuroectodermal tumors have been classified as neuroblastomas,[47] and these tumors are found more frequently in older patients and in atypical sites.

Neuroblastomas are tumors derived from cells of neuroectodermal origin. They are classified clinically into types I to IV and IVs, depending on the primary site and degree of spread. This classification has prognostic significance, and a considerable amount of effort has gone into attempts to biochemically differentiate between the different stages.

Diagnosis of neuroblastomas has relied essentially on the measurement of HVA and HMMA in 24 h urine collections. This method fails to diagnose 5–10% of patients, who are then referred to as "nonsecretors." A wider selection of catecholamine metabolites will enable the diagnosis of additional cases of neuroblastoma. In our experience of 100 sequential cases investigated by HPLC of 24h urines, 96% were detected by HVA alone and 100% by the combination of HVA and dopamine. Even using the older chemical methodology, < 1% of patients were found to be non-secretors when sufficient metabolites were measured. The pattern of urinary metabolite excretion has not proved to be a useful marker in disease staging, although it has been reported that high HMMA excretion is associated with disseminated tumors (stages III, IV, and IVs). In our series, there was no significant difference in the pattern of secretion of HVA, HMMA, and dopamine in patients under 1 year of age and in those over age 1, the former group including a higher proportion of stage I and II tumors.

Plasma HVA and HMMA measurements have not proved to be more useful than urinary determinations. Normal values are found in 12% of all neuroblastoma patients, and the prevalence of normal values increases to 50% in patients with stages I and II.[48]

A large number of biochemical markers have been used in attempts to provide prognostic indicators for neuroblastoma patients. These include the absolute quantity and pattern of urinary catecholamine metabolite excretion, and plasma concentrations of catecholamines (epinephrine, norepinephrine, and DOPA), dopamine β-hydroxylase, L-amino acid decarboxylase, LDH, ferritin, and neurone-specific enolase. Non-biochemical prognostic indicators include age, stage, chromosomal number (ploidy), N-myc oncogene amplification, and expression and reaction with various monoclonal antibodies. Of all the prognostic markers, age, sex, N-myc, and ploidy have been the most successful and the biochemical markers less so.

Screening for Neuroblastoma

Treatment of neuroblastoma remains problematical, and the overall prognosis is relatively poor. Because of this, it has been thought worthwhile to develop population screening programs for the preclinical detection of tumors, as there is a significantly better prognosis for patients with stage I or stage II disease. These programs were first introduced and widely applied in Japan after the development of assays for HMMA and HVA on filter paper collections of urine. Infants were screened at about 6 months of age. Initially, chemical methods were used for HMMA with large numbers of false positives and false negatives, but the use of HPLC overcame these problems. Reports of the Japanese screening programs were highly promising, with early detection and treatment appearing to produce a remarkable improvement in prognosis.

However, screening for neuroblastoma has not received universal acceptance.[49] Neuroblastoma is a tumor which appears to have a high incidence of spontaneous regression, especially tumors appearing in early infancy. This, taken with the fact that following screening there appeared to be a doubling of the incidence of neuroblastoma in Japan, raised the possibility that some of the tumors detected on screening at age 6 months would have spontaneously regressed, and hence that patients were subjected to unnecessary treatment. The only way to resolve the controversy is a large-scale controlled trial. Such a trial is presently underway in North America.

REFERENCES

1. Briggs MH, Brotherton J. Steroid biochemistry and pharmacology. London: Academic Press, 1971:1-22.
2. Gower DB. Biosynthesis of the corticosteroids. In: Makin HLJ, ed. Biochemistry of steroid hormones, 2nd ed. Oxford: Blackwell Scientific Publications, 1984:117-69.
3. Gower DB. Biosynthesis of the androgens and other C19 steroids. In: Makin HLJ, ed. Biochemistry of steroid hormones, 2nd ed. Oxford: Blackwell Scientific Publications, 1984:170-206.
4. Miller WL. Molecular biology of steroid hormone synthesis. Endocrinol Rev 1988;9:295-318.
5. Lieberman S, Greenfield NJ, Wolfson A. A heuristic proposal for understanding steroidogenic processes. Endocrinol Rev 1984;4:128-48.
6. Lieberman S, Prasad VVK. Heterodox notions on pathways of steroidogenesis. Endocrinol Rev; 1990;11:469-93
7. Waterman MR, Simpson ER. Regulation of steroid hydroxylase gene expression is multifactorial in nature. Rec Prog in Horm Res 1989;45:533-63.
8. Biglieri EG, Wajchenberg BL, Malerbi DA, Okeda H, Lema CE, Kater CE. The zonal origins of the mineralocorticoid hormones in the 21-hydroxylation deficiency congenital adrenal hyperplasia. J Clin Endocrinol Metab 1981;53:964-69.
9. Hornsby PJ. The regulation of adrenocortical function by control of growth and structure. In: Anderson DC, Winter J, ed. The adrenal cortex. London: Butterworths, 1985:1-31.
10. Peterson RE. Metabolism of adrenal cortical steroids. In: Christy NP, ed. The human adrenal cortex. New York; Harper and Row, 1971:87-187.
11. Addison GM, Chard C, Price DA. Steroid hormone metabolism. In: Hicks JM, Boeckx RL, eds. Pediatric clinical chemistry. Philadelphia: Saunders, 1984:240-94.
12. Riad-Fahmy D, Read GF, Walker RF, Griffith K. Steroids in saliva for assessing endocrine function. Endocrinol Rev 1982;3:367-95.
13. Dillon MJ, Ryness JM. Plasma renin activity and aldosterone concentration in children. Brit Med J 1975;4:316-19.

14.   Shackleton CHL, Honour JW. Simultaneous estimation of urinary steroids by semi-auto-mated gas chromatography: Investigation of neonates and children with abnormal steroid synthesis. Clin Chim Acta 1976;69:267-83.
15.   Shackleton CHL, Taylor NF, Honour J. An atlas of gas chromatographic profiles of neutral urinary steroids in health and disease. Delft: Packard-Becker BV, 1980.
16.   Strachan T. Molecular pathology of congenital adrenal hyperplasia. Clin Endocrinol 1990;32:373-93.
17.   Narasimhulu S. Heterogeneity of the bovine adrenal steroid 21-hydroxylase. Endocrinol Res 1989;15:67-84.
18.   Speiser PW, Agder L, Ueshiba H, White PC, New MI. Aldosterone synthesis in salt wasting congenital adrenal hyperplasia with complete absence of adrenal 21-hydroxylase. N Engl J Med 1991:145-49.
19.   Murphy JF, Joyce BG, Dyas J, Hughes IA. Plasma 17-hydroxyprogesterone concentration in ill newborn infants. Arch Dis Child 1983;58:532-34.
20.   Knudtzen J, Aakvaag A, Bergsjo P, Markestad Y. Elevated 17-hydroxyprogesterone levels in premature infants. Acta Paediatr Scand 1991;80:96-97.
21.   Pang SY, Wallace AM, Hofman L, Thuline HC, Dorche C, Lyon CT, et al. Worldwide experi-ence in newborn screening for classical adrenal hyperplasia due to 21-hydroxylase defi-ciency. Pediatrics 1988;81:866-74.
22.   Pang S, Hotchkiss J, Drash AL, Levine LS, New MI. Microfilter paper method for 17-alpha-hydroxyprogesterone radioimmunoassay: Its application for rapid screening for congenital adrenal hyperplasia. J Clin Endocrinol Metab 1977;45:1003-8.
23.   Addison GM. Workshop on screening for congenital adrenal hyperplasia (steroid 21-hydroxylase deficiency). J Inher Metab Dis 1986;9 Suppl 1:111-14.
24.   Virdi NK, Rayner PH, Rudd BT, Green A. Should we screen for congenital adrenal hyper-plasia? A review of 117 cases. Arch Dis Child 1987;62:659-62.
25.   Forest MG, Betuel H, David M. Prenatal treatment in congenital adrenal hyperplasia due to 21-hydroxylase deficiency: Update 88 of the French multicentric study. Endocrinol Res 1989;15:277-301.
26.   Speiser PW, Laforgia N, Kato K, Pareira J, Khan R, Yang SY, et al. First trimester prenatal treatment and molecular genetic diagnosis of congenital adrenal hyperplasia. J Clin En-docrinol Metab 1990;70:838-48.
27.   Porter B, Finzi M, Leiberman E, Moses S. The syndrome of congenital adrenal hyperplasia in Israel. Paediatrician 1977;6:100-5.
28.   Zadik Z, Kahana L, Kaufman, M, Bendeleri A, Hachberg Z. Salt loss in hypertensive form of congenital adrenal hyperplasia (11β-hydroxylase deficiency). J Clin Endocrinol Metab 1984;58:384-88.
29.   Honour JW, Dillon MJ, Shackleton CHL. Analysis of steroids in urine for differentiation of pseudohypoaldosteronism and aldosterone biosynthetic defects. J Clin Endocrinol Metab 1982;54:384-88.
30.   Daneman A. Adrenal neoplasms in children. Sem Roentgen 1988;23:205-15.
31.   Grant DB. Virilizing adrenal tumours. In: Forest MG, ed. Androgens in childhood. Paediatric and adolescent endocrinolgy. Basel; Karger 1989;19:236-46.
32.   Honour JW, Price DA, Taylor, NF, Marsden, HB, Grant, DB. Steroid biochemistry of virilising adrenal tumours in childhood. Eur J Paediatr 1984;142:165-69.
33.   Jones KL. The Cushing syndromes. Pediatr Clin North Am 1990;37:1313-32.
34.   Forest MG. Adrenal steroid deficiency states. In: Brook CDG, ed. Clinical paediatric endocri-nology. Oxford; Blackwell Scientific Publications, 1981:396-428.
35.   Clayton RN. Diagnosis of adrenal insufficiency (editorial). Brit Med J 1989;298:271-72.
36.   Dickstien G, Shechechner C, Nicholson W, Rosner I, Shen-Orr Z, Adawi F, et al. Adreno-corticotrophin stimulation test: Effect of basal cortisol level, time of day and suggested new sensitive low dose test. J Clin Endocrinol Metab 1991;72:773-78.
37.   Weinkove C, Anderson DC. Interactions between the adrenal cortex and medulla. In: An-derson DC, Winter JSD, eds. Adrenal cortex. London: Butterworths, 1985:208-34.

38. Gjessing LR. Biochemistry of functional neural crest tumours. Adv Clin Chem 1968;11:81-131.
39. Tuchman M, Morris CL, Ramnaraine ML, Bowers LD, Krivit W. Value of random urinary homovanillic acid and vanillylmandelic acid levels in the diagnosis and management of patients with neuroblastoma: Comparison with 24-hour urine collections. Pediatrics 1985;75:324-28.
40. Nishi M, Miyake H, Takeda T, Takasugi N, Hanai J, Kawai T. Can a patient with neuroblastoma be diagnosed by a single urine sample collected randomly? Oncology 1991;48:31-33.
41. Worthington DJ, Hammond EM, Eldeeb BB, Addison GM, Morris Jones PH, Mann JR. Neuroblastoma: When are urinary catecholamines and their metabolites "normal"? Ann Clin Biochem 1988;25:620-26.
42. Tuchman M, Stoeckeler JS. Conjugated versus "free" acidic catecholamines in random urine samples: Significance for the diagnosis of neuroblastoma. Pediatr Res 1988;23:576-79.
43. Barrand MA, Callingham BA. The catecholamines: Adrenaline, noradrenaline and dopamine. In: Gray CH, James VHT, eds. Hormones in blood, 3rd ed., Vol 5. London: Academic Press, 1983:55-124.
44. Eichler I, Eichler HG, Rotter M, Kyrle PA, Gasic S, Korn A. Plasma concentrations of free and sulfoconjugated dopamine, epinephrine and norepinephrine in healthy infants and children. Klinische Wochenschrift 1989;67:672-75.
45. Hunneman DH, Jonas W, Gabriel, M. Gahr M. Effect of age on homovanillic acid and 4-hydroxy-3-methoxymandelic acid levels in plasma. Eur J Pediatr 1986;145:555-57.
46. Deal JE, Sever PS, Barrat TM, Dillon MJ. Pheochromocytoma: Investigation and management of 10 cases. Arch of Dis Child 1990:65;269-74.
47. Triche TJ. Neuroblastoma and other childhood neural tumours. Pediatr Pathol 1990;7:175-93.
48. Gahr M, Hunneman DH. The value of determination of homovanillic and vanillylmandelic acids in plasma for the diagnosis and follow up in neuroblastoma in children. Eur J Pediatr 1987;146:489-93.
49. Murphy SB, Cohn SL, Craft AW, Woods WG, Sawada T, Castleberry RP, et al. Do children benefit from mass screening for neuroblastoma? Consensus statement from the American Cancer Society Workshop on Neuroblastoma Screening. Lancet 1991;377:344-46.

Disorders of Calcium and Phosphorus Metabolism in Infants and Children

Maria Lourdes A. Cruz, M.D.   Ronald Bainbridge, M.D.
Reginald C. Tsang, M.D.

INTRODUCTION

Calcium (Ca), phosphorus (P), magnesium (Mg), vitamin D, calcitonin (CT), and parathyroid hormone (PTH) form part of an intricate network of systems that maintain the stability of the skeleton and regulate several Ca and P related metabolic activities. The increased need for Ca and P during infancy and childhood requires optimal functioning of the systems of absorption, transport, and assimilation of these minerals. Disorders in any of several steps in these systems may result in prolonged and severe consequences in the affected child. Early recognition of the physical and biochemical signs associated with these disorders, and subsequent treatment, may allow possible diminution of the consequences.

BIOCHEMISTRY AND PHYSIOLOGY

Less than 1% of the total body Ca is in the extracellular compartment, while approximately 98% is in bone. Serum Ca is approximately 50% ionized, 40% protein bound (90% to albumin), and 10% chelated to citrate, phosphate, and other anions. Serum total and ionized calcium (iCa) concentrations are usually tightly regulated within narrow ranges. Ionized Ca concentration is the physiologically active form of Ca and is more tightly regulated than total serum Ca concentrations. A circadian pattern has been described for serum iCa concentration, with a variation of 0.32 mg/dL (0.08 mmol/L), the reference range being 4.8–5.2 mg/dL (1.2–1.3 mmol/L).[1] Season, diet, and race also appear to affect serum Ca concentrations.[2] Binding of Ca to albumin is pH dependent, increasing at higher pH and decreasing at lower pH, thereby effecting changes in serum iCa concentration.[3]

The distribution of total body P is approximately 80% in bone, 9% in skeletal muscle, and 11% in extracellular fluid and other tissues. Less than 1% of body phosphorus is found in serum. Serum P is approximately 55% dissociated, 35% complexed to the cations, sodium, Ca^{2++} and Mg^{2+}, and 10% protein bound. Serum P concentration is not as tightly regulated as serum Ca concentration and varies with nutritional status, age, race, and season.[2] Measurements of serum P include both inorganic and organic phosphates and probably partly explain the wide variation observed in serum P measurements. Serum concentrations of Ca and P are regulated by PTH, vitamin D, CT, and Mg (see Figure 9–1).

Parathyroid Hormone

Parathyroid hormone is an 84 amino-acid polypeptide secreted by the parathyroid glands. The hormonal activity resides in the amino terminal 1-34 fragment. In normal adults, only 5–30% of the circulating immunoreactive hormone is intact PTH; the rest consists of inactive C-terminal fragments.[4] Parathyroid hormone secretion is acutely increased in response to decreases in serum Ca concentration and decreased by increased Ca concentration. Acute changes in serum Mg concentration affect PTH secretion in a manner similar to Ca. However, chronic Mg deficiency inhibits PTH secretion.[5]

Parathyroid hormone regulates both serum Ca and P concentrations through its actions on bone, gut, and kidneys (Figure 9–1). PTH acts synergistically with vitamin D initially on bone to release Ca and P. The mechanism of acute PTH action involves stimulation of osteoclastic activity while inhibiting osteoblastic activity. The intracellular mechanisms involved includes activation of a cyclic adenosine monophosphate (cAMP) dependent system.

The long-term effect of PTH on bone is to stimulate both osteoclast and osteoblast activity, resulting in the characteristic histologic lytic bone changes observed in hyperparathyroidism.[6] Since PTH facilitates the conversion of 25-hydroxy vitamin D (25-OHD) to 1,25-dihydroxy vitamin D [1,25(OH)$_2$D], it is indirectly involved in active intestinal absorption of Ca. The action of PTH on the kidney increases distal tubular Ca reabsorption, and inhibits proximal tubular reabsorption of P, resulting in phosphaturia. Renal tubular reabsorption of amino acids, sodium, and bicarbonate are also inhibited by

PTH. Parathyroid hormone binds to receptors on the basolateral membrane of renal tubular cells, which in turn activates a stimulatory G protein, a subunit of which activates adenylate cyclase to form cAMP. Cyclic AMP triggers a cascade of other intracellular events to effect the changes in tubular reabsorption described above.[7] The net result is a lowering of serum P and increase in serum Ca concentrations (Figure 9–1).

FIGURE 9–1. Effects of Various Calciotropic Hormones on Different Organ Systems and Their Overall Effects on Serum Calcium (Ca) and Phosphorus (P) Concentrations

Parathyroid hormone (PTH) increases bone release of Ca and P and increases renal Ca reabsorption and P excretion, resulting in an overall increase in serum Ca but a decrease in P concentrations. Vitamin D (Vit.D), as 1,25(OH)2D, stimulates intestinal Ca and P absorption, bone Ca and P resorption, and renal Ca and P reabsorption, resulting in an overall increase in serum Ca and P concentrations. Calcitonin (CT) acts mainly to decrease bone resorption and renal reabsorption of Ca and P, resulting in an overall decrease in serum Ca and P concentrations.

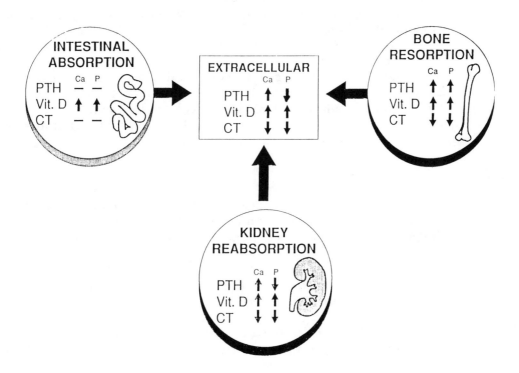

Vitamin D

Most of the body's supply of vitamin D is derived from skin synthesis. Dietary sources of vitamin D assume importance only in children deprived of sun exposure. An intact biliary, pancreatic, and small intestinal system is required for the normal absorption of this fat-soluble vitamin.

Vitamin D_3 is formed in the skin after exposure of its precursor, 7-dehydrocholesterol, to ultraviolet irradiation from sunlight (Figure 9–2). 7-dehydrocholesterol is first converted to previtamin D_3, which is further thermally isomerized to vitamin D. Vitamin D binding globulin (DBG) transports the vitamin D to the liver for further transformation. After intestinal absorption, dietary vitamin D_3 and D_2 are also transported on DBG to the liver. Vitamin D is 25 hydroxylated to 25-hydroxy vitamin D (25-OHD) in the liver. This process is not tightly regulated, allowing for accumulation of 25-OHD, the concentration of which is regarded as an index of body vitamin D status. 25-OHD undergoes further 1-hydroxylation in the proximal renal tubular cell. The enzyme involved in this conversion, 25-OHD 1-hydroxylase, is tightly regulated, and its activity is stimulated by hypocalcemia, hypophosphatemia, and increased PTH concentration, and inhibited by increases in serum Ca, P, and $1,25(OH)_2D$.

1,25-dihydroxy vitamin D is the most physiologically active form of vitamin D. Its primary sites of action are the gut, bone, and kidney, similar to PTH (Figure 9–1). The active transport of Ca across the gut basolateral membrane is facilitated. How $1,25(OH)_2D$ affects gut absorption of P is less clear. In bone, both osteoblast and osteoclast activity are stimulated, with the net result being bone remodelling and increased mineralization. 1,25-dihydroxy vitamin D enhances renal tubular reabsorption of Ca in concert with PTH. Vitamin D status also appears to be affected by season, diet, gender, and race.[2]

Calcitonin

Calcitonin (CT), a 32-amino acid peptide, is produced by the C-cells of the thyroid gland. Its secretion is stimulated by hypercalcemia, hypermagnesemia, gastrin, pancreozymin, and glucagon.[8] Hypocalcemia has the opposite effect.[8]

Calcitonin lowers serum Ca concentration by inhibiting the effect of PTH on bone and by promoting calciuria and phosphaturia via its renal effect (Figure 9–1). However, in the absence of CT, serum Ca remains fairly well regulated, raising questions as to its importance in normal regulation of serum Ca concentration. Serum CT concentrations are increased in the newborn infant and may remain so well into infancy. The exact physiologic significance of this increase is unclear.

FIGURE 9–2. Normal Vitamin D Metabolism

Vitamin D2 from diet, and Vitamin D3 from diet and skin photoconversion, are hydroxylated in the liver to 25-OHD. 25-OHD undergoes further hydroxylation in the kidney to form 1,25(OH)2D which is stimulated by parathyroid hormone (PTH). 1,25(OH)2D is responsible for increasing bone resorption and intestinal calcium and phosphorus absorption. PTH acts synergistically with 1,25(OH)2D to increase bone resorption.

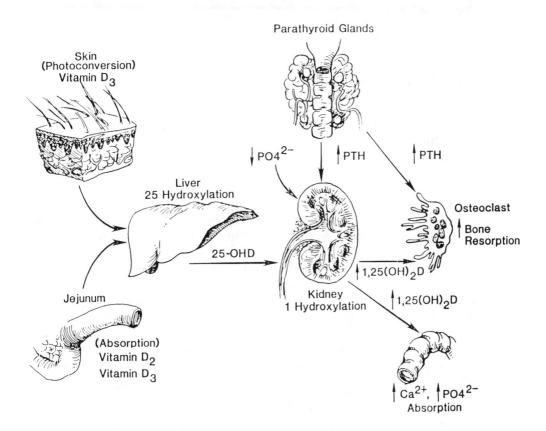

NEWBORN

The third trimester is the time of maximal intrauterine Ca and P accretion. Daily accretion rates of 117–150 mg Ca/kg and 74 mg P/kg have been estimated for near-term fetuses.[9, 10] Interruption of the placental supply of these minerals at the time of delivery therefore predisposes the neonate to hypocalcemia at a time when oral feeds are limited. There is a marked increase in PTH secretion after birth,[11] presumably in response to the sudden decrease in serum Ca concentration at delivery.[12] This may be blunted in preterm infants as compared to term infants; however, PTH secretion appears to increase with increasing postnatal age.

Serum $1,25(OH)_2D$ concentrations rise steadily during the first day of life. The exact mechanism of this occurrence remains unclear, as is its role in regulating neonatal serum Ca concentrations. Serum CT concentrations are increased at birth and decrease after the first few days and weeks of life. Serum Ca concentrations may be inversely related to serum CT concentrations during this period.

CLINICAL SIGNIFICANCE OF DISORDERS OF CALCIUM AND PHOSPHORUS METABOLISM

Some biochemical changes associated with disorders of Ca and P metabolism in infancy and childhood are listed in Table 9–1.

Hypocalcemia

Neonatal hypocalcemia is often defined as a total serum calcium of < 7.8 mg/dL (2 mmol/L) for term infants,[13] or < 7.0 mg/dL (1.75 mmol/L) for preterm infants, and serum ionized Ca < 4.4 mg/dL (1.10 mmol/L).[2, 13]

Traditionally, neonatal hypocalcemia has been classified as either early or late. "Early" neonatal hypocalcemia occurs during the first 48 hours of life, while "late" neonatal hypocalcemia occurs toward the end of the first week of life. In some cases, the distinction between the two conditions may not be clear-cut.

Early neonatal hypocalcemia occurs as a result of the inability of the neonate to adequately compensate for the sudden cessation of placental Ca supply after birth. The usual protective changes observed in calciotropic hormone secretion may be blunted. Preterm infants may not exhibit the surge in PTH secretion observed in term infants at birth,[14] and their restricted oral Ca intake may aggravate the problem. Birth asphyxia may result in an increase in serum CT concentration and may delay enteral feeding, both of which may theoretically aggravate neonatal hypocalcemia.[15] Early neonatal hypocalcemia in infants of diabetic mothers may be related to Mg insufficiency and consequently to impaired PTH secretory activity.[16] In most cases, early neonatal hypocalcemia resolves within the first week of life. Prolonged hypocalcemia should prompt the physician to investigate other, more permanent causes.

Late neonatal hypocalcemia may be a manifestation of a congenital defect, a result of disorders of vitamin D metabolism, or a result of Mg and P mineral disturbance. Congenital hypoparathyroidism is the

TABLE 9-1. Some Biochemical Changes in Disorders of Calcium and Phosphorus Metabolism in Infancy and Childhood

Disorder	Serum Phosphorus Concentration	Parathyroid Hormone Concentration	Serum 1,25(OH)₂D Concentration	Serum 25-OHD Concentration	Urinary Calcium Excretion	Urinary Phosphorus Excretion
HYPOCALCEMIA						
Parathyroid disorders						
Hypoparathyroidism						
Congenital	↑	↓	↓	N	↓	↓
Transient or functional	↑	↓	↓	N	↓	↓
Pseudohypoparathyroidism	↑	↑	↓		↓	↓
Vitamin D disorders						
Vitamin D deficiency	↓	↑	N; ↑	↓	↓; Var	↑
Hepatic disease	↓	↑	N; ↓	↓	↓; Var	↑
Renal disease	↑	↑	↓	N	↓; Var	↓
Vitamin D dependent rickets, type I	↓	↑	Very ↓	N; ↑	↓; Var	↑
Vitamin D dependent rickets, type II	↓	↑	Very ↑	N; ↑	↓; Var	↑
Mineral disorders						
Hypomagnesemia	N	N; ↓	N; ↓	N	↓	N
High phosphate load	↑	↑	↓	N	↓	↑
HYPERCALCEMIA						
Iatrogenic	N	↓	↓	N	↑	↑
Low P intake	↓	↓	↑	N	↑	↓
Hyperparathyroidism	↓	↑	↑	N	↑	↑
Vitamin D intoxication	N; ↑	↓	N; ↑	↑	↑	↑
Subcutaneous fat necrosis	N	↓	N; ↑	N	↑	N
Idiopathic hypercalcemia of infancy	N	↓	N; ↑	N	↑	N
Benign familial hypocalciuric hypercalcemia	N	N; ↑	N; ↑	N	↓	N
Immobilization	N	↓	↓	N	↑	↑

Disorder	Serum Calcium Concentration	Parathyroid Hormone Concentration	Serum 1,25(OHD)₂D Concentration	Serum 25-OHD Concentration	Urinary Calcium Excretion	Urinary Phosphorus Excretion
HYPOPHOSPHATEMIA						
Inadequate P intake	N; ↑	↓; ↑	↑; ↓	N	↑	↓
Hyperparathyroidism	↑	↑	↑	N	↑	↑
Hypophosphatemic rickets	N	N	N; ↓	N	N	↑
HYPERPHOSPHATEMIA						
Parathyroid disorders						
Hypoparathyroidism	↓	↓	↓	N	↓	↓
Pseudohypoparathyroidism	N; ↑	N; ↑	N; ↓	N	N; ↑	N; ↑
Thyrotoxicosis	↑	↓	↓	N	↑	↓
High phosphate intake	↓	↑	↓	N	↓	↑
Renal failure	↓	↑	↓	N	↓	↑

N = normal, Var = variable, ↑ = increased, ↓ = decreased

most significant cause of late-onset hypocalcemia which has to be treated early in life, and is discussed below. Vitamin D problems include insufficient dietary vitamin D intake or production due to liver or renal disease (resulting in decreased intestinal Ca absorption and renal Ca reabsorption), congenital deficiency of renal 1-hydroxylase (Vitamin D dependent rickets, type I), and $1,25(OH)_2D$ resistance (Vitamin D dependent rickets, type II). Of the mineral problems, it is important to detect the presence of hypomagnesemia, whether transient or due to hereditary intestinal Mg malabsorption or renal Mg losses, since hypocalcemia generally cannot be corrected until hypomagnesemia is alleviated. As mentioned earlier, the relationship between hypocalcemia and hypomagnesemia may be related to the important role of Mg in PTH secretion. High phosphate loads, usually dietary (see discussion below), lead to hyperphosphatemia and secondary hypocalcemia.

Treatment consists of Ca supplementation at doses of 30–75 mg elemental Ca/kg/d, titrated to the response of the patient. When tolerated by the patient, we recommend the use of the intravenous form of 10% Ca gluconate (9.4 mg elemental Ca/mL), given *orally* in 4–6 divided doses.[17] Otherwise, Ca gluconate given intravenously must be administered carefully, since it may cause cardiac arrhythmia and skin necrosis. Since most causes of hypocalcemia in the neonate are transient, Ca supplementation is usually not required for long periods.

Hypercalcemia

Hypercalcemia is defined as total serum Ca concentration of > 10.8 mg/dL (2.7 mmol/L), or serum ionized Ca concentration > 5.6 mg/dL (1.4 mmol/L).[2, 13] Increased serum total Ca concentrations are usually associated with increased serum ionized Ca concentrations. Hypercalcemia in the neonate is usually iatrogenic: administration of Ca salts for treatment of hypocalcemia or for prophylaxis during exchange transfusions; the use of thiazide diuretics which depress urinary Ca excretion; and hyperalimentation errors, either excess Ca or insufficient P. Human milk feeding of preterm infants may lead to hypophosphatemia because of the low P content of human milk, and this in turn may cause secondary hypercalcemia.

Other rarer causes of hypercalcemia in the newborn which may have a metabolic or familial basis include: hyperparathyroidism (primary or secondary to maternal hypoparathyroidism, from increased release of Ca from bone); vitamin D intoxication (parents who are food faddists may give large doses of vitamins to their infants); hypercalcemia associated with subcutaneous fat necrosis (usually in asphyxiated, large-for-gestational-age infants; thought to be related to Ca release from fat); idiopathic infantile hypercalcemia (associated with Williams syndrome: elfin facies, developmental delay, failure to thrive, heart disease; may be a vitamin D hyperresponsive state); and benign familial hypocalciuric hypercalcemia, in which the infant may have signs of hyperparathyroidism. In older children, immobilization hypercalcemia may occur.

Treatment consists of correction of the underlying cause: removal of iatrogenic or external causes; Ca and P supplementation of human milk given to preterm infants; surgical removal of hyperparathyroid glands. Treatment of severe hypercalcemia associated with subcutaneous fat necrosis and idiopathic infantile hypercalcemia consists of removal of dietary Ca and vitamin D as well as avoidance of sunlight exposure. In severe cases, hydration, diuresis, and steroids may be required. In familial cases in which patients are asymptomatic, supportive treatment may suffice. Exercise may prevent the occurrence of immobilization hypercalcemia.

Hypophosphatemia

Hypophosphatemia is usually defined as serum P concentrations < 4.8 mg/dL (1.55 mmol/L) in formula fed to infants under 18 months of age.[2] Transient causes include hypophosphatemia induced by respiratory (mechanical ventilation) alkalosis and low dietary P intake. The latter may occur in a preterm infant fed human milk due to the low P content of human milk,[18] and has also be seen in children with high aluminum hydroxide (antacid) intake (aluminum binds P in the gut). Metabolic causes of hypophosphatemia include hyperparathyroidism (decreased renal P reabsorption due to PTH action); renal losses associated with Lowe's syndrome (renal tubular acidosis with proximal tubule P losses, mental retardation, failure to thrive, cataracts, and rickets); and X-linked hypophosphatemia. Management consists of treatment of the underlying causes for transient hypophosphatemia; surgical removal of the parathyroid glands in hyperparathyroidism; and P, Vitamin D, and alkali supplementation in Lowe's syndrome.

Hyperphosphatemia

Hyperphosphatemia in infants up to 18 months of age is defined as serum P concentrations > 8.4 mg/dL (2.7 mmol/L).[2] In older children and adolescents, serum P concentrations > 6.0 mg/dL (2 mmol/L) are considered to be in the hyperphosphatemic range. In contrast to adults, in whom there are many causes of hyperphosphatemia, causes of hyperphosphatemia in infants and children are usually limited to parathyroid disorders (hypoparathyroidism and pseudohypoparathyroidism, both of which demonstrate decreased renal P excretion); thyrotoxicosis (increased bone resorption); increased dietary P load from cow milk based formula and cereals; and renal failure (decreased

P excretion). Treatment consists of treatment of the underlying cause and reduction of exogenous sources of P. The use of intestinal P binders in renal failure may also be needed.

Neonatal Hypoparathyroidism

Neonatal hypoparathyroidism[19] may be transient or permanent. As mentioned earlier, transient neonatal hypoparathyroidism may occur in preterm infants, as well as in infants of insulin-dependent diabetic mothers (IDMs), in whom there may be a blunted PTH response to low serum Ca concentrations. This phenomenon has been termed "functional hypoparathyroidism."[14] About 30% of preterm infants and 50% of IDMs present with hypocalcemia in the first few days of life, and may have signs such as jitteriness, tetany, seizures, or cardiac arrhythmias. Treatment consists of continued provision of adequate Ca supply, either enterally or parenterally, at a dose of about 75 mg elemental Ca/kg/d until Ca homeostatic mechanisms of the infants become functional. This disease entity usually lasts for a few days, after which Ca supplementation may be weaned and eventually discontinued.

Transient neonatal hypoparathyroidism may also occur in infants of untreated hyperparathyroid mothers. Maternal hypercalcemia secondary to excess PTH activity leads to fetal hypercalcemia, which inhibits fetal parathyroid gland hormone production. The management is similar to management of the hypocalcemic preterm infant or infant of a diabetic mother. The disorder may last for several weeks.

Recently, several case reports have identified patients who recovered from transient neonatal hypoparathyroidism, but who redeveloped hypocalcemia when followed to childhood and adolescence.[20, 21] It has been suggested that patients who are thought to have transient hypoparathyroidism should undergo a sodium-EDTA test later in life, after a period of stable eucalcemia, to identify those who would be at increased risk for subsequent development of permanent hypoparathyroidism.[21] Patients with minimally functioning parathyroid glands would theoretically not be able to mount the expected increase in PTH secretion during hypocalcemia induced by the EDTA test. These patients should be followed closely thereafter so that when hypocalcemia recurs, therapy can be reinstituted speedily.

Congenital hypoparathyroidism is a permanent condition accompanied by hypocalcemia. It is associated with agenesis, dysgenesis, or hypoplasia of the parathyroid glands. The disorder may be transmitted as an X-linked or autosomal dominant gene, but may also occur as a sporadic mutation, (so called "idiopathic"). There are no characteristic physical features in congenital hypoparathyroidism, unless it is associated with a genetic disorder such as ring chromosomes. These infants present with unremitting hypocalcemia and very low or undetectable serum PTH concentrations ("hormone deficient hypoparathyroidism") and increased serum P concentrations. The average age of onset of symptoms, however, is during the adolescent years.

It is important to detect and treat the resultant hypocalcemia, especially in infancy, since prolonged and/or severe hypocalcemia may be associated with cardiac arrhythmias, tetany, seizures, and mental retardation. Candida infection of the nails and mouth may occur in one-sixth of patients. A feature of untreated early hypoparathyroidism in later infancy and childhood is dental hypoplasia. Management consists of lifelong vitamin D treatment, usually in the form of $1,25(OH)_2D$ at a dose of $0.03–0.08$ µg/kg/d, preferably given in twice-daily doses. Older children may not require as much vitamin D. This form of vitamin D is used since there is inadequate PTH stimulus for renal conversion of 25-OHD to the active form $1,25(OH)_2D$. Further, the short half-life of the drug allows for ease of management. Ca supplements may also be additionally required. Adequacy of treatment is assessed by normalcy of serum Ca concentrations and return of serum P concentrations to normal.

Pseudohypoparathyroidism is another variant of congenital parathyroid gland dysfunction. In contrast to idiopathic hypoparathyroidism, parathyroid glands in individuals affected by this disorder are hyperplastic and actively secreting increased amounts of PTH. In this disorder, the problem is deficient end-organ responsiveness to PTH ("hormone resistant hypoparathyroidism"). Also in contrast to idiopathic hypoparathyroid individuals, who have no dysmorphic features, individuals with pseudohypoparathyroidism are characteristically short and thickset, with round facies, short necks, and short fingers and toes at birth. Subcutaneous soft tissue calcific nodules, dental hypoplasia, and various degrees of developmental delay and mental retardation may develop later in infancy and childhood.

Diagnosis is based on persistent hypocalcemia in the face of markedly increased (rather than low) serum PTH concentrations, in association with hyperphosphatemia and the above-mentioned physical stigmata. Confirmation of the diagnosis requires an intravenous PTH infusion test in which skeletal and/or renal cell response to PTH is assessed: in normal individuals, urinary cAMP (an index of PTH effect on plasma membrane adenyl cyclase activity) and/or urinary phosphate excretion are increased in response to the PTH challenge.[19] This response is diminished or nearly absent in pseudohypoparathyroid individuals.

As in idiopathic hypoparathyroidism, treatment consists of lifelong treatment with $1,25(OH)_2D$ and Ca.

Neonatal Hyperparathyroidism

Neonatal hyperparathyroidism[19] occurs less often than neonatal hypoparathyroidism and may be primary or secondary. Primary neonatal hyperparathyroidism is usually caused by an autosomal recessive gene, although it may also be familial or occur as part of multiple endocrine adenomatosis. The condition is associated with failure to thrive (poor weight gain and growth), increased serum PTH concentrations, hypercalcemia, hyperphosphaturia leading to hypophosphatemia, and hypercalciuria sometimes leading to nephrocalcinosis. Skeletal demineralization may occur in untreated cases, as Ca is continually "leached" out from bone by excessive amounts of circulating PTH. Surgical removal of the parathyroid glands is crucial; otherwise, the prognosis is poor.

Secondary hyperparathyroidism may occur in infants of mothers with untreated hypoparathyroidism. Hypocalcemia in the mother leads to compensatory fetal parathyroid gland hyperplasia. with subsequent increased PTH secretion. The biochemical findings can be similar to those found in primary hyperparathyroidism, except that infants commonly present with lytic bone lesions with little effect on serum Ca concentrations. The diagnosis is confirmed by identification of hypoparathyroidism in the mother. In most cases, the condition is transient and only requires supportive treatment during the rare hypercalcemic period. Rarely, steroids, furosemide, and calcitonin may be required.

Hyperparathyroidism in Older Children

Hyperparathyroidism in older children[19] is more commonly secondary. Children suffering from liver failure may have reduced conversion of dietary vitamin D_3 to 25-OHD. The resultant poor absorption of Ca leads to hypocalcemia, which in turn stimulates parathyroid gland hyperactivity. In children with chronic renal disease, inadequate or absent renal conversion of 25-OHD to its active form, $1,25(OH)_2D$, leads to hypocalcemia and subsequent secondary hyperparathyroidism.

In these children, skeletal deformities due to rickets (so-called hepatic or renal rickets) may occur. Hyperchloremic acidosis due to excess PTH and increased alkaline phosphatase due to increased bone turnover may be detected. Aminoaciduria and urinary cAMP excretion may also be increased. Detection of increased PTH concentrations is best done with the use of the intact PTH molecule assay.[22] Treatment for secondary hyperparathyroidism is treatment of the primary disorder.

In the occasional instances of primary hyperparathyroidism in childhood, adenomas are the usual etiology. Surgery is the treatment of choice.

Nutritional Causes of Ca and P Disorders

In preterm infants, Ca and P requirements are high. The high require-ments are related to mineral deprivation due to early delivery, poor in-testinal absorption of cow milk based formula, and use of calciuretic medication, especially in sick preterm infants. Inadequate provision of these minerals can increase the risk of hypocalcemia, hypophosphate-mia, hypercalciuria, and rickets in these infants.

The high Ca and P requirements can be partially met by paren-teral solutions and adequately met by most milk formulae specially for-mulated for preterm infants. Additionally, the use of human milk fortified with Ca, P, and protein in preterm infants has been advocated to ensure adequate supply and optimize growth.[18] In parenteral solu-tions, the amounts of Ca and P will determine the stability of the min-erals; a Ca:P ratio of 1.3 to 1.7 is also important to ensure proper Ca homeostasis.[23]

In term infants, the relatively high P content of standard commer-cial formulae (due to the naturally high P content of cow milk from which these formulae are derived) may result in hyperphosphatemia and secondary hypocalcemia. Evaporated milks, in particular, have high P content and readily cause hypocalcemia. Some of these hypocal-cemic infants will develop neonatal tetany and seizures. Commercial milk has been reformulated to improve the Ca : P ratio, and hypocalce-mic tetany is less frequently seen.

The high P and fiber load of many cereals given to infants as first foods could also conceivably cause problems in term infants. Phospho-rus increases Ca-P complexing and may compete with Ca absorption, while phytate and fibers bind Ca within the intestinal lumen. The re-sultant inadequate Ca absorption may lead to hypocalcemia. High serum PTH concentrations have been found in infants fed cereal at age 4 months versus those who were started on cereal at age 6 months, but there was no apparent effect on bone mineral content.[24]

Maternal preferences, beliefs, and habits play a direct and import-ant role in the nutrition of infants, whether the mothers choose to pro-vide human or commercial milk to their babies. Breast-fed infants of mothers who are on macrobiotic diets (food sources limited to grains, cereals, fruits, nuts, and vegetables, with prohibition of foods from ani-mal sources, including dairy products) and who are not supplemented with vitamin D have been documented to have low serum 25-OHD, Ca, and P concentrations and suffer from an increased risk of rickets, es-pecially in temperate climates.[25] Infants of vegetarian mothers who provide dairy products to their infants do not appear to suffer from this problem. Milk from these mothers also appears to be adequate in Ca and P.

Mothers with inadequate sun exposure due to dress customs may also be vitamin D deficient, especially if they are vegetarian; their infants will be susceptible to vitamin D deficiency, particularly if they are likewise shielded from sun exposure. The numerous reports of rickets in countries like Saudi Arabia attest to this phenomenon.[26] Conversely, infants of mothers who believe in taking large amounts of vitamin supplements which contain vitamins A and D are at risk for developing hypercalcemia. Both of these vitamins increase bone resorption with subsequent increase in serum Ca concentrations.

REFERENCE RANGES

Reference values of Ca, iCa, P, PTH, CT, 1,25(OH)$_2$D, 25-OHD, UCa excretion, and TRP are given in Table 9–2. Conversion factors are:

Ca mg/dL × 0.25 = mmol/L
P mg/dL × 0. 323 = mmol/L
Ca mmol/L × 2 = meq/L
P mmol/L × 2 = meq/L
25-OHD ng/mL × 2.4 = nmol/L
1,25(OH)$_2$D pg/mL × 2.4 = pmol/L

REFERENCES

1. Carruthers BM, Copp DH, McIntosh H. Diurnal variation in urinary excretion of calcium and phosphate and its relation to blood levels. J Lab Clin Med 1964;63:959-68.
2. Specker BL, Lichtenstein P, Mimouni F, Tsang R. Calcium-regulating hormone and minerals from birth to 18 months of age: A cross-sectional study. II Effects of sex, race, age, season, and diet in serum minerals, parathyroid hormone, and calcitonin. Pediatr 1986;77:891-96.
3. Root AW, Harrison H. Recent advances in calcium metabolism. J Pediatr 1976;88:1-18, 177-99.
4. Segre GV, Habener JF, Powell D, Tregear GW, Potts Jr, JT. Parathyroid hormone in human plasma: immunochemical characterization and biological implications. J Clin Invest 1972;51:3163-72.
5. Chase LR, Slatopolsky E. Secretion and metabolic efficacy of parathyroid hormone in patients with severe hypomagnesemia. J Clin Endocrinol Metab 1974;38:363-71.
6. Mundy GR, Roodman G. Osteoclast ontogeny and function. In: Peck W, ed. Bone and mineral research, vol 5. Amsterdam: Elsevier, 1987.
7. Chase LR, Aurbach G. Parathyroid functions and the renal excretion of 3',5'-adenylic acid. Proceedings of the National Academy of Sciences 1967;58:418-525.
8. David L, Salle BL, Putet G, Grafmeyer DC. Serum immunoreactive calcitonin in low birthweight infants: Description of early changes; effects of intravenous calcium infusion; relationships with early changes in serum calcium, phosphorus, magnesium, parathyroid hormone, and gastric levels. Pediatr Res 1981;15:803-8.
9. Shaw J. Parenteral nutrition in the management of sick low birthweight infants. Pediatr Clin North Am 1973;20:333-58.
10. Zeigler E, O'Donnel A, Nelson S, Fomon S. Body composition of the reference fetus. Growth 1976;40:329-41.
11. Saggese G, Baroncelli GI, Bertelloni S, Cipolloni C. Intact parathyroid hormone levels during pregnancy, in healthy term neonates and in hypocalcemic preterm infants. Acta Paediatr Scand 1991;80:36-41.

TABLE 9-2. Normal Values (mean ± 1 SD unless otherwise indicated)

	Ca mmol/L (mg/dL)	iCa mmol/L (mg/dL)	P mmol/L (mg/dL)	PTH ng/L pg/mL	CT ng/L pg/mL	1,25(OH)$_2$D pmol/L (pg/mL)	25-OHD nmol/L (ng/mL)	UCa excretion* mg/kg/d	TRP** mmol/L (mg/dL)
Cord Blood	2.55 ± .15 (10.2 ± .60)[1]	1.45 ± .07 (5.83 ± .30)[1]	3.14 ± .23 (9.74 ± .73)[2]	3.4 ± .91[2]	58 ± 19[3]	81.4 ± 23 (33.9 ± 9.8)[2]	31.2 ± 7 (13 ± 3)[4]	—	—
0–18 months[5]									
Black	2.43 ± .15 (9.73 ± .60)	1.31 ± .04 (5.24 ± .18)	2.08 ± .22 (6.47 ± .69)	11.5 ± .4	65 ± 35	168 ± 62 (70 ± 26)	127 ± 43 (53 ± 18)		
White	2.41 ± .15 (9.67 ± .59)	1.30 ± .06 (5.22 ± .25)	2.19 ± .29 (6.78 ± .92)	12.3 ± .5	61 ± 34	137 ± 15 (57 ± 25)	122 ± 41 (51 ± 17)		
Summer	2.36 ± .14 (9.46 ± .56)	1.30 ± .04 (5.21 ± .17)	2.20 ± .26 (6.83 ± .81)	12.5 ± .3	75 ± 35	146 ± 41 (61 ± 17)	127 ± 38 (53 ± 16)		
Winter	2.47 ± .11 (9.91 ± .44)	1.30 ± .04 (5.23 ± .18)	2.08 ± .26 (6.44 ± .80)	11.0 ± .5	46 ± 30	173 ± 62 (72 ± 26)	108 ± 43 (45 ± 18)		
Children	2.35 ± .17 (9.40 ± .70)[6]	1.14 ± .13 (4.59 ± .52)[7]	1.13 ± .22 (3.50 ± .70)[6]	11.0 ± 35[8]	32 ± 22[9]	120 ± 13 (50 ± 5.5)[10]	84 ± 22 (35.2 ± 9.2)[11]	2.4[12]	1.15–2.44 (3.56–7.55)[8]
Summer						73 ± 5 (30.4 ± 2.3)[13]	64 ± 6 (26.5 ± 2.4)[13]		
Winter						56 ± 5 (23.4 ± 2.3)[13]	46 ± 5 (19.4 ± 2.1)[13]		

*Urinary calcium excretion

**Tubular reabsorption of phosphate per liter glomerular filtrate.

Source:

[1] American Journal of Diseases of Children 1988;142:516-18

[2] Pediatric Research, 1992 abstract (in press)

[3] Journal of American College of Nutrition 1990;9:358-62

[4] Journal of Clinical Endocrinology and Metabolism 1987;65:588-91

[5] Journal of Pediatrics 1986;77:891-96

[6] American Journal of Clinical Pathology 1978;69:24-31

[7] Pediatric Research 1973;7:485-93

[8] Archives of Diseases in Childhood 1991;65:1208-11

[9] Pediatric Research 1977;11:112-16

[10] Kidney International 1990;38:528-35

[11] Journal of Pediatrics 1977;91(6):904-8

[12] Archives of Diseases in Childhood 1974;49:97-101

[13] Pediatric Research 1991;30:654A

12. Schedewie HK, Odell WD, Fisher DA, Krutzik SR, Dodge M, Cousins L, Fiser WP. Parahormone and perinatal calcium homeostasis. Pediatr Res 1979;13:1-6.
13. Loughead JL, Mimouni F, Tsang R. Serum ionized calcium concentration in normal neonates. Am J Disease Child 1988;142:516-18.
14. Venkataraman PS, Tsang RC, Chen IW. Pathogenesis of early neonatal hypocalcemia: Studies of serum calcitonin, gastrin, and plasma glucagon. J Pediatr 1987;110:599-603.
15. Tsang RC, Chen I, Hayes W, Atkinson W, Atherton H, Edwards N. Neonatal hypocalcemia in infants with birth asphyxia. J Pediatr 1974;84:428-33.
16. Tsang RC, Kleinman LI, Sutherland JM, Light IJ. Hypocalcemia in infants of diabetic mothers. J Pediatr 1972;80:384-95.
17. Cruz ML, Tsang R. Disorders of calcium and magnesium homeostasis. In: Yeh T, ed. Neonatal therapeutics. St. Louis: Mosby Year Book, 1991.
18. Steichen JJ, Krug-Wispé SK, Tsang R. Breastfeeding the low birth weight infant. Clini Perinatol 1987;14(1):131-71.
19. Tsang RC, Noguchi A, Steichen J. Pediatric Parathyroid Disorders. Pediatr Clin North Am 1979;26(1):223-49.
20. Kooh SW, Binet A. Partial hypoparathyroidism: A variant of transient congenital hypoparathyroidism. Amer J Disease Child 1991;145:877-80.
21. Cruz ML, Mimouni F, Tsang R. Transient hypoparathyroidism. J Pediatr 1992;120:332.
22. Bergenfelz A, Norden NE, Ahren B. Intact parathyroid hormone assay is superior to mid region assay in the EDTA-infusion test in hyperparathyroidism. Clin Chim Acta 1991;197:229-36.
23. Koo WWKK, Tsang R. Mineral requirements of low-birth weight infants. J Am Col Nutrition 1991;10(5):474-86.
24. Bainbridge R, Mimouni F, Tsang RC, Landi T, Crossman M, Harris L. Effect of cereal feeding on bone mineralization in infants. Pediatr Res 1990;27:280A.
25. Dagnelie PC, Vergote F, van Staveren WA, van den Berg H DP, Hautvast J. High prevalence of rickets in infants on macrobiotic diets. Amer J Clin Nutri 1990;51:202-8.
26. Belton NR, Elidrissy ATH, Gaafer TH. Maternal vitamin D deficiency as a factor in the pathogenesis of rickets in Saudi Arabia. In: AW Norman KS DV Herrath, HG Grigoleit, ed. Vitamin D. chemical, biochemical, and clinical endocrinology of calcium metabolism. Berlin: de Gruyter, 1982.

Disorders of Carbohydrate Metabolism in Infants and Children

Denis Daneman, M.B., B.Ch., F.R.C.P.(C)

INTRODUCTION

Abnormalities of carbohydrate metabolism, specifically diabetes mellitus and hypoglycemic disorders, are encountered fairly frequently in the pediatric population. Diabetes mellitus is more common in older children and adolescents, while hypoglycemia occurs more often in the neonate. These disorders are dealt with in this chapter in two sections. The first section discusses diabetes mellitus: its classification, etiology, epidemiology, presentation, and management. The second section covers the hypoglycemic syndromes: their classification, diagnosis, and management.

DIABETES MELLITUS

Diabetes mellitus in children may be classified as Type I or insulin-dependent diabetes mellitus (IDDM); Type II or non-insulin-dependent diabetes mellitus (NIDDM), usually referred to as maturity-onset diabetes in the young (MODY); and other types of diabetes.[1] In children, the latter includes diabetes associated with cystic fibrosis; iron-overload diabetes due to transfusion therapy for thalassemia major or other anemia; and diabetes resulting from drug administration, such as corticosteroids alone or in combination with agents such as L-asparaginase.[2] Disturbances of glucose homeostasis associated with endocrine excess syndromes, such as Cushing's syndrome, pheochromocytoma, and growth hormone excess, are quite uncommon in childhood. Occasionally seen are patients with impaired glucose tolerance in the childhood age group.[3] This may represent the very earliest phase of IDDM or occasionally a hyperglycemic response to the stress of an intercurrent illness. Impaired glucose tolerance of varying severity may also be found in association with a number of syndromes, including Refsum's syndrome, Friedreich's ataxia, Alström's syndrome, Prader-Willi syndrome, Lawrence-Moon-Bardet-Biedl syndrome, Werner's syndrome, and Turner's syndrome.

Insulin-Dependent Diabetes Mellitus

Etiology and Pathogenesis

Presently, evidence strongly suggests that IDDM stems from an autoimmune attack on the β-cells of the islets of Langerhans.[4] The major thrusts of research in this area have focused on attempts to determine which components of the immune system mediate the attack, which factor(s) trigger(s) the reaction, and what allows it to persist until all β-cells have been destroyed. Current wisdom suggests that at least two factors are required for the expression of IDDM: genetic susceptibility and external (environmental) agents. These combine in an as yet undetermined manner to precipitate the immune changes leading to the development of IDDM. MacLaren and others have postulated a series of events, starting with exposure to a foreign antigen and ending with β-cell destruction, to explain the pathogenesis of IDDM.[5, 6] This schema is presented below, but it must be pointed out that, although feasible, it remains unproven.

Most likely, the process leading to IDDM starts as a vigorous immune response to a foreign, and as yet unidentified, antigen which closely resembles a normal component on the β-cell (immune mimickry). These antigens are ingested by macrophages somewhere in the body and present the mimic antigen (in close association with a class II major histocompatibility complex [MHC] molecule) to helper T cells, which in turn are able to secrete interleukins that activate other helper cells, as well as antibody-producing β-cells and cytotoxic T cells. In the pancreas, the sensitized cytotoxic T cells recognize the natural "twin" of the foreign antigen, i.e., the autoantigen on the β-cell wherever it is bound by the ubiquitous class I MHC molecules. Antibodies bind the β-cells as well, impairing them either directly or indirectly by eliciting help from other parts of the immune system, for example, by binding complement. Involvement of macrophages and further stimulation of helper T cells may amplify and sustain the destruction.

As the attack proceeds, the β-cells become progressively damaged, overproducing class I molecules and amplifying the cytotoxic T cell response. The damaged cells also display class II molecules, which should induce the immune system to suppress autoimmunity. However, in IDDM, the opposite occurs: more helper T cells are stimulated. Damage to the β-cells may release sequestered antigens, which even further stimulate the immune system, allowing acceleration of β-cell damage.

In the schema presented above, the immune markers, such as islet cell antibodies (ICA) and insulin autoantibodies (IAA), which are present in the majority of subjects either before or at the time of diagnosis of IDDM, are considered indicators of the immune attack on the β-cells rather than participants in the battle itself.[7-10] The exception to this may be the antibodies directed against the 64,000 molecular weight (64k) protein on the surface of the β-cell (see discussion below).[11]

Immune Markers

Three major antibodies have been identified, either before or at the time of diagnosis of IDDM[12] Their presence supports the immune pathogenesis of IDDM and may be helpful in predicting those individuals likely to develop IDDM in the future. The most studied of these antibodies is the islet cell antibody (ICA), which develops against an islet cell cytoplasmic glycoprotein.[13] This antibody is not specific to the β-cell and is directed at all islet cells. It is detectable at diagnosis in the majority of individuals with IDDM and its presence in non-diabetic individuals is highly predictive of future IDDM. For example, Bottazzo and colleagues have demonstrated that 100% of ICA-positive individuals with titers > 100 JDF units will develop IDDM over a 10-year period of observation.[14] The ICA assay is subject to methodological problems, and international workshops have set up strict assay standards.[15] This assay is likely to be the most appropriate for large-scale screening of first-degree relatives of those with IDDM, or even the population at large. At present, no interventions exist which will predictably prevent the ongoing destruction of the β-cells in the islets, and so population screening with ICA or other antibody assays remains within the realm of research.[13]

Antibodies to the insulin molecule—insulin autoantibodies (IAA)—have been noted prior to the initiation of insulin therapy in at least one-third to one-half of children with new-onset IDDM.[9, 10, 16, 17] These antibodies most likely develop in response to the release of insulin or insulin-degradation products from the β-cell damaged by the immune attack.

Also present in patients with IDDM are antibodies directed at a 64k protein on the surface of the β-cell—anti-64k antibodies. In contrast to the ICA, this is a β-cell specific antigen.[11, 18-21] Of the three antibodies listed, this is the only one found in rodent models of IDDM, the Non-Obese Diabetic mouse and BioBreeding rat. Recently, Baekkeskov and her colleagues identified the 64k protein as the enzyme glutamic acid decarboxylase.[21] The importance of this observation remains to be demonstrated. Difficulties with methods for detecting the 64k antibody make it an unlikely candidate for mass screening at the present time.

Genetic Susceptibility

Susceptibility to the development of IDDM appears to be related to class II or the D group of histocompatibility locus antigens (HLA).[22, 23] Over 95% of those with IDDM have either HLA DR-3 and/or -4 present. The presence of HLA DR-2 appears to confer protection against the development of IDDM. More recently, attention has focused on the DQ region of the D-locus, and specifically on the amino acid at position 57 on the β-chain.[24] The presence at this position of an aspartic acid (ASP) residue appears to protect against the development of IDDM, while a non-ASP residue confers susceptibility. This may be a critical region of the class II molecule responsible for binding the "autoantigen" involved in the pathogenesis of IDDM. Tighter binding in the presence of the non-ASP residue may increase the likelihood of recognition by T cells which mediate the immune attack.[5, 24, 25]

Metabolic Factors

Prior to the clinical expression of IDDM, glucose homeostasis is normal. However, decreased first-phase insulin secretion in response to an intravenous glucose tolerance test has been demonstrated in individuals later presenting with classical IDDM.[26] Furthermore, there are some individuals who have transient hyperglycemia associated with intercurrent illness or glucocorticoid use, months or even years before clinical presentation of IDDM.[3]

Epidemiology

IDDM is considered one of the most common chronic diseases of childhood, affecting 1 in 300 to 600 individuals by the age of 20 years.[27] The incidence of IDDM varies with geographical location, with the lowest incidence being noted in countries closest to the equator and increasing with distance from the equator.[28] This suggests a climatic effect on IDDM incidence. Incidence figures of less than 1 new case per

100,000 population per year in Japan, to 10–15 per 100,000 in North America, to the highest levels of about 30 per 100,000 in Finland have been reported.

IDDM affects both sexes equally and may occur at all ages. However, there is a low incidence in infants and toddlers, a peak in early school-age children, and a second, larger peak in early adolescence, occurring earlier in girls than in boys.[29] Some data also suggest a seasonal effect on IDDM presentation: a larger number of cases present in the winter months (November to March in the Northern Hemisphere) than during the summer. Mini-epidemics of IDDM have been reported, suggesting the possible role of infectious agents in the final triggering process.[30]

The presence of IDDM in a family member increases the risk in other first-degree relatives of developing the disease.[31] Table 10–1 summarizes this risk. Furthermore, HLA-typing can also help predict risk of IDDM: if a sibling of a proband with IDDM is HLA-identical, his or her relative risk is increased 90–100-fold; if only haploidentical, the increase is 35–40-fold; if HLA-nonidentical, the relative risk is not increased above the background population.

TABLE 10–1. Risk of Developing IDDM in First-Degree Relatives

Individual with IDDM	Risk to Offspring/Sibling
Father	6%
Mother	2%
Sibling	5%
Offspring	5%
Both parents	5%
Identical twins	30–50%
Nonidentical twins	5%

Presentation and Diagnosis

Although a few children are identified as having IDDM on routine health visits, most present with a history of a few days to a few weeks of typical symptoms of hyperglycemia: polyuria (nocturia, enuresis); polydipsia; polyphagia; weight loss (often with increased appetite); lethargy; and proceeding to frank ketoacidosis (vomiting, dehydration, abdominal pain, etc.). In our experience, one-quarter to one-third of children present in diabetic ketoacidosis (DKA), defined by a venous pH < 7.30 and serum bicarbonate concentration < 15 mmol/L.[32] Most of the remainder present with ketonuria, but without full-blown acidosis. A small minority present before ketosis develops, and in these the differential diagnosis of MODY or other type of diabetes will depend on observation of the natural history of the disease. Most will progress to obvious insulin dependence.

In the vast majority of children, the diagnosis of IDDM is made by the presence of the classical symptoms in association with glycosuria, hyperglycemia, and ketonuria. Measurement of acid-base and electrolyte status is only necessary to confirm the clinical picture of ketoacidosis. In the absence of ketonuria or if hyperglycemia is an incidental finding, observation of the course of the disorder plus determination of ICA status may be helpful. Glucose tolerance testing is rarely, if ever, required to make the diagnosis of IDDM, but may be helpful with NIDDM (see discussion below).

Approach to the Management of IDDM

Management of the child with newly diagnosed IDDM requires initial correction of the DKA and stabilization of the hyperglycemia, as well as ongoing education and support for the child and his or her family to enable them to carry out effective self-management at home.[33] Long-term care involves helping the child achieve "optimal" metabolic control, preventing the short-term complications of hypoglycemia and ketoacidosis, and early detection and intervention for the long-term micro- and macrovascular complications. Since IDDM requires the acquisition of numerous self-management skills, psychosocial issues must receive substantial attention, both anticipatory guidance and intervention in the event stress arises, either in the form of an intercurrent illness or psychological stress.

Treatment of Diabetic Ketoacidosis

Table 10–2 summarizes briefly the key components of ketoacidosis management. Central to the pathogenesis of DKA is insulin deficiency; increased concentrations of the counter-regulatory hormones (glucagon, epinephrine, cortisol and growth hormone) may exacerbate the hyperglycemia and ketosis, but cannot initiate DKA on their own.[34] Insulinopenia leads to intracellular starvation in the presence of hyperglycemia.

The hyperglycemia causes the osmotic diuresis and accompanying loss of electrolytes (sodium, potassium, phosphate) in the urine. This diuresis will lead ultimately to dehydration. Insulinopenia also leads to lipolysis (and eventually to ketogenesis) and proteolysis. Ketogenesis will produce the metabolic acidosis.

Serum potassium concentrations initially rise, due both to failure to enter the cells and to leeching from the cells in exchange for hydrogen ions. This is followed by decreasing serum concentrations as more potassium is lost in the urine. Because of the osmotic effect of glucose in the intravascular space, blood pressure will be maintained until very late in the process. Similarly, serum sodium concentrations will appear spuriously low, as will the hematocrit. A rising serum sodium concentration suggests extreme free-water loss and severe dehydration.

TABLE 10–2. Treatment of Diabetic Ketoacidosis

1. FLUID REPLETION	Initial fluids to contain normal saline, infused at 10–20 mL/kg body weight/h for the first 1–2 h, and then at 5–10 mL/kg/hr depending on the degree of dehydration. When plasma glucose concentration falls < 15 mmol/L or falls at a rate > 5–10 mmol/h, change to 5% dextrose in 0.2% saline or 3.3% dextrose in 0.3% saline. Chart intake and output very carefully to document ongoing repletion. *Beware of either too slow or too rapid rehydration.*
2. INSULIN REPLACEMENT	As soon as the diagnosis of DKA is made, an IV infusion of regular human insulin is begun at the rate of 0.1 unit/kg/h, switching to 0.02 units/kg/h when the plasma glucose concentration falls < 15 mmol/L. The objective is to maintain glucose concentration in the 6–15 mmol/L range to avoid either hypo- or hyperglycemia. Insulin may also be administered by the intramuscular or subcutaneous route if intravenous infusion is not possible.
3. ALKALI THERAPY	Administration of bicarbonate is indicated only in more severe DKA: pH < 7.20 and serum bicarbonate < 12 mmol/L. The amount of bicarbonate calculated to increase serum concentration to 12–15 mmol/L: half the repletion amount may be given over the first 20–30 min, the rest administered over the following 2–4 h.
4. POTASSIUM REPLACEMENT	After the child has voided, KCl should be added to the IV fluid: eg. 20–30 mmol/L if the concentration is above 4.5 mmol/L, and 30–40 mmol/L if below this concentration.
5. MONITORING	Careful monitoring of the clinical status (level of consciousness, blood pressure, pulse, etc.) as well as assessment of fluid balance is essential with regular measurement of plasma glucose (every hour for the first 4–6 h and every 2 h thereafter), acid-base and electrolyte status (every 4 h until correction has occurred).
6. OTHER FACTORS	All children should be given nothing by mouth at least during the early stages of therapy. The use of nasogastric tubes and urinary catheters can be avoided unless the child is comatose. Precipitating factors (such as intercurrent illness) should be dealt with if present.

Stabilization of the Hyperglycemia and Family Education

Once the ketoacidosis has been corrected, the child is usually started on twice-daily (before breakfast and dinner) injections of an intermediate-acting insulin, with or without addition of a short-acting insulin.[35] We prefer to begin all children on human insulin of either bio- or semisynthetic origin. The intermediate-acting insulin may be either NPH (isophane) or Lente, and the short-acting preparation is regular (soluble/crystalline) insulin. Approximately two-thirds to three-quarters of the daily dose is given in the morning, although the dose must be carefully tailored to individual needs. We increase the dosage slowly to achieve plasma glucose concentrations in the 4–10 mmol/L (~72–180 mg/dL) range before the main meals.

An essential part of the diabetes treatment regimen is a nutritional plan that is balanced in terms of total energy content, types of nutrients (50–55% carbohydrate with an emphasis on complex carbohydrates, 30–35% fat with decreased saturated fat intake, and 15–20% protein), and timing of meals and snacks. The meal plan must also be tailored to individual needs, since noncompliance is virtually assured in any child provided with an inadequate diet. Nutritional counseling requires assurance that the family understands not only the basic meal plan, but also how to adjust the food intake during nonbasal conditions, such as with exercise or during intercurrent illness.

Regular blood glucose and urine glucose and ketone testing is begun, and again is tailored to individual needs.[36] For all children with IDDM, we advise daily blood glucose testing before breakfast and dinner, with additional testing before lunch, at bedtime, and in the early morning hours as indicated. During initial stabilization, the children and their parents are taught how to perform self-monitoring of blood glucose (SMBG) and results are checked by simultaneous capillary specimens sent to the chemistry laboratory. Quality control of the accuracy of SMBG is essential, whether performed by patients or hospital personnel, and whether by visually-read strips or reflectance meters.[37]

During initial stabilization, which may occur either during an initial hospitalization or as an out-patient, depending on the center, the family must be educated in all aspects of diabetes care.[38] This education process is best carried out in a tertiary care center that has extensive experience in the care of children with IDDM. It is also best carried out by a multidisciplinary diabetes health care team which includes, in addition to the responsible physician, a diabetes nurse educator, dietician, behavioral specialist (social worker or psychologist), public health nurses, and laboratory facilities for performance of measurements such as hemoglobin A1c (HbA1c), serum lipids, and thyroid function tests (thyroxine and TSH concentrations).

For most families, the education program will include information about the pathophysiology of diabetes (hyperglycemia and ketoacidosis); administration of insulin and adjustment of insulin dose requirements; performance of SMBG; meal planning; the causes, recognition, and treatment of hypoglycemia; the effect of intercurrent illness on diabetes control and management; and the long-term complications of diabetes. An integral part of the education program is support for the child and family in dealing with the psychosocial impact of the diagnosis. In those families whose educational level is low or whose anxiety about the initial diagnosis is severe, a less intensive educational approach ("survival skills only") at the time of diagnosis is indicated. For all families, however, diabetes education only begins at diagnosis and must continue throughout the lifetime of the individual.

Early Clinical Course

The initial clinical and biochemical abnormalities of IDDM respond dramatically to treatment, usually with correction within 24–36 h of diagnosis. Within a few days to a few weeks of starting insulin therapy, most children enter into the "honeymoon" or partial remission period, during which time stable metabolic control is achieved relatively easily and insulin dose requirements fall.[32] Complete remission (i.e., cessation of the need for insulin therapy) is much less common (< 10%) and leads inevitably to the reinstitution of insulin therapy after a period of weeks to months. The remission period has been presumed to be due to β-cell recovery after correction of the initial severe hyperglycemia. However, changing peripheral insulin sensitivity, food intake (initially high to correct for weight loss) and restored physical activity may all play a role in the expression of this early phase of IDDM in these children.[39]

Attempts have been made to alter the early course of IDDM by the use of immune modulation therapies (e.g., cyclosporine, prednisone, interferon, azothiaprine)[40, 41] Currently, none of these approaches has proved either effective or entirely safe. Since more than 90% of β-cells are presumed to have been destroyed by the time of disease presentation, it is unlikely that this type of therapy will ever be able to completely ameliorate the disease. However, preservation of even a small amount of residual β-cell mass may render the IDDM less severe and thus more easily controlled with current therapy.

Objectives of IDDM Therapy

The overall objective of IDDM therapy should be to achieve normal glucose homeostasis, thereby preventing both the short- and long-term complications of the disorder. However, there are a few problems with this approach:

1. Normoglycemia, or near normoglycemia, is extremely difficult to achieve using either conventional (once or twice daily injections)

or intensive (continuous insulin infusion pumps or multiple daily injections) insulin therapy. In children's diabetes centers, less than 5% of the children with IDDM have HbA1c values within the nondiabetic range after the honeymoon period.[42]

2. Attempts to achieve normoglycemia are associated with a significant (2–10-fold) increase in episodes of severe hypoglycemia.[43, 44]

3. Evidence that very strict metabolic control will decrease or prevent the long-term complications of IDDM remains elusive. Most trials have been conducted over relatively short periods of time or in small numbers of subjects. These studies do not provide convincing evidence on the relationship between long-term diabetes control and complications.

The latter requires completion of large, multicenter trials comparing the effects of conventional and intensive treatment approaches on the long-term outcome of IDDM.[44, 45]

Despite these reservations, the following objectives should be pursued in the treatment of children with IDDM:

1. Control the signs and symptoms of hyperglycemia (polyuria, polydipsia, etc.).

2. Prevent DKA.

3. Avoid all but mild, occasional hypoglycemia that can be easily recognized and treated.

4. Maintain normal growth and physical development.

5. Maintain normal lipid profiles and prevent, wherever possible, the development of obesity.

6. Set realistic goals of therapy for each child.

7. Ensure optimum understanding of IDDM by each child and his or her family.

8. Provide psychosocial support for the child and family.

9. Ensure smooth transition from pediatric to adult diabetes care.

10. Provide surveillance for diabetes-related complications.

Therapeutic goals should guide the family and health care team toward optimal physical and emotional well-being and should be individualized to the specific needs and abilities of each child. For example, less strict blood glucose targets are necessary in infants and younger children with IDDM to prevent hypoglycemia, whereas in highly motivated adolescents and young adults, near normoglycemia occasionally may be feasible. Problems arise when either (a) unrealistic expectations are placed on the child and family, or (b) responsibility for self-management is shifted to the child at too early an age.[46]

Routine Follow-up

All children with IDDM should be seen by their health care team at regular intervals (three to four times a year) in order to evaluate their progress. Attention should focus specifically on diabetes-related issues such as insulin dose requirements, dietary compliance and satisfaction, results of blood glucose measurements performed at home, symptoms and frequency of hypo- and hyperglycemia, intercurrent illnesses and their impact on diabetes control, adequacy of growth and sexual development, and psychosocial adjustment to the diabetes, including school attendance and performance. Physical examination should include height and weight measurement with plotting on appropriate growth curves, blood pressure measurement, fundus examination, palpation of the thyroid gland and liver, and inspection of injection sites.

These routine follow-up visits provide the opportunity to improve understanding of diabetes, make appropriate adjustments in the treatment regimen, and intervene in the event any medical or psychosocial problems are detected. It also allows techniques of insulin injection, SMBG, and meal planning to be assessed. Furthermore, regular measurement of HbA1c and annual measurement of serum cholesterol, triglycerides, and thyroid function can be accomplished at these visits. Urine testing for protein (microalbuminuria, where available) and ophthalmologic examination should be performed annually in children over 12–15 years of age with IDDM of more than 5 years duration.[47]

The specific components of the diabetes treatment regimen include the following:

- insulin therapeutics
- nutritional planning
- exercise and its impact on metabolic control
- monitoring techniques
- hypoglycemia recognition and treatment
- psychosocial issues.

INSULIN. For the child with IDDM, insulin administered by injection is essential for life. Most children are treated with human insulin products given as twice-daily injections of mixtures of intermediate- and short-acting preparations (e.g., NPH plus regular insulin). More intensive therapy, using three or four daily injections or infusion pumps, has not received general acceptance by children and has not yet been shown to improve metabolic control in large clinic populations.[48] Insulin dose must be tailored to the individual needs of each child: there are no easy prescriptions. Insulin requirements change on a dynamic basis in relation to changes in food intake, exercise patterns, etc. We recommend changes in insulin dose based on patterns of blood glucose concentrations observed over 3–5 day periods. More frequent dose adjustment, although possible in some children, may lead to over-insulinization and/or confusion.

DIET. There is no doubt that meal planning is an essential component of diabetes management. The plan for each child must include sufficient caloric intake to meet the needs for normal growth and development. Attention must also be paid to the types of foods and timing of meals and snacks. For very young children (< 4–5 y), a strict meal plan (exchange type diet) will likely be impossible to institute. Rather, these children require a balanced approach to diet, stressing timing of meals, mix of foods and avoidance of hypoglycemia. In older children, a more structured meal plan is an integral part of the diabetes regimen.

EXERCISE. Children with diabetes are at risk from exercise-related hypoglycemia because of the increased glucose utilization by muscle during exercise, combined with their inability to switch off absorption of the subcutaneously administered insulin (and, in fact, the increased absorption due to increased blood flow to the exercising limbs).[49] Care must be taken, therefore, to provide sufficient calories on a daily basis to avoid hypoglycemia during usual amounts of physical activity, with extra calories provided when an extraordinary amount of exercise is planned. Late post-exercise hypoglycemia (i.e., hypoglycemia occurring many hours after completion of the period of exercise) occurs in some individuals. Its presence can be detected and prevented by more frequent glucose monitoring when physical activity changes.

Physical fitness has been shown to have certain salutary effects on those with IDDM. It improves efficiency of glucose utilization, insulin sensitivity, and perhaps also overall morbidity and mortality from the IDDM.

MONITORING METABOLIC CONTROL. Monitoring of metabolic control can be divided into two aspects: self-monitoring of blood and urine glucose concentrations at home, and objective monitoring using specifically HbA1c measurement.[50, 51] All children and their families should be taught to perform self-monitoring of both blood glucose and urine glucose and ketones at home. Emphasis should be placed on accuracy of testing and a plan agreed upon for frequency of each type of testing. For daily monitoring, we prefer blood glucose testing before breakfast and dinner with target concentrations of blood glucose of 4–10 mmol/L (~72–180 mg/dL). Additional testing should be performed as indicated, including more frequent testing following changes in the treatment regimen, during intercurrent illness, to monitor the effects of exercise on the diabetes control, etc. Urine testing for glucose needs only be used to complement the blood testing. Urine ketone testing, however, is essential during intercurrent illness and when blood glucose concentrations are well above the target range (e.g., > 15 mmol/L, > 270 mg/dL).

Debate continues over the best techniques for blood and urine testing. Accuracy, ease of use, affordability, durability, and portability are some of the factors to be considered when choosing self-monitoring techniques. Although many people prefer the reflectance meters, visually-read strips, if properly used, can provide virtually the same accuracy.[37]

HbA1c has become the gold standard measure of long-term metabolic control.[51] The observation that hemoglobin is glycated in proportion to the average blood glucose concentration over the life span of the red cell (90–120 days) provided the long-sought-after objective assessor of diabetes control. Measurement of HbA1c is subject to a number of potential problems, mostly methodological, including failure to remove the labile fraction (pre-HbA1c) prior to measurement, difficulties in comparing measurement by different methods, and lack of availability of appropriate standards.[52] Nevertheless, when measured appropriately, HbA1c allows tracking of metabolic control in individual patients over time. HbA1c measurement does not replace the need for daily self-monitoring, nor, if high, does it indicate what specific changes need to be made in the diabetes regimen.

HbA1c measurement in large clinic populations has shown that very few children or adults with IDDM achieve nondiabetic concentrations.[42, 44] Mean HbA1c concentrations in children's diabetes clinics are, on average, 1.5 to 2 times the mean of the nondiabetic population. A useful formula is that the mean blood glucose concentration in the nondiabetic population is about 5 mmol/L (90 mg/dL) and mean HbA1c approximately 5%. For every 1% increase in HbA1c there is an approximately 1.5–2 mmol/L (~25–35 mg/dL) rise in mean blood glucose concentration. Thus, an HbA1c of 8% reflects a mean glucose of about 9.5–11 mmol/L (~170–200 mg/dL), far from normoglycemia.

Recently, some authors have advocated measurement of fructosamine as an addition to or alternative to HbA1c measurement.[53] This assay is relatively simple, measuring the reduction of nitro blue tetrazolium by 1-amino-1-deoxyfructose. It has been documented to monitor changes in glycemic control over a 1 w interval.[53] Whether this assay provides real benefits over the accurate measurement of blood glucose concentrations remains to be proved.

In addition to monitoring blood glucose at home and regular measurement of HbA1c levels, it is important that all children with IDDM have their serum lipids and thyroid function tests checked on an annual basis. Lipid abnormalities are associated with poor metabolic control, but are also widespread in the population at large.

Hypercholesterolemia and hypertriglyceridemia are additional risk factors for the development of macrovascular complications of IDDM.

HYPOGLYCEMIA. Hypoglycemia is a serious and constant risk in all individuals treated with insulin. It is clear that insulin delivery in IDDM is not physiological; any small change in the diabetes treatment regimen may precipitate hypoglycemia.[43, 54-55] Identifiable causes of hypoglycemia include: excess (intentional or unintentional) insulin administration; missed, delayed, or decreased size of a meal or snack; and insufficient extra caloric ingestion during periods of increased physical activity. Sometimes, the cause of the hypoglycemia may not be identifiable. Symptoms of hypoglycemia include those due to catecholamine responses ("early warning symptoms," including shakiness, anxiety, pallor, hunger, etc.) and those due to neuroglycopenia (abnormal behavior, confusion, convulsion, coma).

Prevention of hypoglycemia depends on the ability to predict changes in the treatment program that may predispose to these episodes. This requires regular blood glucose monitoring and insulin dose decreases when glucose concentrations are below or in the lower part of the target range. Treatment of hypoglycemia involves ingestion of concentrated simple carbohydrate at the first symptoms of a hypoglycemic reaction. For those with significant neuroglycopenia, injection of glucagon or intravenous glucose will rapidly correct the hypoglycemia.

Mild, occasional hypoglycemia is likely to occur in most insulin-treated individuals and probably has no long-term consequences. Severe hypoglycemia, on the other hand, may occasionally have serious neurological consequences and will invariably increase anxiety about the diabetes treatment. These episodes should be avoided as far as possible. Nevertheless, a number of studies demonstrate that about one-third of children with IDDM will have one or more episodes of severe hypoglycemia during their lifetimes.

PSYCHOSOCIAL ISSUES. It is clear that the development of a chronic disorder such as IDDM places significant stress on both child and family.[56-59] In many families, this does not cause any serious consequences; in some, however, the additional burden of dealing with the diabetes routines may lead to psychosocial distress. It is essential that the health care team involved in the care of these children and their families be aware of the role that psychosocial factors play in the achievement of stable diabetes control, and, also the impact of this disorder on normal child and adolescent development. The availability of social workers and psychologists as members of the multidisciplinary diabetes health care is essential in dealing with these problems, both in terms of anticipatory guidance and crisis intervention.

Surveillance for Long-Term Complications

The years before puberty are thought to contribute little, if anything, to the long-term complications of IDDM. This suggests that the clock starts ticking on these complications at about the time when adolescent development begins.[60] This indicates the possible role of sex hormones and/or growth factors in the pathogenesis of the complications. Thus, surveillance for complications need only begin after puberty has begun and a significant duration of diabetes has elapsed. The American Diabetes Association, for example, has suggested that after age 15 years and 5 years duration of diabetes, all IDDM individuals should undergo routine annual ophthalmologic examinations. This includes dilatation of the pupil and careful examination of the fundus, with or without the addition of stereofundus photography or fluorescein angiography. In this way, early background retinopathy can be detected and followed if it progresses towards pre- or frank proliferative retinopathy.

Similarly, all those with IDDM should be screened regularly for the presence of diabetic nephropathy.[61, 62] Traditionally, this has involved blood pressure measurement and use of a dipstick to detect proteinuria. It is evident that blood pressure screening is a vital part of diabetes management: detection and adequate treatment of hypertension has been demonstrated to slow progression of nephropathy. Detection of microalbuminuria, before the onset of frank proteinuria (i.e., stage of incipient nephropathy), has been shown to be a predictor of later development of progressive nephropathy.[63, 64] Whether intervention at this stage in the normotensive adolescent will prevent progression of renal disease remains to be proved.

Macrovascular disease surveillance implies regular measurement of serum lipid concentrations and intervention strategies to maintain these within the normal range if increased. Routine physical examination should also include neurological assessment and foot inspection, especially in those youngsters with long-duration diabetes.

Summary

IDDM is a common and complex metabolic disorder with significant implications for both short- and long-term health. It is clear that a multidisciplinary health care approach is required to assist children and their families in dealing with the medical and psychosocial impact of the disease. This requires a considerable effort both on the part of the health care team and other health professionals involved in providing the services (e.g., laboratory measurements, eye examinations) essential for optimum care.

Non-Insulin-Dependent Diabetes Mellitus (NIDDM) in the Young

NIDDM, although rare before age 30 years, can occur in young people.[65] Two types of presentation have been reported: (1) sporadic cases of NIDDM, and (2) MODY, which implies NIDDM with autosomal dominant inheritance.[65] The frequency of these conditions has been reported to vary from as low as 0.15% of all diabetic patients in Germany, to 4.8% of those with diabetes < 25 years of age in India, to as high as 10% of all cases of youth-onset diabetes among Black Americans in the United States. The frequency with which this condition is misdiagnosed as IDDM is unknown, but is likely relatively low, particularly where there is a strong family history of MODY/NIDDM or when the diabetes is asymptomatic at presentation.

Diagnosis of MODY or sporadic NIDDM in youngsters depends on the presence of abnormal glucose concentrations in the absence of ketosis. Oral glucose tolerance testing is not required if fasting plasma glucose concentrations are above 140 mg/dL (> 7.8 mmol/L) or a random level above 200 mg/dL (> 11.1 mmol/L) is noted. If these criteria are not met and diabetes is suspected, an oral glucose tolerance test may be helpful: diagnosis depends on a 2 h plasma glucose > 200 mg/dL (> 11.1 mmol/L) and at least one other value at 0.5, 1, or 1.5 h > 200 mg/dL.[1]

Treatment of MODY or sporadic NIDDM in young people consists primarily of dietary management, with addition of oral hypoglycemic agents where necessary. Insulin administration should be reserved for those patients who are unable to achieve glycemic targets on diet and oral agents.[66]

Hypoglycemic Disorders

In comparison with older children and adults, glucose homeostasis in newborn infants and young children is in a more precarious state, balanced between obligatory glucose requirements on the one hand and the ability to maintain an adequate supply of glucose during fasting on the other. This is thought to be the result largely of the relatively higher proportion of brain mass to body size in these youngsters.[67] Postabsorptive glucose flux rates in children (35 ± 2 µmol/kg/min) are almost three times as high as in adults (12.8 ± 0.5 µmol/kg/min). Similarly, glucose flux during fasting is also significantly higher (23 ± 3 and 9.8 ± 0.5 µmol/kg/min in children and adults respectively).[68] Despite this increased requirement for glucose, hepatic glycogen content in normal children is enough to meet the demand for up to 18 h. Thereafter, gluconeogenesis becomes the primary source of endogenous glucose production. The relatively smaller muscle mass in newborns and infants relative to body size may also compromise their ability to mobilize sufficient gluconeogenic substrate to maintain their higher glucose requirements.[67]

Fatty acid availability is also of great importance in the maintenance of glucose homeostasis in infants and children.[69] The relatively faster decrease in glucose concentration and increase in ketone body concentrations during fasting in children indicate an acceleration in the normal adaptation to fasting observed in adults.

The higher glucose flux rates, limited gluconeogenic capacity, and rapid rate of fatty acid metabolism in young infants suggest that any abnormalities in the mobilization, interconversion, and utilization of a variety of substrates will place these children at much greater risk for the development of hypoglycemia than is the case in older children and adults.[70]

Definition of Hypoglycemia

The earlier definitions of hypoglycemia in the newborn period were derived from neonates fasted for up to 72 h.[67] Despite ongoing debate as to the exact concentration of plasma glucose that reflects hypoglycemia, and despite inadequate long-term neurodevelopmental studies, the older definitions are no longer considered tenable.

For practical purposes, any neonate or child with a plasma glucose concentration below 2.2 mmol/L (40 mg/dL) should be evaluated for hypoglycemia. Probably, those in whom concentrations between 2.2 and 2.7 mmol/L (40–50 mg/dL) are found should be carefully observed.[70]

Signs and Symptoms of Hypoglycemia

In the neonate and infant, the signs and symptoms of hypoglycemia are likely to be fairly non-specific (e.g., irritability and/or lethargy, hypotonia, feeding problems, cyanosis, apnea or tachypnea, hypothermia, pallor) and easily confused with those of other common conditions, including any central nervous system abnormality, cardiac failure, congenital heart disease, sepsis, respiratory distress syndrome, or other metabolic disturbance such as hypocalcemia. Careful monitoring of plasma glucose concentrations in all newborns has become mandatory over the first hours of life to prevent the development of hypoglycemia.

In older infants and children, the clinical presentation of hypoglycemia may be divided into signs and symptoms arising from catecholamine responses (sweating, weakness, shakiness, tachycardia, anxiety, hunger, pallor) and those from neuroglycopenia (headache, confusion or abnormal behavior, convulsions or coma). Repeated or prolonged episodes of severe hypoglycemia may result in permanent brain damage;

the effects of asymptomatic hypoglycemia on brain development remain uncertain.[71, 72]

Causes of Hypoglycemia in Infants and Children

Table 10–3 presents the disorders associated with hypoglycemia in infants and children based on the etiology of these conditions. In the immediate neonatal period, most episodes of hypoglycemia are transient and associated with either small for gestational age or preterm infants, other stress situations, or infants of diabetic mothers. Persistent neonatal or infantile hypoglycemia is far less common, but usually due to (in descending order of frequency) hyperinsulinism, other hormonal deficiency, or an inborn error of metabolism. After one year of age, ketotic hypoglycemia, a condition seen with declining frequency, is the most common diagnosis.

Abnormal Hormone Secretion

Hyperinsulinism

Hyperinsulinism results in an increase in peripheral glucose utilization (particularly by fat and muscle cells) and a decrease in hepatic glucose production, the latter likely the more important determinant of the hypoglycemia.[70] High insulin concentrations also suppress mobilization of other endogenous substrates, leading to suppression of ketogenesis and proteolysis.

TRANSIENT NEONATAL HYPERINSULINISM. Hypoglycemia in the infant of the diabetic mother (IDM) is the direct result of prolonged maternal hyperglycemia leading to fetal and neonatal hyperinsulinemia.[73] Other defects such as decreased glucagon secretion and delayed induction of gluconeogenic enzymes may exacerbate the hypoglycemia.[73-75] This condition can be prevented by the achievement of meticulous glucose homeostasis in the pregnant mother with diabetes, particularly in the late stages of gestation and during labor and delivery.[76]

Hypoglycemia in infants with erythroblastosis fetalis has been attributed to hyperinsulinism associated with β-cell hyperplasia.[77] The reason for this remains unknown. Similarly, in the Beckwith-Wiedemann syndrome, a rare syndrome characterized by omphalocele, macroglossia, visceromegaly, and abnormal ear creases, transient, and occasionally more persistent, hyperinsulinemic hypoglycemia has been noted.[78]

SUSTAINED HYPERINSULINISM. Most children with sustained hyperinsulinism present within the first year of life, either in the immediate newborn period, when they may appear similar to the IDM (i.e., macrosomia), or later in the first year.[79]

TABLE 10–3. Hypoglycemic Disorders of Infants and Children

Hyperinsulinism
    Transient Neonatal:
        Infant of diabetic mother
        Erythroblastosis fetalis
        Beckwith-Wiedemann syndrome
    Persistent/Sustained:
        Islet cell dysplasia
        Focal/diffuse adenomatosis
        Insulinoma
    Drug-induced:
        Insulin, oral hypoglycemic agents
    Growth hormone deficiency**
    ACTH or cortisol deficiency**
    ? Glucagon deficiency*
    ? Somatostatin deficency
    ? Thyroid hormone deficiency
ABNORMAL SUBSTRATE AVAILABILITY
    Ketotic hypoglycemia**
    Hypoglycemia associated with surgery
ABNORMAL FUEL METABOLISM
    Inborn errors of metabolism***
        Carbohydrate:
            Glycogen storage disease
            Defective hepatic gluconeogenesis
        Amino acids:
            Maple syrup urine disease
        Fatty acids:
            Systemic carnitine deficiency
        Transient or acquired defects
            Small-for-gestational-age infants
        Other causes:
            Reye's syndrome
            Alcohol ingestion
            Salicylates
            Cyanotic congenital heart disease

*Hypoketotic syndromes: suppressed or defective ketogenesis
**Hyperketotic syndromes: "exaggerated" ketogenesis
***Organic acidosis: lactic acidosis, hepatomegaly, associated features

The pathologic findings in children with hyperinsulinism may vary greatly: in many there is a generalized increase in β-cells, either in relation to the pancreatic ducts (nesidioblastosis), scattered singly or in small numbers throughout the pancreas or an increase in the number and size of the islets of Langerhans.[80] In some, pancreatic histology may appear normal.

The preferred term, islet cell dysplasia or dysmaturation, suggests a functional defect in insulin secretion rather than a specific pathologic entity. The fact that spontaneous remission has been reported by a number of authors supports the concept that at least some cases of islet cell dysplasia may be the result of delayed maturation of the mechanisms controlling islet cell embryology and/or insulin secretion.[80, 81]

A distinct insulinoma is extremely uncommon in young children. More common findings include either focal or diffuse increases in islet cells ("adenomatosis") not confined to β-cells.

The pathology of the pancreas in neonates and infants with hyperinsulinism cannot be predicted by either the clinical presentation or by results of dynamic testing (e.g., glucose responses to insulin secretogogues such as tolbutamide or leucine). The relative infrequency of insulinomas in children suggests that imaging techniques (ultrasound, CT scan, magnetic resonance) are unlikely to be helpful in localizing the pathology in more than a small minority of cases.[80, 81]

Initial therapy of sustained hyperinsulinism consists of intravenous glucose infusion to prevent life-threatening hypoglycemia. Inability to control hypoglycemia with infusion rates of 12–15 mg/kg/min of glucose should lead to addition of other agents including glucagon (IV infusion), somatostatin (IV infusion of native somatostatin or SC injection of a long-acting analog) and diazoxide orally.[79, 81] The use of glucagon and somatostatin is confined mainly to preoperative stabilization of these patients. In a few cases, long-acting analogs of these two hormones have been employed over prolonged periods in a effort to avoid surgery.[82]

Diazoxide (10–20 mg/kg/day divided into three equal doses) may control the hyperinsulinism and has been used indefinitely in some cases.[79] In the newborn, diazoxide may cause sodium and water retention with resultant hypertension and cardiac failure; these side-effects may be controlled by the addition of a thiazide diuretic.[83] Other side effects of diazoxide include hypertrichosis, hyperuricemia, and neutropenia. Careful monitoring of blood glucose concentrations will help prevent hyperglycemia-related problems.

In the infant in whom hypoglycemia persists despite intensive medical management, and/or in whom significant side-effects of drug therapy are noted, subtotal (> 95%) pancreatectomy becomes the treatment of choice.[84, 85] Intraoperative ultrasonography may help in localizing areas of adenomatosis. Transient postoperative hyperglycemia, which may necessitate insulin therapy, suggests effective treatment. In a significant number of patients, however, subtotal pancreatectomy fails to control the hyperinsulinism; in these children, further medical or surgical management may be required. Total pancreatectomy will almost certainly result in insulin dependence and malabsorption.

In a proportion of these patients, spontaneous remission has been reported months to years after introduction of medical management.[79] Thus, in children controlled on diazoxide, repeat testing should be carried out at intervals to assess the need for ongoing treatment.

DRUG-RELATED HYPERINSULINISM.   Accidental ingestion of oral hypoglycemic agents may cause hyperinsulinemic hypoglycemia in children. Factitious hypoglycemia due to malicious (i.e., intentional) insulin administration to infants or children has been reported.[86, 87] Measurement of insulin and C-peptide concentrations would be useful in diagnosis: high insulin with undetectable C-peptide concentrations are diagnostic.[87] This should be regarded as a form of child abuse.

Growth Hormone, ACTH, and Cortisol Deficiencies

Children with hypopituitarism (growth hormone deficiency with or without associated ACTH deficiency) have a propensity to develop hypoglycemia. This tends to occur in those hypopituitary children somewhat underweight for height rather than those with the more typical pudgy, relatively overweight appearance.[88] Findings in the neonatal period which may suggest hypopituitarism include the presence of a micropenis in males, hyperbilirubinemia, or midline facial defects such as cleft lip or palate.

The pathogenesis of hypoglycemia in these disorders is uncertain. At the time of hypoglycemia, these children are ketotic, have low insulin concentrations, and low concentrations of the gluconeogenic substrates alanine and glutamine. They also have a blunted glycemic response to administered glucagon. It is likely that growth hormone and ACTH increase hepatic glucose production and decrease peripheral utilization by facilitating fatty acid and amino acid mobilization and by opposing the hepatic effects of insulin.

Hypopituitarism as a cause of hypoglycemia is usually self-limited: children over 3–4 years of age do not require growth hormone to maintain euglycemia. Replacement therapy with growth hormone and hydrocortisone, increasing the latter three- to fivefold during periods of stress, eliminates the hypoglycemia.

Occasionally, children in whom hyperinsulinism and hypopituitarism coexist have been described.[79] The reason remains elusive; perhaps serious hyperinsulinemic hypoglycemia may lead to pituitary infarction.

Hypoglycemia may also complicate the presentation of Addison's disease or other causes of adrenal insufficiency in children. Hypoglycemia is a relatively uncommon feature in the presentation of congenital adrenal hyperplasia.

Other Hormone Deficiencies

Isolated glucagon or somatostatin deficiencies have been proposed as possible mechanisms for hypoglycemia due to hyperinsulinism, i.e., loss of paracrine control of insulin secretion.[89, 90] Proof of these entities remains unconvincing. The role of thyroid hormones in maintenance of glucose homeostasis in infants and children is probably minimal. There are, however, reports of hypoglycemia associated with hypothyroidism, which is reversible with appropriate replacement therapy.

Abnormal Substrate Availability

Ketotic Hypoglycemia

This is the most common cause of hypoglycemia in children presenting beyond the first year of life.[91] Nevertheless, the incidence of this condition has decreased over the past decade. Generally, it presents between 12 months and 4 or 5 years of age and spontaneously remits by 6–8 years.

Normal children exhibit ketonemia, but not symptomatic hypoglycemia, 24–36 h after introduction of a hypocaloric, ketogenic diet (high in fat and low in carbohydrate). In contrast, in children with ketotic hypoglycemic, within 8–16 h after introducing a similar diet, both ketonemia and symptomatic hypoglycemic usually develop.[92] Similar results are found in response to a monitored fast lasting 21–24 h. Ketotic hypoglycemia may be the extreme end of the spectrum of normal responses to fasting in children in this age group.

The pathophysiologic mechanism responsible for this condition is unknown. The importance of hypoalaninemia (alanine is an important gluconeogenic amino acid) and abnormal adrenomedullary responses remains uncertain.[93]

Hypoglycemia usually manifests in these infants in association with an intercurrent illness or during periods of reduced caloric intake. Monitoring for ketonuria at such times may help prevent hypoglycemia. Treatment consists of regular meals high in carbohydrate and protein, particularly during these periods of catabolism.

Hypoglycemia Associated with Surgery

There are numerous reports of hypoglycemia complicating the postoperative period in children.[95, 96] The possible mechanisms include: prolonged preoperative fasting, intra- and post-operative stress with increase demands for energy, and the effects of a variety of medications on glucose production and utilization. The use of intravenous glucose infusions and glucose monitoring will help to prevent this complication.

Abnormal Fuel Metabolism

Inborn Errors of Metabolism

Deficiencies of enzymes important in mobilization, interconversion and utilization of a variety of substrates may be associated with hypoglycemia.[70] These autosomal, recessively inherited errors of carbohydrate, amino acid, or fatty acid metabolism are generally associated with failure to thrive, developmental delay, hepatomegaly, and metabolic (lactic or organic) acidosis.

CARBOHYDRATE: *Glycogen Storage Disease and Disorders of Hepatic Gluconeogenesis.*[97] Deficiency of one of the enzymes responsible for hepatic glycogen synthesis (glycogen synthetase deficiency) or release (deficiency of the debrancher enzyme and defective/deficient activation of hepatic phosphorylase) will cause hypoglycemia by decreasing availability of glucose in the post-absorptive state.

Glycogen storage disease, Type I, due to glucose-6-phosphatase deficiency, is the most common of these inborn errors. Hydrolysis of glucose-6-phosphate is essential for the release of hepatic glucose via either gluconeogenesis or glycogenolysis. Deficiency of the enzyme causes prolonged hypoglycemia early in infancy. The mobilization of glycogen and induction of gluconeogenesis result in the production of lactate rather than glucose leading to lactic acidosis. This metabolic error thus leads to accumulation of hepatic glycogen and fatty infiltration of the liver, the latter being responsible for the marked hepatomegaly. Other features include psychomotor and growth retardation, hyperlipidemia, and hyperuricemia. Diagnosis depends on demonstration of fasting hypoglycemia in association with hepatomegaly and metabolic (lactate) acidosis. A hallmark of Type I disease is an absent glycemic response to glucagon, a potent glycogenolytic hormone. Confirmation of diagnosis depends on direct enzyme determination in a liver biopsy specimen.

Treatment of these conditions is aimed at preventing hypoglycemia. This can be achieved by constant intravenous or intragastric infusion of glucose. This has been translated into frequent daytime feedings with constant nocturnal intragastric infusion or late-evening ingestion of a slow release form of glucose, namely raw cornstarch.[98]

Three other types of glycogen storage disease may also occur in infancy with findings similar to those described for Type I disease: amylo-1,6-glucosidase deficiency (Type 3), hepatic phosphorylase deficiency (Type 6) and phosphorylase kinase deficiency (Type 9).

Deficiency of hepatic fructose-1,6-diphosphatase also results in defective gluconeogenesis. Clinical features are similar to those in glycogen storage disease, Type I. Treatment consists of a diet high in carbohydrate (55–60%), and low in fat (30%). Intravenous glucose infusion may be required during periods of catabolism.

Other enzyme deficiencies associated with carbohydrate metabolism that may lead to hypoglycemia include pyruvate decarboxylase, phosphoenolpyruvate carboxykinase, galactose-1-phosphate uridyl transferase (galactosemia) and fructose-1-phosphate aldolase (hereditary fructose intolerance).

AMINO ACIDS: *Branched chain α-ketoacid dehydrogenase deficiency (Maple Syrup Urine Disease).* Hypoglycemia is noted in patients with Maple Syrup Urine Disease (MSUD) during periods when concentrations of branched-chain amino acids and α-ketoacid are very high, e.g., during illness or other stress.[99] The etiology of the hypoglycemia is unknown. Other defects in amino acid metabolism that may be associated with hypoglycemia include methylmalonic aciduria, glutaric acidemia, and ethylmalonicadipic aciduria. The treatment of these disorders involves limiting intake of the offending amino acid, with caloric supplementation during times of stress.

FATTY ACIDS. A rare group of disorders has been identified in which hypoglycemia occurs in association with hypoketonemia, but not hyperinsulinism. These disorders involve defective β-oxidation of fatty acids. Systemic carnitine deficiency presents with profound hypoglycemia, floppiness, hepatomegaly, encephalopathy, and increased concentrations of free fatty acids, ammonia, and liver and muscle enzymes (creatine kinase and lactic dehydrogenase).[100, 101] The similarity to Reye's syndrome is striking. Another presentation is with cardiac failure alone. Other disorders include distinct or combined abnormalities of medium- or long-chain acyl-coenzyme A dehydrogenases, resulting in accumulation of abnormal fatty acid metabolites.[102, 103]

Many of these children exhibit an enzyme defect in the catabolism of acyl-coenzyme A compounds. Some of the conditions associated with this include propionic, isovaleric, and methylmalonic acidurias and long- and medium-chain acyl dehydrogenase deficiencies. Deficiency in acyl carnitine transferase leads to hypoglycemia, hypoketonemia, and lactic acidosis, but not a Reye's-like syndrome.

Diagnosis depends on finding hypoglycemia in the absence of ketonuria. This suggests the need for measurement of concentrations of insulin, ketone bodies, free fatty acids, lactate, and free and total carnitine. Urine should also be analyzed for volatile and non-volatile organic acids.

The mechanism of hypoglycemia in these disorders is unknown but may relate either to accelerated rates of glucose utilization or to decreased glucose production. Treatment includes frequent feedings and oral carnitine replacement. During periods of catabolism, intravenous glucose infusion may become essential.

Miscellaneous

Small-for-Gestational-Age (SGA) Infants

Many SGA infants develop transient neonatal hypoglycemia. This may be due to a number of mechanisms, including decreased substrate stores, increased demand for substrate due to intercurrent stress, or a delay in induction of the enzyme systems required for gluconeogenesis.

Once identified, SGA infants should have their glucose concentrations monitored carefully over the first days of life to prevent hypoglycemia. Early feeding and/or intravenous infusions of glucose are warranted, particularly in those with significant neonatal illness.

Other Causes

Reye's syndrome often follows a viral illness (influenza A or B, varicella) and may be compounded by the administration of aspirin. Hypoglycemia is prominent in younger children presenting with this condition and can be prevented by administration of glucose.

Salicylate compounds may produce hypoglycemia and ketones by poorly defined means. A history of salicylate ingestion should be sought in all acutely hypoglycemic infants. Ethyl alcohol inhibits hepatic gluconeogenesis and may also produce hypoglycemia. Hypoglycemia in cyanotic congenital heart disease may be due to poor hepatic perfusion, resulting in a decreased rate of hepatic glucose production.

Investigation of Hypoglycemia[104, 105]

The diagnosis of hypoglycemia depends on the accurate laboratory measurement of plasma glucose concentration, and not merely by reagent strips with or without reflectance meters. Demonstration of a plasma glucose concentration below 2.2 mmol/L (40 mg/dL) should trigger further evaluation.

The history and physical examination give important clues to possible etiology. For example, age at presentation is clearly important. In newborns, large-for-gestational-age infants are more likely to be hyperinsulinemic, whereas SGA infants are more prone to substrate deficiency. The finding of a micropenis and hyperbilirubinemia should raise the suspicion of hypopituitarism. Children diagnosed beyond 1 year of age are most commonly suffering from ketotic hypoglycemia.

Although many diagnostic tests have been utilized in the diagnosis of hypoglycemia in infants and children, most often only a thorough history, physical examination, and limited testing are required. The oral glucose tolerance test contributes very little, if anything, to the diagnosis and should not be used in evaluating hypoglycemia in the pediatric population. Of utmost importance is obtaining a so-called "critical blood sample," i.e., a blood specimen taken at the time of hypoglycemia in which not only plasma glucose but also hormones (growth hormone, cortisol, and insulin) and metabolites (ketone bodies, lactate, fatty acids, venous blood gas) are measured. This specimen may be obtained when the infant presents to the emergency room or after performance of a monitored fast in which glucose is measured at regular intervals. In young infants, omission of one or two feedings may be sufficient to produce the hypoglycemia; in older children a fast of up to 24–30 h may be required. In older children, the fast should begin after supper, so that hypoglycemia is likely to occur between 9:00 AM and 6:00 PM the following day. Table 10–4 outlines results of glucose, hormone, and metabolite testing at the time of hypoglycemia in the different diagnostic categories.

TABLE 10–4. Investigation of Hypoglycemia in Childhood Critical Blood Sample

	Hyper-insulinsim	Inborn Error	Ketotic Hypoglycemia	Hormone (GH/ Cortisol Deficiency)
Glucose	↓	↓	↓	↓
Lactate	N	↑	N	N
B-hydroxybutyrate	↓	N	↑	↑
Free fatty acids	↓	N	↑	↑
Growth hormone	N/↑	↑	↑	N/↓
Cortisol	N/↑	↑	↑	N/↓
Insulin	↑*	↓	↓	↓
Associated features	LGA**	Hepatomegaly Developmental/ growth delay Metabolic acidosis Hyperlipidemic Hyperuricemic		Newborn: micropenis hyperbilinubinemia hypothyroidism Older: short stature

*may be within the "usual" physiologic range.
**large for gestational age

The presence of hypoglycemia in the absence of ketonuria/ketonemia is strongly suggestive of hyperinsulinism. In these infants, a glucagon stimulation test (0.03 mg/kg intravenously) performed at the time of hypoglycemia will result in a significant glycemic response (< 1.1–1.7 mmol/L or 20–30 mg/dL increment in the first 10 min).[106] The hyper-responsiveness to glucagon is due to the presence of excess hepatic glucose deposition resulting from the hyperinsulinism. Provocative tests of insulin secretion provide no diagnostic advantage.

Hypoglycemia and hypoketonemia may also be seen in disorders of ketogenesis, i.e., fatty acid oxidation defects. In these children, plasma carnitine concentrations and a search for urinary organic acids may prove helpful.

Hypoglycemia without hepatomegaly but with ketonemia/uria starting after 1 year of age is often indicative of ketotic hypoglycemia. These children will have low plasma insulin concentrations at the time of hypoglycemia, as well as a blunted response to glucagon administration. Growth hormone and ACTH or cortisol deficiency may be confused with ketotic hypoglycemia. These conditions can be excluded by finding normal/increased concentrations at the time of hypoglycemia. If not found, dynamic testing for these hormones may be required.

The combination of hypoglycemia, hepatomegaly, and metabolic acidosis suggests an abnormality of hepatic gluconeogenesis or glycogenolysis. The presence of nonglucose-reducing sugars in the urine points to a diagnosis of galactosemia. The specific defects in gluconeogenesis are best determined by measuring specific enzyme activities in a liver biopsy specimen. Disorders of amino acid and fatty acid metabolism depend on accurate measurement of urinary metabolites and liver (or muscle) biopsy specimens.

To diagnose factitious hypoglycemia, simultaneous insulin and C-peptide measurement will reveal high insulin concentrations in the absence of detectable C-peptide.

Summary

Hypoglycemia is a rare condition in young infants and children beyond the immediate newborn period. Its presence suggests a significant pathological disorder, particularly in the first year of life. A careful history, physical examination, and investigation should help define the different etiologies and allow specific treatment.

REFERENCES

1. National Diabetes Data Group: Classification of diabetes mellitus and other categories of glucose intolerance. Diabetes 1979;28:1039-57.

2. Shuman CR. Diabetes mellitus: Definition, classification and diagnosis. In Galloway J, Potvin J, Shuman C., Diabetes mellitus (9th ed.). Indianapolis: Lilly, 1988:1-14.

3. Schatz DA, Kowa H, Winter WE, Riley WJ. Natural history of incidental hyperglycemia and glycosuria of childhood. J Pediatr 1989;115:676-80.

4. Cahill GF Jr., McDevitt HO. Insulin-dependent diabetes mellitus: The initial lesion. N Engl J Med 1981;304:1454-65,.

5. Atkinson MA, MacLaren NK. What causes diabetes? Scientific American July 1990:62-71

6. Eisenbarth GS. Type I diabetes: A chronic autoimmune disease. N Engl J Med 1986;314:1360-68.

7. Bottazzo GF, Florin-Christensen A, Doniach D. Islet cell antibodies in diabetes mellitus with autoimmune polyendocrine deficiencies. Lancet 1974;ii:1279-83.

8. Palmer JP, Asplin CM, Clemens P, et al. Insulin antibodies in insulin-dependent diabetics before insulin treatment. Science 1983;222:1337-39.
9. Sochett E, Daneman D. Relationship of insulin autoantibodies to presentation and early course of IDDM in children. Diabetes Care 1989;12:517-23.
10. Maclaren NK. How, when, and why to predict IDDM. Diabetes 1988;37:1591-94.
11. Baekkeskov S,Nielsen J, Marner B, et al. Autoantibodies in newly diagnosed diabetic children immunoprecipitate human pancreatic islet cell proteins. Nature (Lond.)1982;298:167.
12. Powers AC, Eisenbarth G. Autoimmunity to islet cells in diabetes mellitus. Ann Rev Med 1985;36:533-44.
13. Eisenbarth GS. Genes, generator of diversity, glycoconjugates, and autoimmune beta-cell insufficiency in type I diabetes. Diabetes 1987;36:355-64.
14. Tarn AC, Dean BM, Schwarz G, et al. Predicting insulin-dependent diabetes. Lancet 1980;i:845-50.
15. Gleichmann H, Bottazzo GF. Progress toward standardization of cytoplasmic islet cell-antibody assay. Diabetes 1987;37:578-84.
16. Arslanian SA, Becker DJ, Rabin B, et al. Correlates of insulin antibodies in newly diagnosed children with insulin-dependent diabetes before insulin therapy. Diabetes 1985;34:926-30.
17. Atkinson MA, Maclaren NK, Riley WJ, et al. Are insulin autoantibodies markers for insulin-dependent diabetes mellitus? Diabetes 1986;35:894-98.
18. Baekkeskov S, Landin M, Kristensen JK, et al. Antibodies to a 64000-Mr islet cell protein precede the clinical onset of insulin-dependent diabetes. J Clin Invest 1987;79:926-34.
19. Christie MR, Daneman D, Champagne P, Delovitch TL. Persistence of serum antibodies to a Mr-64000 islet cell protein after onset of Type I diabetes. Diabetes 1990;39:653-656.
20. Baekkeskov S, Warnock G, Christie M, et al. Revelation of the specificity of 64k autoantibodies in IDDM serums by high-resolution 2-D electrophoresis. Unambiguous identification of 64k target antigen. Diabetes 1989;38:1133-41.
21. Baekkeskov S, et al. Identification of the 64K autoantigen in insulin-dependent diabetes as the GABA-synthesizing enzyme glutamic acid decarboxylase. Nature 1990;347:151-152.
22. Wolf E, Spencer KM, Cudworth AG. The genetic susceptibility to type I insulin-dependent diabetes: Analysis of the HLA-DR association. Diabetologia 1983;24:224-30.
23. Cavander DE, Wagener DK, Rabin BS, et al. The Pittsburgh insulin-dependent diabetes mellitus (IDDM) study. HLA antigens and haplotypes as risk factors for the development of IDDM in IDDM patients and their siblings. J Chron Dis 1984;37:555-68.
24. Todd JA, Bell JI, McDevitt HO. HLA-DQ beta gene contributes to susceptibility and resistance to insulin-dependent diabetes mellitus. Nature (Lond.) 1987;329:599-604.
25. Todd JA. Genetic control of autoimmunity in type I diabetes. Immunology Today 1990;11:122-29.
26. Srikanta S, Ricker AT, McCulloch DK, et al. Autoimmunity to insulin, beta cell dysfunction, and development of insulin-dependent diabetes mellitus. Diabetes 1986;35:139-42.
27. Drash AL. Diabetes mellitus in the child and adolescent. Curr Prob Pediatr 1986;16:417-542.
28. LaPorte RE, Tajima N, Akerblom HK,et al. Geographic differences in the risk of insulin-dependent diabetes mellitus: The importance of registries. Diabetes Care 1985;8(Suppl 1):101-7.
29. Fleegler FM, Rogers KD, Drash AL, et al. Age, sex, and season of onset of juvenile diabetes in different geographic areas. Pediatr 1979;63:374-79.
30. Rewers M, LaPorte RE, Walczak M, et al. Apparent epidemic of insulin-dependent diabetes mellitus in midwestern Poland. Diabetes 1987;36:106-13.
31. Poussier P, Schiffrin A, Ciampi A, et al. The risk of developing disease for siblings of patients with insulin-dependent diabetes mellitus. Clin Invest Med 1991;14:1-8.
32. Sochett EB, Daneman D, Clarson C, Ehrlich RM. Factors affecting and patterns of residual insulin secretion during the first year of type I (insulin-dependent) diabetes mellitus in children. Diabetologia 1987;30:453-59.
33. Drash A. Clinical care of the diabetic child. St. Louis: Yearbook Medical Publishers, Inc., 1987.

34. Foster D, McGarry J. The metabolic derangements and treatment of diabetic ketoacidosis. New Engl J Med 1983;309:159-169.

35. Daneman D, Ehrlich R. Children with insulin-dependent diabetes mellitus. Medicine N Am 1985;15:2926-34.

36. Daneman D, Siminerio L, Transue D, et al. The role of self-monitoring of blood glucose in the routine management of children with insulin-dependent diabetes mellitus. Diabetes Care 1985;8:1-4.

37. Clarson C, Daneman D, Frank M, et al. Self-monitoring of blood glucose: How accurate are children with diabetes at reading Chemstrip bG? Diabetes Care 1985;8:354-58.

38. Wexler P. The social worker and the child with juvenile diabetes mellitus. In Traisman HJS (Ed.), Management of juvenile diabetes mellitus. St.Louis: Mosby, 1980:272-279.

39. Yki-Jarvinen H, Koivisto V. Natural course of insulin resistance in type I diabetes. N Engl J Med 1986;315:224-30.

40. Marks JB, Skyler JS. Immunotherapy of type I diabetes mellitus. J Clin Endocrinol Metab 1991;72:3-9.

41. Dupre J, Stiller CR. Summary and critical evaluation of immunosuppression trials in recent-onset type I diabetes. In Andreani D, Kolb H, Pozzilli P (Eds.), Immunotherapy of type I diabetes. Chichester: Wiley, 1989:137-145.

42. Daneman D, Wolfson D, Becker D, Drash A. Factors affecting glycosylated hemoglobin values in children with insulin-dependent diabetes. J Pediatr 1981;99:847-53.

43. The DCCT Research Group. Diabetes Control and Complications Trial: Results of feasibility study. Diabetes Care 1987;10:1-19.

44. The DCCT Research Group. Epidemiology of severe hypoglycemia in the Diabetes Control and Complications Trial. Am J Med 1991;90:450-59.

45. The DCCT Research Group. Are continuing studies of metabolic control and microvascular complications in insulin-dependent diabetes mellitus justified? The Diabetes Control and Complications Trial. N Engl J Med 1988;318:246-50.

46. Daneman D. When should your child take charge? Diabetes Forecast May 1991:61-66.

47. Position statement of the American Diabetes Association. Eye care guidelines for patients with diabetes mellitus. Diabetes Care 1988;11:745-46.

48. Brink SJ, Stewart C. Insulin pump treatment in insulin-dependent diabetes mellitus: Children, adolescents and young adults. JAMA 1986;255:617-21.

49. Zinman B. Exercise in diabetes treatment. Clinical Diabetes 1983;1:18-22.

50. Skyler JS. Patient self-monitoring of blood glucose. Clinical Diabetes 1983;1:12-17.

51. Nathan DM, Singer DE, Hurxthal K, Goodson JD. The clinical information value of the glycosylated hemoglobin assay. N Engl J Med 1984;310:341-46.

52. Baynes JW, Bunn HF, Goldstein DE, et al. National diabetes data group: Report of the expert committee on glycosylated hemoglobin. Diabetes Care 1984;7:602-6.

53. Sobel DO, Abbassi V. Use of the fructosamine test in diabetic children. Diabetes Care 1991;14:578-83.

54. Daneman D, Frank M, Perlman K, et al. Severe hypoglycemia in children with insulin-dependent diabetes mellitus: Frequency and predisposing features. J Pediatr 1989;115:681-85.

55. Gale E. The frequency of hypoglycemia in insulin-treated diabetic patients. In Serrano-Rios M, Lefebvre P (Eds), Diabetes. Amsterdam: Elsevier, 1985:934-37.

56. Kovacs M, Feinberg TL, Paulauskas R, et al. Initial coping responses and psychosocial characteristics of children with insulin-dependent diabetes mellitus. J Pediatr 1985;106:827-34.

57. Koski M-L. The coping process in childhood diabetes mellitus: A critical review. Acta Paediatr Scand 1980;Suppl 198:1-56.

58. Hauenstein EJ, Marvin RS, Snyder AL, Clarke WL. Stress in parents of children with diabetes mellitus. Diabetes Care 1989;12:18-23.

59. Jacobson AM, Hauser ST, Wolfsdorf JI, et al. Psychologic predictors of compliance in children with recent onset of diabetes mellitus. J Pediatr 1987;110:805-11.

60. Kostraba J, Dorman J, Orchard T, et al. Contribution of diabetes duration before puberty to development of microvascular complications in IDDM subjects. Diabetes Care 1989;12:686-93.

61. Mogensen CE, Christensen CK, Vittinghus E. The stages in diabetic renal disease. Diabetes 1983;32(Suppl 2):64-78.

62. Sochett E, Daneman D. Microalbuminuria in children with insulin-dependent diabetes mellitus. J Pediatr 1988;112:744-48.

63. Mogensen CE, Christensen CK. Predicting diabetic nephropathy in insulin-dependent patients. N Engl J Med 1984;311:1430-32.

64. Cook JJ, Daneman D. Microalbuminuria in adolescents with insulin-dependent diabetes mellitus. Am J Dis Child 1990;144:234-37.

65. Fajans SS. Scope and heterogeneous nature of MODY. Diabetes Care 1990;13:49-64.

66. Winter WE, Maclaren NE, Riley WJ, et al. Maturity-onset diabetes of youth in black Americans. N Engl J Med 1987;316:285-91.

67. Cornblath M, Schwartz R. Disorders of carbohydrate metabolism in infancy, 2nd ed. Philadelphia: WB Saunders, 1976.

68. Haymond MW, Howard C, Ben-Galim E et al. Effects of ketosis on glucose flux in children and adults. Am J Physiol 1983;245:E373-378.

69. Haymond MW, Karl E, Clarke WL et al. Differences in circulating gluconeogenic substrates during short-term fasting in men, women and children. Metabolism 1982;31:33-4.

70. Haymond MW. Hypoglycemia in infants and children. Endocrinology Clinics of North America 1989;18:211-52.

71. Griffiths AD, Bryant GM. Assessment of effects of neonatal hypoglycemia: A study of 41 cases with matched controls. Arch Dis Child 1971;46:819-27.

72. Jacobs DG, Haka-Ikse K, Wesson DE, et al. Growth and development in patients operated on for islet cell dysplasia. J Pediatr Surg 1986;21:1184-89.

73. Pildes RS. Infants of diabetic mothers. N Engl J Med 1973;289:902-904.

74. Williams PR, Sperling MA, Racasa Z. Blunting of spontaneous and amino-acid stimulated glucagon secretion in infants of diabetic mothers (IDM). Diabetes 1975;24:411 (Abstract).

75. Susa JB, Cowett RM, Oh W et al. Suppression of gluconeogenesis and endogenous glucose production by exogenous insulin adminstration in the newborn lamb. Pediatr Res 1979;13:594-98.

76. Rovers G Gargiulo M, Nicolin V. Maximal tolerated insulin therapy in gestational diabetes. Diabetes Care 1980;3489-94.

77. Barrett CT, Oliver TK. Hypoglycemia and hyperinsulinism in infants with erythroblastosis fetalis. N Engl J Med 1968;278:1260-63.

78. Cohen MD, Gorlin RJ, Feingold M et al. The Beckwith-Wiedemann syndrome: Seven new cases. Am J Dis Child 1971;122:515-19.

79. Stanley CA, Baker L. Hyperinsulinism in infants and children. Adv Pediatr 1976;122:515-55.

80. Jaffe R, Hashida Y, Yunis E. Pancreatic pathology in hyperinsulinemic hypoglycemia of infancy. Lab Invest 1980;42:356-65.

81. Aynsley-Green A, Polak J, Bloom S, et al. Nesidioblastosis of the pancreas: Definition of the syndrome and the management of severe neonatal hyperinsulinemic hypoglycemia. Arch Dis Child 1981;56:496-508.

82. DeClue TJ, Malone JI, Bercu BB. Linear growth during long-term treatment with somatostatin analog (SMS 201-995) for persistent hyperinsulinemic hypoglycemia of infancy. J Pediatr 1990;116:747-55.

83. McGraw M, Price D. Complications of diazoxide in the treatment of nesidioblastosis. Arch Dis Child 1985;60:62-64.

84. Schiller M, Krausz M, Meyer S et al. Neonatal hyperinsulinism: Surgical and pathologic considerations. J Pediatr Surg 1980;15:16-20.

85. Gough MH. The surgical treatment of hyperinsulinism in infancy and childhood. Br J Surg 1984;71:75-78.

86. Bauman WA, Yalow RS. Child abuse: Parenteral insulin administration. J Pediatr 1981;99:588-91.

87. Scarlett JA, Mako ME, Rubenstein AH et al. Factitious hypoglycemia: Diagnosis by measurement of serum C-peptide immunoreactivity and insulin binding antibodies. N Engl J Med 1977;297:1029-32.

88. Hopwood NJ, Forsman PJ, Kenny FM, Drash AL. Hypoglycemia in hypopituitary children. Am J Dis Child 1975;129:918-22.

89. Vidnes J, Oyasaeter S. Glucagon deficiency causing severe neonatal hypoglycemia in a patient with normal insulin secretion. Pediatr Res 1977;11:943-49.

90. Kollie LA, Monneus LA, Cejka V. Persistent neonatal hypoglycemia due to glucagon deficiency. Arch Dis Child 1978;53:422.

91. Pagliara AS, Karl IE, Haymond MW. Hypoglycemia in infancy and childhood. J Pediatr 1973;82:558-77.

92. Colle E, Ulstrom RA. Ketotic hypoglycemia. J Pediatr 1964;64:632-51.

93. Senior B. Ketotic hypoglycemia. J Pediatr 1973;82:555-56.

94. Christensen NJ. Hypoadrenalinemia during insulin hypoglycemia in children with ketotic hypoglycemia. J Clin Endocrinol Metab 1974;38:107-12.

95. Kelnar CJH. Hypoglycemia in children undergoing adenotonsillectomy. Br Med J 1976;1:751-52.

96. Shumake LB. Postoperative hypoglycemia in congenital hypertrophic pyloric stenosis. South Med J. 1975;68:223.

97. Hers H-G, Van Hoof F, De Barsy T. Glycogen storage diseases. In: Stanbury JB, Wyngaarden JG, Fredrickson DA, eds. The metabolic basis of inherited disease. New York: McGraw-Hill, 1989.

98. Chen YT, Cornblath, M., Sidbury, J.B. Cornstarch therapy in type I glycogen storage disease. N Engl J Med 1984;310:171-75.

99. Haymond MW, Karl IE, Feigin RD, et al. Hypoglycemia and maple syrup urine disease: Defective gluconeogenesis. Pediatr Res 1973;7:500-8.

100. Glasgow AM, Engel AG, Bier D, et al. Hypoglycemia, hepatic dysfunction, muscle weakness, cardiomyopathy, free carnitine deficiency and long-chain acyl carnitine excess responsive to medium chain triglyceride diet. Pediatr Res 1968;17:319.

101. Engel AG, Banker BQ, Eiben RM. Carnitine deficiency: Clinical, morphological and biochemical observations in a fatal case. J Neurol Neurosurg Psychiat 1977;40:313.

102. Roe CR, Millington DA, Maltby DA, et al. Recognition of medium chain acyl-CoA dehydrogenase deficiency in asymptomatic siblings of children dying of sudden infant death or Reye's-like syndromes. J Pediatr 1986;108:13-18.

103. Stanley CA, Hale DE, Coates PM, et al. Medium chain acyl-CoA dehydrogenase deficiency in children with nonketotic hypoglycemia and low carnitine levels. Pediatr Res 1983;17:877-84.

104. Grupposo PA, Schwartz R. Hypoglycemia in children. Pediatrics in Review 1989;11:117-24.

105. Phillip M, Bashan N, Smith CPA, Moses SW. An algorithmic approach to diagnosis of hypoglycemia. J Pediatr 1987;110:387-90.

106. Finegold DN, Stanley CA, Baker L. Glycemic response to glucagon during fasting hypoglycemia: An aid in the diagnosis of hyperinsulinsim. J Pediatr 1980;96;257-59.

Neurologic and Psychiatric Disorders

Roger J. Packer, M.D.   *Stephen I. Deutsch, M.D., Ph.D.*

INTRODUCTION

Discoveries in the neurosciences have ushered in a new era in the understanding and treatment of childhood neurologic and psychiatric disorders. Elucidations of the biochemical, cellular, and genetic mechanisms of childhood neurologic disease will, no doubt, result in alterations and refinements of treatment. Discussed in this chapter are the pathobiology and rationale for the treatment of some of the more common neurologic and psychiatric diseases of childhood.

EPILEPSY

Clinical Aspects

The epilepsies are recurrent convulsive and nonconvulsive seizures caused by temporary excessive and hypersynchronous discharges of cortical neurons. It has been estimated that one of every 11 people will have at least one seizure by the age of 80, and that 3% of the population have recurrent, unprovoked seizures.[1] The highest incidence of epilepsy occurs in children under 5 years of age, and 1–2 children out of every 1,000 will have recurrent convulsions.

A variety of different conditions, such as breathholding spells, vasovagal episodes, gastroesophageal reflux, and psychogenic disorders, may mimic epilepsy, so correct clinical diagnosis is the cornerstone of appropriate management. Clinical manifestations of epilepsy include generalized motor involvement (tonic, clonic, or tonic-clonic), staring episodes with or without automatisms, partial motor movements, or loss of postural tone. These manifestations often vary within an individual patient.

Although a variety of different classification systems exists, the most widely recognized is the schema developed by the International League Against Epilepsy (ILAE).[2] The ILAE classification utilizes two broad categories of seizures: those arising in one cerebral hemisphere primarily accompanied by focal electroencephalographic abnormalities (partial or focal seizures) and those with clinical and electrocortical manifestations of involvement of both cerebral hemispheres from onset (generalized seizures). Distinction between seizure types is often blurred and arbitrary, as focal seizures with rapid secondary generalization may mimic generalized seizures. The clinical manifestation of seizures may also depend on the age of the patient. Appropriate classification requires inclusion of the age of onset and remission of the epileptic seizure, the interictal neurologic status of the patient, the etiology and trigger mechanism of the attacks, the interictal and ictal EEG, the response to antiepileptic medication, the remission rate and the genetics of the seizure type.

Although diagnosis is clinical, electroencephalography remains the primary tool for evaluating patients and abetting classification. In general, focal epileptiform activity indicates a partial or localized epilepsy, in contradistinction to generalized epileptiform discharges, which suggest generalized epilepsy. Interictal electroencephalographic abnormalities are seen in probably no more than 50% of patients on the initial electroencephalogram.[1] Multiple recordings performed with various stimulation techniques, such as hyperventilation and sleep deprivation, or with more refined recording techniques may increase this yield to as high as 90%.

Neuroimaging studies are useful in the understanding of epilepsy, but in themselves are rarely diagnostic. Magnetic resonance imaging has proven more sensitive than CT in detecting small cerebral lesions related to epilepsy.[3] Neuroimaging is indicated in all children with partial seizures and possibly the majority of children with recurrent generalized seizures. Other neuroimaging studies such as positron emission tomography and single photon emission computed tomography (SPECT) are presently primarily research techniques. However, since these techniques may show interictal metabolic abnormalities in patients with otherwise normal neuroimaging studies, they may become more clinically useful in the future.[3]

Pathophysiology

The major cellular events involved in the generation of epileptogenic foci are slowly unfolding.[4] During epileptiform discharges there are marked abnormalities in ion transport, with shifts in the ratio between extracellular and intracellular potassium, sodium, and calcium. A variety of neurotransmitters have been implicated in the epileptogenic process, including gamma-amino-butyric-acid, glycine, glutamate, and catecholamines. Determination of which of these events are primary and which are secondary remains to be elucidated. These cellular events all result in the electrical synchronization necessary for the epileptic foci to spread and become clinically evident.

Treatment

The effective treatment of epilepsy is highly dependent on appropriate diagnosis of the type of epilepsy present and an understanding of the natural history of the disease. Some forms of childhood epilepsy, such as febrile seizures, have a relatively stereotypical presentation, a limited period of expression, and may not require treatment. Other forms of childhood epilepsy, including "benign rolandic epilepsy" and absence seizures, carry excellent prognoses and excessive treatment may be more damaging than the epilepsy itself. Anticonvulsant medication remains the cornerstone of treatment for most childhood epilepsies. The mechanisms of action of anticonvulsant drugs are incompletely understood and consist of an interplay between their effects on neurotransmitter action, repetitive neuronal firing mechanisms, neuronal networks, and cellular ionic transport.[5, 6] The combination of these effects and the pharmacokinetic properties of the drugs determines their spectrum of action and clinical efficacy.

The decision to treat a patient must be based on the likelihood of recurrent seizures, potential side effects of the drugs, the consequence of further seizures on the patient's life, and the probability that treatment will effectively reduce the risk of future seizures. Estimates of the rate of recurrence of seizures within the first year after a single unprovoked convulsion are hard to come by, and an incidence ranging between 16% and 62% has been suggested.[7] Recurrence seems more likely if the patient is neurologically abnormal or if there is a strong family history of recurrent unprovoked convulsions. A partial seizure or an abnormal interictal electroencephalogram also seems to increase the likelihood of epilepsy.

Role of Laboratory in Treatment

Assessment of drug concentrations has become an integral part of the management of children with epilepsy. However, there is an increasing tendency to rely too heavily on drug concentrations in patient care decisions. Monitoring of drug concentrations is an important adjunct to the management of epileptic patients. However, drug concentrations should be considered as an aid and a guide, not the prime determinant of patient management. Some patients experience excellent seizure control on relatively low concentrations of drugs, while others tolerate concentrations which are above the accepted normal range and require such dosages for adequate seizure control (see Table 11–1). Drug concentrations are especially useful for patients on two or more drugs. Assays for the more commonly used drugs, including phenobarbital, phenytoin, carbamazepine, valproate, and possibly ethosuximide should be available on an immediate basis, 24 h per day, at centers caring for many patients with epilepsy.

TABLE 11–1. Therapeutic Profile of Common Anticonvulsants

Drug	Serum Half-Life (h)	Therapeutic Drug Concentrations (ug/mL)
Phenobarbital		15–35
Neonates	63–98	
Infants	47 ± 8	
Children (< 15 years)	37–73	
Adults	64–141	
Phenytoin		10–20
Neonates	7–140*	
Infants and Children	11.6–31.5*	
Adults	7–42*	
Carbamazepine		8–12
Neonates	8–37	
Infants and Children	3–32	
Adults	11–22	
Valproic Acid		50–100(120?)
Neonates	10–67	
Infants and Children	4–10	
Adults	12–16	
Ethosuximide		40–100
Infants and Children	15–68	
Adults	50–60	

*At therapeutic drug concentrations. Lower at low doses.

Although obtaining of multiple serum specimens at different times after a drug is taken would be optimal to determine the pharmacokinetic aspects of an anticonvulsant, the approach is rarely practical. More commonly, to avoid the problem of erratic initial absorption, trough drug concentrations are monitored to aid in determining appropriate drug dosages. In general, the metabolism of an anti-epileptic drug is faster in children than adults. However, in the neonatal period, metabolism may be relatively slower, requiring modification of dosage. Toxicity, especially sedation, may be related to either drug accumulation of anticonvulsants with long half-lives or peak concentrations of an individual drug. In these cases, measurements of "peak" drug concentrations at a time when absorption should be maximum or multiple drug concentrations to determine the elimination of a drug may be useful.

Another important role of the laboratory is the monitoring of the effect of a given drug on other organs. Routine monitoring of hematologic and hepatic function for patients taking drugs such as carbamazepine and valproate is recommended, although their utility is poorly substantiated.

Partial and Secondarily Generalized Seizures

Phenytoin, carbamazepine, phenobarbital, and primidone are essentially equally as effective in control of partial and secondarily generalized seizures.[1, 5] One drug may be effective when the other drug is not. Other agents, such as valproate and clonazepam, may also be effective. These drugs differ substantially in their side effects and pharmacokinetic properties; these differences are most useful in determining the best choice of drug for an individual patient.

Phenytoin

Phenytoin exerts its effects by varying mechanisms including alterations in ionic transport, changes in neurotransmitter action (including the enhancement of gamma-amino-butyric acid), decreases in neuronal repetitive firing, and the facilitation of neuronal network inhibitory mechanisms.[5] The drug may either be given by oral or intravenous routes. The oral absorption of phenytoin is slow and variable with maximum blood concentrations occurring within 4 to 8 hours.[5, 7, 8] Absorption in the neonatal/early infancy period is often incomplete and unreliable. Another problem with oral delivery of the drug in infants is the variable concentration of oral suspensions, as phenytoin may precipitate in the bottom of the bottle. The drug is 90% bound to plasma proteins in adults, but to a lesser extent in neonates. It is taken up in brain within minutes after intravenous administration.

Calculation of the appropriate daily dose of phenytoin in an individual patient can be difficult, as the metabolism of the drug changes with age and is dependent on serum concentrations.[5, 7, 8]

Phenytoin is primarily metabolized in the liver and elimination follows Michaelis-Menten pharmacokinetics, so that enzymes responsible for eliminating the drug become saturated at higher dosages. The half-life of the drug becomes longer as the plasma concentration increases. At higher plasma values, a small increase in dosage will result in progressively greater plasma concentrations. The steady-state half-life of phenytoin is quite long in the neonates (ranging up to 57 h) and progressively declines over the first few months of life. Initially, dosages in the range of 5–8 mg/kg/d are needed in children and adolescents, although much higher oral dosages are usually required in the neonatal period. Therapeutic blood concentrations range between 10 and 20 ug/mL. However, there is a great degree of variability for a given patient, and some patients will tolerate and respond to much higher concentrations.

Since a large number of drugs have been reported to interact with phenytoin, monitoring of drug concentrations is needed for patients on multiple medications.

The most frequently encountered symptoms of phenytoin toxicity include nausea, sedation, tremor, and slow cognition.[7] Increased seizures have been reported in patients with increased phenytoin concentrations; however, some patients tolerate drug concentrations well above the accepted safe range with little or no toxicity and improved seizure control. In addition, diphenylhydantoin at drug concentrations in the normally accepted effective range may precipitate minor motor seizures and a pseudo-degenerative clinical picture. The actual effect of phenytoin on intellectual status of children is unsettled and demonstrable cognitive sequelae are mild and difficult to reproduce in studies. Long-term effects of phenytoin on the cerebellum have been suggested. In children, especially girls, troublesome side effects include hirsutism, coarsening of facial features, and gingival hyperplasia. These side effects usually relegate phenytoin to a secondary role in the management of females (and some males) with seizures. Phenytoin also has teratogenic side effects and use in pregnancy is to be avoided, when possible.

Carbamazepine

Carbamazepine is available only in an oral preparation. Gastrointestinal absorption is somewhat unpredictable, but seems relatively good at all ages, with maximum absorption occurring 4–8 h after intake.[5, 7, 9] Distribution of the agent is uniform and the half-life of the drug is initially long (greater than 24 h), but falls in children to a mean of 9 h after chronic use. As is the case with phenytoin, carbamazepine is metabolized primarily in the liver. Carbamazepine interacts with many drugs. The effects of drug interactions between carbamazepine and other drugs which are metabolized by the liver are somewhat less predictable than is the case for phenytoin.

Carbamazepine affects sodium and potassium membrane permeability at a cellular level.[5] It also affects the release of various neurotransmitters, although the specific mechanism of biochemical action (if there is one) is poorly characterized. It has varied effects on neuronal firing mechanisms.

Initial side effects of carbamazepine include ataxia, nausea, and lethargy.[5, 7] These side effects usually disappear after chronic administration. Inappropriate release of antidiuretic hormone may occur. Dose-related bone marrow depression and hepatic toxicity are the most common severe side effects of medication. Low white-cell counts occur relatively frequently with the drug, but a reduction in drug dose is necessary only when there is a progressive, severe fall in counts. Severe aplastic anemia and hepatotoxic reaction are idiosyncratic. Monitoring of liver functions and blood counts in patients taking the drug is recommended, although its utility is unproven.

Monitoring of drug concentrations is a useful adjunct to carbamazepine use, as best seizure control has been reported with drug concentrations ranging between 8 and 12 ug/mL.[5, 7] Once again, there is a great deal of patient variability, with some patients tolerating higher concentrations of the drug and others experiencing good seizure control at lower drug concentrations.

Due to the lack of cosmetic side effects, lack of sedation, and little disturbance of cognitive functions, carbamazepine has been used widely in pediatrics.[5, 7] It has become a drug of choice for most children (especially girls) with partial and secondarily generalized seizures. However, since it has to be given more frequently than phenytoin due to its relatively short half-life, compliance becomes a more pressing issue with this drug.

Phenobarbital

Phenobarbital is the anticonvulsant with the longest experience of use.[10] It can be used orally, intravenously, or, in rare cases, intramuscularly. Phenobarbital is readily and completely absorbed after oral administration and reaches peak concentrations after 1–3 h.[10] It is evenly distributed throughout tissues and has an extremely long elimination half-life. This is especially true in neonates, where the half-life may be greater than 96 h. However, in later infancy and childhood, the half-life usually falls significantly (usually in the 40–50 h range). After intravenous injection, the drug is delivered to brain, but at a somewhat slower rate than is phenytoin.

Phenobarbital has a direct effect on neuronal excitability and synaptic transmission.[5] It has a variety of pharmacologic effects which are primarily postsynaptic and include enhancement of gamma-aminobutyric acid, antagonism of the excitatory effects of glutamate, and direct effects on ion conductance.

The drug dosage needed to obtain adequate serum concentration varies widely with age. In neonates and young children, 4–5 mg/kg/day may be needed to maintain adequate drug concentrations, whereas dosages in the 1–3 mg/kg range are needed in older children and adults. The range of effective serum concentrations of the drug is quite wide (15–35 ug/dL). Similarly, the side effects of the drug may occur at varied serum concentrations.

The most common side effects of phenobarbital include somnolence and ataxia.[10] As many as 40% of infants and children may experience a paradoxical effect, with increased irritability, behavioral abnormalities, and hyperactivity. This effect may or may not be dose related. Chronic use of the drug seems to cause difficulty in cognition. Some researchers have postulated a permanent effect on cognitive abilities after chronic use of the drug, but this is far from conclusively proven.[11] The detrimental effects on cognition and behavior have resulted in a secondary role for phenobarbital in the management of most childhood epilepsies. However, it probably remains the safest proven effective therapy for febrile seizures.

One phenobarbital derivative, mephobarbital, has been utilized because of anecdotal reports of its lower incidence of associated hyperactivity.[10] Mephobarbital is rapidly metabolized to phenobarbital, and it seems most likely that the utility of mephobarbital is related to lower overall phenobarbital concentrations than an intrinsic effect of the drug.

Primidone

Primidone is administered orally. The drug is metabolized to phenobarbital and phenylethylmalonamide (Pema). The primidone and its two major metabolites all have independent anticonvulsive activity.[5] It is unclear which derivative (or derivatives) is effective in controlling seizures in an individual patient. More frequent doses of the drug result in higher primidone levels and possibly better control of associated generalized seizures. Dosage is usually increased slowly due to problems with oversedation. The appropriate switch-over dose between phenobarbital and primidone is variable, and to obtain phenobarbital equivalent concentrations, doses of primidone 3–9 times greater than phenobarbital are necessary.

Monitoring drug concentrations in patients on primidone can be difficult. Seizure control usually best correlates with the phenobarbital concentrations, but both the primidone and the Pema concentrations have been related to seizure control. Side effects are similar to those of phenobarbital.

Generalized Seizures

Although a variety of drugs, such as phenytoin, phenobarbital and carbamazepine, are effective against generalized tonic-clonic seizures, valproate is probably the single most effective drug.[1] A variety of different benzodiazepine derivatives may also be effective, especially in myoclonic seizures. Ethosuximide is probably equally effective as valproate for the treatment of absence seizures.

Valproate

Valproate is presently available only in an oral preparation. Although the drug may be used in a short-acting preparation, it is most commonly used in a long-acting preparation which is well absorbed.[6, 12] The longer acting, slower release form of valproate has a half-life of somewhere between 15 and 20 h. The drug is bound to plasma proteins, is lipophilic, and has a wide volume of distribution. Valproate is more slowly eliminated in neonates, but reaches adult metabolism by approximately 3 months of age.[13]

Valproate's main mechanism of action seems to be the enhancement of neurotransmission at gamma-amino-butyric-acid synapses.[6] It also decreases brain aspartic acid concentrations and increases the concentration of glycine.

Valproate is usually started in a relatively low dose of 10 mg/kg/d and is slowly increased to 30–50 mg/kg/d. Blood concentration measurements are somewhat useful, as concentration of 50–100 ug/dL are usually needed for seizure control. However, higher drug values can, at times, be tolerated and can be somewhat more efficacious. There are extensive interactions between valproate and other antiepileptic drugs. It tends to increase phenobarbital concentrations and decrease measured concentrations of phenytoin. However, since it competes with phenytoin for protein-binding sites, there may be a relative increase in free phenytoin. Ethosuximide concentrations tend to rise when valproate is added. Drug concentrations of valproate are usually lowered by the concomitant use of other anticonvulsants.

Some side effects of valproate are related, while others are not.[12] The drug may cause a decrease in appetite and gastrointestinal side effects, including cramping and diarrhea. However, it may also cause an increase in appetite and weight gain, especially in adolescent girls. The two major side effects of valproate are bone marrow suppression and hepatotoxicity. Thrombocytopenia is usually dose related, but an idiosyncratic aplastic anemia may also occur.

Mildly increased transaminase concentrations and mild increase of ammonia are common in patients taking valproate. These increases tend to be dose related. However, fatal idiosyncratic hepatotoxicity (irreversible upon cessation of the drug) may occur. This has been primarily reported in children under age 2 y, although occasionally older children may have similar sequelae. Potential hepatic toxicity has limited the use of the drug in younger children, except in extreme circumstances. The use of carnitine has been proposed as a useful adjunct for patients with dose-related hepatic dysfunction or unexplained lethargy or somnolence. However, the efficacy of this drug remains unproven. Fatal pancreatitis with associated disseminated intravascular coagulopathy may also occur with valproate.

Because of these side effects, patients require serial monitoring of blood counts, including platelet counts, and liver function tests while on valproate. However, such monitoring probably is not helpful in cases of idiosyncratic toxicity. Since valproate has little detrimental effect on cognition, it has become the drug of choice for many older children with generalized epilepsy.

Ethosuximide

Ethosuximide is given orally.[12] It is a member of a family of drugs including phensuximide and methsuximide. Although these other suximide derivatives may have a slightly broader spectrum of activity, they are usually utilized as second-line drugs.

Ethosuximide is absorbed rapidly, with maximum plasma concentrations occurring at 3 h. It is primarily metabolized in the liver and tends to have a relatively long elimination half-life of 30–60 h. It can be given once daily; however, because of intestinal side effects, it is usually prescribed 2 times a day.

The mechanism of action of ethosuximide is poorly characterized.[6] It does seem to have effects on ionic transport, and concentrations of gamma-hydroxy-butyric acid are decreased after chronic treatment with the drug.

The drug usually reaches a steady state 5–12 d after initiation of dose. Effective blood concentrations tend to range in the 40–100 ug/mL dose. Dose-related side effects include nausea, abdominal discomfort, and anorexia. A variety of idiosyncratic side effects may occur, but they tend to be relatively infrequent. The drug may cause deleterious effects on behavior and cognition. However, because of the relative infrequency of severe side effects, it probably remains the drug of choice for simple absence seizures of childhood.

Benzodiazepines

The benzodiazepines are a group of drugs including diazepam, clonazepam, clorazepate, and lorazepam.[5, 10] These drugs may be effective in many types of epilepsy. They all are rapidly absorbed from the gastrointestinal tract. They are widely distributed within body tissues and because of this distribution initially have a relatively short half-life. However, conversion to active metabolites such as N-dimethyl-diazepam results in products with a long half-life (50–120 h). The half-life tends to increase with age.

The benzodiazepines induce a wide variety of antiepileptic changes.[5] Almost all neurotransmitters are altered in some way by benzodiazepine administration. There are also specific receptors in the nervous system for the benzodiazepines, and it is probable that at least some of the efficacy of these drugs is related to these receptors.

Acute use of benzodiazepines may cause respiratory depression and hypotension. Chronic use is associated with drowsiness, incoordination, irritability, and hypotonia. Cognitive impairment and behavioral disturbances may also occur.

Status Epilepticus

The treatment of status epilepticus deserves separate mention.[14] A variety of drugs can be used to treat status epilepticus, and there is reason to believe that rapid control will result in fewer long-term sequelae. The benzodiazepines are the most rapidly effective drugs in the treatment of status. However, their use can induce depression of respiration and hypotension. Diazepam has a relatively short half-life, as its effects usually are limited to approximately 30 min. Lorazepam has a longer half-life (4–8 h) and is probably equivalent to diazepam in efficacy. The acute monitoring of benzodiazepine drug concentrations is usually not useful in the management of status epilepticus.

Phenytoin has almost as rapid an onset of action as the benzodiazepine derivatives. It has a relatively long half-life and does not cause significant central nervous system depression. For these reasons it is the drug of choice when monitoring the level of consciousness is of major importance in patients with recurrent seizures. Doses of 18–20 mg/kg will result in drug concentrations of 18–26 ug/mL, levels which are often needed for the control of status epilepticus. Acute monitoring of drug concentrations post-infusion can be a useful adjunct to treatment of patients receiving phenytoin.

Phenobarbital is also used frequently in patients with status epilepticus. However, it has a less rapid onset of action than the benzodiazepines or phenytoin. It also depresses consciousness and respiration, especially when used after a benzodiazepine. Usually doses of 10–30 mg/kg are needed for seizure control. Monitoring of drug concentrations also can be useful in the determination of optimum dose of the drug.

MIGRAINE HEADACHES

Headaches are extremely common in pediatric patients. The term "headache" covers a wide variety of symptoms and has many different causes.[15] Migraine is a specific form of headache that may occur in up to 5% of patients by age 15. Half of all individuals who develop migraine headaches have their first attack before age 20. In children, the classical migraine headache is uncommon, and a variety of different criteria have been proposed for diagnosing childhood migraine. In essence, a diagnosis is made in a child who has recurrent headaches, often associated with nausea or vomiting, that are throbbing and relieved primarily by rest.[16] There is usually a family history of migraine and auras may occur, but are less frequent than in adults. The episodes may be triggered by specific phenomena, such as anxiety, fatigue, stress, menses, and diet (chocolate, nitrites, and monosodium glutamate). By definition, patients will have no other reason for the headaches.

Despite the common nature of this disorder, the underlying pathophysiology of migraine headaches has never been fully elucidated.[17] Abnormalities of regional cerebral blood flow have been documented in patients with migraine. Initially, there is a period of cortical hypoperfusion which may be associated with an aura or other focal neurologic deficits; rebound hyperperfusion has not been documented.

The role of neurotransmitters as a cause or a sequelae of this vascular change remains unclear. Serotonin has been most commonly implicated as the major neurotransmitter involved in migraine attacks. This is because serotonin is known to cause vasoconstriction in certain vascular structures and vasodilation in others. However, a direct relationship with serotonin has never been proven, and other neurotransmitters, including the prostaglandins, prolactin, and gamma-aminobutyric acid, have also been implicated in migraine. Others have postulated that migraine is a state of central neuronal hyperexcitability and that a variety of different excitatory amino acids cause an activation of neuronal depolarization.

Treatment

As can be expected, given the uncertainty concerning the pathogenesis of migraine attacks, treatment has been primarily empiric.[18] In general, most patients with infrequent headaches do not require any specific treatment.[18] At times, avoidance of situations or foods that trigger migraine can decrease the frequency of attacks. Other forms of non-pharmacological treatment include psychotherapy and biofeedback.

In adults, medications that acutely abort the attack, such as ergotamine and various combinations of ergotamine derivatives, are most commonly used. These drugs seem to be useful only early in the course of the migraine (best used during the aura), and since most children do not have well defined auras or cannot determine when their headaches are beginning, their use in pediatrics is quite limited. Ergotamines are well absorbed after oral dosage, but plasma concentrations after rectal administration are higher.

If migraines are frequent enough to require treatment, most pediatric patients respond best to chronic prophylactic treatment. There is no such thing as a best medication for migraine. Results seem as dependent on the enthusiasm of the caregiver as on the drug itself.

Propranolol is probably the most widely used prophylactic agent for migraine.[18] Its effects include prevention of arterial dilatation via blocking beta receptors, blocking of catecholamine-induced platelet aggregation, decreased platelet adhesiveness, and prevention of epinephrine release. Patients are usually begun at 10–20 mg/d, and dosage is increased until the symptoms are relieved or bradycardia occurs. Drug concentration monitoring usually is not useful, and the best measure of potential toxicity is probably pulse rate taken approximately 45 min after an oral dose.

Cyproheptadine can also be used as prophylaxis.[18] It has both antihistamine and calcium channel-blocking properties. Again, dosage is variable and the drug is usually slowly increased until there are symptoms of sedation. Patients usually begin on approximately 4 mg a day, in divided dosages, and the dose is increased as tolerated.

Recently calcium channel blockers have been used in patients with migraine.[18] In fact, some report that these drugs are the treatment of choice in patients with migraine. Their use in pediatrics has been limited to date, and the overall safety of these drugs and how they should be used is poorly documented. Similarly, nonsteroidal anti-inflammatory drugs have been widely used in adults. Their safety, especially in regard to long-term gastrointestinal side effects, is poorly documented in children.

Amitriptyline has also been used in children with migraine, especially in those patients who seem to have a mixed-headache syndrome. Measurement of blood concentrations may be helpful, but it is usually as effective to monitor dose-related side effects, including dizziness, dry mouth, visual blurring, and urinary retention. Antiepileptics, such as phenytoin and phenobarbital, also have been recommended for the prevention of migraine.[17] A relationship between drug concentrations and efficacy has not been shown.

Methysergide is a drug with known antiserotoninergic effects. Although it is an effective drug in treating migraine, its long-term use may cause retroperitoneal, pleural, and cardiac fibrosis. Use in pediatrics has been quite limited.

MOVEMENT DISORDERS
(excluding Gilles-de-la-Tourette's Syndrome)

Movement disorders are not an uncommon accompaniment of many neurologic illnesses.[19] A variety of different movements may occur, including tremor, myoclonus, chorea, athetosis, and dystonia. Multiple types of abnormal movements may occur in the same patient. Appropriate treatment is dependent on correct clinical diagnosis. The neuronal pathways involved in the control of movement are extremely complex. The motor cortex, brainstem, cerebellum, and spinal cord all play a role in the coordination of movements. However, the basal ganglia or its direct connections are the areas most commonly implicated as the cause of movement disorders. The neuronal pathways that course through the basal ganglia and their interactions are extremely complex and involve a variety of neurotransmitters, including dopamine, serotonin, gamma-amino-butyric acid, glutamic acid, epinephrine, and acetylcholine. Treatment is usually aimed at modulating a believed imbalance between neurotransmitters. Although these neurotransmitters and their roles are increasingly being elucidated, most treatment remains empiric.

Dystonia/Choreoathetosis

Symptomatic treatment for dystonia in cases where localized treatment with drugs such as botulinum toxin is not possible usually involves anticholinergic drugs.[20] Monitoring of drug concentrations is usually unnecessary in these conditions, as these anticholinergic drugs are slowly increased until there is evidence of undue toxicity, usually sedation. Some patients will benefit from additive treatment with benzodiazepine derivatives, levodopa, or bromocriptine. Other drugs which are at times effective include carbamazepine, tetrabenazine, clonazepam, and baclofen.

Choreoathetosis may also respond to pharmacological treatment. Therapy with different agents probably working by different mechanisms, such as haloperidol, diazepam, and valproate has been reported to be beneficial. Drug concentration monitoring for patients on these medications usually is not particularly helpful. The use of phenothiazine derivatives and drugs such as haloperidol is limited by the potential long-term side effects of these drugs on movement, including the development of acute and tardive dyskinesias.

TOURETTE'S SYNDROME

Clinical Aspects

Tourette's syndrome (TS), first described in 1885, is characterized by tics, i.e., rapid, repetitive and purposeless contractions of muscle groups. Typically, the tics first present in the facial region and often progress in a cephalo-caudal fashion to involve other muscle groups. Phonic tics are included in the syndrome and consist of barks, grunts, sniffling, and other guttural noises. Vocal tics can also include words and phrases. Coprolalia (i.e., the explosive utterance of obscenities) is one of the more dramatic features of TS and occurs with a frequency of about 30%. Motor tics tend to precede vocal tics. The symptoms tend to wax and wane in severity throughout the course of the disorder. Recently, investigators have been impressed with the phenomenological experience of patients with TS, especially descriptions of the "inner tension" associated with efforts to suppress the "irresistible" urge to tic and the relief experienced following discharge of a tic.

A major survey of school children in Monroe County, New York, suggested that a low estimate of the prevalence of TS is 28.7 cases per 100,000 pupils.[21] The data also suggested that milder presentations of TS exist in the community; for example, only 18 of 41 identified children required pharmacotherapy. In this survey, 56.4% of the biological relatives of 39 probands about whom family history could be obtained had tics or TS.

Tourette's syndrome (TS) is a disorder with a childhood onset. Family history studies have shown that there is an increased risk of TS and chronic multiple tics (CMT) in biological relatives of probands with TS.[22, 23] CMT appears to be a variant expression of TS. Moreover, a vertical pattern of transmission of a single major locus with two alleles emerged from the family history studies as responsible for susceptibility to TS and CMT. The most likely mode of inheritance is an autosomal dominant one with a greater degree of penetrance in affected males; males may be affected as much as four times more frequently as females.

Obsessive-compulsive disorder (OCD) can coexist with TS or be another alternative phenotypic expression of the genotype for TS. The frequency of coexisting OCD in 27 probands with TS was 52%,[22] and it is likely that OCD is an alternative expression of TS. A genetic relationship between Attention Deficit/Hyperactivity Disorder (ADHD) and TS[22] has not been proven. Although 60% of 27 TS probands demonstrated coexisting ADHD, there was no enrichment of ADHD among biological relatives of TS probands who did not also manifest ADHD. In the absence of biological markers, the genetic relatedness of ADHD and TS is hard to study because attentional problems, hyperactivity, and impulsiveness may be the earliest manifestations of TS itself. Also, coexistence of the two disorders may be a function of the high prevalence rate of ADHD in the general population rather than a genetic relatedness.

Pathophysiology

The substantia nigra, basal ganglia, and their interconnections with the frontal cortex are probable sites of anatomic involvement in TS.[22] Diminished concentrations of immunoreactive dynorphin in the globus pallidus was reported in a study of a single patient with TS.[24] This finding supports anatomic involvement of the basal ganglia in the pathophysiology of TS. Moreover, a report of increased concentrations of immunoreactive dynorphin in CSF of patients with TS has stimulated interest in a pathological role for this neuropeptide.

The pathophysiology of TS is not likely to be confined to an abnormality of a single retrotransmitter system. The possible effectiveness of clonidine, an alpha$_2$-adrenergic agonist, in the treatment of TS would implicate noradrenergic mechanisms.[25] The potential relatedness of OCD to TS and the salutary effects of selective serotonin-reuptake blockers in the treatment of OCD have stimulated interest in serotonergic abnormalities.[22] Dopaminergic mechanisms are implicated by the salutary therapeutic effects of D-2 dopamine receptor antagonists and the reported lowered CSF levels of homovanillic acid (HVA) at baseline and after probenecid loading in patients with TS.[22]

Diminished presynaptic dopaminergic activity may also result in postsynaptic dopamine receptor supersensitivity. This increased sensitivity of postsynaptic dopamine receptors would explain the therapeutic action of D-2 receptor antagonists and agents that dampen presynaptic dopaminergic activity. Moreover, hypersensitive dopamine receptors could explain the heightened sensitivity of some patients to exacerbation of their tics following psychostimulant administration.

Treatment

A dopamine antagonist administered in low, individually titrated doses (especially haloperidol or pimozide) is the mainstay of the pharmacotherapy of TS.[26, 27] Clinical trials with more selective D-2 dopamine receptor antagonists are especially promising. Neuroleptic medications do not totally remit tics, but are effective in reducing the severity of the symptomatology by as much as 80% in as many as 80% of affected patients.

Haloperidol has been the most widely used drug. Typically, maximal daily dosages of haloperidol are below 10 mg. Children are very sensitive to the extrapyramidal and sedative side effects of haloperidol; limitations to dosing may also result from subtle side effects such as cognitive blunting, depression, and school phobia. In young children, haloperidol is begun at 0.25 mg/d, and dosage adjustments, if necessary, are made about weekly.

Pimozide may be associated with fewer side effects than haloperidol.[26, 27] Moreover, pimozide, a diphenylbutylpiperidine compound, possesses the additional property of blockade of voltage-sensitive calcium ion channels,[28] which may be very relevant to its therapeutic action in TS.

Calcium channel antagonists (especially of the dihydropyridine class) have been reported to be therapeutically effective in a few cases when administered alone or in combination with a neuroleptic medication.[29, 30] Dampening of noradrenergic transmission by low doses of clonidine may be effective in about 50% of patients.[25] When effective, the onset of clonidine's therapeutic action may emerge slowly over the course of months. Moreover, clonidine may influence preferentially a different profile of symptoms than neuroleptic medications, especially the inner tension associated with the disorder.

Although psychostimulants may exacerbate tics, some authors advocate their adjunctive administration with neuroleptic medications.[27, 31] The rationale for psychostimulant administration is twofold: psychostimulants address the ADHD often associated with TS, and they antagonize the unpleasant side effects of sedation and depression associated with neuroleptic medication. The availability of selective serotonin-reuptake blockers, their salutary therapeutic effects in OCD, and the high frequency of coexisting OCD in patients with TS have stimulated interest in trials in patients with TS and OCD. There is also some provocative data showing that opiate antagonists may reduce the frequency of motor and phonic tics.[32]

OBSESSIVE-COMPULSIVE DISORDER

Clinical Aspects

The phenomenology of obsessive-compulsive disorder (OCD) in childhood shows a marked continuity between the presentations in childhood and adulthood.[31] Children experience their rituals and/or preoccupations as unreasonable, causing substantial interference with their lives. Rituals occur more frequently than obsessions, although they often coexist, and "pure" ritualizers can be identified (i.e., patients whose rituals were executed without accompanying mental content). "Washing," "repeating" and "checking" rituals are most common; obsessions tend to focus on avoidance of dirt and contamination, danger to self and family, and religiosity.

The emergence of OCD in the presence of a "compulsive" personality disorder is relatively rare in children. In one series of patients, children had a higher than expected presentation of coexisting developmental disability.[31] Consistent with the literature on adults, other associated disorders include depression (probably secondary to OCD) and anxiety. Even in children, rituals are performed secretively, delaying their recognition by parents by about 4–6 m. Also, parents frequently participate in the rituals; they often prepare checklists and provide reassurance that everything is orderly.

OCD occurs in the first-degree biological relatives of about 25% of patients. The pattern of symptoms in affected family members differs from that in probands. A minimum estimate for the lifetime prevalence rate of 0.4% is postulated.[33]

Pathophysiology

A variety of converging evidence implicates a neurologic abnormality, especially one that may involve the basal ganglia as its anatomic focus, in the pathophysiology of OCD. Tics and "soft signs" suggestive of neurodevelopmental delay occur in a high percentage of children with OCD.[34] Moreover, in one series, choreiform movements occurred in about one-third of children with OCD.[34] The genetic relatedness of TS and OCD has already been discussed. OCD also has been described in patients with demonstrable basal ganglia lesions, for example after a wasp sting, carbon monoxide poisoning, and the encephalitis lethargica epidemic of 1916–1917.[34] A Positron Emission Tomography (PET) scan study observed increased glucose utilization in the caudate nuclei of 14 OCD patients with and without coexisting major depression, in comparison to a group of 14 unipolar depressed patients and 14 controls.[34] This PET scan result was not replicated in a group of 18 adults with childhood-onset OCD compared with 18 controls;[34] however, in the latter study, elevated metabolic rates were observed in frontal cortex and cingulate gyri of the OCD patient group.

There are known interconnections between the frontal cortex and basal ganglia, and their interruption may be the basis of the palliative effects of capsulotomy and cingulectomy in the neurosurgical treatment of severe OCD. The volume of the caudate nucleus was shown to be reduced bilaterally in a computerized tomographic (CT) scan study comparing 10 male patients with childhood-onset OCD and 10 male controls.[35] Finally, an association between Sydenham's chorea and OCD has provided further evidence of basal ganglia involvement in the pathophysiology of OCD.[36]

Pharmacologic studies suggest a selective behavioral supersensitivity of postsynaptic serotonin receptors in patients with OCD.[37] It has been postulated that the value of selective serotonin reuptake blockers in the pharmacotherapy of OCD may reside in their ability to "down-regulate" postsynaptic serotonin receptors with prolonged administration. Clinically, the anti-obsessional effects of selective serotonin-reuptake blockers emerge after several weeks, consistent with the time course of serotonin receptor down-regulation, whereas the inhibition of serotonin transport occurs immediately. The relevance of serotonergic transmission to the pathophysiology of OCD is supported by studies showing a lowered number of ^{3}H-imipramine binding sites on the platelets of untreated OCD patients, an inverse correlation between CSF 5-hydroxyindoleacetic acid (5-HIAA) concentrations and illness severity at baseline, and a correlation between reduction in platelet serotonin concentrations and clinical improvement with clomipramine treatment.[33, 36, 38, 39]

Treatment

In a double-blind controlled study with a crossover design, clomipramine was shown to be superior to placebo in the treatment of early-onset OCD in 19 patients.[40] The anti-obsessional effect required several weeks to emerge and appeared to be independent of depressive symptoms at baseline. Consistent with this latter impression, clomipramine was a more effective anti-obsessional agent than desipramine, a secondary tricyclic antidepressant, in the treatment of children and adolescents.[41, 42] Similarly, fluoxetine, a selective serotonin-reuptake blocker, was reported to be efficacious in the treatment of 4 out of 8 patients with early-onset OCD.[40] Although clomipramine can attenuate symptoms of OCD in short-term clinical trials, it is still too early to know if pharmacologic intervention alters the long-term prognosis of this disorder.

There is no relation between the anti-obsessional effect of clomipramine and its plasma concentrations or those of its metabolites.[33] After 5 weeks of active treatment with clomipramine (dose range 75–200 mg/day), plasma levels of the demethylated metabolite are about 2.5 times greater than the parent compound. The demethylated metabolite is capable of significant blockade of norepinephrine reuptake; thus, the actions of clomipramine *in vivo* may be less selective for serotonergic transmission. Whereas a decrease in platelet serotonin content was associated with a positive response to treatment with clomipramine, there was no association between a drug-induced decrease in platelet serotonin concentration and plasma tricyclic concentrations. These data argue against a simple pharmacokinetic explanation for the anti-obsessional effects of clomipramine. Moreover, in contrast to major depressive disorder, the monitoring of plasma clomipramine concentrations may not be helpful in the treatment of early-onset OCD.

ATTENTION-DEFICIT HYPERACTIVITY DISORDER

Clinical Aspects

The behavioral syndrome referred to as Attention-Deficit Hyperactivity Disorder (ADHD) in the latest revision of the *Diagnostic and Statistical Manual* (DSM-III-R, 3rd ed.) of the American Psychiatric Association is characterized by developmentally inappropriate motor restlessness, impulsiveness, distractibility, and inattention. By definition, the onset of the disorder is before age 7; in fact, its recognition usually occurs when a child enters first grade and must conform to the demands of a structured classroom setting. A subtle neurological substrate is thought to account for the disorder in many children. Target behaviors should be observed in different situations.

The literature on this disorder is vast and has been plagued by inconsistent definitional criteria for its identification. The literature has referred to this behavioral syndrome as attention-deficit disorder with and without hyperactivity, hyperkinetic syndrome of childhood, and minimal brain disorder, among other designations. Depending on the investigation, these terms were more or less restrictive with respect to the diagnostic criteria used for enrolling study patients. For purposes of this review, both ADHD and attention-deficit disorder, with and without hyperactivity, will be employed consistent with the definitions appearing in the DSM-III-R and its earlier version, DSM-III, respectively.

The disorder is often associated with an academic skills disorder or other specific developmental disorders.

Pathophysiology

The initial enthusiasm that measurement of neurotransmitter metabolites in urine and plasma, especially urinary excretion of 3-methoxy-4-hydroxyphenylglycol (MHPG), would clarify the pharmacologic action of the psychostimulants in attention-deficit hyperactivity disorder (ADHD) has waned.[43, 44] MHPG is a principal metabolite of norepinephrine, and its reduced urinary excretion in patients treated with dextroamphetamine focused attention on a possible pathophysiologic abnormality of noradrenergic transmission. Hypoperfusion of the striatal region in ADHD has been suggested.[45] Methylphenidate has been shown to increase striatal blood flow significantly. PET studies demonstrate the potential importance of a circuit involving the frontal cortex, caudate nucleus, globus pallidus, and thalamus in ADHD. Adults who have childhood histories of hyperactivity, who have persisting difficulty with inattention and restlessness as adults, and who are also the biologic parents of children with attention-deficit disorder with hyperactivity also demonstrated diminished glucose utilization.[46]

The two primary psychostimulants used in patients with ADHD, methylphenidate and d-amphetamine, are indirect-acting dopamine agonists releasing prejunctional stores of neurotransmitter. Although their clinical effects are similar, methylphenidate and d-amphetamine appear to act on two distinct pools of presynaptic dopamine. Methylphenidate releases dopamine from reserpine-sensitive vesicles, whereas d-amphetamine releases "newly synthesized" dopamine.

Treatment

Estimates suggest that as many as 700,000 American children receive stimulant medication; methylphenidate is most frequently prescribed for hyperactivity. Initially, there was enormous optimism that the measurement of methylphenidate blood concentrations and the clinical application of pharmacokinetic data would account for responders and nonresponders and reduce or eliminate toxicity, respectively. However, this has not proved to be true.

Absorption of the drug is essentially complete after an oral dose, although much of the parent compound is hydrolyzed before reaching the systemic circulation. Peak serum concentrations are attained in about 1–2 h, and elimination half-lives range from 2.3 to 4.2 h. In addition to its metabolism to ritalinic acid, which is inactive, methylphenidate is para-hydroxylated to an "active" metabolite; however, the significance of the para-hydroxylated metabolite is doubtful because of its low penetrability across the blood-brain barrier.[45, 49]

There is as much as fourfold inter-individual variability with respect to methylphenidate serum levels at 1, 2, and 3 h after an oral dose. Variability does not seem to be related to meals or activity levels, so methylphenidate can be administered with meals in order to avoid stomach aches and anorexia. In addition, serum methylphenidate levels vary within the same individuals on different days. Thus, marked intra-individual variability limits the clinical utility of serum concentrations. Serum concentrations obtained at various time intervals after an oral dose do not correlate with behavioral changes, as measured by teachers and parents or in the laboratory.[48, 49]

In a large study of children with attention-deficit disorder with hyperactivity (ADDH) evaluated in a normal classroom setting, methylphenidate (10–65 mg/d) was shown to "normalize" a variety of target behaviors at 4 and 8 weeks of treatment.[50] Methylphenidate also improves aspects of the mother-child interaction, even in preschool-age children with ADHD. In general, methylphenidate seems to diminish off-task and noncompliant behaviors of the children, while also diminishing the use of commands and directives by the mothers.[47]

An investigation comparing two dose concentrations of methylphenidate (0.3 and 1.0 mg/kg) found that the higher dose was optimal for effecting behavioral improvement, whereas the lower dose resulted in the greatest improvement in a short-term memory task performed in the laboratory.[51] These results heightened early concern that distinct methylphenidate dose-response relations existed for behavioral improvement, academic performance, and cognition. However, most clinical studies have suggested that academic performance and learning of most children does not worsen at doses of methylphenidate above 0.3 mg/kg.[52] In fact, dose-dependent positive effects of methylphenidate on academic performance (at doses of 0.15, 0.3, and 0.6 mg/kg) have been shown.[53]

Chronic treatment does not accelerate methylphenidate metabolism. Tolerance to the beneficial effects of methylphenidate on behavior is not observed. An upward adjustment of dose other than that needed to account for body growth is usually not required.[54]

The issue of stimulant-associated side effects is especially important in view of the fact that in some settings, 3–6% of school-age children are receiving this class of medication.[55] There have been serious concerns that behavioral side effects occurring in school interfere with learning and socialization. The rate of occurrence of side effects has been examined in 83 children who participated in a placebo-controlled crossover study of active dose concentrations of methylphenidate of 0.3 and 0.5 mg/kg twice a day.[55] Serious adverse effects, including tic, dizziness, headache, worsening hyperactivity, and "excessive speech and disjointed thinking," forced 3.6% of the children to terminate the protocol. Insomnia, decreased appetite, stomach aches and headaches occurred significantly more frequently in children receiving the drug. Parental ratings suggested that a small but significant number of children experienced decreased appetite and insomnia in the high-dose methylphenidate condition: 13% and 18% of the children were rated by parents as showing severe decreased appetite and insomnia in the 0.5 mg/kg condition, compared to 1% and 7% in the placebo condition, respectively.

Interestingly, according to the teacher ratings of a subsample of 53 of the 83 children, medication resulted in a decrease of the following "side effects": staring/daydreaming, sadness, and anxiety. Compared with placebo, fewer than half of the children experienced significant side effects. The study also demonstrated a high rate of occurrence of similar side effects in the children receiving placebo. There was no evidence to support concerns that behavioral side effects interfere with school performance. The data do, however, support the importance of clinical monitoring of the emergence of side effects. The higher dose (0.5 mg/kg BID) seemed appropriate for less than 25% of the sample, because of the accompanying side effects.

MAJOR DEPRESSIVE DISORDER

Clinical Aspects

From a developmental psychodynamic perspective, there has been controversy as to whether the necessary psychic structures, especially the superego, are developed sufficiently in children for them to manifest a full depressive syndrome. The controversy was resolved in the late 1970s, when it was reported that prepubertal children with major depression could be identified using unmodified adult criteria for the disorder.[56] The phenomenology of major depressive disorder (MDD) in prepubertal children is similar to that of adults; these children show persistence of dysphoria and loss of interest, depressive ideation, and objective symptoms of appetite and sleep disturbances.[57] The magnitude of the clinical problem is large. In one study, about 7% of pediatric inpatients and between 30% and 60% of outpatients attending a child psychiatry clinic met criteria for MDD.[58] A failure to recognize MDD and intervene therapeutically can have disastrous consequences for the development of these children.

There are emerging data suggesting a strong genetic contribution to the presentation of very early-onset affective disorder. Data suggest that an inverse relation may exist between age of onset and pedigree "loading."[59] Moreover, an earlier age of onset of MDD may be associated with recurrences and a more probable bipolar disorder outcome in adulthood. There has been no obvious Mendelian pattern to the inheritance of affective illness, nor is the nature of what is inherited known (i.e., single gene vs. polygenic influences).

Pathophysiology

Neuroendocrine investigations of prepubertal depressives confirm the existence of biological abnormalities; moreover, these abnormalities often persist following resolution of the depressive episode, suggesting that they may serve as genetic trait markers. The principal neurotransmitters which are implicated in the pathophysiology of depression are norepinephrine, serotonin, and acetylcholine. Abnormalities of growth hormone secretion (after stimulation tests) have also been noted.[60]

Prepubertal depressives do not show the electroencephalographic (EEG) abnormalities during sleep (rapid eye movement) that are seen in polysomnographic studies of adult depressive (i.e., decreased REM latency, decreased slow-wave sleep time, increased REM density, and shift in the distribution of REM during the night). The abnormalities in the sleep EEGs of adult depressives are among the most robust of the "biological markers" associated with psychiatric disorders.[61] MDD in childhood may also be distinguishable from the same descriptive condition in adulthood by its lowered responsiveness to pharmacotherapy with tricyclic antidepressants.[62] Conceivably, the lowered tricyclic antidepressant-responsiveness of prepubertally depressed children is a function of a greater genetic "loading" of, and more severe form of illness in, these patients.

Treatment

The recognition of MDD in childhood stimulated systematic evaluation of the therapeutic efficacy of imipramine and other antidepressant medications. The results of these studies emphasize the potential importance of monitoring plasma levels of drug concentrations and pharmacokinetic considerations in the pharmacotherapy of these children. The relation between plasma drug concentration and imipramine efficacy has been documented.[63] A relation appears to exist between reduction in the severity of depression and both the concentration of total drug and desipramine in the plasma. There is not an obvious relationship between response and plasma concentrations of the parent compound alone.

However, the monitoring of plasma concentrations of imipramine and its metabolites has not resulted in improved strategies or guidelines for initial dosing. This is due to wide interindividual variability in steady-state plasma concentrations. Monitoring of plasma concentrations of imipramine and its demethylated metabolite confirms compliance and assists in dosage regulation, enabling the avoidance of subtherapeutic or "toxic" plasma concentrations. Plasma concentrations of imipramine and desipramine greater than 150 ng/mL are usually needed for response.[64] Drug concentrations above 400 ng/mL may result in a toxic-confusional state, which may be difficult to distinguish from the depressive symptoms.[63] At times, dosage escalation to the therapeutic range is limited by prolongation of the PR interval, increased heart rate, orthostatic hypotension, irritability, chest pain, and a behavioral syndrome of forgetfulness and perplexity. There is some evidence to suggest that adolescents are less responsive than younger children.[65]

Nortriptyline, the demethylated metabolite of amitriptyline, is the other tricyclic antidepressant whose therapeutic efficacy in the treatment of prepubertal depression has been studied systematically.[66] Secondary demethylated metabolites are predominantly "blockers" of the presynaptic reuptake of norepinephrine. The selection of nortriptyline in these studies was guided, in part, by the data suggesting that desipramine, the secondary demethylated metabolite, was primarily responsible for imipramine's action. Other reasons for the selection of nortriptyline included its safety (especially cardiac safety) in the geriatric population when plasma concentrations are maintained within a "therapeutic" range, and the existence of predictive kinetics for establishing the effective maintenance dose in adults.

Plasma nortriptyline concentrations obtained 24 h after a single oral test dose can be used to predict the daily maintenance dose that would result in steady-state levels between 60 and 100 ng/mL in children and adolescents.[67] This dose range correlates best with response. This predictive approach, based on single-dose kinetics, is useful in identifying "slow" metabolizers who would be at risk for the development of toxic side effects. Plasma concentrations of nortriptyline of less than 100 ng/mL are associated with little cardiotoxicity.[67] There have been recent studies that question the efficacy of both imipramine and nortriptyline in prepubertal children and adolescents with MDD.[68]

In summary, there are a variety of therapeutic agents used in child psychiatry. Their indications, desired therapeutic concentrations, and maintenance doses are given in Table 11–2.

TABLE 11–2. Therapeutic Profile of Commonly Used Agents in Child Psychiatry

Drug Class	Indication	Therapeutic Drug Concentration (ug/mL)	Maintenance Dose
Antidepressants			
Imipramine	Depression	0.125–0.225	Max. dosage 5 mg/kg/d
	Hyperactivity	N/A*	Mean dosage 80 mg/d
	Sleep Disorders	N/A*	10–50 mg at bedtime
	Pavor Nocturnus and Somnambulism	N/A*	
	Enuresis	N/A*	75 mg at bedtime
Nortriptyline	Depression	0.060–0.100	20–50 mg/d
Clomipramine	Obsessive-Compulsive Disorder	N/A*	75–200 mg/d
Desipramine	Hyperactivity	N/A*	Max. dosage 5 mg/kg/d
Stimulants			
Methylphenidate	Attention-Deficit Hyperactivity Disorder	Uninformative	10–60 mg/d
Dextroamphetamine	Attention-Deficit Hyperactivity Disorder	N/A*	2.5–40 mg/d
Alpha$_2$-Adrenergic Agonist			
Clonidine	Tourette's Syndrome	N/A*	0.05–0.6 mg/d
Neuroleptic Medication			
Haloperidol	Tourette's Syndrome	N/A*	0.5–10 mg/d
	Schizophrenia	N/A*	1.5–2.4 mg/d
	Pervasive Developmental Disorder, Infantile Autism	N/A*	0.5–3.0 mg/d
Pimozide	Tourette's Syndrome	N/A*	2.0–12.0 mg/d

*N/A = not applicable

REFERENCES

1.   Scheuer ML, Pedley, TA. The evaluation and treatment of seizures. NEJM 1990;323:1468-1474.
2.   Commission on Classification and Terminology of the International League Against Epilepsy. Proposal for revised classification of epilepsies and epileptic syndromes. Epilepsia 1989;30:389-99.
3.   Theodore WH, Dorwart R, Holmes, M, et al. Neuroimaging in refractory partial seizures: Comparison of PET, CT, and MRI. Neurology 1986;36:750-9.
4.   Delgado-Escueta AV, Ward AA, Woodbury DM, Porter, RJ. New wave of research in the epilepsies. In: Delgado-Escueta AV, Ward AA, Woodbury DM, Porter RJ, eds., Advances in neurology. New York: Raven Press, 1986;44:3-55.
5.   Fairgold CL, Browning RA. Mechanisms of anticonvulsant drug action: I. Drugs primarily used for generalized tonic-clonic and partial epilepsies. Eur J. Ped 1987;146:2-7.
6.   Faingold CL, Browning, RA. Mechanisms of anticonvulsant drug action: II. Drugs primarily used for absence epilepsy. Eur J. Pediat 1987;146:8-14.
7.   Ramsey RE. The use of phenytoin and carbamazepine in the treatment of epilepsy. Neurology Clinics, Epilepsy 1986;4:585-600.
8.   Woodbury DM. Absorption, distribution and excretion—Phenytoin. In Levy RH, Dreifuss FE, Mattson RH, et al., eds., Antiepileptic drugs. New York: Raven Press, 1989:177-96.
9.   Morselli PL. Absorption, distribution and excretion—Carbamazepine. In: Levy RH, Deifuss FE, Mattson RH, et al., eds., Antiepileptic drugs. New York: Raven Press, 1989:473-90.
10. Vining EPG. The use of barbituates and Bbnzodiazepines in the treatment of epilepsy. Neurology Clinics, Epilepsy 1986;4:617-32.
11. Farwell JR, Lee YJ, Hirtz DG, et al. Phenobarbital for febrile seizures: Effects on intelligence and seizure recurrence. NEJM 1990;322:364-9.
12. Wallace SJ. Use of ethosuximide and valproate in the treatment of epilepsy. Neurology Clinics, Epilepsy 1986;4:601-16.
13. Levy RH, Shen, DD. Absorption, distribution and excretion—Valproate. In: Levy RH, Dreifuss FE, Mattson RH, et al., eds., Antiepileptic drugs. New York: Raven Press, 1989:583-600.
14. Leppik IE. Status epilepticus. Neurology Clinics, Epilepsy 1986;4:633-44.
15. Olesen J. The classification and diagnosis of headache disorders. Neurology Clinics, Headaches 1996;8:793-99.
16. Prensky AL. Migraine and migrainous variants in pediatric patients. Pediatr. Clin North Am 1976;23:461-70.
17. Moskowitz MA. Basic mechanisms in vascular headache. Neurologic Clinics, Headaches 1990;8:801-16.
18. Raskin NH. Modern pharmacology of migraine. Neurology Clinics, Headaches 1990;8:857-66.
19. Young AB, Penny JB. Neurochemical anatomy of movement disorders. Neurologic Clinics, Symposium on Movement Disorders 1984;2:417-33.
20. Fahn S, Jankovic J. Practical management of dystonia. Neurologic Clinics, Symposium on Movement Disorders 1984;2:55-750.
21. Caine ED, McBride MC, Chiverton P, Bamford KA, Rediess S, Shiao J. Tourette's syndrome in Monroe Country school children. Neurology 1988;38:472-5.
22. Chappell PB, Leckman JF, Pauls D, Cohen DJ. Biochemical and genetic studies of Tourette's syndrome: Implications for treatment and future research. In: Deutsch SI, Weizman A, Weizman R, eds., Application of basic neuroscience to child psychiatry. New York: Plenum Publishing, 1990:241-60.
23. Pauls DL, Leckman JF. The inheritance of Gilles de la Tourette's syndrome and associated behaviors. Evidence for autosomal dominant transmission. N Engl J Med 1986;315:993-7.
24. Haber SN, Kowall NW, Vonsattel JP, et al. Gilles de la Tourette's syndrome: A postmortem neuropathological and immunohistochemical study. J Neurol Sci 1986;75:225-41.

25. Cohen DJ, Detlor J, Young JG, Shaywitz BA. Clonidine ameliorates Gilles de la Tourette syndrome. Arch Gen Psychiatry 1980;37:1350-7.

26. Shapiro AK, Shapiro E, Eisenkraft GJ. Treatment of Gilles de la Tourette syndrome with pimozide. Am J Psychiatry 1983;140:1183-6.

27. Shapiro AK, Shapiro E, Fulop G. Pimozide treatment of tic and Tourette disorders. Pediatrics 1987;79(6):1032-9.

28. Gould RJ, Murphy KMM, Reynolds IJ, Snyder SH. Antischizophrenic drugs of the diphenylbutylpiperidine type act as calcium channel antagonists. Proc Natl Acad Sci USA 1983;80:5122-5.

29. Berg R. A case of Tourette syndrome treated with nifedipine. Acta Psychiatr Scand 1985;72:400-1.

30. Alessi NE, Walden M, Hsieh PS. Nifedipine-haloperidol combination in the treatment of Gilles de la Tourette's syndrome: A case study. J Clin Psychiatry 1989;50:103-4.

31. Sverd J, Gadow KD, Paolicelli LM. Methylphenidate treatment of attention-deficit hyperactivity disorder in boys with Tourette's syndrome. J Am Acad Child Adolesc Psychiatry 1989;28(4):574-9.

32. Sandyk R, Iacono RP, Crinnian C, Bamford CR, Consroe PF. Effects of naltrexone in Tourette's syndrome (Abstract). Ann Neurol 1986b;20:437.

33. Flament MF, Whitaker A, Rapoport JL, et al. Obsessive compulsive disorder in adolescence: An epidemiological study. J Am Acd Child Adolesc Psychiatry 1988;27(6):764-71.

34. Swedo SE, Rapoport JL. Neurochemical and neuroendocrine considerations of obsessive-compulsive disorders in childhood. In: Deutsch SI, Weizman A, Weizman R, eds., Application of basic neuroscience to child psychiatry. New York: Plenum Publishing, 1990:275-84.

35. Luxenberg JS, Swedo SE, Flament MF, Friedland RP, Rapoport J, Rapoport SI. Neuroanatomical abnormalities in obsessive-compulsive disorder detected with quantitative X-ray computed tomography. Am J Psychiatry 1988;145:1089-93.

36. Swedo SE, Rapoport JL, Cheslow DL, et al. High prevalence of obsessive-compulsive symptoms in patients with Sydenham's chorea. Am J Psychiatry 1989;146:246-9.

37. Zohar J, Mueller EA, Insel TR, Zohar-Kodouch RC, Murphy DL. Serotonergic responsivity in obsessive-compulsive disorder. Comparison of patients and healthy controls. Arch Gen Psychiatry 1987;44:946-51.

38. Weizman A, Carmi M, Hermesh H, et al. High-affinity imipramine binding and serotonin uptake in platelets of eight adolescent and ten adult obsessive-compulsive patients. Am J Psychiatry 1986;143:335-9.

39. Flament MF, Rapoport JL, Murphy DL, Berg CJ, Lake CR. Biochemical changes during clomipramine treatment of childhood obsessive-compulsive disorder. Arch Gen Psychiatry 1987;44:219-25.

40. Flament MF, Rapoport JL, Berg CJ, et al. Clomipramine treatment of childhood obsessive-compulsive disorder: A double-blind controlled study. Arch Gen Psychiatry 1985;42:977-83.

41. Leonard HL, Swedo S, Rapoport JL, et al. Treatment of childhood obsessive compulsive disorder with clomipramine and desmethylimipramine: A double blind crossover comparison. Psychoparm Bull 1988;24:93-5.

42. Liebowitz MR, Hollander E, Fairbanks J, Campeas R. Fluoxetine for adolescents with obsessive-compulsive disorder (letter). Am J Psychiatry 1990;147(3):370-1.

43. Zametkin AJ, Rapoport JL. Neurobiology of attention deficit disorder with hyperactivity: Where have we come in 50 years? J Am Acad Child Adolesc Psychiatry 1987;26:676-86.

44. Elia J, Borcherding BG, Potter WZ, Mefford IN, Rapoport JL, Keysor CS. Stimulant drug treatment of hyperactivity: Biochemical correlates. Clin Pharmacol Ther 1990;48:57-66.

45. Lou HC, Henriksen L, Bruhn P, Borner H, Nielsen JB. Striatal dysfunction in attention deficit and hyperkinetic disorder. Arch Neurol 1989;46:48-52.

46. Zametkin AJ, Nordahl TE, Gross M, et al. Cerebral glucose metabolism in adults with hyperactivity of childhood onset. N Engl J Med 1990;323:1361-6.

47. Barkley RA. The effects of methylphenidate on the interactions of preschool ADHD children with their mothers. J Am Acad Child Adolesc Psychiatry 1988;27:336-41.

48. Gualtieri CT, Wargin W, Kanoy R, et al. Clinical studies of methylphenidate serum levels in children and adults. J Am Acad Child Psychiatry 1982;21(1):19-26.

49. Gualtieri CT, Hicks RE. Neuropharmacology of methylphenidate and a neural substrate for childhood hyperactivity. Psychiatric Clinics of North America 1985;8(4):874-92.

50. Abikoff H, Gittleman R. The normalizing effects of methylphenidate on the classroom behavior of ADDH children. J Abnormal Child Psychology 1985;13(1):33-44.

51. Sprague R, Sleator E. Methylphenidate in hyperkinetic children: Differences in dose effects on learning and social behavior. Science 1977;198:1274-6.

52. Rapport MD, Stoner G, DuPaul GJ, Birmingham BK, Tucker S. Methylphenidate in hyperactive children: Differential effects of dose on academic, learning, and social behavior. J Abnormal Child Psychology 1985;13(2):227-44.

53. Pelham WE, Bender ME, Caddell J, Booth S, Moorer SH. Methylphenidate and children with attention deficit disorder: Dose effects on classroom academic and social behavior. Arch Gen Psychiatry 1985;42:948-52.

54. Safer DJ, Allen RP. Absence of tolerance to the behavioral effects of methylphenidate in hyperactive and inattentive children. J Pediat 1989;115:1003-8.

55. Barkley RA, McMurray MB, Edelbrock CS, Robbins K. Side effects of methylphenidate in children with attention deficit hyperactivity disorder: A systemic, placebo-controlled evaluation. Pediatrics 1990;86:184-92.

56. Spitzer RL, Endicott J, Robins E. Research diagnostic criteria: Rationale and reliability. Arch Gen Psychiatry 1978;35:773-82.

57. Puig-Antich J, Blau S, Marx N, Greenhill LL, Chambers W. Prepubertal major depressive disorder. A pilot study. J Am Acad Child Psychiatry 1978;17:695-707.

58. Kashani J, Barber G, Bolander F. Depression in hospitalized pediatric patients. J Am Acad Child Psychiatry 1981;20:123-34.

59. Freimer N, Weissman MM. The genetics of affective disorder. In: Deutsch SI, Weizman A, Weizman R, eds., Application of basic neuroscience to child psychiatry. New York: Plenum Publishing, 1990:285-96.

60. Puig-Antich J, Goetz R, Davies M, et al. Growth hormone secretion in prepubertal major depressive children: II. Sleep related plasma concentrations during a depressive episode. Arch Gen Psychiatry 1984a;41:463-6.

61. Puig-Antich J. Affective disorders in children and adolescents: Diagnostic validity and psychobiology. In: Meltzer HY, ed., Psychopharmacology: The third generation of progress. New York: Raven Press, 1987:843-59.

62. Geller B, Cooper TB, McCombs HG, Graham D, Wells J. Double-blind placebo-controlled study of nortriptyline in depressed children using a "fixed plasma level" design. Psychopharmacol Bull 1989;25:101-8.

63. Preskorn SH, Bupp SJ, Weller EB, Weller RA. Plasma levels of imipramine and metabolites in 68 hospitalized children. J Am Acad Child Adolesc Psychiatry 1989;28:373-5.

64. Puig-Antich J, Perel JM, Lupatkin W, et al. Imipramine in prepubertal major depressive disorders. Arch Gen Psychiatry 1987;44:81-9.

65. Ryan ND, Puig-Antich J, Cooper T, et al. Imipramine in adolescent major depression: Plasma level and clinical response. Acta Psychiatr Scand 1986;73:275-88.

66. Geller B, Perel JM, Knitter EF, Lycaki H, Farooki ZQ. Nortriptyline in major depressive disorder in children: Response, steady-state plasma levels, predictive kinetics, and pharmacokinetics. Psychopharmacology Bulletin 1983;19:62-5.

67. Geller B, Cooper TB, Chestnut EC, Anker JA, Price DT, Yates E. Child and adolescent nortriptyline single dose kinetics predict steady state plasma levels and suggested dose: Preliminary data. J Clin Psychopharmacol 1985a;5:154-8.

68. Geller B, Cooper TB, Graham DL, Marsteller FA, Bryant DM. Double-blind placebo-controlled study of nortriptyline in depressed adolescents using a "fixed plasma level" design. Psychopharmacology Bulletin 1990;26(1):85-90.

Autoimmune Disorders of Childhood

Robert N. Lipnick, M.D., F.A.A.P., F.A.C.R.

RHEUMATIC DISORDERS OF CHILDREN

There are over 50 different diseases that may affect the musculoskeletal system (joints, bones, and muscles), as well as internal organs and skin. In the United States, approximately 250,000 children suffer from juvenile rheumatoid arthritis (JRA), while systemic lupus erythematosus (SLE) and dermatomyositis follow in relative frequency.

This chapter deals with juvenile rheumatic diseases and their laboratory diagnosis, recognizing that most of these disorders are characterized not by specific laboratory tests, but by a constellation of signs and symptoms and by radiographic abnormalities of bones and joints.

PATTERNS OF PRESENTATIONS

1. Acute mono- or oligoarthritis (affecting one or a few joints)

2. Acute polyarthritis

3. Chronic mono- or pauciarthritis

4. Chronic polyarthritis

5. Non-articular "rheumatism" (symptoms arising from periarticular tissues or muscles)

6. Arthritis associated with skin disease

7. Arthritis associated with gastro-intestinal disease

8. Arthritis associated with pleuro-pulmonary disease

9. Arthritis associated with infection

10. Arthritis associated with hematologic and neoplastic disorders

11. Systemic disease associated with vasculitis

12. Arthritis associated with endocrine, biochemical, or metabolic disorders

13. Hereditary diseases of connective tissue

JUVENILE RHEUMATOID ARTHRITIS

JRA is the most common rheumatic disorder in the pediatric population. JRA may not represent a single disease but rather a syndrome of diseases. Current evidence implicates an autoimmune pathogenesis. Genetic, environmental, and immunoregulatory factors are believed to be involved in the pathogenic process. JRA is primarily a synovial disease (i.e., affecting the joint lining), with secondary pathological changes occurring in the synovial fluid, cartilage, periarticular tissues, and bone. The synovium becomes inflamed, causing pain and swelling in one or several peripheral joints. Fibroblasts, blood vessels, and chronic inflammatory cells proliferate, and the resulting granulation-tissue pannus extends over the surface of the articular cartilage, eroding and destroying it. The destructive changes may extend to articular and periarticular bone and to periarticular soft tissue, leading to joint deformities.

The pathogenic process may extend well beyond the border of synovial tissue and involve other tissues. Clinically, the patient may have overwhelming fatigue, morning stiffness lasting many hours, high fever, rash, swelling of joints, pericarditis, uveitis, and other signs of acute or chronic disease.

SYSTEMIC LUPUS ERYTHEMATOSUS

SLE is an episodic, multisystem disease characterized by widespread inflammation of the blood vessels and connective tissue and the presence of circulating autoantibodies. Its clinical manifestations are extremely variable, and its natural history is unpredictable. Untreated, SLE is often progressive and leads to death. SLE is regarded as a prototype of autoimmune diseases in humans. Although it remains a disease of uncertain etiology, many scientific observations are consistent with the hypothesis that SLE results from altered immunologic responsiveness on a background of a genetic predisposition to the disease.

The basic pathologic lesions of SLE are immune complex and autoantibody deposition in vessels and other tissues, resulting in fibrinoid necrosis, inflammatory cellular infiltrates, and sclerosis of collagen. The fibrinoid material is eosinophilic with hematoxylin-eosin stain and is deposited within the interfibrillar ground substance of the connective tissues. Vascular endothelial thickening is another characteristic of SLE. Capillaries, venules, and arterioles are all involved. Secondary changes include vascular obstruction and development of thrombosis.

Children with SLE may present with disease that ranges from an acute, rapidly fatal onset to an insidious onset with a long history of slowly unfolding exacerbations. There is enormous variability in the character and severity of the presenting signs and symptoms. Any organ in the body may be involved. A single system may be affected at onset; however, it is more usual to find multisystem disease. A lupus-like syndrome may be induced by many drugs, especially the following: antiarrhythmics (procainamide, quinidine); anticonvulsants; antihypertensive agents (hydralazine, methyldopa); and D-Penicillamine.

NEONATAL LUPUS SYNDROME

Children of mothers who have SLE may develop manifestations of lupus in the neonatal period that are mediated by the transplacental passage of maternal IgG autoantibodies. The neonatal lupus syndrome (NLS) is more common in females than in males.

The affected infant demonstrates a transiently positive ANA and diminished serum complement concentrations. In the majority of these babies, there is no associated clinical disease and the serological abnormalities regress within several weeks to months after birth, in accordance with the normal half-life of maternal IgG (24–28 days). The clinical manifestations include rash, complete congenital heart block, hepatomegaly, thrombocytopenia, and neutropenia.

IgG autoantibodies which cross the placenta and enter the fetal circulation are apparently responsible for the observed infant pathology. Anti-Ro antibodies are most characteristic of the syndrome, although anti-La antibodies may be found in some individuals. The latter infants usually do not have complete congenital heart block.

JUVENILE DERMATOMYOSITIS

Juvenile dermatomyositis (JDM) is a multisystem disease characterized by acute and chronic nonsuppurative inflammation of striated muscle and skin. Early in its course, the disease is marked by the presence of a vasculitis, and later by the development of calcinosis. The average

age of onset is approximately 6 y, with a sex ratio of female to male of 1.7 to 1.

The etiology and pathogenesis of JDM remains unknown, although it is probably multifactorial in etiology. Potential pathogenic mechanisms include abnormalities of cellular immunity resulting in T-lymphocyte mediated destruction of striated muscle and deposition of immune complexes in muscle tissue. JDM has also been described in association with immunodeficiency and infection. Immunoglobulin G (IgG), immunoglobulin M (IgM), and the third component of complement (C3) can be found deposited in the vessel walls of skeletal muscle. A dermatomyositis-like disease has been described in some children with agammaglobulinemia in association with ECHO virus infection, and occasionally in patients with selective IgA deficiency and C2 deficiency. In addition, increased titers of serum antibodies to coxsackie virus B and toxoplasma have been reported.

Dermatomyositis usually presents in childhood with a combination of easy fatigue, malaise, muscle weakness, rash, and fever. Clinical expression and progression of the disease are variable.

The distinctive pathologic lesions of JDM involve the striated muscles, skin, and gastrointestinal tract. The main pathologic feature of the disease is muscle necrosis. Characteristic but nonspecific changes include disruption of the myofibril and tubular system, central nuclear migration, prominent nuclei, and basophilia. Concomitant degeneration and regeneration of muscle fibers result in variation in fiber size. Areas of focal necrosis are replaced during the healing phase by fibrous and fat tissue.

Routine laboratory studies are of little diagnostic help in the child with JDM. Nonspecific tests of inflammation such as the ESR and C-reactive protein tend to correlate with the degree of clinical inflammation or to be of no clinical usefulness.

Leukocytosis and anemia are uncommon at onset, except in the child with associated GI bleeding. Urinalysis is usually normal, although a few children have microscopic hematuria. There are no specific abnormalities of serum immunoglobulin concentrations. Children with JDM usually lack circulating rheumatoid factor. Antinuclear antibodies (ANAs) have been reported in patient serum at a frequency varying from 10 to 50%.

The three most helpful laboratory abnormalities are increased serum concentrations of the muscle enzymes, abnormal electromyographic changes, and specific histopathologic abnormalities on muscle biopsy. The serum muscle enzymes are important for diagnosis and for monitoring the effectiveness of therapy. Some individual variation in the pattern of enzyme increases occurs in JDM, and therefore it is recommended that CK, aspartate aminotransferase (AST), and aldolase be measured to provide a reliable baseline. The height of increase is variable but ranges from 20 to 40 times normal for CK and AST.

Rarely, children have no increase in the serum concentration of CK during the acute phase of the disease, while other children have a persistent increase of this enzyme late in the course of disease, without any other clinical indication of muscle inflammation. In the latter instance, evaluation of serum CK in family members may reveal an unrelated, but unsuspected, genetic abnormality. Lactic dehydrogenase (LDH) and alanine aminiotransferase (ALT) are increased in many children with JDM, but are less specific. Serum concentrations of all of these enzymes are increased in a wide variety of other conditions, such as muscle trauma, motor neuron diseases, vasculitis, metabolic disorders, toxins, and infections. Very large increases are most commonly associated with JDM and, to a somewhat lesser extent, with muscular dystrophy.

SPONDYLOARTHROPATHIES

The spondyloarthropathies (SAS) consist of a group of inflammatory arthropathies that affect the joints of the axial skeleton as well as peripheral joints. The four disorders classified as a spondyloarthropathy include juvenile ankylosing spondylitis (JAS), psoriatic arthritis, arthritis associated with inflammatory bowel disease, and Reiter's syndrome. They differ from JRA in many ways. Inflammation of the joints of the axial skeleton (spine and sacroiliac joints) and inflammation of the entheses (sites of attachment of ligaments and tendons on to bone) are common in children with a spondyloarthropathy, while uncommon in JRA. There is a high frequency of Human Leukocyte Antigen (HLA) B27 among patients with a spondyloarthropathy.

Juvenile Ankylosing Spondylitis

Juvenile ankylosing spondylitis is a chronic, progressive, inflammatory disorder of unknown etiology involving the sacroiliac joints, spine, and large peripheral joints. Ninety percent of cases occur in males, with the usual age at onset being the second or third decade of life. There is a strong genetic predisposition to ankylosing spondylitis, with several family members often involved. Ninety percent of patients with ankylosing spondylitis have HLA-B27. The gene that determines this specific cell surface antigen may be linked to other genes that determine pathologic autoimmune phenomena or that lead to an increased susceptibility to infectious or environmental antigens. There is no specific immunological diagnostic test.

The disease begins with the insidious onset of low back pain and stiffness, usually worse in the morning. Symptoms of the acute disease

TABLE 12–1. Laboratory Abnormalities in the Rheumatic Diseases of Childhood

Abnormality	Juvenile Rheumatoid Arthritis — Polyarthritis	Oligoarthritis	Systemic Onset	Systemic Lupus Erythematosus	Dermatomyositis	Scleroderma	Vasculitis	Rheumatic Fever
Anemia	+	–	+	+	+	+	+	+
Leukopenia	–	–	–	+++	–	–	–	–
Thrombocytopenia	–	–	–	+	–	–	–	–
Leukocytosis	+	–	+++	–	+	–	+++	+
Thrombocytosis	+	–	+	–	+	–	+	+
Antinuclear antibodies	–	+	–	+++	+	+	+	–
Anti-DNA antibodies	–	–	–	+++	–	–	–	–
Rheumatoid factors	+	–	–	+	–	+	+	–
Anti-streptococcal antibodies	–	–	–	–	–	–	–	+++
Hypocomplementemia	–	–	+	+++	–	–	+	–
Elevated hepatic enzyme levels	+	–	+	+	+	+	+	–
Elevated muscle enzyme levels	–	–	–	+	+++	+	+	–
Abnormal urinalysis	+	–	+	+++	+	+	+	–

– = absent,   + = minimal,   ++ = moderate,   +++ = severe

TABLE 12–2. Characteristics of Synovial Fluid in the Rheumatic Diseases

Group	Condition	Synovial Complement	Color/Clarity	Viscosity	Mucin Clot	WBC Count	PNM%	Miscellaneous Findings
Non-inflammatory	Normal	N*	Yellow/Clear	N	N	<200	<25	
	Traumatic arthritis	N	Xanthochromic//Turbid	N	N	<2,000	<25	Debris
	Osteoarthritis	N	Yellow/Clear	N	N	1,000	<25	
Inflammatory	SLE	N – ↓	Yellow/Clear	↓	N	5,000	10	LE cells
	Rheumatic fever		Yellow/Cloudy	↓	Fair	5,000	10–50	
	Juvenile rheumatoid arthritis	N – ↓	Yellow/Cloudy	↓	Poor	15,000–20,000	75	
	Reiter's syndrome	N – ↑	Opaque	↓	Poor	20,000	80	Reiter's cells
Pyogenic	Tuberculosis arthritis	N – ↑	Yellow/Cloudy	↓	Poor	25,000	50–60	Acid-fast bacteria
	Septic arthritis	↑	Serosanguinous/Turbid	↓	Poor	80,000–200,000	75	Low glucose, bacteria

* N = Normal

include pain and tenderness in the sacroiliac joints and spasm of the paravertebral muscles. Findings in advanced disease include ankylosis of the sacroiliac joints and spine, loss of lumbar lordosis, cervical kyphosis, and decreased chest expansion. Twenty-five percent of patients will have iritis. Carditis, with or without aortitis, is seen in 10% of patients.

Hypergammaglobulinemia, rheumatoid factors, and antinuclear antibodies are not present in the sera of patients with ankylosing spondylitis. During phases of active disease, elevated sedimentation rate and a mild anemia may be observed.

Juvenile Psoriatic Arthritis

Juvenile psoriatic arthritis (JPsA) is a chronic, recurrent, polyarthritis in children younger than 16 years, preceded by, accompanied by, or followed within 15 years by psoriasis. Psoriasis is a common disease, affecting 1 to 2 percent of the Caucasian population and has its onset in childhood in one-third of patients. Approximately 5–7% of patients with psoriasis have arthritis. The onset of arthritis may be acute or insidious and is often preceded by skin disease. The joints most commonly affected in patients with JPsA are knees, ankles, and wrists. Pitting of nails is seen in 75% of children, but onycholysis is uncommon. Other systemic manifestations may include uveitis, fever, pericarditis, and mitral valve prolapse.

In early disease, synovial histologic findings are indistinguishable from those of JRA. However, in chronic JPsA, histologic study shows increased fibrosis of capsule and arterial walls and less prominent synovial hypertrophy in comparison to JRA. Laboratory evaluation usually demonstrates an increased erythrocyte sedimentation rate, absence of rheumatoid factor, and ANA positivity in 17–50% of patients. Hyperuricemia is occasionally seen in patients with severe skin disease. Synovial fluid examination reveals a white blood cell count of 5000–40,000/mL; these are predominately polymorphonuclear cells (PMNs).

Reiter's Syndrome

Reiter's syndrome is classically defined as a clinical triad consisting of arthritis, urethritis, and conjunctivitis. However, the arthritis is frequently accompanied by only one of the other characteristic manifestations. Fever, malaise, and weight loss occur commonly with acute arthritis. The urethritis is nonspecific and often asymptomatic. The conjunctivitis is mild, but 20–50% of patients develop iritis. Balanitis circinata, painless oral ulcerations, and keratoderma blennorrhagicum (thick ketatotic lesions of the palms and soles) are mucocutaneous manifestations. Complications involve spondylitis and carditis.

Most patients have a mild leukocytosis. The urethral discharge is purulent, and smear and culture are usually negative for *Neisseria gonorrhea*. Synovial fluid is sterile, with a white cell count of 2,000–50,000/mL, mostly PMNs.

The cause of Reiter's syndrome is not known. Some cases have been associated with sexual contact. Several infectious agents, including shigella, salmonella, gonococci, mycoplasma, chlamydia, yersinia, and campylobacter have been associated with Reiter's syndrome. Eighty percent of patients with Reiter's syndrome have HLA-B27.

TABLE 12–3. Laboratory Abnormalities in the Common Forms of Spondyloarthropathy Compared to Juvenile Rheumatoid Arthritis

Laboratory Abnormalities	Spondyloarthropathies			Juvenile Rheumatoid Arthritis
	Juvenile Ankylosing Spondylitis	Juvenile Psoriatic Arthritis	Reiter's Syndrome	
Acute phase response	+	+	+	+++
Anemia	+	+	+	+++
Leukocytosis	−	+	+	+
Rheumatoid factors	−	−	−	+
Antinuclear antibodies	−	+	−	+++

− = absent,   + = minimal,   ++ = moderate,   +++ = severe

INFLAMMATORY BOWEL DISEASE

Inflammatory joint disease constitutes one of the most common extraintestinal complications of both ulcerative colitis and Crohn's disease, occurring in 10–20% of such children.

There are two types of arthritis accompanying inflammatory bowel disease, one that is characteristically a nondeforming, nonerosive polyarthritis, and one in which inflammation of the sacroiliac joints occurs. The former is correlated with activity of the gut inflammation and occurs slightly more frequently in girls than in boys. The latter is independent of enteric disease activity, is associated with HLA-B27, and occurs most frequently in teenage boys. In a child with arthritis, in whom weight loss, unexplained fever, abdominal pain, hematochezia, marked abnormalities of the inflammatory indices, or hypoalbuminemia occur, the diagnosis of inflammatory bowel disease should be considered, because joint disease may precede other manifestations of bowel disease by many months.

Laboratory studies are of little assistance in differentiating JRA from the spondyloarthropathies, except that in the latter group RF is absent and HLA-B27 is frequently present. The high frequency of ANA in JRA contrasts with its corresponding low frequency in the spondyloarthropathies.

PROGRESSIVE SYSTEMIC SCLEROSIS

Progressive Systemic Sclerosis (PSS) is a disease of unknown cause characterized by abnormally increased collagen deposition in the skin and internal organs. The course is usually slowly progressive, but it can be rapidly progressive and fatal because of involvement of internal organs such as the lungs, heart, kidneys, and gastrointestinal tract. There may be vascular abnormalities in the lungs and kidneys.

Biopsy of involved skin reveals thinning of the epidermis with loss of rete pegs, atrophy of the dermal appendages, hyalinization and fibrosis of arterioles, and a striking increase of compact collagen fibers in the reticular dermis. Synovial tissue findings range from an acute inflammatory lymphocytic infiltration to diffuse fibrosis with relatively little inflammation. The histologic changes seen in muscle include interstitial and perivascular inflammatory infiltration followed by fibrosis and myofibrillar necrosis, atrophy, and degeneration.

In patients with renal involvement, the histologic appearance of the kidney is similar to that of malignant hypertensive nephropathy, with intimal proliferation of the interlobular arteries and fibrinoid changes in the intima and media of more distal interlobular arteries and of afferent arterioles.

Polyclonal hypergammaglobulinemia is frequently present in patients with progressive systemic sclerosis. The fluorescent antinuclear antibody test is positive in 70% of cases and shows a speckled or nucleolar pattern. A specific antinuclear antibody found only in PSS is anti-SCL 70.

VASCULITIS

The vasculitides represent a spectrum of pathologic and clinical disease ranging from acute, overwhelming necrotizing vasculitis to chronic, indolent vascular inflammation. No verifying pathogenetic mechanism has yet been defined for the vasculitides, but most are probably immunologically mediated disorders.

Polyarteritis nodosa represents one entity in a spectrum of inflammatory diseases involving arteries and veins. It is a multisystem disease characterized by acute inflammation and fibrinoid necrosis of small and medium-sized vessels. The etiology of the vascular inflammation is unknown, although infections and hypersensitivity mechanisms have been suggested because similar arterial lesions are seen in serum sickness-like illnesses following allergic reactions to drugs, after bacterial infections, and in patients who have circulating hepatitis B surface antigen (HBsAg).

The clinical manifestations of polyarteritis nodosa depend on the site and extent of arteries affected and may involve the brain, heart, kidneys, intestinal tract, or peripheral nerves. Aneurysm formation or thrombosis may occur, and the inflammatory process may involve adjacent veins. In the healing stage, fibrotic obliteration of vessel lumina may occur, leading to local and distal vascular insufficiency.

Polyarteritis may occur as a disease on its own. However, it is sometimes difficult to distinguish this disease from other forms of vasculitis, such as hypersensitivity angiitis, allergic granulomatous angiitis (with asthma and eosinophilia), or Wegener's granulomatosis (necrotizing granulomatosis of the respiratory tract, disseminated angiitis, and focal glomerulonephritis). Vasculitis also occurs in association with other rheumatic disorders, such as acute rheumatic fever and systemic lupus erythematosus. There are no characteristic diagnostic tests for this group of diseases, which are characterized by vascular inflammation, aside from *biopsy* of affected vessel. The biopsy will demonstrate the vascular involvement, initially with edema of the *intima* and adjacent media, with subsequent infiltration of acute inflammatory cells, fibrinoid necrosis, and disruption of the elastica. The diagnosis may be suggested by the following histologic clues: the size of the vessels involved, the presence of vascular lesions of the same or different ages, and the presence of giant cells.

SYSTEMIC AND JOINT DISORDERS ASSOCIATED WITH INFECTIONS

Many of the systemic arthritic disorders may be associated with as yet unrecognized infections in genetically susceptible individuals (e.g., juvenile rheumatoid arthritis, systemic lupus erythematosus). Ankylosing spondylitis has been linked to Klebsiella infection. Other disorders associated with clearly identified infectious agents are acute rheumatic fever (streptococcus) and the arthritis and tenosynovitis associated with Neisseria infections. In some disorders, arthritis may be present, but culture of synovial fluid or blood is unrewarding and serologic tests to determine exposure to infectious agents must be carried out.

The presence of specific infection may be established by finding antibodies to microorganisms such as the streptococcus, (i.e., anti-streptolysin-O titer), hepatitis virus, or the spirochete *Borrelia borgdorferi* responsible for Lyme disease. Antibodies to this specific spirochete may be found in serum or synovial fluid. Erythema nodosum may be associated with systemic bacterial or fungal infections. Septic arthritis due to organisms within the joint may be diagnosed by appropriate culture of the synovial fluid. Some organisms, such as staphylococcus, streptococcus, and E. coli, are relatively easy to culture.

Neisseria gonorrhea may be difficult to culture without appropriate labora tory precautions. Tuberculous infection of bones or joints may be difficult to diagnose without open biopsy and culture of synovium. Osteomyelitis or discitis (infection in the disc of the spine arising from vertebral end plate) may require culture by needle aspirate or bone biopsy.

ACUTE RHEUMATIC FEVER

Acute rheumatic fever (ARF) is a childhood rheumatic disease that many physicians believed had only historical significance. However, in 1985, this belief was contradicted unexpectedly when a series of epidemics was reported in several widely diverse geographic regions of the United States.

Acute rheumatic fever typically occurs in children age 4–9 y, although it may also occur in teenagers. The illness appears to be slightly more common in girls than in boys. The illness begins initially as a B-hemolytic streptococcal pharyngitis, followed two to three weeks later by migratory joint pain, fever, and palpitations or fatigue. Chorea may occur, but the onset is usually several months following the pharyngitis. The revised Jones Criteria provide diagnostic guidance (see Table 12–4). Treatment usually involves penicillin prophylaxsis, non-steroidal anti-inflammatory drugs, and, for severe cases, steroids. Phenothiazides may be used in children with chorea.

TABLE 12–4. Jones Critera (revised) for Diagnosis of Rheumatic Fever*

Major Manifestations	Minor Manifestations
Carditis	Fever
Polyarthritis	Arthralgia
Chorea	Previous rheumatic fever or rheumatic heart disease
Erythema Marginatum	Prolonged PR interval
Subcutaneous Nodules	Increased ESR or CRP

Plus: Supporting evidence of preceding streptococcal infection:

Increased titers of antistreptolysin-O or other streptococcal antibodies

Positive throat culture for group A Hemolytic streptococci

Recent scarlet fever

*A definite diagnosis is established with two major criteria or with one major and two minor criteria plus evidence of prior streptococcal infection.

Laboratory findings may be of great help in many cases of ARF, because approximately 40% of patients have an asymptomatic pharyngitis, and thus 2–4 w later, when the patient is first seen, a throat culture may show normal flora and no streptococci. In such cases, markedly increased antistreptolysin-O (ASO) and anti-streptococcal deoxyribonuclease B titers which later return to normal provide supporting evidence of a recent streptococcal infection. Increased sedimentation rate or C-reactive protein is usually present. A prolonged PR interval on EKG is supportive evidence of rheumatic heart disease.

LYME DISEASE

Lyme disease was first recognized in 1975 as a distinct clinicopathologic entity by Steere et al.[10] based on the investigation of a cluster of children with arthritis in Lyme, Connecticut. Until 1983 there was no serologic test available to aid in the diagnosis. Since then, a spectrum of disease manifestations, including a characteristic skin lesion (erythema chronicum migrans), arthritis, and neurologic and cardiac abnormalities, has been shown to be associated with the tick-borne organism *Borrelia burgdorferi*. The serologic test for the antibody response to *B. burgdorferi* has been proposed as the best laboratory method for diagnosis of disease.

Initially, indirect immunofluorescent antibody (IFA) measuring both IgM and IgG was used, but most laboratories now use the enzyme-linked immunosorbent assay (ELISA), measuring both IgM and IgG. Some laboratories will perform Western Blot analysis to confirm an equivocal ELISA result. Several years ago, a group of investigators reported 17 patients with signs and symptoms of Lyme disease with negative serologic testing by IFA, ELISA, and Western Blot who had a specific T-cell blastogenic response to *B. burgdorferi*.

Concern about interlaboratory variability of results and lack of standardization of assays for the detection of the antibody response to *B. burgdorferi* prompted one investigator to send serum specimens from 17 employees working in an area known to be infested with *Ixodes dammini*, the tick vector of *B. burgdorferi*, to four different laboratories in Minnesota. Six employees tested positive for antibodies to *B. burgdorferi* in at least one laboratory, with no employee testing positive in all four laboratories. There is a need for standardization of the assays and the availability of national reference material. The results of serologic testing should not be relied on as the sole criteria in making the diagnosis of Lyme disease.

ACUTE PHASE REACTANTS

Erythrocyte Sedimentation Rate (ESR)

The rate of fall in milliliters per hour of red blood cells (RBCs) by the Westergren Method (ESR) is frequently utilized to document inflammation and also in following the course of chronic rheumatic disorders such as JRA, SLE, JDM, and vasculitis. RBCs in inflammatory disorders tend to form stacks (rouleaux) that partly result from increased concentration of fibrinogen and thus sediment more rapidly. Falsely low sedimentation rates are found in sickle cell disease, anisocytosis, spherocytosis, polycythemia, and heart failure. Prolonged storage of blood or tilting of the calibrated tube will increase the ESR.

C-Reactive Protein (CRP)

CRP is an acute phase reactant serum protein that is present in low concentration in normal serum. It was originally identified by its ability to give a precipitin reaction with pneumococcal C-polysaccharide. CRP concentrations rise rapidly under an inflammatory stimulus and then fall when inflammation subsides. In systemic lupus erythematosus and scleroderma, CRP concentrations are inappropriately low unless infection is present. CRP testing may be performed on freeze-stored serum, its major advantage compared to ESR testing.

In summary, laboratory testing is very valuable in the differential diagnosis of rheumatic diseases in childhood.

TABLE 12–5. Pediatric Diseases Associated with a Positive Rheumatoid Factor

Rheumatic Diseases	Non-Rheumatic Diseases
JRA	Viral (e.g., EBV)
SLE	Chronic active hepatitis
Scleroderma	Chronic infections (e.g., TB, Malaria)
Vasculitis	Subacute bacterial endocarditis
	Malignancy (e.g., Leukemia, Lymphoma)
	Sarcoidosis
	Chronic pulmonary disease
	Post-vaccination

TABLE 12–6. Pediatric Diseases Associated with a Positive Antinuclear Antibody

Rheumatic Diseases	Non-Rheumatic Diseases
SLE	Drugs:
JRA	Anticonvulsants (e.g., Phenytoin)
Dermatomyositis	Anithypertensives (e.g., Hydralazine)
Scleroderma	Antiarrhythmics (e.g., Procainamide)
	Infections:
	Syphilis
	Hepatitis
	Mononucleosis
	Malignancy (e.g., Leukemia, Lymphoma)
	Inflammatory Bowel Disease

The author would like to thank George C. Tsokos, M.D., for his critical review and Sterling McQueen for excellent assistance in the preparation of this manuscript.

SUGGESTED READING

1. Cassidy JT, Petty RE. Textbook of pediatric rheumatology, 2nd ed. New York: Churchill Livingstone, 1990.

2. Lipnick RN, Tsokos GC. Immune abnormalities in the pathogenesis of juvenile rheumatoid arthritis. Clin Exp Rheum 1990;8:177-86.

3. Szer IS, Jacobs JC. Systemic Lupus Erythematosus in childhood. In: Lahita RG, ed., Systemic Lupus Erythematosus, 1st ed. New York: Churchill Livingstone, 1987: 383-412.

4. Pachman LM. Juvenile Dermatomyositis. Pediatr Clin North AM 1986; 33:1097-117.

5. Southwood TR, Petty RE, Malleson PN, et al. Psoriatic arthritis in children. Arthritis Rheum 1989;32:1007-13.

6. Petty RE, Malleson PN. Spondyloarthropathies of childhood. Pediatr Clin North AM 1986;33:1079-96.

7. Suarez-Almazor ME, Catoggio LJ, Maldonado-Cocco, et al. Juvenile Progressive Systemic Sclerosis: Clinical and serologic findings. Arthritis Rheum 1985;28:699-702.

8. Bisno AL. The resurgence of Acute Rheumatic Fever in the United States. Annu Rev Med 1990;41:319-29.

9. Luger SW, Krauss E. Serologic tests for Lyme Disease. Arch Intern Med 1990;150:761-63.

10. Steere AC, Malawista SE, Snydman DR, et al. Lyme arthritis: An epidemic of oligoarticular arthritis in children and adults in three Connecticut communities. Arthritis Rheum 1977; 20:7-17.

CHAPTER 13

The Laboratory and Adolescent Medicine

John T. Repke, M.D. Sue Ellen Carpenter, M.D.
Michele D. Wilson, M.D.

GENERAL ADOLESCENT MEDICINE

Introduction

In 1984 there were 36 million individuals between age 10 and 19 y in the United States. The American Academy of Pediatrics' Committee on Practice and Ambulatory Medicine recommends that a health assessment visit occur every two years during adolescence if the individual is healthy. Some adolescent medicine specialists suggest a more frequent schedule of brief yearly assessments. As part of the health assessment, a history and physical examination are performed and selected laboratory tests are routinely done.[1]

Hematology

Anemia

Iron-deficiency anemia is a common disorder during adolescence, occurring in approximately 8% of females and 3% of males. Several factors contribute to its high prevalence. Adolescents are growing rapidly and therefore have increased iron requirements. They often consume a diet of poor nutritional value and low iron content. Female adolescents lose iron with menstruation. Yet most teenagers with iron-deficiency anemia appear healthy, since the degree of anemia generally is not severe. They may have subtle difficulties such as behavior problems, decreased attention span, or poor school performance.

Screening for anemia is recommended as part of routine health care. At minimum, a hemoglobin and/or hematocrit should be obtained at the initial visit with a teenager and again at the end of puberty. In order to screen for iron-deficiency anemia, ideally one would obtain a hemoglobin, hematocrit, red cell indices and red cell distribution width. A hematocrit alone is often performed, since it can be performed easily in a physician's office or clinic. The micro-hematocrit measurement of capillary blood can be used. Blood is inserted into two heparinized microcapillary tubes and centrifuged. The test has an acceptably high sensitivity but a low specificity; thus, it is an acceptable screening test for anemia. Alternatively, the hemato-crit can be measured by automated counting devices in the laboratory using venous blood. Hemoglobin can be measured by spectrophoto-metric methods. The mean cell volume can be determined directly by Coulter-type counter.

Iron stores can be markedly depleted without anemia. The iron stores decrease initially, as demonstrated by a low-serum ferritin. Next, the serum iron decreases, the iron-binding capacity increases, and the serum transferrin decreases. As the condition continues, erythrocytes become small, as evidenced by a low mean cell volume, and they have a low hemoglobin concentration. The red cell distribution width, which is a measure of the variability of the mean cell volume, increases and is a sensitive measure of iron deficiency states. Protoporphyrin accumu-lates when there is inadequate iron for heme synthesis. Thus, increased concentrations of erythrocyte protoporphyrin indicate iron depletion.

In determining reference ranges for hematologic values during adolescence, it is important to consider age, sex, race, and sexual maturity rating (see Table 13–1). Normal hemoglobin and hematocrit values for females remain fairly constant, while the values for males are more dependent on sexual maturity rating. Hematocrit values for black versus white adolescents are 1%–3% lower on average.[2]

Sickle Cell Screening

If a black adolescent has not previously been screened, he or she should receive a sickle cell screening test during adolescence. An in-dividual who is found to carry the trait should be fully informed of its importance prior to childbearing.

TABLE 13–1. Changes in Hematocrit Values by Pubertal Stages and Race

Pubertal Stage	Race	MALES		FEMALES	
		Mean (%)	SD (%)	Mean (%)	SD(%)
STAGE 1	Black	37.7	2.5	37.3	2.6
	White	39.5	2.4	39.1	3.0
STAGE 2	Black	38.4	2.5	38.9	3.2
	White	39.8	3.0	39.2	2.1
STAGE 3	Black	39.7	2.4	39.0	3.7
	White	40.9	2.6	39.6	2.6
STAGE 4	Black	41.1	2.7	38.4	3.5
	White	42.3	2.5	39.2	2.4
STAGE 5	Black	42.7	3.1	38.7	2.8
	White	43.8	2.7	39.2	3.0

Adapted from Daniel, WA. Hematocrit: Maturity relationship in adolescence. Pediatrics, 1973;52:338.

Cholesterol and Lipid Screening

Coronary artery disease is the major cause of death in the United States. The atherosclerotic process that leads to coronary artery disease begins early in life. Hyperlipidemia and hypercholesterolemia are important risk factors for the development of the disease.

The indications for cholesterol screening in children and adolescents has been the subject of debate, as studies have demonstrated that cholesterol levels during childhood and adolescence do not track consistently into adulthood.

The National Heart, Lung and Blood Institute's Expert Panel on Blood Cholesterol Levels in Children and Adolescents convened to examine the issues related to cholesterol screening in children.[3] The Panel and the American Academy of Pediatrics have recommended that selective rather than universal screening be performed. Furthermore, testing should be performed as part of routine health care. Screening is recommended for a child or adolescent when there is a family history of premature cardiovascular disease, when one or both parents have high serum cholesterol, or when the individual has another known risk factor for atherosclerosis and coronary heart disease.

Serum cholesterol is generally the suggested initial screening test (see Table 13–2). If the serum cholesterol is high (≥ 200 mg/dL; 5.18 mmol/L), a lipoprotein analysis should be done. If the cholesterol value is borderline (170–199 mg/dL; 4.40–5.15 mmol/L), a repeat cholesterol should be obtained. When the average of the two values is high (≥ 200 mg/dL; 5.18 mmol/L) or borderline, a lipoprotein analysis is suggested.

TABLE 13–2. Classification of Total and LDL-Cholesterol
Concentrations [values presented in mg/dL (mmol/L)]

Category	Total Cholesterol	LDL-Cholesterol
Acceptable	< 170 (4.4)	< 110 (2..85)
Borderline	170–199 (4.4–5.15)	110–129 (2.85–3.34)
High	≤ 200 (5.18)	≤ 103 (3.37)

If there is a documented history of premature cardiovascular disease in a parent or grandparent, a lipoprotein analysis should be performed initially, since many of these individuals will have lipoprotein
abnormality. Two separate specimens are obtained and the values
averaged. If the average LDL-cholesterol is acceptable (< 110 mg/dL;
2.85 mmol/L), education alone is recommended, with repeat testing
performed in 5 y. If the LDL-cholesterol is borderline (110–129 mg/dL;
2.85–3.34 mmol/L), a Step-One Diet should be prescribed which
reduces the intake of saturated fatty acids and cholesterol and repeat
testing should be done in 1 y. If the LDL-cholesterol is high (≥ 130
mg/dL; 3.37 mmol/L), a Step-One Diet is recommended; if the diet is
unsuccessful as determined by repeat lipoprotein analysis at 3 m, the
patient should advance to a Step-Two Diet which further limits dietary
intake of saturated fatty acids and cholesterol.

Drug therapy should be considered in children age 10 y or older if
adequate trial of diet therapy is unsuccessful. Referral to a lipid
specialist is indicated in this situation.

Substance Use

Drug use commonly occurs during adolescence. The National Institute
on Drug Abuse conducts a yearly survey of high school seniors to
assess the prevalence of drug use among adolescents. For the class of
1989, 50.9% had used an illicit drug at some time and 19.7% had used
an illicit drug in the last 30 days.[4] Substance use represents a range of
usage from experimentation to drug addiction and dependency. Common complaints that alert the clinician to the possibility of substance
abuse include poor school performance, personality change, family dis-
cord, legal problems, injuries, or physical effects secondary to acute or
chronic drug use. The interview and the use of standardized screening
questionnaires are important components of the assessment. Drug
testing can prove useful in carefully selected situations. The indications for drug testing and the manner in which the sample is obtained
remain controversial. One must carefully consider the ethical issues
prior to undertaking drug testing. It is crucial to know which drugs the
laboratory can detect and to what degree of accuracy.

There are many laboratory techniques available for drug testing. When drug testing is indicated, a screening test is usually done initially followed by a confirmatory tests. Immunoassay techniques are used for screening purposes. This method employs a drug-specific antibody reaction. A limitation of this test is that antibodies can cross-react with related drugs and yield a false-positive result. Enzyme multiplied immunoassay (EMIT) is a commonly used screening test and is less costly than other tests. Radioimmunoassay (RIA) is also available, but has the disadvantages of requiring greater analysis time and using radioactive materials. Fluorescent polarization technique is an alternative screening method.

Confirmation of a positive screening test by a second, more specific measure—chromatography—is recommended. Chromatography involves separation of various components of the specimen followed by identification of the different substances. Thin-layered chromatography (TLC) can detect many drugs of abuse. Although this method is often used, interpretation of the results requires a very skilled individual. False-positive and false-negative results can occur. A combination of gas-liquid chromatography with mass spectrometry (GC/MS) is the gold standard for drug testing. It is a highly specific and sensitive method which requires very advanced technology. Substances present in the sample are ionized and separated. Drugs detected are compared to the mass spectra for known substances in a reference library.[5] The threshold concentrations of drugs used for screening and confirmation has been debated.[6]

Urinalysis/Urine Culture

A urinalysis should be obtained at the initial visit with a teenager and again at the end of puberty. It serves as a screening tool for urinary tract infection, diabetes mellitus, and renal disease. For sexually active males, examination of the urine is a screening tool to detect urethritis (see the section of this chapter entitled "Male Reproductive Health"). Routine urinalysis includes dipstick tests for glucose, protein, occult blood, and pH. A dipstick leukocyte esterase test for pyuria is also available. Urine specific gravity is measured with refractometer. Additionally, microscopic examination should be performed, looking for red blood cells, white blood cells, bacteria, casts and crystals. Most asymptomatic adolescents with isolated proteinuria will not have serious renal pathology; many will have orthostatic proteinuria. Increased urine pH > 7 can be a marker for *Proteus* urinary tract infection. Urine culture is indicated if there is pyuria, defined as > 10 white blood cells per high-power field, bacteria on microscopic examination, or if the patient has signs or symptoms suggestive of either lower or upper urinary tract infection.

Urinary tract infection (UTI) is defined as the presence of bacteria in urine taken directly from the bladder. Manifestations of UTI include dysuria, frequency, urgency, nocturia, voiding of small volumes, incontinence, suprapubic or pelvic pain, gross hematuria, or change in appearance or odor of urine. In females, urinary tract infection must be distinguished from vaginitis or cervicitis. UTI is extremely rare in male adolescents. Fever and/or flank pain suggest renal involvement. Laboratory evaluation of UTI includes microscopic examination of fresh or gram-stained urine. The hemocytometer is a more accurate but less commonly used technique to inspect for pyuria. Pyuria is a very sensitive indicator of UTI. Bacteriuria, defined as > 1 bacteria per oil-immersion field of uncentrifuged urine or > 10 organisms on spun urine, correlates with ≥ 105 colony-forming units per mL but will miss infections with a lower colony count. If a urinary tract infection is suspected on initial assessment, one can either perform standard quantitative cultures plus antimicrobial sensitivity in the microbiology laboratory, or use the dip-slide method of culturing. The dip-slide method utilizes an agar-coated slide which is dipped into urine and allowed to grow overnight at room temperature. Standard cultures are done by inoculating plates with a known volume of urine and examining the plates for growth 24 and 48 h later. The dip-slide is a very sensitive and specific test, limited in its usefulness only by the fact that it is made of a selective media from which unusual pathogens might not be recovered. Any growth from urine obtained by catheterization is significant. The standard teaching is that growth of 10^5 bacteria per milliliter from a clean-catch, midstream urine specimen is indicative of UTI. One should lower the threshold from 10^5 to 10^2 organisms if the patient is symptomatic or has pyuria.[7] The most common uropathogens are *Escherichia coli*, *Staphylococcus saprophyticus*, *Klebsiella pneumoniae*, and *Proteus mirabilis*. Rarely, other gram-negative rods such as *Pseudomonas aeruginosa* or *enterococci* are recovered.[8]

Infectious Mononucleosis

Although many young children have subclinical or mild Epstein-Barr virus (EBV) infection, clinically apparent acute infectious mononucleosis (IM) develops most commonly in adolescents and young adults. EBV infection is more prevalent in lower socioeconomic status groups where 50–85% of children have positive serology by age 4 y, while only 14–50% of middle and upper socioeconomic status children have positive serology by college age. The incubation period for infectious mononucleosis is 5–7 w. Its common manifestations include fever, malaise, lymphadenopathy, tonsillopharyngitis, splenomegaly, hepatomegaly, and abdominal pain. Palatine petechiae, periorbital edema, and rash may also be present.[9] Hematologic findings of IM include lymphocytosis > 50% of the total white blood cell count and atypical lymphocytes

> 10% of all leukocytes. Other laboratory abnormalities include neutropenia and moderate increases of serum transaminases.

Laboratory tests can corroborate the diagnosis of IM. Heterophile antibody tests are the standard means by which the diagnosis is made. The heterophile antibody test measures the titer of agglutinating antibody to sheep or horse (horse is more commonly used) erythrocytes after absorption with guinea pig kidney homogenate. These heterophile antibodies may be detected during the first week of infection but peak during second and third week. Sheep and beef agglutination tests remain positive for 3–6 m; horse agglutination remains positive for as long as 18 m. The rapid slide test is the most frequently utilized heterophile test, and it is positive in over 90% of older children and adolescents with acute infectious mononucleosis.

When the patient has severe symptoms suggestive of IM but lacks heterophile antibodies, the clinician may decide to perform specific serologic tests for Epstein-Barr virus.[10] The presence of IgM antibody to EBV-capsid antigen can make the diagnosis of acute mononucleosis with good reliability, although cross-reactivity with the rheumatoid factor does arise. IgG antibody to EBV-capsid antigen is present in acute disease, but it remains positive for years and therefore cannot be used to distinguish acute from previous infection. Other tests include detection of early antigen antibody response to diffuse or restricted components of EBV-early antigen. Antibodies to EBV-nuclear antigen develop in the late phase of the disease.

Mycoplasma pneumoniae

Mycoplasma pneumoniae is a frequent cause of respiratory infections in teens, accounting for 30–50% of pneumonias in college-age populations. Illness may begin with fever, malaise, and headache. Cough usually develops 3–5 d later. Other signs and symptoms include chills, pharyngitis, chest pain, coryza, nausea and vomiting. Physical exam shows lymphadenopathy, pharyngitis, and abnormal lung findings such as rales, rhonchi, and wheezing. The peak incidence occurs in early adolescence, between 10–14 y.

The organism *Mycoplasma pneumoniae* can be recovered by culture technique from the nasopharynx or oropharynx. Because it takes 2–3 w for the organism to grow, cultures are not helpful clinically. The cold agglutinin reaction which demonstrates IgM autoantibodies that agglutinate red blood cells at 4° C may be increased to a titer > 1:32 in 75% of individuals with *Mycoplasma pneumoniae* but is not very specific. Complement fixation titers measure specific serum antibodies to *Mycoplasma pneumoniae* and will demonstrate a fourfold rise from the onset of illness until 1–3 w later. The treatment is oral erythromycin or tetracycline, 500 mg four times a day for 10 days.

Group A β-hemolytic Streptococci

Group A β-hemolytic streptococcal infection is frequent among teenagers. The clinical presentation can include high fever, exudative pharyngitis, tender anterior cervical lymph nodes, scarlatiniform rash, headache, vomiting, and abdominal pain. The diagnosis is more likely if there is a history of contact with an individual harboring streptococci. By contrast, Group A β-hemolytic streptococci is less probable if the patient has cough, coryza, and rhinitis.

Until recently, throat cultures were the standard technique by which to diagnose streptococcal pharyngitis. Many rapid diagnostic kits are now available that detect Group A β-hemolytic streptococcal antigen from throat swab samples. The tests require 5–60 min to perform. These tests use acid or enzyme extraction technique to remove the Group A carbohydrate from the throat swab sample, followed by latex agglutination. Rapid diagnostic tests are very specific so that false positives are unlikely. Nevertheless, they are less sensitive, so that false negatives occur in 15–40% of cases. Given the high specificity and relatively low sensitivity, many experts suggest using the rapid diagnostic test first. It is generally recommended that if rapid diagnostic tests are used, positive results result in prompt treatment. Thus, rapid diagnosis leads to rapid treatment and a quicker clinical response. If results are negative, culture should be performed and need for treatment is based on culture results.[11, 12] Cultures are usually prepared on a blood agar plate with bacitracin disks.

Serologic evidence occurs late in the disease process and therefore titers are beneficial in the diagnosis of late, nonsuppurative complications of Group A β-hemolytic streptococci but not in diagnosis of acute infection.

The recommended treatment of Group A β-hemolytic streptococcal infection is oral penicillin V, 125–250 mg three or four times a day for 10 d, or a single, intramuscular injection of benzathine penicillin G, 1.2 million units if the patient is over 60 lb. The alternative treatment for the penicillin allergic individual is oral erythromycin ethyl succinate, 40–50 mg/kg/d divided four times a day, or erythromycin estolate, 20–30 mg/kg/d in 2–4 divided doses (maximum daily dose of 1 gram).

Male Reproductive Health

Screening sexually active teenage males for sexually transmitted diseases is a common, although not universal, practice. Some experts screen high-risk teens only, while others believe that all young people are at increased risk. In the asymptomatic male, the first-catch urine specimen is a valuable yearly screening test for urethritis.[13] The first-catch urine specimen consists of the initial 10–20 mL of voided urine. The urine is then centrifuged and the sediment is resuspended and examined microscopically for trichomonads and white blood cells. The finding of > 10 white blood cells on high-power (400x) field is significant pyuria and suggests the presence of urethritis. Alternatively, cultures for *Neisseria gonorrhoeae* and either cultures or rapid diagnostic tests for *Chlamydia trachomatis* can be performed for screening purposes.

Yearly syphilis serology is recommended for high-risk males. The decision as to whether to perform testing for hepatitis B will be based on consideration of the individual's risk factors and the prevalence of disease in the target population. The indications for human immunodeficiency virus (HIV) testing is controversial and should only be done with appropriate informed consent following discussion of risks and benefits.

Homosexual males are at increased risk for sexually transmitted diseases. Urethral, rectal, and pharyngeal cultures for *Neisseria gonorrhoeae* and *Chlamydia trachomatis* should be obtained on a yearly basis. An annual syphilis serology should be performed. Screening for hepatitis B is advocated and, if the individual is surface antibody and antigen negative, immunization is advised. One should consider HIV testing in homosexual teens. In addition, these individuals are at increased risk for intestinal infections, including *Shigella*, *Campylobacter*, *Entamoeba histolytica*, *Giardia lamblia*, cytomegalovirus, hepatitis A, hepatitis B, and hepatitis C.

Sexually active males may develop urethritis manifested by urethral discharge, dysuria, or pruritus at the distal urethra. Asymptomatic urethritis is common. *Neisseria gonorrhoeae*, *Chlamydia trachomatis* and *Ureaplasma urealyticum* cause most infections. If a urethral discharge is present, gram stain of secretions is valuable. The finding of gram-negative diplococci on gram stain of urethral exudate is an extremely specific and sensitive test for *Neisseria gonorrhoeae*. When there is a urethra exudate, it can be sent for gonococcal culture. If not, one should insert a thin swab a minimum of 2 cm into the urethra to obtain culture material. The sample is inoculated onto selective media, typically modified Thayer-Martin media, and placed in a 5% or 10% CO_2 environment to grow. Growth of oxidase-positive, gram-negative diplococci with specific sugar fermentation pattern confirms the presence of *Neisseria gonorrhoeae*. Because of the emergence of increasing resistance, testing for antimicrobial susceptibility and β-lactamase production should be conducted.

The detection of *Chlamydia trachomatis* by culture technique requires that one obtain an endourethral sample. Tissue culture and rapid diagnostic tests are frequently used to diagnose *Chlamydia trachomatis*. *Trichomonas vaginalis* is much less common in males than in females. If one suspects its presence, a wet preparation of secretions should be examined for the motile, flagellated protozoan.

ADOLESCENT GYNECOLOGY

Dysfunctional Uterine Bleeding

Sometimes adolescents present with heavy, prolonged, or very irregular periods. Most perimenarcheal cycles are anovulatory, but they are reasonably regular (21–45 d) and blood loss is modest. These cycles represent estrogen withdrawal bleeding. Follicular stimulating hormone (FSH) stimulates follicular growth and estradiol is produced. The negative feedback mechanism is intact, and as estradiol concentrations rise, FSH is suppressed and the follicle becomes atretic without ovulation. The estradiol concentration subsequently declines and withdrawal bleeding occurs.

The most common cause of dysfunctional uterine bleeding in early adolescence is delayed maturation of the negative feedback system which results in higher than normal FSH concentrations with prolonged estrogen stimulation of the endometrium and excessive proliferation. Irregular shedding of the heavily developed endometrium may lead to heavy uterine blood loss. However, this is a diagnosis of exclusion. Evaluation of the disorder includes pelvic examination to rule out pelvic infection, uterine anomalies or myomas, or a vaginal foreign body (i.e., tampon retention). The initial laboratory evaluation includes a hematocrit with reticulocyte count to assess the severity and chronicity of anemia. A serum human chorionic gonadotropin (HCG) assay is performed to exclude pregnancy as a cause of dysfunctional bleeding. At the time of pelvic examination, cervical cultures are performed for gonorrhea and Chlamydia if pelvic infection is considered a possible etiology.

Bleeding which is heavy enough to require hospitalization, particularly when it occurs in the first menstrual cycle, is more likely to be associated with a bleeding diathesis. In this case, there is usually a history consistent with a bleeding tendency. Nonetheless, all patients should have a bleeding time, prothrombin time, activated partial thromboplastin time, and platelet count. Other endocrinologic disorders which can present as dysfunctional uterine bleeding include diabetes mellitus, thyroid disease, Cushing's syndrome, Addison's disease, hyperprolactinemia, chronic anovulation, and incipient ovarian failure as it progresses through anovulation prior to complete cessation of function (such as that associated with prior chemotherapy or radiation therapy). Therefore, glucose, thyroid stimulating hormone (TSH), thyroxine, T_3 resin uptake, luteinizing hormone (LH), FSH, prolactin, testosterone, dehydro-3-epiandrosterone sulfate (DHEAS), and progesterone concentrations should be obtained prior to therapy in order to make a specific diagnosis.

Oligomenorrhea

Patients who are more than two years from menarche and having fewer than six cycles per year, especially if ovulatory symptoms are not present, require a thorough endocrinologic evaluation. The laboratory evaluation usually includes serum prolactin, thyroid function tests, FSH, LH, and androgens if hirsutism is present. The most common cause of oligomenorrhea in later adolescence is chronic anovulation syndrome, also known as polycystic ovary syndrome (PCO).

Secondary Amenorrhea

Any adolescent with the abrupt loss of menstrual cycles for 4 m after regular cycles have been established should be evaluated. Stress and pregnancy are the most common causes of secondary amenorrhea. The possibility of pregnancy, severe weight loss or gain, increased athletic activity, disruption of the school or home environment, and oral contraceptive use should be sought historically. The laboratory evaluation includes FSH, LH, androgens, prolactin, thyroid function tests, and a pregnancy test.

Patients who have premature ovarian failure characterized by an FSH in a menopausal range on two occasions approximately 2 w apart must be screened for polyendocrine immune syndrome. This syndrome can include hypoadrenalism, hypoparathyroidism, thyroiditis, and pernicious anemia. Therefore, a screening laboratory evaluation including TSH, calcium, phosphorous, hemoglobin, and 8:00 AM and 4:00 PM serum cortisol is performed at the time of diagnosis and annually thereafter. Antimicrosomal antibodies, antithyroglobulin antibodies, adrenal antibodies and parietal cell antibodies are available as adjunct screening for auto-immune disorders. Patients with secondary amenorrhea on the basis of anorexia nervosa should have a complete blood count and serum electrolytes as well as thyroid function tests if these were not included in the initial screening, as they are frequently abnormal.

Hirsutism

An adolescent who presents with a complaint of hirsutism should be assessed historically including recent changes in the amount of hair, location of new hair, relation of hair growth to the onset of puberty, presence of acne, anabolic steroid ingestion, weight gain, voice changes, changes in scalp hair distribution, and presence of acanthosis nigricans as well as family history of hirsutism, glucose intolerance, menstrual irregularity or infertility, and ethnic background. The degree of hirsutism is assessed and recorded in the physical examination. The

Ferriman-Gallwey score is a useful tool for objective measurement.[14] The history of virilization should raise the question of the presence of an androgen producing tumor, adrenal enzyme deficiency, or intersex disorder. The abrupt onset of such changes increases the suspicion of a tumor. Signs of virilization include temporal hair recession, deepening of the voice, clitoral enlargement, or changes in body fat and muscle distribution.

The laboratory is utilized to define the etiology of the patient's hirsutism. The initial evaluation should include serum concentrations for testosterone, DHEAS, LH, FSH, and prolactin. A baseline concentration of 17-hyroxyprogesterone and progesterone obtained in the follicular phase in a menstruating patient is also recommended to rule out late-onset congenital adrenal hyperplasia. In adolescents, free testosterone is drawn because, at initial presentation, total testosterone concentrations are normal, but subtly increased testosterone production decreases circulating sex hormone binding globulin, and increased free testosterone can be measured before total testosterone becomes increased. If virilization is present or a tumor is suspected, serum concentrations of DHEA and androstenedione are added to the initial screening. DHEAS > 7 mg/mL (18.2 μmol/L, androstenedione > 500 mg/100 mL or testosterone > 200 ng/dL (6.94 nmol/L) (depending on the laboratory normal values) raises the suspicion of a tumor or intersex disorder.[15] Because of the possibility of ruling out androgen-secreting tumors which are extremely small, it is recommended that several measurements of the abnormal androgen be obtained that reach a value of 2.5 times greater than the upper limit of normal for the laboratory. Karyotyping is performed on adolescents with significant virilization, especially when associated with vaginal or uterine agenesis, a serum testosterone in the male range, or an increased FSH. Some patients with mild hirsutism have seemingly normal serum androgen concentrations. These patients probably have increased free testosterone as well as increased skin sensitivity to androgens. The degree of skin sensitivity may be reflected in the measurement of the concentration of the androstanediol glucuronide which, although not an androgen itself, is a metabolite of the conversion of testosterone to dihydrotestosterone. Dihydrotestosterone is the active androgen at the level of the skin.

If the stigmata of Cushing's syndrome are present, a 24 h urine specimen is collected for urinary free cortisol and an 8:00 AM serum cortisol concentration after a bedtime dose of 1 mg dexamethasone should be obtained. If the serum concentration of cortisol is not suppressed below 5 μg/dL (13.8 nmol/L) or urinary free cortisol is abnormal, formal dexamethasone suppression testing is performed.[16] If hyperprolactinemia is present, a pituitary adenoma should be excluded; however, some patients with chronic anovulation syndrome

(PCO) have an associated increase in prolactin. Patients with a concentration of 17-hydroxyprogesterone measured in the follicular phase > 2 ng/mL (6.06 nmol/L) should have an adrenal corticotropic hormone (ACTH) stimulation test performed.[17] Baseline serum 17-hydroxyprogesterone and progesterone concentrations are measured, the patient is given 0.25 mg ACTH at time 0, and concentrations of 17-hydroxyprogesterone and progesterone are repeated at 30 min. The rise seen in late-onset congenital adrenal hyperplasia is typically > 6.5 ng/dL/min. In some referral populations, deficiency of 3-β-hydroxy-steroid dehydrogenase has been found to be an important cause of hirsutism. The patients usually present with an increased baseline DHEAS, but with a normal testosterone. Detection of 3-β-hydroxy-steroid dehydrogenase deficiency requires the measurement of baseline and 60 min 17-hydroxyprogesterone and DHA in comparison to the standards developed by Pang and colleagues.[18]

The diagnosis of PCO is made by exclusion of all other clinical entities associated with hirsutism. Reference values must be established within the individual laboratory; however, the LH-to-FSH ratio is above 2.5. An increased LH-to-FSH ratio may occur secondary to androgen excess of other causes. Intermittent sampling may also miss the abnormal gonadotropin ratio. The diagnosis is usually made based on the combination of increased testosterone, an increased LH to FSH ratio, history of anovulatory cycles, and signs of androgen excess. In clinical research centers, confirmatory dynamic testing for PCO may be obtained, such as exaggerated LH and normal FSH response to gonadotropic releasing hormone (GnRH) or an increased androstenedione or testosterone response to HCG stimulation; however, these stimulation tests are not required in usual clinical practice. As our understanding of the abnormalities in carbohydrate metabolism associated with chronic anovulation (HAIR-AN) syndrome increases, the demand for glucose tolerance testing and insulin concentrations will grow.

Anorexia Nervosa and Bulimia Nervosa

Anorexia nervosa is a common illness of adolescent girls. The illness does occur in boys, but is much more rare. The diagnosis of anorexia nervosa is based on the clinical presentation of (1) body weight 15% below what is expected, (2) intense fear of gaining weight or becoming fat, (3) a perceptual distortion that one's body is fat despite being obviously underweight.[19] In girls, the disease is invariably accompanied by amenorrhea. The amenorrhea sometimes precedes weight loss. Patients with other medical or neurologic reasons for extreme weight loss do not fear weight gain and do not have the perceptual disorder of anorexia nervosa.

Laboratory evaluation helps to assess the severity of the medical condition of patients with anorexia nervosa. Most patients, although they may appear emaciated and have cool cyanotic extremities, have undergone starvation over a long period of time. They tolerate dramatic physical and biochemical irregularities remarkably well due to adaptation over time. However, severe hypokalemic and alkalosis associated with self-induced vomiting or laxative and diuretic abuse can cause fatal arrhythmias. These patients often have increased serum bicarbonate, hypochloremia, and hypokalemia. Profound hypokalemia is an indication for emergency admission. On admission, an electrocardiogram and chest X-ray are mandatory for further evaluation of the patient's medical status.[20]

Most patients with anorexia nervosa have anemia of chronic illness characterized by a normocytic, hypochromic peripheral blood smear. This may be accompanied by other derangements of hematopoiesis, such as leukopenia and relative lymphocytosis. These abnormalities do not require specific treatment, as weight gain will correct them over time. Many anorexics will have low serum cholesterol, although most anorexic patients will have hypercholesterolemia, possibly secondary to hypothyroidism and/or hypoestrogenism. Carotinemia is also observed in malnourished, anoretic patients and is associated with excessive dietary intake of carrots or other yellow vegetables. Low serum albumin and calcium are other possible manifestations of malnutrition. Abnormal liver enzymes reflect fatty degeneration of the liver and can be observed in the emaciated phase as well as during refeeding.[21]

There are several endocrine manifestations of anorexia nervosa. The amenorrhea, whether primary or secondary, is hypothalamic in nature. It is characterized by very low FSH, LH, and estradiol. These values fall into the prepubertal range, and loss of pulsatility of GnRH and LH has been documented. In boys, testosterone drops dramatically and can be associated with azoospermia. Recovery occurs with weight gain and patients pass through the classic early pubertal phase of nighttime LH release before restoration of normal adult pulsatility. Return to ovulatory cycles often requires weight gain to 10% above the ideal body weight and seems to require relief of psychological stress as well. However, fertility is not impaired in patients who fully recover.

Cortisol and growth hormone may be normal or slightly increased. Abnormal thyroid function tests are characterized by low plasma T_3, increased reverse T_3, and low-normal T_4. No abnormalities in prolactin secretion have been described. The abnormalities in gonadotrophin secretion, thyroid function, and cortisol secretion may suggest the presence of a primary hypothalamic defect. However, the return of normal pituitary function with successful therapy implies these abnormalities are secondary to weight loss.[22]

In adolescents who experience the onset of anorexia nervosa in early puberty, growth failure can occur. An X-ray for bone age is helpful in assessing growth potential. Patients who are chronically malnourished can develop osteoporosis due to hypoestrogenemia.[23] Bone densitometry is performed to assess the need for estrogen replacement therapy. Although it is preferable to allow menstrual cycles to resume spontaneously through nutritional rehabilitation, the development of osteoporosis warrants prompt intervention.

Bulimia nervosa is a disorder characterized by recurrent binge eating and purging. Purging can occur via self-induced vomiting, laxative or diuretic abuse, fasting, or rigorous exercise. These activities are accompanied by persistent overconcern with body shape and weight and a feeling of loss of control over the behavior involved.[24] Patients with isolated bulimia nervosa are not usually malnourished, as are patients with anorexia nervosa.

The biochemical abnormalities associated with vomiting and laxative or diuretic abuse include hypokalemia, increased serum bicarbonate and hypochloremia. With laxative abuse, metabolic acidosis occasionally occurs instead. Fasting which produces dehydration can lead to aldosterone secretion and further renal loss of potassium. Patients who binge and vomit may have increased serum amylase due to parotid gland enlargement. Cardiomyopathy accompanied by increased liver enzymes and erythrocyte sedimentation rate is associated with ipecac intoxication.[25]

Pelvic Masses

Pelvic masses in adolescents may be detected by the patient due to increasing abdominal girth or present with abdominal pain due to adnexal torsion or cyst formation. Pelvic ultrasound and magnetic resonance imaging (MRI) yield the most useful radiologic information identifying the character of pelvic masses. Computed tomography (CT) of the abdomen is traditionally used to assess the upper abdomen and periaortic lymph nodes for ovarian tumor metastasis. Laboratory evaluation of pelvic masses includes a complete blood count with differential and an erythrocyte sedimentation rate (ESR) for patients with suspected tubo-ovarian abscess and an HCG to rule out intrauterine or ectopic pregnancy. Choriocarcinoma, hydatidiform mole, and benign or malignant germ cell tumors of the ovary also elaborate HCG. The endodermal sinus tumor and embryonal cell carcinoma may secrete α-fetoprotein. Struma ovarii, mature thyroid tissue, is sometimes present as a component of benign cystic teratoma and can cause hyperthyroidism. TSH and T_4 should be measured when symptoms are present. CA-125 was the first tumor marker to be defined with a monoclonal antibody against epithelial ovarian cancer. More than 80% of ovarian cancer patients have CA-125 antigen concentrations > 35 units/mL, compared with 1% of normal individuals.[26] CA-125 can be used to follow the progress of therapy in patients with epithelial tumors. However, CA-125 is particularly poor as a screening marker in adolescents because it can be positive in patients with endometriosis or pelvic inflammatory disease, and these entities are much more frequent than ovarian cancer in the adolescent population.

ADOLESCENT PREGNANCY

Adolescent pregnancy is a major health care issue in the United States. The United States has the highest adolescent pregnancy rate of industrialized nations. While some of the major problems relating to adolescent pregnancy are social and educational, a considerable part of our health care costs are in the area of actual clinical care. While the laboratory requirements for the management of adolescent pregnancy are not significantly different from that of adult pregnancy, there are certain areas that require emphasis. The teenager who is pregnant carries with her many of the same pregnancy-related risks as her adult counterpart. Added to these, however, are not infrequently a deprived socioeconomic background leading to disorders of nutrition, as well as being epidemiologically in a group that is at increased risk for acquiring sexually transmitted diseases, having low-birth-weight infants, and developing preeclampsia.

Initial Laboratory Profile

Upon registration in an obstetric care facility, the pregnant teenage patient will find herself being screened in many ways. Part of this initial screening will include a Papanicolaou smear (Pap smear). While cervical cancer is not particularly prevalent in patients in this age, it is becoming increasingly clear that sexually active adolescents are at increased risk for exposure to human papilloma virus. Cytologic screening of the cervix can alert the clinician to the presence of this virus and, where indicated, lead to the performance of colposcopy and a more thorough investigation of cervical histology.

Also, sexually active adolescents not infrequently have more than one sexual partner, or have sexual partners who themselves have more than one sexual partner. This places the adolescent at greater risk for acquiring other sexually transmitted diseases, including syphilis, gonorrhea, Chlamydia, and HIV. A cervical sample can be used to screen for gonorrhea and Chlamydia, while a simple blood test can be used as an initial screen for exposure to syphilis. Screening for these diseases is particularly important, as all of them may be associated with adverse perinatal events. Gonorrhea has clearly been shown to be associated with increased rates of post-delivery infections, and while the significance of Chlamydial infections on pregnancy outcome are controversial,[27] there is no question that exposure to Chlamydia can result in conjunctivitis and pneumonia in the newborn.

The finding of positive syphilis serology is extremely important, as the ramifications of this finding for both mother and infant are significant. There is current controversy as to what the optimal method of screening should be and whether it should include not only first-trimester and third-trimester screening, but intrapartum screening and newborn screening as well. Also, based on recent findings, there is some question as to whether the rapid plasma reagin (RPR) test is sufficient, or whether a fluorescent Treponemal antibody test should become standard in high-risk populations.[28] This issue may not be settled for several years. Our current policy is to screen pregnant women at the time of their first prenatal visit and again in the third trimester. Women who have had no prenatal care are screened on arrival in Labor and Delivery.

Another very important part of prenatal screening now includes determination of HIV antibody status. In our institution, this is done only with the informed consent of the patient, and screening is offered to all individuals in our adolescent clinic. The decision to offer screening to all patients seeking prenatal care is well-founded epidemiologically.[29-32] While there is no cure for HIV infection, there are developing protocols which may serve to reduce mother-to-fetus transmission, thus making screening a worthwhile consideration.

In addition to the above tests, other routine laboratory tests are ordered at the initial visit. A complete blood count is performed, with the most frequent finding being a low hemoglobin and hematocrit, suggestive of iron deficiency anemia. On occasion, this initial screening of hemoglobin and hematocrit has lead to the diagnosis of diseases such as immune thrombocytopenia or leukemia. In patients of African-American, Asian, or Mediterranean descent, special attention should be paid to blood cell morphology and indices, or a hemoglobin electrophoresis should be performed to rule out the possibility of sickle cell disease or thalassemia.

A serum specimen is sent to the blood bank for determination of blood group and Rh type, as well as for screening for atypical antibodies. This information is vitally important for the management of the remainder of the pregnancy. Atypical blood group antibodies have been responsible for repeated miscarriage and hydrops fetalis. Rh negative women must be evaluated very carefully to determine whether or not they will require antepartum administration of Rh immunoglobulin.

Also, at the first visit, immunity status with regard to rubella and occasionally other viral and protozoal illnesses may be determined.

Mid-Trimester Screening

In addition to the routine testing described above, other tests may be offered to women in the middle trimester of their pregnancy. The first of these is offered at approximately 16 w gestation and is the screening test for neural tube defects, namely maternal serum α-fetoprotein. The occurrence of neural tube defects does not seem to be age related, and therefore adolescents will benefit as much from this test as their adult counterparts. A single blood test may be drawn at approximately 16 w of gestation, and a result is generally reported as multiples of the mean (MOM). A result of less than 2.5 MOM, after correction for gestational age, is generally interpreted as normal. AFP concentrations may be lower among diabetics and in very obese individuals, and the laboratory should be able to adjust for these factors in calculating the final MOM result. Results coming back higher than this can be followed up with another serum specimen. If the second specimen is reported as normal, the screening procedure ends. If the second specimen also reveals an increase, then further evaluation using ultrasound and possibly amniocentesis with determination of amniotic fluid α-fetoprotein (AFAFP) may be required (see Figure 13–1.) Amniotic fluid acetylcholinesterase is also measured and is a much more specific test than AFAFP in detecting neural tube defects. Additionally, very low concentrations of α-fetoprotein have been associated with an increased incidence of Down syndrome.

First trimester and mid-trimester cytogenetic testing may also be available for those adolescents who have either a family history or a previous pregnancy history suggesting the need for such testing. Chorionic villus sampling, a procedure done in the first trimester, usually at approximately 10–11 w gestation, will allow for determination of fetal karyotype as well as detection of certain metabolic disorders. This may also be done via amniocentesis at approximately 16–17 w gestation. While it is rare that adolescents require such testing, it does occasionally happen, and the collaboration of Maternal and Fetal Medicine specialists with Laboratory Medicine personnel is crucial.

Third Trimester Screening

In the routine, uncomplicated adolescent pregnancy, certain screening tests are repeated and others added as the patient approaches 28 w gestation. A repeat complete blood count is obtained in order to determine whether or not there has been adequate iron intake during the pregnancy or whether further iron supplementation is necessary. A repeat blood type and atypical antibody screen is sent as well. A follow-up serologic test for syphilis is also an important part of this screening procedure, as is a pelvic examination with culturing once again for the

FIGURE 13–1. Mid-Trimester Maternal Screening

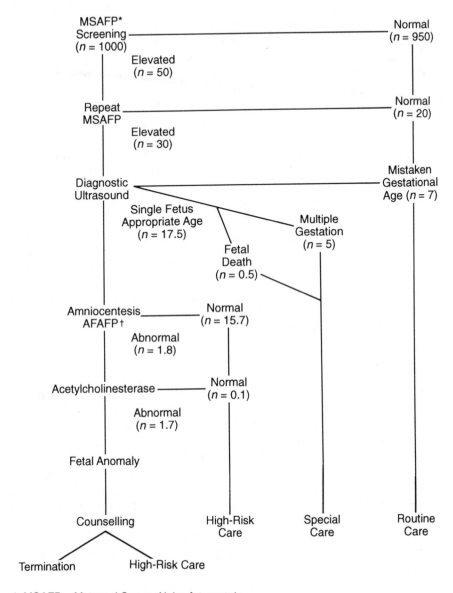

MSAFP* Screening (n = 1000)

Normal (n = 950)

Elevated (n = 50)

Repeat MSAFP

Normal (n = 20)

Elevated (n = 30)

Diagnostic Ultrasound

Mistaken Gestational Age (n = 7)

Single Fetus Appropriate Age (n = 17.5)

Multiple Gestation (n = 5)

Fetal Death (n = 0.5)

Amniocentesis AFAFP†

Normal (n = 15.7)

Abnormal (n = 1.8)

Acetylcholinesterase

Normal (n = 0.1)

Abnormal (n = 1.7)

Fetal Anomaly

Counselling

High-Risk Care

Special Care

Routine Care

Termination

High-Risk Care

* MSAFP = Maternal Serum Alpha-fetoprotein

† AFAFP = Amniotic Fluid Alpha-fetoprotein

presence of gonococcal and/or Chlamydial infection. Not all centers routinely screen for Chlamydia; this depends primarily on the population of patients that they serve and the availability of relatively inexpensive test kits, utilizing either culture (most expensive) or fluorescent antibody slide test kits or enzyme assay kits.

Also at 28 w gestation, all adolescents are screened for gestational diabetes. There is some controversy as to whether this test is necessary as a routine screening test for women under age 25 y,[33] but since the test is relatively easy to do and relatively inexpensive, our clinic has chosen to employ it routinely. Also at this time, a screening test for hepatitis B is performed. While the issue of cost effectiveness of routine hepatitis B screening has not been completely resolved, there is data to suggest that in high-risk populations it is a very worthwhile test.[34] The information gained from such testing can be extremely important with respect to newborn management and the need for hepatitis B immunoglobulin in hepatitis B vaccine administration.

Finally, in the pregnant teenage patient whose pregnancy has remained uncomplicated throughout its term, one final series of tests is performed on arrival in Labor and Delivery. A hemoglobin and hematocrit is obtained once again, as is a blood group and antibody screen. This may be sent to the blood bank of the hospital, where it is held in the event that blood products would be needed during the patient's delivery process.

Pathologic Conditions

The above laboratory utilization applies to the uncomplicated teenage pregnancy. However, as mentioned at the beginning of this section, teenagers are more likely to be at risk for the development of infections and preeclampsia, and are at increased risk for preterm delivery.

Screening for infection can be initiated with the sexually transmitted disease screening described above. However, many adolescents will present in premature labor or with preterm premature rupture of membranes which may or may not be related to sexually transmitted diseases. Under these circumstances, it is very important that the patient be fully evaluated for evidence of intraamniotic infection or infection of other sites. Included would be cervical cultures and cultures of the amniotic fluid, looking specifically for sexually transmitted infections as well as Group B streptococcal infection or colonization. Group B streptococcal colonization is of great importance, since Group B streptococcal sepsis remains the leading cause of neonatal sepsis and death in nurseries within the United States. Culture remains the best test for Group B streptococcal colonization, although more rapid techniques are sorely needed. This is important because early identification of Group B streptococcal colonization in the absence of frank infection can lead to clinical intervention with antibiotics. This may result in prolongation of pregnancy or reduced morbidity from premature delivery. Additional information can be obtained from urinary culture, since urinary tract infections, particularly infections of the upper urinary tract, have been associated with an increased incidence of preterm delivery.

In patients presenting close to term with suggestions of infection, an amniotic fluid sample may also be sent for analysis for fetal lung maturity. This most commonly consists of a request for a lecithin:sphingomyelin ratio and for presence or absence of phosphatidylglycerol. The availability of this test around the clock can significantly aid the clinician in making important decisions regarding delivery.

Premature labor is a clinical condition frequently encountered with teenage pregnancy. Since premature labor frequently can be secondary to infection, once again the utilization of the laboratory to rule out the possibility of infection as quickly and as accurately as possible is crucial to correct clinical decision making. The ability to rapidly determine the chemical evidence for probable fetal lung maturity can also play a crucial role in deciding how aggressively to try and prevent the continuation of uterine activity.

When the above information has been gathered, if a decision has been made to try to inhibit labor, the role of the laboratory will remain important. Betamimetic agents such as ritodrine hydrochloride or terbutaline sulfate are the most commonly employed agents (tocolytics) for the initial prevention of preterm labor. Each of these agents is metabolically active and can result in profound disturbances of electrolyte and chemistry profiles. Betamimetics can raise serum glucose, raise plasma insulin, and lower serum potassium. Magnesium sulfate, another tocolytic, may result in a profound drop in measurable serum calcium, sometimes making it difficult for the clinician to interpret true calcium balance. In this circumstance, availability of ionized calcium measuring techniques can be helpful, although they are rarely necessary.

Preeclampsia, formerly and perhaps more commonly called toxemia of pregnancy, is also a particularly important problem for teenagers. Epidemiologically, we know that younger women having their first child represent a high-risk group for the development of preeclampsia. Preeclampsia is defined as the development of hypertension with proteinuria, edema, or both, usually occurring after the 20th week of gestation. The clinical assessment of the patient with suspected preeclampsia is extremely important. However, also of great importance is the development of the laboratory profile of such a patient. The initial laboratory evaluation of the patient with preeclampsia would include a complete blood count, electrolytes, with specific attention to serum creatine and urea nitrogen, and a chemistry profile with specific attention paid to alanine amino transferase, aspartate aminotransferase, lactic acid dehydrogenase, and uric acid.

Some 24 hr urinary tests may also be helpful in assisting the clinician in making the diagnosis of preeclampsia and determining its severity. Specifically, these would include determination of urinary creatine clearance, total urinary protein per 24 h, and 24 h urinary calcium excretion. Each of these results will help the clinician better determine the nature and severity of the patient's illness. In mild preeclampsia, all of these values may be normal, with the exception of the urinary protein being slightly increased, usually > 300 mg/L/24 h. As disease severity increases, one can expect to see an increase in urinary protein, a decrease in creatine clearance, a rise in serum creatine with a rise in blood urea nitrogen, an increase in uric acid, and an increase in liver function tests. In very severe cases, thrombocytopenia and hypofibrinogenemia can also occur in the clinical setting of disseminated intravascular coagulation (DIC), and more sophisticated tests can be utilized.[35]

To make a correct diagnosis of preeclampsia is extremely important. Next in importance is determining its severity, since this will necessitate further decision making regarding timing of delivery. In the patient with severe preeclampsia, the general rules are for stabilization of the patient and her fetus, followed by attempts at expeditious delivery. Once this decision has been made, most patients are given magnesium sulfate for the purposes of preventing the progression of preeclampsia to eclampsia. Antihypertensive agents may also be required. During this critical period, close laboratory assessment of these patients is essential. This includes careful attention being paid to electrolytes and chemistries, as well as to coagulation factors. In patients receiving magnesium sulfate, serum magnesium concentrations are frequently followed at 6–12 h intervals as an adjunct to clinical assessment of the patient. In general, the patient in this clinical situation will be considered to have therapeutic serum magnesium concentrations at approximately 4–6 mEq/L (2–3 mmol/L).

In some cases, preeclampsia can be accompanied by premature separation of the placenta (abruptio placentae), which is an obstetric emergency. This can cause an acceleration of the disseminated intravascular coagulopathy process, which can result in significant fetal-maternal blood exchange. This can be of extreme importance in mothers who are Rh negative, requiring that a laboratory perform an assessment of the percentage of fetal cells in the maternal circulation so that an appropriate amount of Rh immunoglobulin can be given. In general, 300 µg of Rh immunoglobulin will be sufficient to cover a 30 mL fetal-maternal blood exchange (15 mL fetal red cells).

SUMMARY

The laboratory plays an important supportive role in general adolescent medicine, assisting the clinician in primary health care provision. The role of the laboratory has greatly expanded and, in fact, has become crucial in the management of simple and complicated endocrine disorders of adolescence. The laboratory evaluation of the pregnant patient can be as complicated as the patient herself. The adolescent, because of the high-risk nature of her pregnancy, has benefited from our expanded use of the clinical laboratory. As the clinician's ability to diagnose and manage various conditions improves, there is no doubt that the role of the laboratory as the physician's partner in clinical management will continue to expand.

REFERENCES

1. Marks A, Fisher M. Health assessment and screening during adolescence. Pediatr 1987;80(suppl):135-58.
2. Friedman IM, Goldberg E. Reference materials for the practice of adolescent medicine. Pediatr Clin North Am 1980;27(1):198.
3. Adolescent Medicine 1991;17(no. 12):1-7.
4. Johnston LD, O'Malley PM, Bachman JG. Illicit drug use by American high school seniors in 1989. News and Information Services of the University of Michigan, Feb. 13, 1990.
5. Turner CE, Elsohly MA, Martin DM. Laboratory and psychiatric aspects of drug abuse testing. In: Giannini AJ, Slaby AE, eds., Drugs of abuse. Oradell, New Jersey: Medical Economics Co., 1989.
6. Soldin SJ, Morales AJ, D'Angelo L, Bogema SC, Hicks JM. The importance of lowering the cut-off tests for benzoylecgonine/cocaine. Clin Chem 1991;37:993.
7. Stamm WE, Counts GW, Running KR, Fihn S, Turck M, Holmes KK. Diagnosis of coliform infection in acutely dysuric women. N Engl J Med 1982;307:463-8.
8. Johnson JR, Stamm WE. Diagnosis and treatment of acute urinary tract infections. Infect Dis Clinics N America 1987;773-91.
9. Sumaya CV, Ench Y. Epstein-Barr virus infectious mononucleosis in children: I. Clinical and general laboratory findings. Pediatr 1985;75:1003-10.
10. Sumaya CV, Ench Y. Epstein-Barr virus infectious mononucleosis in children: II. Heterophile antibody and viral-specific responses. Pediatr 1985;1011-9.
11. Centor RM, Meier FA, Dalton HP. Throat culture and rapid tests for diagnosis of group A streptococcal pharyngitis. Ann Int Med 1986;105:892-9.
12. Denny FW. Current problems in managing streptococcal pharyngitis. J Peds 1987;111:797-806.
13. Adger H, Sweet RL, Shafer MA, Schachter J. Screening for *Chlamydia trachomatis* and *Neisseria gonorrhoeae* in adolescent males: Value of first catch urine examination. Lancet 1984;2:944-5.
14. Ferriman D, Gallwey JD. Clinical assessment of body hair growth in women. J Clin Endocrinol Metab 1961;21:1440.
15. Emans SJH, Goldstein DP. Pediatric and adolescent gynecology, 3rd ed. Boston: Little, Brown 1990:258.
16. Rebar RW. Practical evaluation of hormonal studies. In: Jaffe RB, Yen SSC, eds., Reproductive endocrinology, 2nd ed. Philadelphia: W.B. Saunders, 1986:683-733.

17.   Azziz R, Zacur HA. 21-hydroxylase deficiency in female hyperadrogenism: Screening and diagnosis. J Clin Endocrinol Metab 1989;69:577.
18.   Pang S, Lerner A, Stoner E, et al. Late onset adrenal steroid 3-beta hydroxysteroid dehydrogenase deficiency: I. A cause of hirsutism in pubertal and prepubertal women. J Clin Endocrinol Metab 1985;60:428.
19.   DSM III-R. The American Psychiatric Association 1987:63.
20.   Andersen AE. Practical comprehensive treatment of anorexia nervosa and bulimia. Baltimore: Johns Hopkins University Press 1985:67.
21.   Halmi KA, Falk Jr. Common physiological changes in anorexia nervosa. Int J Eating Disorders 1981;1:16-27.
22.   Frohman LA, Krieger DT. Neuroendocrine physiology and disease. In: Felig P, Baxter JD, Broadus AE, Frohman LA, eds., Endocrinology and metabolism, 2nd ed. New York: McGraw-Hill, 1987:234-5.
23.   Brotman AW, Sturn TA. Osteoporosis and pathologic fractures in anorexia nervosa. Am J Psych 1985;142:495.
24.   DSM-III R. The American Psychiatric Association. 1987:63.
25.   Halmi KA, Eating disorders. In: Talbott JA, Hales RE, Yudofsky SC, eds., Textbook of psychiatry. Washington, DC: The American Psychiatric Press 1988:761.
26.   Bast RC Jr, Klug TL, St. John E, et al. A radio immunoassay using a monoclonal antibody to monitor the course of epithelial ovarian cancer. N Engl J Med 1983;309:883.
27.   Investigators of the Johns Hopkins Study of Cervicitis and Adverse Pregnancy Outcomes. Association of *Chlamydia trachomatis* and *Mycoplasma hominis* with intrauterine growth retardation and preterm delivery. Am J Epidemiol 1989;129:1247-57.
28.   Dorfman DH, Glaser JH. Congenital syphilis presenting in infants after the newborn period. N Engl J Med 1990;323:1299-302.
29.   Barbacci M, Dalabetta GA, Repke JT, et al. Human immunodeficiency virus infection in women attending an inter-city prenatal clinic: Ineffectiveness of targeted screening. Sexually Trans Dis 1990;17:122-6.
30.   The Johns Hopkins—Georgetown Working Group on HIV Infection in Pregnant Women and Newborns. A policy proposal for information and testing. JAMA 1990;264:2416-20.
31.   Repke JT, Townsend TR, Coberly JS, et al. Sero prevalance of human immunodeficiency virus type I among pregnant women. Am J Perinatol (in press).
32.   Barbacci M, Repke JT, Chaisson RE. Routine prenatal screening for HIV infection. Lancet 1991;337:709-11.
33.   Marquette GP, Klein VR, Repke JT, Neibyl JR. Cost effective criteria for glucose screening. Obstet Gynecol 1985;66:181-4.
34.   McQuillan GM, Townsend TR, Johannes CB, et al. Prevention of perinatal transmission of hepatitis B virus: The sensitivity, specificity, and predictive value of the recommended screening questions to detect high risk women in an obstetric population. Am J Epidemiol 1987;126:484-91.
35.   Proietti AB, Johnson MJ, Proietti FA, Repke JT, Bell WR. Assessment of fibrin(ogen) degradation products in preeclampsia using immunoblot, ELISA and latex-bead agglutination. Obstet Gynecol 1991;77:696-700.

Lawrence Sweetman, Ph.D.   Julian C. Williams, M.D., Ph.D.

INTRODUCTION

It is estimated that there are 10^5 genes in the human genome, and more than 5000 human genetic diseases have been delineated to date. In only 10% of these has the protein abnormality been identified. Until recently, with the advent of "reverse genetics," the vast majority of those with known protein defects have been characterized initially through analytic techniques on accumulated metabolites and are termed "inborn errors of metabolism." From a knowledge of the accumulated metabolite and biochemical pathways, the enzymatic defect has been subsequently proven. Thus, the identification and characterization process itself tends to select for defects in intermediary metabolism which are enzymatic and usually inherited as autosomal or sex-linked recessive traits. Hereditary abnormalities in structural, receptor, or developmental proteins are much more difficult to characterize at the protein level and are not routinely diagnosed by standard analytic or clinical chemistry techniques.

While 1–2% of all human births are afflicted by chromosomal or single gene disorders, a much smaller percentage are associated with inborn errors of metabolism. The incidence of individual diseases is only estimated, as in most cases true frequencies have not been determined by newborn screening programs or population studies of gene frequency. Thus, as a rule *metabolic diseases are underdiagnosed.* The estimated incidence ranges from about 1:10,000 for phenylketonuria (PKU) and medium-chain acyl-CoA dehydrogenase (MCAD) deficiency to 1:500,000–1:1,000,000 for the rare disorders. Nevertheless, the number of distinct diseases (approximately 600, with approximately 20–30 new diseases reported every year) makes for a rather large aggregate occurrence, especially in large medical centers.

The economic and social impact of these diseases on the health care system is several orders of magnitude larger in countries with well-developed programs for control of infectious disease and perinatal mortality, as patients with inborn errors of metabolism have a disproportionately high frequency of acute hospital admissions and chronic complications such as mental retardation.

Unfortunately, the clinical manifestations of genetic metabolic disease are extremely diverse, and without a high index of suspicion, the correct diagnosis is rarely made on the initial clinical presentation. If the patient is fortunate enough to survive the first illness, the diagnosis may be made upon repeated hospitalizations.

While it is impractical to list all known clinical symptoms of metabolic disease, some generalities can be enumerated:

1. Since inborn errors of metabolism are rare, the common diseases should be ruled out first. However, if the routine diagnostic tests are normal, the patients' symptoms not entirely congruent with the suspected diagnosis, or the response to treatment inappropriate, the possibility of inherited metabolic disease should be considered.

2. Mental retardation without a known history of perinatal morbidity, meningitis, or trauma is suspicious, and progressive retardation is due to metabolic errors until proven otherwise.

3. Failure to thrive, if not attributable to psychosocial deprivation, hormonal disturbances, or gastroenterologic/renal disease may be a manifestation of metabolic disorders.

4. Many of the hereditary enzyme deficiencies involve catabolic enzymes and, as detailed below, the normal catabolic response to infection/fasting will result in an exaggerated physiologic response. An inappropriately severe response to minor infection/fasting or failure to respond to appropriate treatment should be suspect, especially if associated with chemical abnormalities such as hypoglycemia, hyperammonemia, excessive ketoacidosis/lactic acidosis, or deficient ketosis.

5. Hepatosplenomegaly, multi-focal bone abnormalities, myopathy and/or muscle weakness, and hepatic dysfunction may be manifestations of genetic/metabolic disease.

Unfortunately, few of the inborn errors of metabolism can be diagnosed by routine clinical chemistry tests, although abnormalities, particularly in urinalysis or electrolyte balance, may suggest the need for further specific tests. Microscopic examination of tissue biopsies may be more helpful for some disorders, but again are not generally diagnostic. Specific diagnosis is dependent on two processes:

1. The use of sophisticated analytic techniques such as high-performance liquid chromatography (HPLC), gas chromatography (GC), or gas chromatography/mass spectrometry (GCMS) for the identification of abnormal metabolites.

2. The specific assay of enzyme activity in tissue samples, or occasionally, body fluids.

These two processes are, with the exception of amino acid analysis by high pressure ion exchange chromatography, not generally available in most hospitals, medical centers, or commercial laboratories. Diagnosis is dependent on the acumen of the clinician and the clinical pathologist or laboratory scientist and the referral of samples to the appropriate specialized laboratory. An essential requisite for diagnosis is the collection of appropriate samples with the recognition that the greatest accumulation of abnormal metabolites occurs at the height of catabolism, i.e., upon presentation and before the administration of intravenous glucose. Thus, blood and urine specimens should be collected and stored upon presentation, or as soon as possible thereafter, for future analysis.

The recent advent of molecular genetic techniques has altered this diagnostic schema for some diseases. For those disorders whose causative gene has been cloned or restriction fragment length polymorphisms (RFLPs) have been identified, molecular diagnosis may be utilized based on symptom recognition or the identification of abnormal metabolites in physiologic fluids. Although currently these tests are performed only generally in research laboratories, they soon will be generally available and are amenable to newborn screening programs.

Genetic metabolic diseases can be crudely categorized into those with chronic, slowly progressive manifestations and those with acute, life-threatening symptoms. Although the correspondence is imperfect, they also can be similarly divided into those diseases with the accumulation of large molecules which are endogenously synthesized (chronic diseases) and small molecules (acute diseases), many of which are derived from dietary components.

The catabolic effects of fasting/infection will increase the degradation of small molecules and the flux of their breakdown products. This is pronounced for those molecules (protein, triglycerides, and glycogen) which are the storage forms of the metabolic fuels (amino acids, fatty acids, and glucose, respectively) necessary for energy production.

Those disorders which are due to a deficiency of an enzyme in the catabolic pathway of one of these small molecules will then manifest a sudden increase in the accumulation of toxic intermediates and, consequently, acute symptoms.

Treatment of those chronic, slowly progressive disorders which are due to the accumulation of large molecules is primarily symptomatic and supportive, without alteration of the inevitable, downhill course. Catabolic defects in the degradative pathways of small molecules are more amenable to therapeutic intervention. If the offending molecule is "essential," i. e., derived from the diet and not endogenously synthesized, dietary restriction of intake may be effective. Acute crises may be treated by dialysis of the accumulated, toxic small molecules. Catabolic increases of the flux of these small molecules resulting in accumulation of toxic metabolites may be suppressed by supplying exogenous fuel such as intravenous glucose. In some cases, such as the organic acidemias and urea cycle defects, endogenous detoxification mechanisms can be augmented by supplying exogenous glycine, carnitine, or benzoate.

LYSOSOMAL STORAGE DISEASES

The lysosomal storage diseases are due to genetic deficiencies of the hydrolases of the lysosome which normally degrade the complex macromolecules of the cell. Many of these macromolecules are glycoprotein and glycolipid components of cell membranes.

The majority of lysosomal enzyme deficiencies involve exoglycosidic hydrolases which cleave a terminal carbohydrate residue. Failure to remove a terminal carbohydrate results in a block in degradation of the entire macromolecule and its accumulation within the lysosome. The resulting lysosomal hypertrophy presumably inhibits other lysosomal degradative processes, distorts intracellular structure and, upon lysis, results in cell death.

The majority of these diseases can be categorized into three groups, named for the stored materials: the mucopolysaccharidoses, glycolipidoses, and glycoproteinoses.[1-3] All of these disorders have slowly progressive symptoms; are inherited as autosomal recessive traits, with a few exceptions; and often can be prenatally diagnosed by enzyme assay. The incidence of these disorders averages about 1:100,000. They can occur in all ethnic groups, and some occur in very high incidence in specific groups, such as Gaucher and Tay-Sachs disease in Ashkenazi Jews. Tentative diagnosis is established by clinical symptoms and analysis of stored materials in urine and tissues. Diagnostic confirmation is by hexoseaminidase A assay in fibroblasts, leukocytes, tissues, or, occasionally, body fluids.

The mucopolysaccharide storage diseases are due to the accumulation of mucopolysaccharides (MPS) which are polymers of monosaccharides containing sulfate, amino, and carboxyl groups.[4] These macromolecules are predominantly synthesized in connective tissues and accumulation in these sites accounts for the symptoms of coarse facial features, dysostosis multiplex, and restriction of joint motion. Storage in other tissues accounts for hepatosplenomegaly, corneal clouding, and/or mental retardation. Table 14–1 lists the disorders, inheritance pattern, and symptoms, as well as the specific enzyme deficiency and accumulated metabolite.

In association with the correct symptoms, a tentative diagnosis can be assigned upon demonstration of MPS accumulation, usually in urine. An acid turbidity test or an MPS spot test with toluidine blue will indicate an increased MPS concentration. Thin-layer chromatography or electrophoresis (see Figure 14–1A) will allow identification of the MPS species and selection of the appropriate enzyme assay for specific diagnosis.

The glycolipidoses present with more diverse symptoms.[5] In general, bone/joint abnormalities and corneal clouding do not occur. Organomegaly is present in some, but not all, disorders. Mental retardation and/or focal neurologic deficits are frequently, but not universally, present. Table 14–2 lists these disorders with their respective symptoms, stored material, and enzymatic deficiency. Although methods exist for analysis of the accumulated glycolipid in tissues, these techniques are not readily available and frequently lack sufficient sensitivity to be easily applied to the analysis of blood and urine. Thus, specific diagnosis is dependent on enzymatic assay of leukocytes, fibroblasts, tissues, or, in some cases, plasma/serum.

The glycoproteinoses are due to a deficiency of a glycosidase or aminohydrolase necessary for the degradation of the oligosaccharide chains of glycoproteins. The clinical symptoms overlap those of the MPS storage disorders and the glycolipidoses. Presumptive diagnosis is based on analysis of the accumulated oligosaccharides in urine by thin layer-chromatography (see Figure 14–1B) or HPLC with confirmation by enzyme assay (Table 14–2).

PEROXISOMAL DISORDERS

Peroxisomal disorders can be grouped as in Table 14–3 according to whether there are greatly diminished number or absence of peroxisomes with multiple enzyme defects, as in group 1; normal peroxisomes with single enzyme deficiencies, as in group 2; and abnormal peroxisomes with more than one enzyme defect, as in group 3.[6] The disorders and their biochemical abnormalities are listed in Table 14–3. More detailed descriptions of representative disorders from groups 1 and 2 follow.

TABLE 14–1. Mucopolysaccharidoses (MPS)

Disorder	Urine Excretion of Mucopolysaccharides	Primary Enzyme Deficiency	Clinical Features
Hurler syndrome (MPS-I)	Dermatan sulfate Heparan sulfate	α-L-iduronidase	Excessive growth in infancy followed by severe dwarfing thereafter, hernias, hepatosplenomegaly, progressive clouding of cornea, limitation of joint mobility, deterioration of mental function and coarseness of facial features, rhinorrhea, hydrocephalus, deafness, cardiac murmurs. Death usually occurs in the first decade of cardiorespiratory causes.
Scheie syndrome (MPS I-S)			Progressive clouding of cornea and joint limitation, aortic insufficiency, normal intelligence, normal stature.
Hurler-Scheie Compound (MPS I-H/I-S)			Features intermediate between Hurler and Scheie syndromes.
Hunter Syndrome (MPS II) Severe	Dermatan sulfate Heparan sulfate	Iduronide sulfatase	Dwarfing, deafness, retinal degeneration, hepatosplenomegaly, hernias, progressive limitation of joint mobility and deterioration of mental function, cardiac murmurs, clear cornea, cutaneous nodules. Death usually occurs in the second decade.
Mild			Same general features as severe Hunter syndrome, but mental deterioration much slower. Survival well into adult life.
Sanfilippo syndrome A (MPS III-A) B (MPS III-B) C (MPS III-C) D (MPS III-D)	Heparan sulfate	Heparan N-sulfatase N-acetyl-α-D-glucosaminidase Acetyl CoA:α-glucosaminide-N-acetyl-transferase N-acetyl-α-D-glucosaminide-6-sulfatase	Clear cornea, severe deterioration of mental function prior to school age, minimal organomegaly and shortening of stature. No differences in clinical features between the various types.

TABLE 14–1 Continued

Morquio syndrome (MPS IV) Morquio A	Keratan sulfate	N-acetylgalactosaminide-6-sulfatase	Severe dwarfing, pectus carinatum, kyphoscoliosis, genu valgum (prominent joints, some of which may be lax), mild corneal clouding, normal intelligence. May have cervical cord compression because of cervical spine dislocation, thin enamel.
Morquio B		ß-galactosidase	Similar to Morquio A syndrome, but dysostosis multiplex is milder and enamel is normal.
Maroteaux-Lamy syndrome (MPS VI) Severe	Dermatan sulfate	Arylsulfatase B (N-acetyl-galactosaminide-4-sulfatase)	Normal or excessive growth during infancy followed by severe dwarfing, limitation of joint mobility, corneal clouding, coarsening of facies, hepatosplenomegaly, hernias, cardiac murmurs, deafness, normal intelligence.
Mild			Skeletal features and growth retardation less prominent than in severe Maroteaux-Lamy syndrome.
ß-Glucuronidase	Dermatan sulfate Heparan sulfate	ß-glucuronidase	Variable features including coarse facies, hepatosplenomegaly, hernias, corneal clouding, dysostosis multiplex and mental retardation.

Modified from Williams & Howell[4] with permission.

FIGURE 14–1A. Electrophoresis of Urinary Mucopolysaccharides (performed according to Wessler[17])

Lanes 1 and 5: Standards, top to bottom, heparan sulfate, dermatan sulfate, and chondroitin sulfate. **Lane 2:** Normal urine. **Lane 2':** Normal urine with added dermatan sulfate. **Lane 3:** Urine from Sanfilippo with high heparan sulfate. **Lane 3':** Same urine with added dermatan sulfate. **Lane 4:** Urine from Morquio with high keratan sulfate. **Lane 4':** Same urine with added dermatan sulfate.

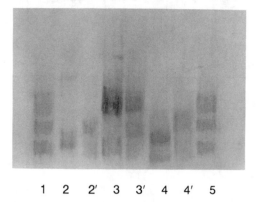

1   2   2'   3   3'   4   4'   5

FIGURE 14–1B. Thin-layer Chromatography of Urinary Oligosaccharides (performed according to Humbel & Colart[18])

Lane 1: GM1 gangliosidosis   **Lane 2:** Glycogen storage disease type III   **Lane 3:** Mucolipidosis type III
Lane 4: Fucosidosis   **Lane 5:** Mannosidosis

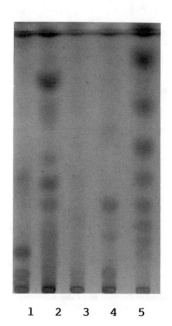

1   2   3   4   5

TABLE 14-2. Glycolipidoses and Glycoproteinoses

Disorder	Characteristic Clinical Features	Enzyme Deficiency	Enzyme Diagnosis in:	Confirmatory Tests
G_{M2}-gangliosidoses	Dementia, myoclonic seizures, blindness, and macular cherry-red spots predominate in early-onset forms; cerebellar ataxia and spinal muscular atrophy predominate in late-onset forms. Ashkenazi Jewish predilection (alpha-locus forms).	Hexosaminidase a. Alpha-locus disorders: Hexosaminidases A (and S) (Tay-Sachs disease and variants). b. Beta-locus disorders: Hexosaminidase A and B (Sandhoff disease and variants). c. Activator-locus disorders: Hexosaminidase A activator (AB-variant).	a. Serum, leukocytes, cultured skin fibroblasts, urine. b. Serum, leukocytes, cultured, skin fibroblasts, urine. c. Cultured skin fibroblasts.	Membranous cytoplasmic bodies in rectal ganglion cells (all types). Excessive urinary oligosaccharides in beta-locus disorders.
G_{M1}-gangliosidoses	Infantile form gives encephalopathy, hepatosplenomegaly, bone and joint involvement, often cherry-red spots; in a late-infantile form, encephalopathy predominates; in later onset form (Morquio type B), skeletal involvement predominates.	G_{M1}-ganglioside beta-galactosidase.	Leukocytes, cultured skin fibroblasts.	Excess urinary oligosaccharides in characteristic pattern.
Fabry disease	Purple 1- to 3-mm macular-maculopapular skin lesions, painful neuropathy, renal disease; X-linked (incompletely) recessive inheritance; vascular involvement may occur (lymphedema, stroke).	α-galactosidase A	Plasma or serum, leukocytes, cultured skin fibroblasts.	Characteristic histologic and histochemical appearance of biopsied skin lesions.

TABLE 14-2 Continued

Disease	Clinical features	Enzyme / biochemical defect	Diagnostic tissue source	Pathology
Gaucher disease	Infantile form: severe hepatosplenomegaly and severe encephalopathy; juvenile form: milder nervous system involvement, variable splenomegaly; "adult" form (may begin in childhood): splenomegaly (thrombocytopenia), bone involvement, nervous system unaffected, Ashkenazi Jewish predilection.	Cerebroside beta-glucosidase (glucocerebrosidase)	Cultured skin fibroblasts, leukocytes.	Characteristic foam cells in bone marrow.
Niemann-Pick disease	Type A: severe infantile hepatosplenomegaly and severe encephalopathy, often cherry red spots, Ashkenazi Jewish predilection; Type B: hepatosplenomegaly in childhood without encephalopathy; Type C: Childhood encephalopathy with variable organ enlargement; Type D: infantile hepatosplenomegaly in Nova Scotia Acadians.	a. Sphingomyelinase (Deficient in types A, B; often partially deficient in "type C"). b. Abnormal cholesterol esterification in type C.	a. Cultured skin fibroblasts, leukocytes (Types A, B). b. Cultured skin fibroblasts.	Characteristic foam cells in bone marrow (all types). Types C and D: Characteristic membranous bodies by electron microscopy in rectal, skin, or conjunctival biopsy. Types C, D: Elevated sphingomyelin in liver biopsy.
Metachromatic leukodystrophy	Late infantile form: dementia, spasticity, optic atrophy, neuropathy.; juvenile forms: similar but later onset; adult form: dementia predominates; multiple sulfatase deficiency: infantile neurologic deterioration with seizures, ichthyosis, and mucopolysaccharidosis-like face and bone changes.	a. Arylsulfatase A (sulfatide sulfatase) (late-infantile, juvenile, and adult forms). b. Arylsulfatase A activator (usually resembles juvenile form clinically). c. Arylsulfatase A and at least ten other sulfatases (multiple sulfatase deficiency).	a. Serum, leukocytes, cultured skin fibroblasts, urine. b. Cultured skin fibroblasts. c. Cultured skin fibroblasts.	Metachromatic cells and demyelination by light microscopy, tuffstone bodies by electron microscopy in myelinated nerve from skin or sural nerve biopsy.
Krabbe leukodystrophy	Infantile encephalopathy, seizures, optic atrophy, neuropathy; rare later-onset forms.	Cerebroside beta-galactosidase (galactocerebrosidase).	Serum, leukocytes, cultured skin fibroblasts.	Demyelination and needle-like inclusions by electron microscopy on nerve biopsy.

TABLE 14-2 Continued

Farber disease	Early infantile painful arthropathy; subcutaneous nodules near joints, tendon sheaths, and pressure points; hoarseness; often hepatomegaly.	Acid ceramidase	Cultured skin fibroblasts, leukocytes.	Characteristic light and electron microscopic picture of biopsied skin lesions.
Fucosidosis	Infantile form: retardation, spasticity, seizures, coarse facies, hepatosplenomegaly, cardiomegaly, dysostosis multiplex, clear cornea. Juvenile form: retardation, coarse facies, dysostosis multiplex, minimal hepatosplenomegaly, angiokeratoma.	α-fucosidase	Plasma or serum, leukocytes, cultural skin fibroblasts.	Excess urinary oligosaccharides in characteristic pattern.
Mannosidosis α form	Mild and severe forms with earlier onset in the latter. Slightly coarse facies, hepatosplenomegaly, dysostosis multiplex, cataracts, hernias, progressive retardation.	α-mannosidase	Plasma or serum, leukocytes, cultured skin fibroblasts	Excess urinary oligosaccharides in characteristic pattern.
β form	Mental retardation with delayed speech, scrotal angiokeratoma, mildly coarse facies, mild dysostosis multiplex. Few patients known and physical findings vary.	β-mannosidase	Plasma or serum, leukocytes, cultured skin fibroblasts	Excess urinary excretion of a disaccharide in humans.

TABLE 14-2 Continued

Aspartylglycosaminuria	Early onset infections and diarrhea with childhood manifestation of speech delay and progressive retardation, cardiac murmurs, macroglossia, cataracts, hypotonia, loose joints and dysostosis multiplex.	Aspartylglycosaminidase	Plasma or serum, leukocytes, cultured skin fibroblasts.	Excess urinary aspartylglucosamine and complex glycopeptides.
Schindler disease	Mental retardation, progressive neurodegeneration with cortical blindness and myoclonic seizures.	α-galactosidase B (α-galactosaminidase)	Plasma or serum, leukocytes, cultured skin fibroblasts.	Excess urinary excretion of O-linked oligosaccharides.
Sialidosis				
Type I	Macular cherry red spot, punctate lens apacities, decreasing visual acuity, myoclonic seizures, ataxia, mild retardation, juvenile onset.	Neuraminidase	Plasma or serum, leukocytes, cultured skin fibroblasts.	Excess urinary excretion of oligosaccharides in characteristic pattern.
Type II	Earlier onset, coarse facies, increased head circumference, short stature, cataracts, corneal clouding, hepatosplenomegaly, hernias, dysostosis multiplex, moderate retardation.			
I-Cell disease				
Mucolipidosis II	Early onset of coarse facies, dysostosis multiplex, hernias, hepatosplenomegaly, clear corneas, cardiac murmurs, and progressive mental retardation. A later onset form with milder symptoms is termed mucolipidosis III or pseudo-Hurler polydystrophy.	UDP-N-acetylglucosamine: glycoprotein N-acetylglucosaminylphosphotransferase.	Leukocytes and cultured skin fibroblasts	Increased plasma and urine lysosomal enzyme activities with a concomitant decrease in fibroblast lysosomal enzymes. Increased urinary oligosaccharides in a characteristic pattern.

Modified from Johnson[5] with permission.

TABLE 14–3. Peroxisomal Disorders

Group 1:	Multiple enzyme defects with reduced numbers of peroxisomes
	Zellweger cerebrohepatorenal syndrome Neonatal adrenoleukodystrophy Infantile Refsum disease
Group 2:	Single enzyme defects with normal peroxisomes
	X-linked adrenoleukodystrophy: VLCFA acyl-CoA synthase deficiency with increased VLCFA
	Acatalasemia: Catalase deficiency
	Hyperoxaluria type I: Glyoxylate alanine aminotransferase deficiency with increased oxalic, glycolic, and glyoxylic acids
	3-Oxoacyl-CoA thiolase deficiency (Pseudo-Zellweger syndrome) Acyl-CoA oxidase deficiency Bifunctional enzyme deficiency
	Refsum disease: Phytanic acid alpha-hydroxylase deficiency with increased phytanic acid.
Group 3:	More than one enzyme defect with abnormal peroxisomes Rhizomelic chondrodysplasia punctata Zellweger-like syndrome

X-linked Adrenoleukodystrophy

This is an example of a group 2 single deficiency of very-long-chain fatty acid (VLCFA) acyl-CoA synthase in peroxisomes which are normal in structure and number. This enzyme is required for the catabolism of the VLCFA—i. e., straight-chain C24:0, C25:0, and C26:0 fatty acids—which occurs mainly in peroxisomes, and its deficiency results in increased VLCFA in plasma lipids.[6] The severe childhood form results in progressive demyelination and neurological deficit with adrenal insufficiency. The adult form presents with adrenal insufficiency and slowly progressive paraparesis. Although adrenal hormone replacement can correct the adrenal insufficiency, the neurological manifestations are not yet treatable, although some beneficial response has been seen with a diet low in fatty acids and supplemented with glycerol trioleate and trierucate. As an X-linked disorder, only males are affected. About 85% of female heterozygotes can be diagnosed by increased VLCFA.

Zellweger Syndrome

This is an example of a group 1 disorder in which peroxisomes are absent or greatly reduced in number, which results in multiple enzyme deficiency.[7] This is due to a number of different defects in the biogenesis of peroxisomes.

The classical Zellweger cerebrohepatorenal syndrome reflects the multiorganic effects of a deficiency of peroxisomes. Symptoms include dysmorphic features, severe muscular hypotonia, mental retardation, impaired liver function, eye abnormalities, renal cysts, and chondrodysplasia resulting in early death. The biochemical abnormalities include a combination of many of the abnormalities of the single enzyme defects. Among these are increased VLCFA in plasma lipids, decreased plasmalogen synthesis and concentrations in tissues, increased phytanic acid, increased intermediates of bile acid synthesis, and increased pipecolic acid.

Rhizomelic Chondrodysplasia Punctata

This is representative of group 3 disorders with peroxisomes present but with abnormal structures and more than one enzyme deficient. Plasmalogen synthesis is decreased and phytanic acid oxidation is impaired. The oxidation of VLCFA is normal.

CARBOHYDRATE DISORDERS

Numerous disorders affecting carbohydrate metabolism have been identified, including transport defects such as pentosuria and glucose-galactose malabsorption, the intestinal disaccharidase deficiencies of sucrase-isomaltase and lactase, erythrocyte abnormalities of anaerobic glycolysis, enzyme deficiencies resulting in the accumulation of toxic monosaccharide phosphates, disorders of glucose homeostasis, and those resulting in lactate accumulation.[8] Many are quite rare. The relatively more common diseases resulting in significant morbidity/mortality are described below.

The nervous system has obligate requirements for glucose and elaborate hormonal and enzymatic mechanisms have evolved for glucose homeostasis with fasting. Glucose is stored as glycogen for release when glucose concentrations diminish from the post-absorptive phase and, under most conditions, enough glycogen is available for 24 hours. Maintenance of glucose concentrations is then dependent on gluconeogenic synthesis from amino acids, lactate, and glycerol. Enzymatic deficiencies of glycogen synthesis and degradation and of gluconeogenesis may result in hypoglycemia with its associated effects. These disorders are inherited as autosomal recessive traits in general and occur with an approximate incidence of 1:100,000 in all ethnic groups, excepting certain inbred populations. Besides the obvious effects of hypoglycemia on the brain, symptomatology of the glycogen storage diseases (GSD) is directly manifested in liver, muscle, or both. Van Gierke disease (GSD I) is due to the hepatic deficiency of glucose-6-

phosphatase, an enzyme necessary for the release of free glucose as the ultimate step in glycogen degradation. Symptoms include hepatomegaly, hypotonia, growth failure, platelet dysfunction resulting in epistaxis and easy bruising, and the neurologic effects of hypoglycemia. Metabolic abnormalities also include lactic acidosis, hypercholesterolemia, hypertriglyceridemia, and hyperuricemia. Untreated, hepatic adenomas are common, with progression to carcinoma frequently occurring in older patients. Diagnosis requires assay of glucose-6-phosphatase and/or its required transport proteins in liver tissue. Treatment is fairly simple and effective by avoiding fasting with frequent feedings, nocturnal nasogastric drip of carbohydrate or enteral formulas, and/or supplementation with complex carbohydrates such as starch. With treatment, the majority of symptoms and secondary metabolic abnormalities normalize or significantly improve. Debrancher enzyme deficiency (GSD III) has similar but less severe symptoms, i.e., hepatomegaly, fasting hypoglycemia, and hypertriglyceridemia. Lactic acidosis and hyperuricemia do not occur, and the hypoglycemia appears only after longer fasting than in GSD I. Presumably, this is due to the availability of glucose released by phosphorylase from the termini of the glycogen molecule before it reaches a branch point.

Many patients with debrancher deficiency also have muscle weakness with hypotonia and develop a chronic progressive myopathy in the later decades of life. Enzymatic diagnosis of this disorder can be accomplished in leukocytes, fibroblasts, and muscle and liver tissue. Hepatic phosphorylase deficiency (GSD VI) and the deficiency of its activator enzyme, hepatic phosphorylase B kinase, have minimal symptomatology, with hepatomegaly being constant. Usually no treatment is necessary except for frequent feedings in those few patients with mild hypoglycemia in childhood. The rarest of the hepatic glycogenosis is brancher deficiency (GSD IV), with an incidence of about 1:500,000. Rather than hepatomegaly and hypoglycemia, the major symptom is progressive hepatic cirrhosis, resulting in failure to thrive and death at an early age. Enzyme deficiency can be confirmed in multiple tissues and the only available treatment is liver transplantation. Post-transplant, enzyme deficiency in non-hepatic organs such as skeletal and cardiac tissue continues and may result in myopathy with time.

Although muscle symptoms are minor manifestations of the aforementioned glycogen storage diseases, a major muscle glycogenesis is McArdle disease (GSD V), or muscle phosphorylase deficiency. Patients are usually asymptomatic until puberty for unknown reasons, and then present with severe muscle cramps and myoglobinuria with strenuous exercise. Myoglobinuria may results in renal failure. Avoidance of strenuous exercise is the major treatment modality, although fructose and a diet high in protein have been suggested to be of benefit. In the fourth and fifth decades of life, a chronic progressive myopathy may occur.

Diagnosis is by the absence of lactate production in a forearm ischemic exercise test, abnormal muscle histology, or enzyme assay. Phosphofructokinase deficiency, a very rare disorder, has similar findings, with the added component of a mild hemolytic anemia. Pompe disease (GSD II), also known as α-glucosidase or acid maltase deficiency, differs from the other glycogenesis in that it is due to a defective lysosomal rather than a cytosolic enzyme. As such, symptoms are not related to a deficiency of glucose in affected tissues but to the progressive accumulation of glycogen inside lysosomes. Patients present with severe hypotonia and cardiomegaly in the first year of life and succumb to cardiac failure by age two. Milder variants may not manifest until adulthood, with a progressive skeletal myopathy.

Other disorders of glucose homeostasis are those affecting the gluconeogenic process. Deficiency of pyruvate carboxylase, which converts pyruvate to oxaloacetate as the first step in pyruvate's transformation to glucose, results in hepatomegaly and the neurologic sequelae of recurrent hypoglycemia, i. e., psychomotor retardation, seizures, and hypotonia. Metabolic abnormalities include increased pyruvate, lactate, alanine, and ketone bodies. Continuous provision of glucose corrects the metabolic abnormalities, as does the accepted treatment of avoiding fasting. Fructose-1, 6-diphosphatase deficiency has similar symptoms, abnormal laboratory findings, and treatment. The diseases can be separated by assay of the respective enzymes in liver, kidney, or intestinal tissue or, in the case of pyruvate carboxylase, also in fibroblasts and leukocytes.

Another mechanism of toxicity in defects of carbohydrate metabolism is the accumulation of monosaccharide phosphates. In hereditary fructose intolerance due to a deficiency of fructose-1-phosphate aldolase, ingestion of fructose results in emesis, hypoglycemia, seizures, coma, disseminated intravascular coagulation, and acute hypotension. Chronic symptoms include failure to thrive, hypotonia, hepatomegaly and cirrhosis, and a renal Fanconi syndrome. Strict avoidance of fructose corrects all abnormalities with an excellent prognosis. Although this disorder is very rare, accumulation of galactose-1-phosphate in galactosemia is more common, with an incidence of about 1:50,000. Unlike hereditary fructose intolerance, for which the defective enzyme must be measured in liver or intestinal tissue, in galactosemia the pertinent enzyme, galactose-1-phosphate uridyltransferase, can be measured in all tissues, including erythrocytes. Thus, it is amenable to newborn screening programs by direct assay or by measuring the accumulated metabolites galactose-1-phosphate, galactose, and galactitol. The symptoms are those of severe hepatic dysfunction, failure to thrive, renal Fanconi syndrome, susceptibility to *E. coli* sepsis, mental retardation, and cataracts. Treatment depends on elimination of galactose from the diet, predominantly in the form of lactose derived from milk products. With treatment from the neonatal period, outcome is good, although intelligence is minimally decreased and females have varying degrees of ovarian failure.

Unlike the previously discussed inborn errors of metabolism with secondary accumulation of lactic acid and pyruvate associated with low plasma glucose concentrations, the primary disorders of lactate and pyruvate accumulation have significant neuromuscular pathology not due to hypoglycemia.[9] Pyruvate dehydrogenase converts pyruvate to acetyl-CoA and is the entry point of glycolysis to the tricarboxylic acid cycle. Its deficiency causes pyruvate accumulation and the concomitant increase of lactate.

Complete deficiency results in early-onset psychomotor retardation, hypotonia with hyperreflexia, poor coordination, and optic atrophy. Partial deficiency may be manifested in childhood with intermittent ataxia, encephalopathy, and mild chronic motor dysfunction. Enzyme deficiency can be determined in multiple tissues. Unfortunately, there is no treatment with significant efficacy.

Another major group of diseases resulting in lactic acidosis are the mitochondrial myopathies due to defects in the respiratory chain enzymes. Symptoms are extremely diverse and include abnormalities of muscle and brain function, short stature, cardiomyopathy, renal tubular dysfunction, endocrinopathy, and hepatic dysfunction. Various syndromes such as Leigh, Kearns-Sayre, myoclonic epilepsy with ragged red fibers, mitochondrial encephalomyelopathy, lactic acidosis, stroke, and Leber hereditary optic atrophy are part of this group. Some disorders have Mendelian inheritance, but as some of the mitochondrial proteins are encoded by mitochondrial genes, some have a maternal inheritance pattern. Diagnosis of these diseases may be aided by the dyad of lactic acidosis and neuromuscular dysfunction and confirmed by abnormal muscle histology, mitochondrial electron microscopy, enzyme assay, and mitochondrial DNA structure. There is no known treatment which significantly alters symptoms or prognosis, although a low-carbohydrate diet is frequently advocated.

AMINO ACID DISORDERS

These are defined as those inherited metabolic disorders with an abnormal concentration of one or more amino acids in physiologic fluids caused by either a deficiency of an enzyme or a defect in renal transport. A deficiency of an enzyme generally results in increases of an amino acid in plasma, urine, and/or cerebrospinal fluid.

Analysis of amino acids in plasma is more diagnostic than analysis of urine because the reference range of amino acid concentrations in plasma is relatively narrow and increases or decreases are readily quantified. Reference ranges of amino acid concentrations in urine are much wider, and since generalized amino acidurias are frequent in sick children, it is difficult to reliably detect specific increases of amino acids. A defect in renal transport results in excretion of increased amounts of amino acids in urine, while plasma amino acid concentrations are generally normal. For these disorders, analysis of urine is more informative than plasma. Analysis of amino acids in physiological fluids is most commonly done by cation exchange chromatography with post-column ninhydrin colorimetric detection.[10] Reference ranges for amino acids are age-dependent and have been extensively tabulated elsewhere.[11]

Table 14–4 summarizes the abnormal concentrations of amino acids in plasma and/or urine that are diagnostic for a large number of amino acid disorders. The differential diagnosis frequently depends on a pattern of amino acid increases and/or decreases rather than on the concentration of a single amino acid. In addition to abnormal concentrations of amino acids, many of the disorders have abnormal excretions of organic acids derived from the amino acids, providing a complementary method of diagnosis (see Table 14–5). Six of the more important amino acid disorders in Table 14–4 are discussed in more detail below.

PKU and Hyperphenylalaninemia

The best known disorder of amino acid metabolism is classical PKU (phenylketonuria), with an incidence of about 1:10,000 in Caucasian newborns; it is very rare in black infants. PKU is due to a deficiency of phenylalanine hydroxylase, a liver-specific enzyme which converts phenylalanine to tyrosine. Phenylalanine is increased in plasma (> 1,200 umol/L). Untreated PKU results in severe mental retardation.

With newborn screening and prompt treatment with a phenylalanine-restricted diet continuing lifelong, mental development is grossly normal although specific defects in spatial perceptual relationships and mathematic ability are found. Phenylalanine in plasma is routinely measured to monitor treatment. High concentrations of phenylalanine in maternal PKU cause severe fetal damage and therefore dietary treatment should be continued during pregnancy.

Hyperphenylalaninemia with modest increases of phenylalanine without phenylketonuria occurs with less severe deficiency of phenylalanine hydroxylase and generally may not require rigid dietary treatment. Approximately 1–2% of hyperphenylalaninemia is caused by defects in the synthesis or metabolism of tetrahydrobiopterin, a cofactor for phenylalanine hydroxylase. The diagnosis requires analysis of urinary pteridines.

TABLE 14–4. Amino Acid Disorders: Pathological Levels of Amino Acids

Disorder	Amino Acid	Abnormal Levels*	
		Plasma	Urine
DISORDERS OF AROMATIC AMINO ACID METABOLISM			
Hyperphenylalaninemia			
Phenylketonuria (PKU): Phenylalanine			
Hydroxylase Deficiency	Phenylalanine	inc	inc
Biopterin Disorders	Phenylalanine	inc	inc
Tyrosinemia			
Transient Neonatal	Tyrosine	inc	inc
Hepatorenal (Type I)	Tyrosine	inc	inc
	Methionine	inc	
	Other amino acids		inc
Oculocutaneous (Type II)	Tyrosine	inc	inc
Nonspecific Liver Damage	Tyrosine	inc	inc
	Methionine	inc	inc
Hawkinsinuria	Tyrosine	inc	
	Hawkinsin		inc
DISORDERS OF NEUTRAL AMINO ACID METABOLISM			
Maple Syrup Urine Disease			
Classic	Valine	inc	inc
	Alloisoleucine	present	present
	Isoleucine	inc	inc
	Leucine	inc	inc
	Alanine	dec during severe episodes	
Intermittent, Variable, Intermediate, Thiamine-responsive	Above branch-chain amino acids increased during episodes, but may be normal to slightly increased between episodes.		
Dihydrolipoyl Dehydrogenase (E3) Deficiency	Branched-chain amino acids may be norm or slightly elevated.		
3-Hydroxyisobutyryl-CoA Deacylase Deficiency	S-(2-carboxypropyl-cysteine		inc
	S-(2-carboxypropyl)-cysteamine		inc
Non-ketotic Hyperglycinemia	Glycine	inc	inc
		(also inc in CSF)	
Sarcosinemia	Sarcosine	inc	inc
Hartnup Disorder	Neutral amino aids	norm to dec	inc
DISORDERS OF BASIC AMINO ACID METABOLISM			
Hyperlysinemia	Lysine	inc	inc
	Pipecolic acid	inc	
Saccharopinuria	Lysine	inc	inc
	Saccharopine	inc	inc
Lysinuric Protein Intolerance	Lysine	norm to dec	inc
	Arginine	norm to dec	inc
	Ornithine	norm to dec	
	A number of amino acids	inc	

*inc = increased, dec = decreased, norm = normal

Continued

TABLE 14-4 Continued

Disorder	Amino Acid	Abnormal Levels*	
		Plasma	Urine
Alpha-aminoadipic Aciduria	Alpha-aminoadipic acid	inc	inc
Hyperornithinemia-gyrate Atrophy	Ornithine	inc	inc
Hyperornithinemia-Hyperammonemia-Homocitrullinuria (HHH) Syndrome	Ornithine	inc	norm
	Homociturulline	norm	inc
Histidinemia	Histidine	inc	inc

DISORDERS OF UREA CYCLE

Common finding: Glutamine and alanine increased when hyperammonemic.

N-Acetylglutamate Synthetase	Amino acids	norm	norm
	Orotic acid	norm	norm
Carbamoyl Phosphate Synthase	Amino acids	norm	norm
	Orotic acid	norm	norm
Ornithine Carbamoyltransferase Deficiency	Amino acids	norm	norm
	Orotic acid		inc
Citrullinemia	Citrulline	inc	inc
	Orotic acid	inc	inc
Argininosuccinate Lyase Deficiency	Argininosuccinic acid	inc	inc
	Orotic acid		inc
Argininemia	Arginine	inc	inc
	Orotic acid		inc
	Lysine, ornithine, cystine		inc

DISORDERS OF IMINO ACID METABOLISM

Hyperprolinemia			
Type I	Proline	inc	inc
	Hydroxyproline	norm	inc
	Glycine	norm	inc
Type II	Proline	inc	inc
	Hydroxyproline	norm	inc
	Glycine	norm	inc
	Δ'-pyrroline-5-carboxylic acid	inc	Inc
	Δ'-pyrroline-3-hydroxy-5 carboxylic acid		inc
Hyperhydroxyprolinemia	Hydroxyproline	inc	inc
Prolidase Deficiency	Iminodipeptides of proline and hydroxyproline		inc
Neonatal Iminoglycinuria	Proline, hydroxyproline, and glycine	norm	inc to age 6 mos
Familial Renal Iminoglycinuria	Proline		inc
	Hydroxyproline		inc
	Glycine		inc

* inc = increased, dec = decreased, norm = normal

Continued

TABLE 14-4 Continued

Disorder	Amino Acid	Abnormal Levels*	
		Plasma	Urine

DISORDERS OF SULFUR AMINO ACID METABOLISM

Disorder	Amino Acid	Plasma	Urine
Homocystinuria			
Cystathionine Beta-Synthase Deficiency	Homocystine	inc	inc
	Cysteine-homocysteine mixed disulfide	inc	inc
	Methionine	inc	inc
	Cystine	norm to dec	
	Cystathionine	norm to dec	
Cobalamin Disorders: cblC, dblD, cblE & cblG and B$_{12}$ deficiency	Homocystine	inc	inc
	Cysteine-homocysteine mixed disulfide	inc	inc
	Methionine	norm to dec	
	Cystathionine		norm to dec
5,10-Methylenetetrahydrofolate Reductase Deficiency	Homocystine	inc	inc
	Methionine	norm to dec	
	Cystathionine		norm to inc
Cystathioninuria	Cystathionine	norm to inc	inc
Hypermethioninemia	Methionine	inc	
	Methionine sulfoxides	Inc	
3-Mercaptolactic-Cysteine Disulfiduria	3-Mercaptolactic-cysteine mixed disulfide		inc
Sulfite Oxidase Deficiency	S-Sulfocysteine		inc
	Cystine	norm to dec	
Cystinuria	Cystine	norm	inc
	Dibasic amino acids (lysine, ornithine, arginine)	norm	inc
Cystinosis	Cystine	norm	norm
		(inc in lysosomes of tissues)	

DISORDERS OF BETA- AND GAMMA-AMINO ACID METABOLISM

Disorder	Amino Acid	Plasma	Urine
Hyper-Beta-Alaninemia	Beta-alanine	inc	inc
Beta-Aminoisobutyric Aciduria	Beta-aminoisobutyric acid	norm to slightly inc	inc
Gamma-aminobutyric Acid Amino-transferase Deficiency	gamma-aminobutyric	inc	
	Beta-alanine	inc	
	Gamma-aminobutyric, beta-alanine, and homocarnosine also inc in CSF.		
Carnosinase Deficiency	Carnosine	inc	inc
	Anserine		inc
Homocarnosinosis	Homocarnosine	norm	norm
		(inc in CSF)	

*inc = increased, dec = decreased, norm = normal

TABLE 14–5. Organic Acidurias: Pathological Excretions of Organic Acids

Disorder	Compound	Typical Abnormal Excretions (mmol/mol Creatinine)
DISORDERS OF AROMATIC AMINO ACID METABOLISM		
Phenylketonuria	Phenylpyruvic	300–1000
	Phenyllactic	200–1000
	2-Hydroxyphenylacetic	50–2000
Tyrosinemia		
Transient Neonatal, Oculocutaneous, and Hepatorenal Forms	4-Hydroxyphenylpyruvic	140–2000
	4-Hydroxyphenyllactic	100-5000
	4-Hydroxyphenylacetic	140–500
	N-acetyltyrosine	30–200
Hepatorenal Only	Succinylacetone	20–700
Hawkinsinuria	4-Hydroxycyclohexylacetic	10–70
	5-Oxoproline	1300–9000
	4-Hydroxyphenylpyruvic	170–1600
	4-Hydroxyphenyllactic	1000–5000
Alcaptonuria	Homogentisic	1000–5000
DISORDERS OF BRANCHED-CHAIN AMINO ACID METABOLISM		
Maple Syrup Urine Disease	2-Oxoisocaproic	400–4400
	2-Oxo-3-methylvaleric	500–2500
	2-Oxoisovaleric	300–800
	2-Hydroxyisovaleric	850–3600
	2-Hydroxyisocaproic	3–80
	2-Hydroxy-3-methylvaleric	60–400
Dihydrolipoyl Dehydrogenase (E3) Deficiency	Lactic	1000–30,000
	2-Oxoglutaric	150–1100
	2-Oxoisocaproic	0–200
	2-Oxo-3-methylvaleric	0–15
	2-Oxoisovaleric	0–3
	2-Hydroxyisovaleric	0–400
	2-Hydroxyisocaproic	0–70
	2-Hydroxy-3-methylvaleric	0–70
Isovaleric Acidemia	Isovalerylglycine	2000–9000
	3-Hydroxyisovaleric	1000–2000
	4-Hydroxyisovaleric	20–300
3-Methylcrotonyl-CoA Carboxylase Deficiency	3-Hydroxyisovaleric	1700–59,000
	3-Methylcrotonylglycine	400–1000
Biotin-Responsive Multiple Carboxylase Deficiency		
Holocarboxylase Synthetase Deficiency	3-Hydroxyisovaleric acid	250–3600
	3-Methylcrotonylglycine	30–260
	Methylcitric	15–200
	3-Hydroxypropionic	45–1300
	Lactic	100–75,000
Biotinidase Deficiency	Same as above, but generally smaller elevations.	
3-Methylglutaconic Aciduria		
3-Methylglutaconyl-CoA Hydratase Deficiency	3-Methylglutaconic	500–1000
	3-Hydroxyisovaleric	150–250
	3-Methylglutaric	5–10
Normal Hydratase	3-Methylglutaconic	25–600
	3-Methylglutaric	10–85
3-Hydroxy-3-Methylglutaric Aciduria	3-Hydroxy-3-methylglutaric	200–11,000
	3-Methylglutaconic	140–10,000
	3-Methylglutaric	14–1000
	3-Hydroxyisovaleric	60–4000
	3-Methylcrotonyglycine	0–400

Continued

TABLE 14-5 Continued

Disorder	Compound	Typical Abnormal Excretions (mmol/mol Creatinine)
3-Oxothiolase Deficiency		
Mitochondrial Branched-Chain 3-Oxo-thiolase Deficiency	2-Methyl-3-hydroxybutyric	200–4400
	2-Methylacetoacetic	0–650
	Tiglylglycine	0–1000
Cytosolic 3-Oxothiolase Deficiency or Succinyl-CoA: 3-Oxoacid-CoA Transferase Deficiency	3-Hydroxybutyric	Large
	Acetoacetic	Large
Propionic Acidemia	Methylcitric	150–2800
	3-Hydroxypropionic	20–2000
	Propionylglycine	0–450
	3-Hydroxyvaleric	0–1200
Methylmalonic Acidemia: Mutase Deficiency and Cobalamin Disorders	Methylmalonic	150–15,500
	(Plus same metabolites as propionic acidemia)	
Malonyl-CoA Decarboxylase Deficiency	Malonic	50–4000
	Methylmalonic	0–80
3-Hydroxyisobutyric Aciduria	3-Hydroxyisobutyric	130–400
DISORDERS OF DIBASIC AMINO ACID METABOLISM		
2-Oxoadipic Aciduria	2-Oxoadipic	20–220
	2-Hydroxyadipic	50–220
Glutaric Aciduria Type I	Glutaric	500–12,000
	3-Hydroxyglutaric	60–3000
	Glutaconic	0–360
Hyperornithinemia-Hyperammonemia-Homocitrullinuria (HHH) Syndrome	Orotic	30–500
Lysinuric Protein Intolerance	Orotic	1–640
DISORDERS OF THE UREA CYCLE		
N-Acetylglutamate Synthetase, Carbomoyl Phosphate Synthase, and Argininos-succinate Lyase Deficiency	No abnormalities or organic acids	
Ornithine Carbamoyltransferase Deficiency and Citrullinemia	Orotic	10–1300
	Uracil	30–500
Argininemia	Orotic	500–1000
DISORDERS OF PYRIMIDINE METABOLISM		
Orotic Aciduria	Orotic	1400–5600
Dihydropyrimidine Dehydrogenase Deficiency	Uracil	100–1100
	Thymine	35–850
DISORDERS OF FATTY ACID OXIDATION		
Long-chain Hydroxyacyl-CoA Dehydrogenase Deficiency	3-Hydroxydecanedioic	Increased
	3-Hydroxydodecanedioic	Increased
	3-Hydroxytetradecanedioic	Increased
	3-Hydroxy-unsaturated dicarboxylic, saturated and unsaturated dicarboxylic	Increased
Long-chain Acyl-CoA Dehydrogenase Deficiency	Suberic	0–20
	Sebacic	0–20
	Dodecamedioic and tetadecanedioic may be elevated	
Medium-Chain Acyl-CoA Deydrogenase Deficiency	Octanoic	2–20
	5-Hydroxyhexanoic	15–700
	7-Hydroxyoctanoic	4–300
	Adipic	5–5200
	Suberic	6–5000

Continued

TABLE 14–5 Continued

Disorder	Compound	Typical Abnormal Excretion (mmol/mol Creatinine)
	Octenedioic	0–250
	Sebacic	0–5000
	Decenedioic	0–750
	Hexanoylglycine	2–730
	Phenylproionylglycine	1–90
	Suberylglycine	6–2200
Short-Chain Acyl-CoA Dehyrogenase Deficiency	Ethylmalonic	180–1150
	Methylsuccinic	20–60
	(Dicarboxylic aids variably elevated.)	
Multiple Acyl-CoA Dehydrogenase Deficiency (Glutaric Aciduria Type II)	Glutaric	0–22,000
	Ethylmalonic	10–1400
	Adipic	0–1600
	Suberic	0–200
	2-Hydroxyglutaric	180–8250
	Isovalerylglycine	0–1000
	Isobutyrylglycine	0–200
	2-Methylbutyrylglycine	0–200
	(Short-chain fatty acides may be elevated.)	
Normals Fed Medium-Chain Triglycerides	Adipic	200–320
	Suberic	10–620
	Sebacic	0–750
	5-Hydroxyhexanoic	0–220
	7-Hydroxyoctanoic	25–150
MISCELLANEOUS DISORDERS		
4-Hydroxybutyric Aciduria	4-Hydroxybutyric	130–7600
	3, 4-Dihydroxybutyric	5–225
Fumarase Deficiency	Fumaric	3000–4000
2-Oxoglutaric Dehydrogenase Deficiency	2-Oxoglutaric	150–1250
Mevalonic Aciduria	Mevalonolactone, mevalonic acid	1000–56,000
5-Oxoprolinuria	5-Oxoproline	4000–30,000
Canavan's Disease	N-Acetylaspartic	1000–7000
D-Glyceric Aciduria	D-Glyceric	10,000–20 ,000
Hyperoxaluria Type I	Oxalic	90–350
	Glycolic	> 100
	Glyoxylic	> 10
Hyperoxaluria Type II	Oxalic	90–350
	L-Glyceric	150–450
Glyceroluria	Glycerol	90,000–190,000
Lactic Acidemia	Lactic	100–30,000
	Pyruvic	50–10,000
	2-Hydroxybutyric	10–1000
	4-Hydroxyphenyllactic	50–500
Intestinal Bacterial Overgrowth	Lactic (D)	45–6000
	3-Hydroxypropionic	100–6400
	4-Hydroxyphenylacetic	100–2000
	3-Hydroxybutyric	100–50,000
Ketosis	Acetoacetic	50–20,000
	3-Hydroxyisobutyric	50–3000
	3-Hydroxyisovaleric	50–1000
	3-Hydroxy-2-methylbutyric	10–200
	Adipic	15–450
	Suberic	0–100

Pathological values from authors' experience and review of the literature.

Tyrosinemia

Tyrosine is transaminated to 4-hydroxyphenylpyruvic acid, which is then further oxidized and cleaved to fumaric acid and acetoacetic acid in liver. The most common form of tyrosinemia is transient neonatal tyrosinemia, especially among premature infants, and resolves with time. The two major inherited disorders of tyrosine metabolism are hepatorenal (type I) and oculocutaneous (type II).

The more severe form, hepatorenal tyrosinemia, is due to a deficiency of fumarylacetoacetate hydrolase, which cleaves the tyrosine catabolite fumarylacetoacetate. There is a secondary deficiency of 4-hydroxyphenylpyruvic acid oxidase, resulting in increased tyrosine and its phenolic acid metabolites. Fumarylacetoacetate is converted to succinylacetone, which is uniquely found in hepatorenal tyrosinemia and useful for differential diagnosis.

Other secondary abnormalities include increased methionine in plasma, a generalized amino aciduria, increased δ-aminolevulinic acid in urine, and increased α-fetoprotein in plasma. The amino acid pattern of increased tyrosine and methionine is not specific for hepatorenal tyrosinemia, but may also occur with severe liver damage due to a variety of causes, including galactosemia and hereditary fructose intolerance. The patients frequently present in infancy with chronic hepatic failure, and development of hepatomas is common. The preferred treatment is liver transplantation.

Oculocutaneous tyrosinemia presents with keratoses of the palms and digits and corneal ulcers, with highly increased tyrosine in the plasma. Some patients have mild mental retardation. This disorder is due to a deficiency of the soluble liver tyrosine aminotransferase, which prevents the normal formation of 4-hydroxyphenylpyruvic acid and its further catabolism in liver. Tyrosine is transaminated in peripheral tissues by aspartate aminotransferase, which results in excretion of the phenolic acid metabolites. Methionine is not increased in this form of tyrosinemia. Treatment with a diet low in phenylalanine and tyrosine can greatly reduce plasma tyrosine concentrations and reverse the oculocutaneous symptoms.

Maple Syrup Urine Disease (MSUD)

MSUD is caused by a deficiency of branched-chain α-ketoacid dehydrogenase, which decarboxylates the branched-chain α-ketoacids derived from transamination of valine, leucine, and isoleucine to acyl-CoA products. In addition to increases of the branched-chain keto and hydroxy acids, the branched-chain amino acids are also increased due to the reversibility of the transaminase reaction. The increased keto acid derived from isoleucine undergoes spontaneous keto-enol tautomerism to form a diastereoisomer which is also transaminated, forming alloisoleucine, which is unique to MSUD. There is a range of severity in the deficiency of the complex, with classical MSUD having complete deficiency and severe life-threatening neonatal ketoacidosis, vomiting, lethargy, and hypotonia. Without treatment, this may progress to coma and death and, if not fatal, results in mental retardation. Treatment requires a special diet severely restricting the intake of the branched-chain amino acids and monitoring of plasma branched-chain amino acid concentrations. Partial enzyme deficiencies result in a range of milder symptoms presenting in infancy or childhood with ketoacidotic episodes and lesser, or even intermittent, increases of the branched-chain amino acids in plasma. These may be treated with mild protein restriction or, in the mildest forms, may require protein restriction only during acute episodes. Thiamine pyrophosphate is a cofactor for the dehydrogenase complex, and some patients are responsive to large doses of thiamine.

Nonketotic Hyperglycinemia

Glycine is normally metabolized to ammonia, carbon dioxide, and hydroxymethyl tetrahydrolfolate by the glycine cleavage system present in brain and liver. Deficiency of this system results in nonketotic hyperglycinemia with increased glycine in plasma, urine, and cerebrospinal fluid. The diagnosis is best made by determining the ratio of glycine in cerebrospinal fluid to that in plasma (normal = 0.03), which is increased tenfold to about 0.3 in this disorder. The diagnosis may be complicated by the existence of transient neonatal hyperglycinemia with increased cerebrospinal fluid to plasma glycine ratios which normalize with time. Nonketotic hyperglycinemia generally presents in the neonatal period with seizures and hypotonia and usually progresses to coma and death. Survivors have little psychomotor development, often develop spastic quadriparesis and die during the first year of life. No effective treatment has been found.

Homocystinuria

Deficiency of cystathionine synthase, which is the most common cause of homocystinuria, results in increased homocystine and cysteine-homocysteine mixed disulfide in plasma and urine with *increased* methionine and decreased cystine in plasma. Common clinical symptoms are subluxation of the lenses, mental retardation, psychiatric disorders, thromboembolism, arterial sclerosis, and osteoporosis. More than a third of the patients are responsive to large doses of pyridoxine, which decreases the homocysteine concentrations.

The relatively rare defects in homocysteine remethylation, such as the disorders of cobalamin metabolism listed in Table 14-4, result in increased amounts of homocystine and cysteine-homocysteine mixed disulfide in plasma and urine, with normal or decreased methionine in plasma.

Cystinuria

Cystinuria is a relatively common disorder of amino acid transport, affecting about 1:7,000. Cystine and the dibasic amino acids are transported in the renal tubule by a common transport mechanism. A deficiency results in normal concentrations of amino acids in plasma, but greatly increased cystine, lysine, ornithine, and arginine in urine (see Figure 14–2). Because of limited solubility, cystine forms renal stones. Treatment is aimed at minimizing stone formation through diluting the urine with a large water intake, alkalinizing the urine to increase cystine solubility, or treatment with penicillamine, which decreases urinary cystine by forming cysteine-penicillamine mixed disulfide, which is more soluble than cystine.

UREA CYCLE DISORDERS

The urea cycle detoxifies ammonia by forming urea and is required for the synthesis of arginine.[12] Deficiencies of any of the six enzymes of the cycle result in hyperammonemia, a low blood urea nitrogen, a secondary increase of glutamine and alanine and decreased arginine in plasma (except for argininemia). The clinical presentation may be acute illness in the first few days of life, with lethargy, vomiting, and coma. The onset may occur later with similar symptoms. Neurological damage often results from severe hyperammonemia. The differential diagnosis of the urea cycle disorders includes analysis of organic acids to rule out organic acidurias which can also cause hyperammonemia. The abnormalities of amino acids found in urea cycle disorders are listed in Table 14–4.

N-Acetylglutamate Synthetase and Carbamoyl Phosphate Synthetase

A deficiency of either of these first two enzymes of the urea cycle does not cause a specific abnormality of amino acid concentrations nor of orotic acid. Their tentative diagnosis depends on excluding other causes of hyperammonemia, and their definitive diagnosis requires assay for enzyme deficiency in liver biopsies.

Ornithine Carbamoyl Transferase Deficiency

This disorder also lacks specific abnormalities of amino acid concentrations, but may be associated with decreased citrulline concentra-

FIGURE 14–2. Amino Acid Chromatogram of Urine from a Patient with Cystinuria
(performed according to Slocum & Cummings[10])

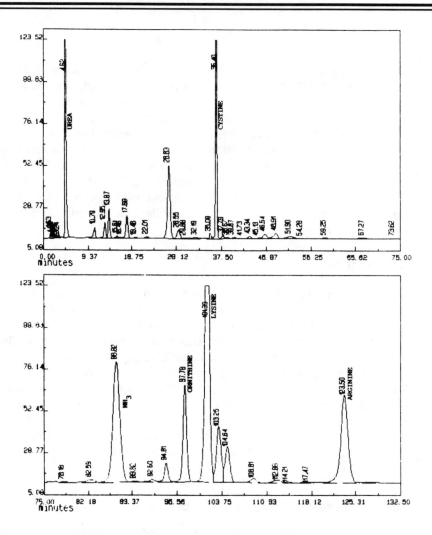

tion. Increased orotic acid excretion due to increased pyrimidine synthesis from accumulated carbamoyl phosphate is present. This is an X-linked disorder. Female heterozygotes for this deficiency may also present with symptoms of hyperammonemia. An interesting method of carrier detection is the finding of increased orotic acid and orotidine in urine after a single dose of allopurinol.

Citrullinemia

This disorder is characterized by large increases of citrulline in plasma and urine due to the deficiency of argininosuccinic acid synthase as well as increased orotic acid in urine.

Argininosuccinic Aciduria

A deficiency of argininosuccinase results in highly increased argininosuccinic acid in plasma and urine and, occasionally, increased orotic acid in urine. Argininosuccinic acid spontaneously forms two anhydrides, resulting in three peaks in the amino acid analysis which coelute with normal amino acids, making their quantification difficult. Citrulline is also moderately increased in this disorder.

Argininemia

A deficiency or arginase causes a large increase of arginine in plasma and urine as well as increased orotic acid in urine. The increased arginine in urine is accompanied by increased lysine, ornithine, and cystine due to competition in reabsorption of these amino acids.

The treatment of the urea cycle disorders involves restriction of dietary protein to reduce the formation of ammonia and supplementation with citrulline or arginine for carbamoyl phosphate synthetase and ornithine carbamoyl transferase deficiency, and arginine for citrullinemia and argininosuccinase deficiency to prevent arginine deficiency. Dialysis is of benefit during episodes of acute decompensation. Additional treatment with benzoate removes nitrogen as hippuric acid or treatment with phenylacetic acid removes nitrogen as phenylacetylglutamine.

ORGANIC ACID DISORDERS

Organic acids are defined as any acids that are not amino acids and thus encompass a very wide range of chemical functional groups, many different areas of metabolism, and hundreds of compounds found in physiological fluids.

Many of the amino acid disorders have abnormalities in organic acids as well as amino acids, and therefore analysis of organic acids gives diagnostic information that is complementary to the analysis of amino acids. For the general analysis of organic acids for diagnostic purposes, urine is the preferred physiological fluid, but there are areas of metabolism such as fatty acid oxidation that might be better diagnosed by analysis of organic acids in plasma. Analyses of organic acids generally have been done by organic solvent extraction of acidified urine, formation of trimethysilyl derivatives, and quantitative or semi-quantitative gas chromatographic or gas chromatography/mass spectrometric analysis.[13, 14] Because of the enormous complexity of organic acids in urine, it is very difficult to unambiguously identify acids by gas chromatographic retention times alone, and GCMS is essential. With the availability of relatively inexpensive bench-top GCMS, the preferred method is quantitative analysis using specific mass spectral fragment masses.[15] Quantification is more important because many compounds originally thought to be "abnormal" metabolites are now known to be metabolites normally present in small amounts. Diagnosis therefore frequently depends upon determining an increase of normal organic acids rather than the presence or absence of an organic acid.

In the diagnosis of the organic acidurias, it is generally a pattern of organic acids that is diagnostic rather than in increase of a single organic acid. This is especially true of many disorders of branched-chain amino acid metabolism where deficiencies of sequential enzymes in a pathway have many abnormal metabolite increases in common. Table 14–5 lists the typical diagnostic increased acids for a wide variety of organic acidurias. The degree of increase of many acids is very dependent on the clinical status of the patient, and when in good clinical control, the diagnostic acids may be minimally increased or even normal in some disorders. Reference ranges for the urinary organic acids of normal subjects are not well established and to some extent are dependent on the methods used, so each laboratory should establish its own reference ranges. Approximate reference ranges for children have been published.[15] Once a patient has been diagnosed with a specific organic aciduria, the role of the laboratory is to provide accurate determinations of specific organic acids in order to monitor therapy with diet or vitamins. In addition to the summary of diagnostic concentrations of urinary organic acids in Table 14–5, five of the more important organic acidurias are discussed in greater detail below.

Isovaleric Acidemia

This is a disorder of the catabolism of leucine caused by a deficiency of isovaleryl-CoA dehydrogenase, which normally metabolizes isovaleryl-CoA to 3-methylcrotonyl-CoA. The accumulated isovaleryl-CoA is hydrolyzed to some extent to free isovaleric acid, which can be increased in plasma and urine; its odor of "sweaty feet" may be quite noticeable during acute episodes. The most diagnostic finding is an increase in the metabolite isovalerylglycine, which is continuously excreted in very large amounts. When patients are clinically ill, additional diagnostic metabolites are 3-hydroxyisovaleric and 4-hydroxyisovaleric acids.

About half of the patients present in the neonatal period with acute episodes of vomiting, ketoacidosis, and lethargy proceeding to coma and often death. Other patients present with intermittent episodes during the first year of life, often precipitated by infection or increased protein intake. Treatment during episodes includes procedures appropriate for many organic acidurias, namely glucose infusion to correct dehydration and to provide calories to reduce catabolism. Treatment during remission is generally with moderate restriction of normal dietary protein. Specific therapies that are beneficial are administration of carnitine, which reduces the toxic concentrations of isovaleryl-CoA by formation of isovalerylcarnitine and excretion in the urine, and/or treatment with glycine, which increases the detoxification of isovaleryl-CoA to isovalerylglycine. The management and clinical status of the patients can be monitored by the concentration of isovaleric acid in plasma and urine.

Propionic Acidemia and Methylmalonic Acidemia

Propionic acid is derived from a variety of precursors, including isoleucine, valine, methionine, and threonine, odd-chain fatty acids and cholesterol, and from intestinal flora. It is metabolized by propionyl-CoA carboxylase to methylmalonyl-CoA, which in turn is metabolized to succinyl-CoA by methylmalonyl-CoA mutase. A deficiency of propionyl-CoA carboxylase causes propionic acidemia, while a deficiency of methylmalonyl-CoA mutase or a defect in the synthesis of its cobalamin cofactor, adenosylcobalamin, causes methylmalonic acidemia. The same increased metabolites occur in both propionic acidemia and methylmalonic acidemia, except that methylmalonic acid is highly increased only in the latter. The most diagnostic organic acid increased in propionic acidemia is methylcitrate, which is formed by citrate synthase. Another less specific metabolite is 3-hydroxypropionate. Propionylglycine is also increased during episodes.

The steps in isoleucine catabolism between tiglyl-CoA and propionyl-CoA are reversible, and during acute episodes a large number of intermediates and their secondary metabolites may be increased. These include tiglylglycine, 2-methyl-3-hydroxybutyric, and 3-hydroxyvaleric acids. In methylmalonic acidemia due to defects of cobalamin metabolism, the increase of methylmalonate is less than in mutase deficiency. The disorders cblA and cblB are defects in the synthesis of adenosylcobalamin. Disorders that affect the synthesis of both adenosylcobalamin and methylcobalamin, i. e., cblC, cblD, and cblF, result in combined methylmalonic acidemia and homocystinuria (See Table 14–4).

Additional biochemical abnormalities of propionic acidemia and methylmalonic acidemia include severe hyperammonemia and ketosis during episodes and a secondary increase of glycine. Most patients present with a severe acidotic episode in the neonatal period and/or with infections or excessive protein intake. Treatment consists of restriction of dietary precursors of propionic acid, namely the essential amino acids valine and isoleucine, and administration of carnitine, which prevents secondary carnitine deficiency due to loss of carnitine as propionylcarnitine in urine. Some patients with methylmalonic acidemia due to cblA or cblB respond to high doses of vitamin B_{12} with decreased concentrations of methylmalonic acid in plasma and urine. Treatment of propionic acidemia is monitored by determining concentrations of propionic acid in plasma and urine, while that of methylmalonic acidemia is monitored by measuring methylmalonic acid in plasma and urine.

Multiple Carboxylase Deficiency

This is due to either of two disorders of the metabolism of the vitamin biotin. Biotin is activated to biotinyl-AMP by holocarboxylase synthetase, which then attaches the biotin covalently to the epsilon-amino group of a lysine in all four biotin-dependent carboxylases: acetyl-CoA carboxylase, propionyl-CoA carboxylase, 3-methylcrotonyl-CoA carboxylase, and pyruvate carboxylase. When the carboxylases are degraded in normal protein turnover or when protein-bound biotin in the diet is digested, the product biocytin (biotinyl-lysine) is cleaved by biotinidase to free biotin, which can then be utilized for synthesis of new biotin-containing carboxylases.

A deficiency of holocarboxylase synthetase or biotinidase causes a deficiency of all four carboxylases. The most diagnostic metabolites are 3-hydroxyisovaleric acid and methylcrotonylglycine, which result from the deficiency of 3-methylcrotonyl-CoA carboxylase. A modest increase of methylcitric and 3-hydroxypropionic acid results from the dysfunction of propionyl-CoA carboxylase, but these are generally much lower than in patients with propionic acidemia. Increased lactic acid results from the deficiency of pyruvate carboxylase. Patients with holocarboxylase synthetase deficiency generally present in the neonatal period with severe metabolic acidosis and ketosis. Those who present later and those with biotinidase deficiency have symptoms of biotin deficiency, such as an erythematous skin rash and alopecia. Biotinidase-deficient patients often have conjunctivitis and periorificial rashes, ataxia, developmental regression, nerve deafness, and optic nerve atrophy. All of the patients with biotinidase deficiency and most of those with holocarboxylase synthetase deficiency show normalization of organic acid metabolites and clinical symptoms with large doses of biotin (10 or more mg/day), making this a very effective treatment.

Glutaric Aciduria Type I

Glutaryl-CoA derived from the catabolism of lysine, hydroxylysine, and tryptophan are normally metabolized by glutaryl-CoA dehydrogenase to crotonyl-CoA. Patients with a deficiency of this enzyme have glutaric aciduria type I. Glutaric acid is usually highly increased in urine of these patients and is accompanied by a lesser increase of 3-hydroxy-glutaric acid which is specific to this disorder (see Figure 14–3). However, some patients have little or no increase of glutaric acid. Glutaric aciduria type II is a defect in the transfer of electrons from a number of dehydrogenases, including glutaryl-CoA dehydrogenase and the fatty acid oxidation acyl-CoA dehydrogenases through electron transfer flavoprotein into the mitochondrial electron transport chain. That disorder may have an increase in glutaric acid, but it is not accompanied by 3-hydroxyglutaric acid but rather by 2-hydroxyglutaric acid, a number of dicarboxylic acids and acylglycines.

FIGURE 14–3. *Lower view:* Gas chromatography-mass spectrometry total ion chromatogram of urine from a patient with glutaric aciduria type I (performed according to Sweetman[15]) *Upper left view:* Mass spectrum of the diTMS derivative of glutaric acid. *Upper right view:* Mass spectrum of the triTMS derivative of 3-hydroxy-glutaric acid.

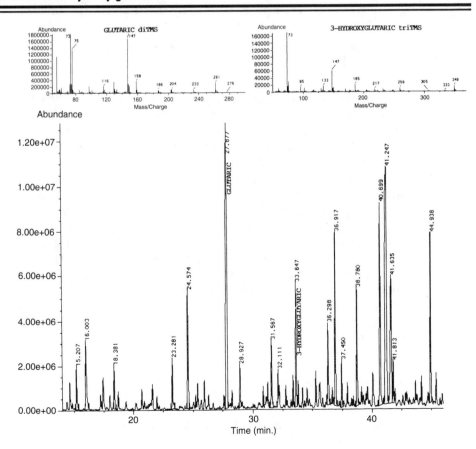

Glutaric aciduria type I causes severe neurological problems during the first year of life, with dystonia and dyskinesia due to neuronal degeneration of the caudate and putamen. Dietary restriction of lysine and tryptophan may be of some benefit prior to the onset of irreversible neurological symptoms.

FATTY ACID DISORDERS

Long-chain fatty acids are a major substrate for energy production in skeletal and cardiac tissues under most physiologic conditions. During fasting, fatty acids and their metabolic products, ketone bodies, become a major fuel for most tissues. Even the normally glucose-dependent brain can adapt to ketone utilization after prolonged fasting induces the necessary enzyme.

Thus, logically one can predict that dysfunction of enzymes necessary for metabolism of fatty acids will manifest as two major symptom groups:

1. Hypotonia, weakness, myopathy, cardiac failure, or cardiomyopathy

2. Hypoglycemia, hepatic failure, or encephalopathy associated with fasting.[16]

The major metabolic flux of long-chain fatty acids is through the beta-oxidation system of the mitochondria present in all cells except the mature erythrocyte. Access of the fatty acid to the beta-oxidation enzymes requires a carnitine-dependent transport system to cross the mitochondrial membrane.

Fatty acids are activated to acyl-CoAs at the outer mitochondrial membrane, converted to acylcarnitines by carnitine palmitoyl transferase (CPT) I, transported across the inner mitochondrial membrane by a translocase, and the fatty acid acyl-CoA regenerated by CPT II. The fatty acid acyl-CoA then undergoes beta-oxidation to generate acetyl-CoA, which is a substrate for energy production in the tricarboxylic acid cycle and for ketone body synthesis. Thus, a failure of energy production or ketone body synthesis from fatty acids can result from a deficiency of:

1. Carnitine

2. CPT I

3. Translocase

4. CPT II

5. Any of the enzymes of the beta-oxidation

Beta-oxidation itself proceeds through a series of steps (acyl-CoA dehydrogenase, enoyl-CoA hydratase, hydroxyacyl-CoA dehydrogenase, and ketoacyl-CoA thiolase) resulting in the release of acetyl-CoA and a fatty acid acyl-CoA derivative which is shorter by two carbon groups. As the fatty acid is shortened, a different series of enzymes performing the same catalytic function, but with different chain length specificity, is required. The enzymes of beta-oxidation are generally categorized as long-chain acyl-CoA dehydrogenase (LCAD), medium-chain acyl-CoA dehydrogenase (MCAD), short-chain acyl-CoA dehydrogenase (SCAD), long-chain enoyl-CoA hydratase, etc.

There are no known genetic defects of carnitine biosynthesis, but low concentrations of carnitine can result from dietary deficiency, malabsorption, liver disease, or increased renal loss. Functional carnitine deficiency can also result when concentrations of total carnitine are normal but free carnitine is low, due to its sequestration in the acylated form. This secondary carnitine deficiency occurs when acyl-CoA accumulates as in the organic acidemias or enzymatic defects in the fatty acid oxidation.

Defects in carnitine transport across the plasma membrane are termed primary carnitine deficiency and classified into myopathic and systemic clinical presentations. The myopathic form manifests as progressive skeletal muscle weakness with a lipid storage. Serum carnitine is normal but muscle carnitine is low, suggesting an abnormality in the muscle transporter. Response to carnitine replacement is variable. Systemic carnitine deficiency is characterized by low serum and tissue carnitine concentrations and is very responsive to supplemental carnitine.

Symptoms of cardiomyopathy, muscle weakness, hypotonia, hypoglycemia, hypoketonemia, and coma implicate a transporter deficiency in many tissues including heart, skeletal muscle, and liver. A single patient with a defective carnitine/acylcarnitine translocase has been identified.[19] Symptoms and signs included hypoglycemia, decreased ketogenesis, low serum free carnitine with increased long-chain acylcarnitine, hyperammonemia, muscle weakness, and mild hypertrophic cardiomyopathy.

SUMMARY

Although inborn errors of metabolism are individually rare, the large number of disorders and the referral patterns to tertiary care institutions result in these genetic diseases commonly being a part of differential diagnoses. As the signs and symptoms of metabolic disease are distressingly vague and routine clinical chemistry tests rarely indicative of a specific diagnosis, the clinician is frequently dependent on the guidance of specialists in laboratory medicine. It is their expertise in the newer technologies such as gas chromatography /mass spectrometry, high-performance liquid chromatography, enzymatic analysis, and recombinant DNA which is essential to the selection of appropriate tests and the interpretation of the results. This review does not discuss the technologies themselves, but rather focuses on the major groups of enzymatic deficiencies, their clinical manifestations, diagnostic tests, and interpretation of abnormalities.

The disorders of lysosomal and peroxisomal catabolic function primarily manifest with slowly progressive symptoms which may affect multiple organ systems or single tissues. Diagnosis is usually dependent on a specific enzymatic analysis of the suspected deficiency, although electron microscopic examination of tissues or analysis of accumulated metabolites may be useful. Treatment is supportive and specific interventional therapy rarely available. Conversely, enzymatic deficiencies of intermediary metabolism frequently manifest acutely due to their important role in physiologic homeostasis and the vastly changing flux of substrate through these pathways under catabolic conditions. These disorders may be classified according to substrate type, i. e., carbohydrate, fatty acid, or amino acid, the latter including amino acidopathies, organic acidemias/acidurias, and the urea cycle defects. Treatment of these diseases focuses on decreasing substrate flux through the affected pathway via dietary restriction or avoidance of catabolic states. Specific therapy with a vitamin cofactor or drugs increasing excretion of toxic metabolites is available in some instances. Diagnosis primarily depends on analysis of accumulated metabolites due to the enzymatic deficiency, which may then be confirmed by direct measurement. Extensive tables listing these metabolites, their usual values, and the corresponding enzyme have been provided to aid in interpretation and diagnosis.

REFERENCES

1. Scriver CR, Beaudet AL, Sly WS, Valle D. The metabolic basis of inherited disease, 6th ed. New York: McGraw-Hill, 1989.
2. Watts RWE, Gibbs WA. Lysosomal storage diseases: Biochemical and clinical aspects. London: Taylor and Francis, 1986.
3. Durand P, O'Brien JS. Genetic disorders of glycoprotein metabolism. Berlin: Springer-Verlag, 1982.
4. Williams JC, Howell RR. Mucopolysaccharidoses. In: Conn RB, ed., Current diagnosis, 7th ed. Philadelphia: WB Saunders, 1985:758-761.
5. Johnson WB. Sphingolipidoses. In: Conn RB, ed., Current diagnosis, 7th ed. Philadelphia: WB Saunders, 1985:770-77.
6. Moser HW, Moser AB. Measurement of saturated very long-chain fatty acids in plasma. In: Hommes FA, ed., Techniques in diagnostic human biochemical genetics: A laboratory manual. New York: Wiley-Liss, 1991:177-91.
7. Lazarow PB, Moser HW. Disorders of peroxisome biogenesis. In: Scriver CR, Beaudet AL, Sly WS, Valle D, eds., The metabolic basis of inherited disease, 6th ed. McGraw-Hill, 1989:1479-1509.

8.   Williams JC, Howell RR. Hereditary disorders of carbohydrate metabolism. In: Conn RB, ed., Current diagnosis, 7th ed. Philadelphia: WB Saunders, 1985:752-58.

9.   Zeviani M, Bonilla E, De Vivo DC, Di Mauro S. Mitochondrial diseases. Neurol Clin 1989;7:123-56.

10. Slocum RH, Cummings JG. Amino acid analysis of physiological samples. In: Hommes FA, ed., Techniques in diagnostic human biochemical genetics: A laboratory manual. New York: Wiley-Liss, 1991:87-126.

11. Bremer HJ, Duran M, Kamerling JP, Przyrembel, Wadman SK. Disturbances of amino acid metabolism: Clinical chemistry and diagnosis. Baltimore: Urban & Schwarzenberg, 1981.

12. Brusilow SW, Horwich AL. Urea cycle enzymes. In: Scriver CR, Beaudet AL, Sly WS, Valle D,, eds., The metabolic basis of inherited disease, 6th ed. New York: McGraw-Hill, 1989;629-63.

13. Goodman SI, Markey SP. Diagnosis of organic acidemias by gas chromatography-mass spectrometry. Laboratory and research methods in biology and medicine (Vol. 6). New York: Alan R. Liss, Inc., 1981.

14. Chalmers RA, Lawson AM. Organic acids in man. London: Chapman and Hall, 1982.

15. Sweetman L. Organic acid analysis. In: Hommes FA, ed., Techniques in diagnostic human biochemical genetics: A laboratory manual. New York: Wiley-Liss, 1991:143-76.

16. Tanaka K, Coates PM. Fatty acid oxidation: Clinical, biochemical and molecular aspects. New York: Alan R. Liss, 1990.

17. Wessler E. Analytic and preparative separation of acidic glycosaminoglycans by electrophoresis in barium acetate. Anal Biochem 1968;26:439-44.

18. Humbel R, Collart M. Oligosaccharides in urine of patients with glycoprotein storage diseases. 1. Rapid detection by thin-layer chromatography. Clin Chim Acta 1975;60:143-45.

19. Stanley CA, Boxer J, Deleeuw S. Mitochondrial inner membrane acylcarnitine translocase deficiency in an infant with an inborn error of fatty acid oxidation. Pediatr Res 1991;29:1178.

Disorders of Lipid and Lipoprotein Metabolism in Children and Adolescents

Nader Rifai, Ph.D., F.A.C.B.   *Peter O. Kwiterovich, Jr., M.D.*

INTRODUCTION

Coronary heart disease (CHD), the leading cause of death in the western world, is responsible for more than 550,000 deaths in the United States each year. It has been estimated that the direct and indirect costs of CHD surpass $50 billion a year. This disease is multifactorial in nature. Epidemiologic findings such as those from the Framingham study have demonstrated that high blood pressure, cigarette smoking, and increased plasma total cholesterol and low density lipoprotein cholesterol (LDL-C) concentrations are "determinant" risk factors of CHD.[1] Other factors that associate with this disease include obesity, male gender, sedentary life style, stress, family history of early myocardial infarction, and decreased plasma high density lipoprotein cholesterol (HDL-C) concentration (< 35 mg/dL [0.91 mmol/L]).

Autopsies performed on young American soldiers killed in action in Korea[2] and Vietnam[3] revealed atherosclerotic lesions. These findings indicated that atherosclerosis, the major cause of CHD, is a process that begins early in life and progresses silently for decades. Coronary artery lesions were also found in aortas beginning at age 3 years[4] and in coronaries starting at age 10 years.[5] Findings from the Bogalusa heart study have demonstrated a correlation between systolic blood pressure, higher total and LDL cholesterol but lower HDL-C concentrations, and the degree of coronary and aortic atherosclerosis in children and adolescents.[6] In the Pathobiological Determinants of Atherosclerosis in Youth (PDAY) Study, post-mortem cholesterol and thiocyanate concentrations predicted the extent of coronary and aortic atherosclerosis, respectively, in autopsies of those aged 14 to 34 years.[7] Therefore, a direct relation between determinant risk factors and the extent of the atherosclerotic lesions in youth seems to exist.

Furthermore, children in countries with an increased incidence of CHD were reported to have higher cholesterol concentrations than children of countries with low incidence.[8] About 5% of American children aged 5 to 18 years have cholesterol concentrations > 200 mg/dL (5.18 mmol/L). In addition, findings from the Muscatine and Princeton School studies have demonstrated that serum cholesterol and lipoprotein cholesterol concentrations cluster in families and display a moderate degree of longitudinal tracking.[9-11] Therefore, those individuals who are in the highest rank order of the population for total and lipoprotein cholesterol concentrations tend to remain in a high rank. The identification of children with high risk of developing CHD at early age offers the possibility of early treatment and prevention of this disease.

The relation between lipids and lipoproteins and early CHD is particularly striking in families with premature CHD.[12] About one-third of the offspring born to parents from families with CHD before age 55 years have hypercholesterolemia or hypertriglyceridemia. Of those born to a parent with angiographically documented early CHD, about half will have a dyslipidemia. More recently, work from the Bogalusa heart study has indicated that measurements of apolipoprotein B-100 (apo B-100), the major protein of low density lipoproteins (LDL), and apo A-I, the major protein of high density lipoproteins (HDL), may be more sensitive indicators of identifying dyslipidemic children born to a parent with premature CHD.[13]

In patients with inherited dyslipidemia, clinical symptoms of CHD usually appear in the fourth or fifth decade of life. By the time most individuals develop the symptoms, the atherogenic process is far advanced and arterial blood flow is markedly diminished. However, clinical manifestations of CHD can develop in children and adolescents with the rare disease homozygous familial hypercholesterolemia.

This chapter describes lipoprotein composition and metabolism; disorders of lipoprotein metabolism, with special emphasis on hypercholesterolemia and increased LDL-C concentrations; screening; the role of the clinical laboratory in the diagnosis and follow-up of children with these disorders; and clinical management of these disorders.

LIPOPROTEIN COMPOSITION

Lipoproteins are particles that have in their core hydrophobic, non-polar lipids (triglyceride and cholesterol esters), which are coated with native surfactants (phospholipids and free cholesterol) and specific proteins called apolipoproteins.[14] The association of the core lipids with the phospholipid and protein coat is non-covalent, occurring primarily through hydrogen bonding and Van der Waals forces. This binding of lipid to protein is loose enough to allow the ready exchange of lipids between serum lipoproteins and between serum and cell membrane lipoproteins, yet tight enough to allow the native lipoprotein complexes to be separated by a variety of analytical techniques.

Lipoproteins are separated into five major classes according to their physical and chemical properties (Table 15–1). Lipoproteins separated by ultracentrifugation are classified by their densities as: (1) chylomicrons, (2) very low density lipoproteins (VLDL), (3) intermediate density lipoproteins (IDL), (4) LDL, and (5) HDL. HDL can be further divided by density into two subpopulations, HDL_2 and HDL_3. As discussed later in this chapter, the two subfractions of HDL seem to differ in their metabolic roles and clinical significance.

Lipoproteins differ in density because they consist of different proportions of triglyceride, cholesterol, phospholipids, and apolipoproteins. In the fasting state, most of the plasma triglyceride is present in VLDL. In the non-fasting state, chylomicrons contribute significantly to the triglyceride level; LDL carry 70% of total plasma cholesterol while HDL contain the lowest amount of plasma triglyceride and about 20% of plasma cholesterol.

The lipoproteins also can be separated by electrophoresis on agarose, cellulose acetate, or paper.[15] At a pH of 8.6, HDL migrate with the α globulins, LDL with the β globulins, and VLDL between the α

TABLE 15–1. Characteristics of Human Plasma Lipoprotein

Variable	Chylomicron	VLDL	IDL	LDL	HDL
Density, Kg/L	< 0.95	0.95–1.006	1.006–1.019	1.019–1.063	1.063–1.210
Electrophoretic mobility	Origin	Pre-beta	Between beta and pre-beta	Beta	Alpha
Molecular Weight	$0.4–30 \times 10^9$	$5–10 \times 10^6$	$3.9–4.8 \times 10^6$	2.75×10^6	$1.8–3.6 \times 10^5$
Diameter, nm	> 70	25–70	22–24	19–23	4–10
Lipid-protein ratio	99:1	90:10	85:15	80:20	50:50
Major lipids	Exogenous triglycerides	Endogenous triglycerides	Endogenous triglycerides, esters cholesteryl esters	Cholesteryl	Phospholipids
Major proteins	A-I B-48 C-I C-II C-III	B-100 C-I C-II C-III E	B-100 E	B-100	A-I A-II

VLDL = very low density lipoproteins, IDL = intermediate density lipoproteins, LDL = low density lipoproteins, and HDL = high density lipoproteins.

and β globulins, the so-called pre-β globulins. IDL form a broad band between β and pre-β globulins. Chylomicrons stay at the point of application. The lipoproteins are still occasionally referred to by their electrophoretic locations, such as pre-β lipoprotein (VLDL).

Apolipoproteins are the protein components of lipoproteins. The characteristics of the major apolipoproteins are summarized in Table 15–2.[14, 16, 17] Each class of lipoprotein has a variety of apolipoproteins in differing proportions, with the exception of LDL which predominantly contain apo B-100. Apo A-I is the major protein in HDL. Apo C-I, -II, -III, and E are present in various proportions in all lipoproteins except LDL.

Apo A-I and apo A-II constitute about 90% of total HDL protein, with an apo A-I to A-II ratio of about 3:1. In addition to being an important structural component of HDL, apo A-I is a co-factor for lecithin cholesterol acyltransferase (LCAT), a plasma enzyme that transfers a fatty acid from phosphatidylcholine to cholesterol, forming cholesteryl ester and lysophosphatidylcholine. Some evidence suggests that apo A-II may inhibit LCAT and/or activate hepatic triglyceride lipase. Apo A-IV, is a component of newly secreted chylomicrons, but is not a major constituent of chylomicron remnants, VLDL, LDL, and HDL. The function of apo A-IV is unknown.

TABLE 15–2. Classification and Properties of Major Human Plasma Apolipoproteins

Apolipoprotein	Molecular Weight (d)	Chromosomal Location	Function	Lipoprotein Carrier(s)
Apo A-I	29,016	11	Cofactor LCAT	Chylomicron, HDL
Apo A-II	17,414	1	Not known	HDL
Apo A-IV	44,465	11	Activates LCAT (?)	Chylomicron, HDL
Apo B-100	512,723	2	Secretion of triglyceride from liver binding protein to LDL receptor	VLDL, IDL, LDL
Apo B-48	240,800	2	Secretion of triglyceride from intestine	Chylomicron
Apo C-I	6,630	19	Activates LCAT(?)	Chylomicron, VLDL, HDL
Apo C-II	8,900	19	Cofactor LPL	Chylomicron, VLDL, HDL
Apo C-III 0–2	8,800	11	Inhibits Apo C-II activator of LPL	Chylomicron, VLDL, HDL
Apo E	34,145	19	Facilitates uptake of chylomicron remnant and IDL	Chylomicron, VLDL, HDL

VLDL = very low density lipoproteins, IDL = intermediate density lipoproteins, LDL = low density lipoproteins, HDL = high density lipoproteins, LCAT = lecithin cholesterol acyltransferase, and LPL = lipoprotein lipase.
From: Rifai N. Lipoproteins and apolipoproteins: Composition, metabolism, and association with coronary heart disease. Arch Path Lab Med 1986;110:694–701. Copyright 1986, American Medical Association. Adapted with permission. Also Kwiterovich PO Jr. Diagnosis and management of familial dyslipoproteinemia in children and adolescents. Pediatr Clin North Am 1990;37:1489-523.

Apo B exists in two forms: apo B-100 and apo B-48. The two proteins are known to be translation products of a single structural gene.[18] Apo B-100, a single polypeptide of over 4,500 amino acids, is a full-length translation product of the apo B gene. Apo B-100 is primarily made in the liver and excreted into plasma on VLDL. Apo B-100 is the major apolipoprotein of LDL, the product of VLDL catabolism. In the fasting state, most of the apo B is apo B-100. For each molecule of LDL or VLDL, there is one molecule of apo B-100. Apo B-48 contains 2151 amino acids and is homologous to the amino terminal portion of apo B-100. Apo B-48 results from the post-transcriptional modification of messenger RNA, in which a single base substitution produces a stop codon corresponding to residue 2153 of apo B-100. Apo B-48 is made in the intestine and is the major apo B component of chylomicrons. Both apo B-100 and B-48 play an important role in regulating lipoprotein secretion (VLDL and chylomicrons, respectively). Apo B-100 is the ligand that enables LDL to be taken up by the LDL receptor (see also discussion below).

Apo C-I, C-II, and C-III are associated with all lipoproteins except LDL. Apo C-I, the smallest of the C apolipoproteins, is reported to activate LCAT *in vitro*. Apo C-II plays an important role in the metabolism of triglyceride-rich lipoproteins (VLDL and chylomicrons) by activating lipoprotein lipase (LPL), an enzyme that hydrolyses the triglyceride in the lipoproteins. Apo C-III exists in at least three polymorphic forms, due to differences in sialic acid content. The precise metabolic function of apo C-III is unknown, but it may inhibit LPL and/or activate LCAT.

Apo E is a constituent of chylomicrons, VLDL, and HDL. It is present in several polymorphic forms due to different amino acid substitutions. Apo E plays a central role in the metabolism of triglyceride-rich lipoproteins. It regulates and facilitates lipoprotein uptake in the liver through (1) the interaction of chylomicron remnants with chylomicron remnant receptors, and (2) the binding of VLDL remnants to the LDL (B, E) receptor.

LIPOPROTEIN METABOLISM

The pathways of lipoprotein metabolism are complex.[14, 19, 20] They can be divided conceptually into exogenous and endogenous systems that transport lipids of dietary and hepatic origin, respectively (Figures 15–1 and 15–2), the intracellular LDL receptor pathway (Figure 15–3), and reverse cholesterol transport (Figure 15–4).

Exogenous Pathway

In the intestine, triglyceride and cholesterol from the diet are incorporated into chylomicrons, which are secreted into lymph and from there

FIGURE 15–1. Exogenous Lipoprotein Metabolism Pathway

TG = triglyceride, CE = cholesterol ester, FC = free cholesterol, PL = phospholipids, HDL = high density lipoproteins, FA = fatty acid, LPL = lipoprotein lipase, B = apolipoprotein B-48, A = apolipoprotein A-I, C = apolipoprotein C-II, E = apolipoprotein E.

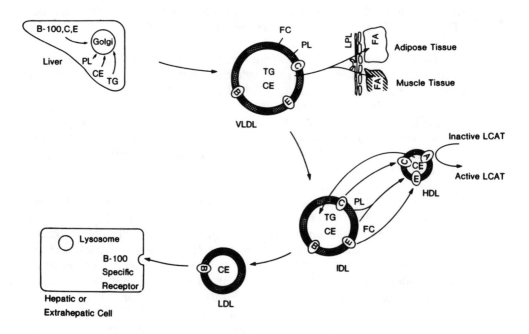

From: Rifai N. Lipoproteins and apolipoproteins: Composition, metabolism, and association with coronary heart disease. Arch Path Lab Med 1986;110:694-701. Copyright 1986, American Medical Association. Reproduced with permission

enter the bloodstream (Figure 15–1). LPL is attached to the luminal surface of endothelial cells that line capillaries of adipose and muscle tissue. Apo C-II is transferred from HDL to chylomicrons, where it enables LPL to hydrolyse chylomicron triglyceride, producing free fatty acids. The fatty acids may either be taken up into muscle cells, where they are used for energy, or into adipose cells, where they are resynthesized into triglyceride and stored for future use. As the triglyceride core in the chylomicron core is depleted, some of the surface material such as phospholipid, and apolipoproteins, are transferred to HDL, and a chylomicron remnant particle is produced. These remnants retain core cholesterol ester, apo B-48, and apo E. The remnants then bind via apo E to chylomicron remnant receptors to the surface of hepatic cells and are then internalized. The cholesterol from these remnants can downregulate 3-hydroxy-3-methylglutaryl coenzyme A reductase (HMG-CoA reductase), the rate-limiting enzyme of cholesterol biosynthesis.

Endogenous Pathway

The liver synthesizes triglycerides from carbohydrates and fatty acids (Figure 15–2). When dietary cholesterol, derived from the receptor-mediated uptake of chylomicron remnants, is insufficient, the liver synthesizes its own cholesterol by increasing the activity of HMG-CoA

FIGURE 15–2. Endogenous Lipoprotein Metabolism Pathway

TG = triglyceride, CE = cholesterol ester, FC = free cholesterol, PL = phospholipids, HDL = high density lipoproteins, LDL = low density lipoproteins, IDL = intermediate density lipoproteins, VLDL = very low density lipoproteins, FA = fatty acid, LPL = lipoprotein lipase, LCAT = lecithin cholesterol acyltransferase, B = apolipoprotein B-100, A = apolipoprotein A-I, C = apolipoprotein C-II, E = apolipoprotein E.

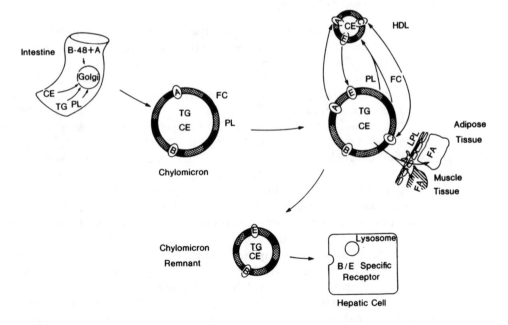

From: Rifai N. Lipoproteins and apolipoproteins: Composition, metabolism, and association with coronary heart disease. Arch Path Lab Med 1986;110:694-701. Copyright 1986, American Medical Association. Reproduced with permission.

reductase. The endogenously made triglycerides and cholesterol are then packaged into VLDL for export.

After excretion from the liver, the VLDL particles acquire apo C-II from HDL and then interact with LPL in tissue capillaries, releasing most of their triglycerides as free fatty acids to be used for energy or storage. As the sizes of VLDL particles diminish through this interaction, their densities increase and the particles are converted into IDL.

Surface material from IDL, including some phospholipids, free cholesterol, and apolipoproteins, are transferred to HDL, and cholesterol ester is transferred from HDL to IDL. The net result of the coupled lipolysis and the cholesterol ester exchange reactions is the replacement of much of the triglyceride core of IDL with cholesterol esters. IDL then undergoes a further conversion in which most of the remaining triglycerides are removed, probably by hepatic triglyceride lipase on the surface of the liver, and all apolipoproteins except B-100 are transferred to other lipoproteins. The resultant particles, which contain mostly cholesterol ester in the core and apo B-100 at the surface, are LDL. A variable fraction of IDL is not converted to LDL, but is taken up into hepatocytes via the LDL (B, E) receptors.

Low Density Lipoprotein Receptor Pathway

The lysine and arginine residues in apo B-100 of LDL bind to high-affinity receptors in coated pits on plasma membranes of hepatic and extra-hepatic cells (Figure 15–3).[20] LDL are then internalized and an endosome formed. The LDL receptors are recycled back to the cell surface, while the LDL particles in the endosome migrate toward the Golgi-endoplasmic reticulum-lysosome region. Once the LDL are delivered to the lysosomes, their apo B-100 component is degraded to small peptides and amino acids, and their cholesterol esters are hydrolyzed to free cholesterol and fatty acids. The free cholesterol has regulating functions in that it inhibits the activity of HMG-CoA reductase and downregulates the production of LDL receptors. Both of these actions apparently occur through the interaction of a derivative of cholesterol, hydroxycholesterol, with specific (and homologous) areas in the regulatory portions of the reductase gene and the LDL receptor gene.

LDL can also be taken up and degraded by a low-affinity process. This mechanism is not saturable, and as the plasma LDL concentrations increase, more LDL are taken up by this route. The non-receptor mediated mechanism is not regulated, and LDL continue to enter, leading to an excess accumulation of cholesteryl esters. For example, when this happens in macrophages and in other scavenger cells, these cells may be converted to "foam cells," which are considered the earliest components of the atherosclerotic lesion. It has been estimated that normally about two-thirds of LDL are degraded by the high-affinity

FIGURE 15–3. Low Density Lipoprotein Receptor Pathway

LDL = low density lipoproteins, ACAT = acyl-CoA cholesterol acyltransferase, HMG-CoA reductase = 3-hydroxy-3-methylglutaryl coenzyme A reductase. Because of the presence of apolipoprotein B-100 on its surface, LDL particle is recognized by a specific receptor in a coated pit and taken into the cell in a coated vesicle (top right). Coated vesicles fuse together to form an endosome. The acidic environment of the endosome causes LDL particle to dissociate from the receptors, which return to the cell surface. The LDL particles are taken to a lysosome where apolipoprotein B-100 is broken down into amino acids and cholesterol ester is converted to free cholesterol for cellular needs. The cellular cholesterol level is self-regulated. Oversupply of cholesterol will lead to: (1) decrease rate of cholesterol synthesis by inhibiting HMG-CoA reductase, (2) increased storage of cholesteryl esters by activating ACAT, and (3) inhibition of manufacturing new LDL receptors by suppressing the transcription of the receptor gene into messenger RNA.

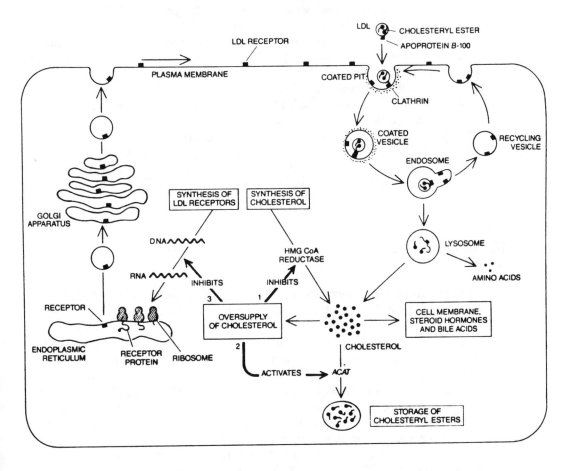

From: Brown MS and Goldstein JL. How LDL receptors influence cholesterol and atherosclerosis. Sci Am 1984;251:58-66. Copyright 1984 by Scientific American, Inc. All rights reserved. Reproduced with permission.

receptor pathway, with the remainder removed by the non-receptor mediated pathway.

Reverse Cholesterol Transport Pathway

HDL are secreted as nascent particles from either liver or intestine (Figure 15–4). These disc-like particles are round and flat and consist primarily of phospholipid in the core, surrounded by apo A-1.

Through the action of LCAT and its co-factor, apo A-1, free cholesterol is removed from peripheral tissues (Figure 15–4) and esterified by the transfer of a fatty acid from lecithin to cholesterol. In the process, HDL particle is converted from a disc to a sphere that contains cholesteryl ester in its core. The cholesteryl ester may be transferred up to VLDL (IDL) by a cholesteryl ester transfer protein (CETP) or taken up directly by the liver by an HDL receptor.

While LDL are the major products resulting from the catabolism of VLDL, some conversion of HDL subfractions also occurs during this process. Surface material from the triglyceride-rich particles are transferred to HDL3 circulating in the plasma, which are subsequently converted to cholesterol ester-rich HDL2 by the action of LCAT. It has been shown that *in vitro* HDL2 was converted back to HDL3 in the presence of hepatic lipoprotein lipase.[21] HDL2 can carry twice as many cholesterol molecules per unit of apolipoprotein compared to HDL3. Thus, they can be viewed as a doubly efficient vehicle for the transfer of cholesterol from the peripheral tissues back to the liver.

PEDIATRIC LIPID AND LIPOPROTEIN CHOLESTEROL CONCENTRATIONS

As a result of their complex metabolism, the plasma concentrations of lipids, lipoproteins, and apolipoproteins are distributed over a wide range of values. Mean serum cholesterol concentration increases from about 66 mg/dL (1.71 mmol/L) at birth to about 155 mg/dL (4.02 mmol/L) at age 3. Approximately half of serum cholesterol at birth is carried in HDL. The LDL-C concentration increases rapidly in the first weeks of life as LDL become the major carrier of serum cholesterol. At age 5, LDL-C concentration is about 97 mg/dL (2.5 mmol/L) and HDL-C is about 54 mg/dL (1.4 mmol/L). Serum total and lipoprotein cholesterol concentrations of males and females in the first two decades of life are presented in Tables 15–3 and 15–4.[22] Later in life, males will have higher LDL-C but lower HDL-C than females, a lipoprotein profile that places males at greater risk of CHD.

FIGURE 15–4. Reverse Cholesterol Transport Pathway

HDL = high density lipoproteins, LDL = low density lipoproteins, IDL = intermediate density lipoproteins, HTL = hepatic lipoprotein lipase, LCAT = lecithin cholesterol acyltransferase, CETP = cholesteryl ester transfer protein, apo E = apolipoprotein E. Cholesterol is removed from macrophages and other arterial wall cells by an HDL-mediated process. The LCAT esterifies the cholesterol content of HDL to prevent it from reentering the cells. Cholesterol esters are delivered to the liver by either one of three pathways: (1) cholesterol esters are transferred from HDL to LDL by CETP and enter the liver through the specific LDL receptor pathway; (2) cholesterol esters are selectively taken from HDL by HDL receptors and HDL particles are returned to circulation for further transport; or (3) HDL have accumulated apo E and therefore the particles can enter the liver through remnant receptors.

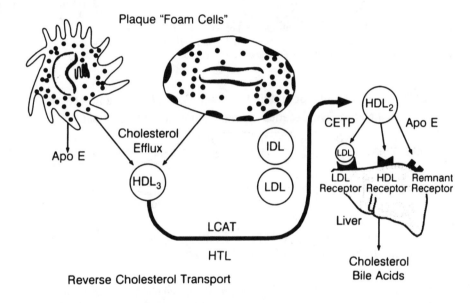

From: Gwynne JT. High density lipoprotein cholesterol levels as a marker of reverse cholesterol transport. Am J Cardiol 1989;64:10G-17G. Reproduced with permission.

DISORDERS OF LIPOPROTEIN METABOLISM

For the purpose of identifying children and adolescents more likely to have an inherited disorder of lipoprotein metabolism, cutpoints have been established above the 95th percentile for increased cholesterol, LDL-C, and triglyceride and the below the 5th percentile for low HDL-C (Tables 15–3 and 15–4).

TABLE 15–3. Serum Lipid Concentrations of Males and Females in the First Two Decades of Life [values in mg/dL(mmol/L)]

Age/Sex	Cholesterol			Triglyceride		
	5th	50th	95th	5th	50th	95th
0–4 y						
Female	112 (2.90)	156 (4.04)	200 (5.18)	34 (0.38)	64 (0.72)	112 (1.27)
Male	114 (2.95)	155 (4.01)	203 (5.26)	29 (0.33)	56 (0.63)	99 (1.12)
5–9 y						
Female	126 (3.26)	164 (4.25)	205 (5.31)	32 (0.36)	60 (0.68)	105 (1.19)
Male	121 (3.13)	160 (4.14)	203 (5.26)	30 (0.34)	56 (0.63)	101 (1.14)
10–14 y						
Female	124 (3.21)	160 (4.14)	201 (5.21)	37 (0.42)	75 (0.85)	131 (1.48)
Male	119 (3.08)	158 (4.09)	202 (5.23)	32 (0.36)	66 (0.75)	125 (1.41)
15–19 y						
Female	120 (3.11)	158 (4.09)	203 (5.26)	39 (0.44)	75 (0.85)	132 (1.49)
Male	113 (2.93)	150 (3.89)	197 (5.10)	37 (0.42)	78 (0.88)	148 (1.67)

Data compiled from: Lipid Metabolism Branch, Division of Heart, Lung, and Blood Institute. The Lipid Research Clinics population studies data book, Vol I: The prevalence study. Bethesda, MD: National Institutes of Health, 1980. [NIH Publication No. 80-1527]

TABLE 15–4. Serum Lipoprotein Concentrations of Males and Females in the First Two Decades of Life [values in mg/dL (mmol/L)]

Age/Sex	LDL-C			VLDL-C			HDL-C		
	5th	50th	95th	5th	50th	95th	5th	50th	95th
5–9 y									
Female	68 (1.76)	100 (2.59)	140 (3.63)	1 (0.03)	10 (0.26)	24 (0.62)	36 (0.93)	53 (1.37)	73 (1.89)
Male	63 (1.63)	93 (2.41)	129 (3.34)	0	8 (0.21)	18 (0.47)	38 (0.98)	56 (1.45)	75 (1.94)
10–14 y									
Female	68 (1.76)	97 (2.51)	136 (3.52)	2 (0.05)	11 (0.28)	23 (0.60)	37 (0.96)	52 (1.35)	70 (1.81)
Male	64 (1.66)	97 (2.51)	133 (3.44)	1 (0.03)	10 (0.26)	22 (0.57)	37 (0.96)	55 (1.42)	74 (1.92)
15–19 y									
Female	59 (1.53)	96 (2.49)	137 (3.55)	2 (0.05)	12 (0.31)	24 (0.62)	35 (0.91)	52 (1.35)	74 (1.92)
Male	62 (1.61)	94 (2.43)	130 (3.37)	2 (0.05)	13 (0.34)	26 (0.67)	30 (0.78)	46 (1.19)	63 (1.63)

HDL = high density lipoproteins, LDL = low density lipoproteins, VLDL = very low density lipoproteins. Data compiled from: Lipid Metabolism Branch, Division of Heart, Lung, and Blood Institute. The Lipid Research Clinics population studies data book, Vol I: The prevalence study. Bethesda, MD: National Institutes of Health, 1980. [NIH Publication No. 80-1527]

Primary versus Secondary Hyperlipidemia

Upon making the diagnosis of hyperlipidemia in a given child, the hyperlipidemic status should be evaluated as to whether it is primary or secondary to one of a variety of metabolic diseases. The diagnosis of primary hyperlipidemia can only be made after secondary causes are ruled out. The secondary causes of hyperlipoproteinemia in children and adolescents are listed in Table 15–5.[23] The secondary causes most commonly seen in the first year of life are glycogen storage disease and congenital biliary atresia. Hypothyroidism, nephrotic syndrome, and diabetes mellitus are more prevalent metabolic causes later in childhood. However, exogenous factors such as dietary and alcohol intake, oral contraceptives, pharmacological agents (steroids, isotretinoin [Accutane], β-blockers, etc.) are the main secondary causes of hyperlipidemia in the first two decades of life.[16, 23]

TABLE 15–5. Causes of Secondary Hyperlipidemia and Hyperlipoproteinemia in Children and Adolescents

Disorder	Cause
Exogenous	Alcohol Contraceptives Steroid therapy Isotretinoin (Accutane®)
Endocrine and Metabolic	Acute intermittent prophyria Diabetes mellitus Hypopituitarism Hypothyroidism Lipodystrophy Pregnancy
Storage Disease	Cystine storage disease Gaucher's disease Glycogen storage disease Juvenile Tay-Sachs disease Niemann-Pick disease Tay-Sachs disease
Renal	Chronic renal failure Hemolytic-uremic syndrome Nephrotic syndrome
Hepatic	Benign recurrent intrahepatic cholestasis Congenital biliary atresia
Acute and Transient	Burns Hepatitis
Others	Anorexia nervosa Idiopathic hypercalcemia Klinefelter's syndrome Progeria (Hutchinson-Gilford syndrome) Systemic lupus erythematosus Werner's syndrome

From: Kwiterovich PO Jr. Disorders of lipid and lipoprotein metabolism. In Rudolph AM (Ed.), Rudolph's pediatrics, 19th ed. Norwalk, CT: Appleton-Lange, 1991:361-75. Reproduced with permission.

Familial Dyslipoproteinemia

Historically, lipoprotein phenotypes reflecting lipoprotein metabolic disorders were classified according to Fredrickson and co-workers (Table 15–6). However, these disorders can now be approached based on the four metabolic pathways discussed above (Figures 15–1 to 15–4).[14, 16, 19] Defects in these pathways leading to hyperlipidemia may be

TABLE 15–6. Classification of Hyperlipidemia

Frederickson Type	Lipid Elevation	Lipoprotein Elevation	Prevalence in Childhood
I	Triglyceride	Chylomicrons	Rare
IIa	Cholesterol	LDL	Common
IIb	Cholesterol Triglyceride	LDL VLDL	Uncommon
III	Cholesterol Triglyceride	beta-VLDL (cholesterol- rich VLDL remnant)	Very rare
IV	Triglyceride	VLDL	Uncommon
V	Triglyceride Cholesterol	VLDL Chylomicrons	Very rare

LDL = low density lipoproteins, VLDL = very low density lipoproteins.
From: Diagnosis and treatment of primary hyperlipidemia in childhood: A joint statement for physicians by the Committee on Atherosclerosis and Hypertension in Childhood of the Council on Cardiovascular Disease in the Young and the Nutrition Committee, American Heart Association. Circulation 1986;74:1181A-8A. Copyright 1986, American Heart Association. Reprinted with permission.

related to (1) increased production of lipoproteins; (2) abnormal intra-vascular processing, e.g., enzymatic hydrolysis of triglyceride; and (3) defective cellular uptake of lipoproteins. Finally, a significant decrease in production and/or an increase in removal of lipoproteins can lead to a marked *reduction* in lipid concentrations.

Exogenous Triglyceride Pathway
(Figure 15-1)

Deficiency in Lipoprotein Lipase Activity

A deficiency in the LPL activity causes severe hyperchylomicronemia (triglyceride as high as 10,000 mg/dL (113 mmol/L). The LPL is needed to hydrolyze triglyceride, and convert chylomicrons, the tri-glyceride-rich particles, to chylomicron remnants. The massive accumulation of chylomicrons in the bloodstream indicates the inability to catabolize dietary fat. VLDL-C concentration is usually normal and HDL-C and LDL-C concentrations are low (Type I). The diagnosis of LPL deficiency is made by determining the enzyme activity in plasma after the administration of heparin. The concentration of apo C-II, the activator of LPL, in these patients is normal. Patients with this disorder generally present in the first decade of life with eruptive xanthomas, lipemia retinalis, and colicky abdominal pain. Overt pancreatitis can develop. LPL deficiency is an extremely rare autosomal recessive disorder (< 1 in 100,000). Several insertions and deletions in the LPL gene that cause the deficiency in the activity of this enzyme have been described.[24]

Deficiency in Apolipoprotein C-II

Deficiency in the LPL cofactor apo C-II produces hypertriglyceridemia that ranges in severity from 800 mg/dL (9.04 mmol/L) to 10,000 mg/dL (113 mmol/L).[24] Total cholesterol concentration in these patients varies considerably, from 151 to 980 mg/dL (3.91 to 25.38 mmol/L). However, HDL-C and LDL-C concentrations are below the 5th percentile at approximately 36 mg/dL (0.93 mmol/L) and 65 mg/dL (1.68 mmol/L), respectively.[16, 24] The LPL activity is very low or absent, secondary to an almost undetectable concentration of apo C-II. As in LPL deficiency, patients with this disorder are not at risk of premature CHD, but recurrent pancreatitis in adulthood can be life threatening. Apo C-II deficiency is a rare disease and is inherited in an autosomal recessive mode. Several mutations in the apo C-II gene have been shown to produce this disorder.[24]

Endogenous Triglyceride Pathway Overproduction of Very Low Density Lipoprotein (Figure 15-2)

Familial Combined Hyperlipidemia (FCH)

About 10–15% of patients with premature CHD (under the age of 55 years) have this disorder. The adult kindred members with FCH may have increased LDL-C alone (> 190 mg/dL [4.92 mmol/L]) (Type IIa), increased triglyceride alone (> 250 mg/dL [6.48 mmol/L]) (Type IV), or increases in both parameters (Type IIb).[16] The overproduction of VLDL-apo B-100 in these patients causes LDL-apo B-100 concentration to be increased. Therefore, even in patients with Type IV, who have normal LDL-C, the ratio of LDL-C to LDL-apo B-100 is decreased (small, dense LDL). Furthermore, FCH patients often have decreased HDL-C, particularly if hypertriglyceridemia is present. This disorder is inherited in an autosomal dominant mode, with an incidence of 1 in 100 individuals. There is a delayed expression of FCH before age 20, but children from families with premature CHD can present with increased cholesterol or triglyceride, or both lipids may be increased.

Hyperapobetalipoproteinemia

Up to a third of patients with premature CHD have a lipoprotein phenotype, hyperapobetalipoproteinemia (hyperapoB). This disorder is characterized by an increased LDL-apo B-100 concentration with normal or moderately increased LDL-C values.[25] In these patients, total cholesterol and triglyceride concentrations are often normal but can be increased, and HDL-C and apo A-I are usually low. Although the exact defects have not yet been established, it appears that an increased hepatic synthesis of VLDL and apo B-100, which leads to the formation of small, dense LDL, and a decreased removal of dietary fat contribute to the formation of hyperapoB. The exact mode of inheritance and the prevalence of hyperapoB also remain uncertain. However, one third of children of a parent who had premature CHD and hyperapoB will also have hyperapoB. HyperapoB may also occur in families with FCH.

Familial Hypertriglyceridemia (FHT) (Type IV)

Production of large VLDL with an abnormally high triglyceride content is responsible for this disorder. Patients with FHT have increased VLDL cholesterol and triglyceride and normal LDL-C and apo B-100 serum concentrations; therefore, there is no increase in the conversion of VLDL to LDL. The HDL-C in FHT patients is decreased, probably secondary to the hypertriglyceridemia. Patients with FHT could develop glucose intolerance, hyperuricemia, obesity, and peripheral vascular disease later in life.[16] FHT is inherited in an autosomal dominant mode with a delayed expression; about 1 in 5 children born to affected parents manifest the phenotype early in life.

Both Exogenous and Endogenous Pathways (Figures 15-1 & 15-2)

Type V Hyperlipoproteinemia

Patients with this rare disorder have a marked hypertriglyceridemia resulting from increased chylomicrons and VLDL. Clinical findings include eruptive xanthomas, lipemia retinalis, pancreatitis, and abnormal glucose tolerance with hyperinsulinism.[16] Although this disorder is not usually expressed in childhood, several affected preadolescents have been described. The exact etiology of this disorder is unknown. It can either be due to an increased production or a decreased removal of VLDL or to a combination of both.

Dysbetalipoproteinemia (Type III)

This disorder is very rare in children and is caused by a defect in the removal of both chylomicron remnants and VLDL remnants.[16, 26] Serum cholesterol and triglyceride concentrations in dysbetalipoproteinemic patients are often increased to an equal degree and HDL-C and LDL-C are decreased.[16] The VLDL-C to serum triglyceride ratio in these patients is > 0.3 (normal: 0.15–0.25). Premature vascular disease and xanthomas can occur, but the yellow deposits in the crease of the palms are very characteristic of this disorder. This disease is caused by a defect in apo E resulting in faulty binding of apo E to both the chylomicron remnant and LDL (B, E) receptors on the hepatic cells; the increased concentration of triglyceride-rich particles is due to their faulty removal. As discussed earlier, apo E exists as three major isoforms, E2, E3, and E4. Apo E3 is the most common allele and apo E2 is the rarest. Most patients with dysbetalipoproteinemia are homozygotic for the apo E2 allele. The presence of the E2E2 phenotype is a necessary but insufficient cause of dysbetalipoproteinemia; overproduction of VLDL must also be present for the full-blown "Type III syndrome" to be expressed.

Low Density Lipoprotein Receptor Pathway (Figure 15-3)

Familial Hypercholesterolemia (Type IIa)

This disorder is inherited as an autosomal dominant and expressed in a heterozygous or homozygous mode with complete expression of high LDL-C at birth. Family studies to confirm the increased LDL-C concentration are essential to substantiate the diagnosis of familial hypercholesterolemia (FH). Heterozygous FH is a commonly seen genetic metabolic disorder with an incidence of 1 in 200–500 individuals in the United States. At birth, patients with heterozygous FH will have LDL-C concentrations higher than the 95th percentile (41 mg/dL [1.06 mmol/L]). After 1 year of age, FH heterozygotes often have total and LDL cholesterol concentrations over the 99th percentile (230 mg/dL [5.96 mmol/L] and 160 mg/dL [4.14 mmol/L], respectively). The HDL-C in these patients is often below average. Some develop tendon xanthomas during the second decade of life, but most heterozygous FH children are asymptomatic. CHD often occurs in the forties in men and in the fifties in women.

The prevalence of homozygous FH is 1 in 1,000,000. Patients will have cholesterol concentrations of 500–1000 mg/dL (12.95–25.90 mmol/L) and usually develop planar xanthomas by the age of 5 years. Angina pectoris, myocardial infarction, and aortic stenosis ordinarily occur before age 20.[16, 23]

FH is the result of a defect in the removal of LDL and therefore a large concentration of these particles accumulates in circulation. The defects include reduced or absent LDL binding because of defective or absent LDL receptors or defective internalization of the bound LDL particles. A number of different mutations in the LDL receptor gene which affect normal synthesis, transport, binding to LDL and internalization of the LDL receptor have been identified in FH.[27]

Familial Defective Apolipoprotein B-100

A mutation in the apo B-100 gene causes a substitution of glutamine for arginine at the residue 3500 in apo B-100 polypeptide, resulting in a reduced positive charge of the ligand and a decreased affinity of LDL to its negatively charged receptor. Therefore, patients with this disorder will have an increased LDL-C due to inadequate removal of LDL from circulation by normal receptors. The incidence of this disorder in children is unknown at present.

Reverse Cholesterol Transport Pathway
(Figure 15-4)

Familial Hypoalphalipoproteinemia

Low HDL-C (below the 5th percentile) and normal lipid and LDL-C concentrations are the characteristics of this syndrome.[16] Although adult patients with this disorder are clinically normal, they are at increased risk of developing CHD. The exact etiology of this disorder is unknown; however, it may involve decreased production or increased catabolism of HDL or apo A-I. This disorder is relatively uncommon in children.

Defects in Decreased Synthesis of Apolipoprotein A-I

Mutations such as a rearrangement at the apolipoprotein gene locus that inactivates both apo A-I and C-III, a deletion of the entire locus, or an insertion in the apo A-I gene will lead to decreased synthesis and an abnormally low serum concentration of apo A-I.[28] Homozygotic patients have no detectable serum apo A-I and traces of HDL-C. Their risk of developing premature CHD is high and they have corneal clouding. Heterozygotes have HDL-C concentrations that are about 50% of normal.

Defects in Increased Catabolism of Apolipoprotein A-I
(Tangier Disease)

This disorder is characterized by both a severely reduced serum concentration of HDL and abnormal HDL composition.[29] Apo A-I, which is also markedly decreased, is synthesized by intestinal cells but rapidly catabolized in plasma. The composition and concentration of the other lipoproteins are abnormal as well. Total and LDL cholesterol concentrations in these patients are below the 5th percentile (112 mg/dL [2.90 mmol/L] and 65 mg/dL [1.68 mmol/L], respectively) and triglyceride is normal or slightly increased. These patients have significant deposition of cholesteryl esters that results in relapsing peripheral neuropathy, splenomegaly and enlarged orange-yellow tonsils. Although the incidence of Tangier disease in children is very rare, children as young as 3 years have been diagnosed with this disorder.

SCREENING AND DIAGNOSIS ("WHO")

Traditionally, hypercholesterolemia in children and adolescents has been defined as a total or LDL cholesterol concentration higher than the 95th percentile (200 mg/dL [5.18 mmol/L] and 130 mg/dL [3.37 mmol/L], respectively). The National Cholesterol Education Program (NCEP) Expert Panel on Blood Cholesterol Levels in Children and Adolescents of the National Institutes of Health[30] and the American Academy of Pediatrics (AAP)[31, 32] used a similar definition of "high cholesterol" (≥ 200 mg/dL) and high LDL-C cholesterol (≥ 130 mg/dL) in children and adolescents from families with hypercholesterolemia or premature CHD. A "borderline" cholesterol concentration was defined as 170–199 mg/dL (4.40–5.15 mmol/L) and "borderline" LDL-C concentration 110–129 mg/dL (2.85–3.34 mmol/L). Borderline values are above the 75th percentile for both analytes.

The NCEP Expert Panel on Blood Cholesterol Levels in Children and Adolescents actually referred to cholesterol values < 170 mg/dL (4.40 mmol/L) and LDL-C values < 110 mg/dL (2.85 mmol/L) as "desirable." Children tend to have higher HDL-C concentrations than adults. Therefore, it is important to determine LDL-C and HDL-C concentrations before classifying the child as hypercholesterolemic.

Cholesterol screening to diagnose hypercholesterolemia is currently recommended for all adults in the United States.[33] However, for children, such a screening program remains highly controversial. According to the NCEP and the AAP,[30-32] only children above age 2 with a family history of hypercholesterolemia (≥ 240 mg/dL [6.22 mmol/L]) or early documented CHD (at 55 years of age or less), myocardial infarction, angina pectoris, peripheral vascular disease, cerebrovascular disease, or sudden cardiac death should be screened for hypercholesterolemia. However, several studies have demonstrated the deficiency of the selective approach and have advocated general screening for children.[34-37] The results of the Bogalusa heart study actually demonstrated that by using the selective screening criteria, only 50% of white children and 20% of black children with high LDL-C concentration (above the 95th percentile, at about 130 mg/dL [3.37 mmol/L]) were detected.[34] However, general screening is expensive, time consuming, and will generate a large amount of work in respect to follow-up. Furthermore, a significant number of children with high cholesterol concentrations will not remain hypercholesterolemic as adults.

Another possible yet unpopular approach is not to do screening at all, but to recommend a prudent low-fat diet, such as the Step-One diet of the American Heart Association (AHA), for all children (Table 15–7).[30, 31] Such an approach would not engender anxiety, labeling, or overzealous treatment; however, it would miss completely those children with significant hypercholesterolemia, who are most at risk for adult CHD.

TABLE 15–7. Current Fat Intake in American Children and Adolescents
and the American Heart Association Step-One and Step-Two Diets

Nutrients	Current Intake	Step One	Step Two
Total Fat			
(% of total calories)	35–36%	< 30%	< 30%
Saturated Fat	14%	< 10%	7%
Polyunsaturated Fat	6%	10%	10%
Monounsaturated Fat	13–14%	10–15%	10–15%
Cholesterol (mg/day)	193–296	< 300	< 200

Adapted from: National Cholesterol Education Program, Lipid Metabolism Branch, Division of Heart, Lung, and Blood Institute. The Report of the Expert Panel on Blood Cholesterol Levels in Children and Adolescents (draft). Bethesda, MD: National Institutes of Health, 1991.

Laboratory Methods for the Diagnosis and Management of Lipoprotein Disorders ("HOW")

The determination of lipid and lipoprotein concentrations is essential in the diagnosis and management of hyperlipoproteinemia. Furthermore, these tests are used in the assessment of CHD risk. Increased concentration of total cholesterol, LDL-C, and apo B-100 and decreased concentration of HDL-C and apo A-I are associated with increased risk of developing premature CHD.

Accurate determination of serum lipids, lipoproteins, and apolipoproteins is dependent on the control of both analytical and preanalytical factors. Preanalytical variations result from differences in life style of patients, altered lipid metabolism due to disease, source of the blood specimen, and conditions of specimen collection. Components of variation can be classified as biological, behavioral, clinical, variability in specimen collection and handling, and analytical.

The NCEP Laboratory Standardization Panel (LSP) issued specific recommendations to minimize the effect of preanalytical factors on lipid and lipoprotein testing.[38, 39] The panel recommends the following:

1. An individual's lipid and lipoprotein profile should only be measured when the individual is in a metabolic steady state.

2. Subjects should maintain their usual diet and weight for at least 2 weeks prior to the determination of their lipids or lipoproteins.

3. Multiple measurements within 2 months, at least 1 week apart, should be performed before making a medical decision about further action.

4. Patients should not perform vigorous physical activity within the 24-h period prior to testing.

5. Fasting or non-fasting specimens can be used for total cholesterol testing. However, a 12-h fasting specimen is required for triglycerides and lipoproteins.

6. The patient should be seated for at least 5 min before specimen collection.

7. The tourniquet should not be kept on more than 1 min during venipuncture.

8. Total cholesterol, triglyceride, and HDL-C concentrations can be determined in either serum or plasma. When EDTA is used as the anticoagulant, plasma should be immediately cooled to 2–4° C to prevent changes in composition and values should be multiplied by 1.03.

9. For total cholesterol testing, serum can be transported either at 4° C or frozen. Storage of specimens at –20° C is adequate for total cholesterol measurement. However, specimens must be stored frozen at –70° C or lower for triglyceride and lipoprotein and apolipoprotein testing.

10. Blood specimens should always be considered potentially infectious and therefore must be handled accordingly.

No specific recommendations were made by the panel concerning apolipoprotein testing. However, similar steps to those described should be taken to help minimize preanalytical sources of variation in apolipoprotein measurements.

The principles of the most commonly used methodologies in clinical laboratories for the determination of total, HDL, and LDL cholesterol, triglyceride, and apolipoproteins are briefly discussed in this chapter. Additional information is available in clinical chemistry textbooks.

Electrophoretic Separation of Lipoproteins

Electrophoresis separates lipoproteins according to their charges and allows the visual examination of their patterns.[15] Such an examination can be useful in the diagnosis of the various types of hyperlipoproteinemia. Although this technique is easily performed and requires simple equipment, it is a qualitative or a semi-quantitative method at best. In addition, lipoprotein electrophoresis cannot differentiate normal from abnormal lipid transport because only the ester bonds of triglyceride and cholesterol are stained; free cholesterol and phospholipids remain unstained. Therefore, patients with biliary cirrhosis would have a normal electrophoretic pattern in spite of a cholesterol concentration > 1000 mg/dL (25.9 mmol/L). Lipoprotein electrophoresis should always be coupled with quantitative measurements of plasma lipids and lipoproteins.

Measurement of Total Cholesterol Concentration

According to proficiency surveys (College of American Pathologists Comprehensive Proficiency Surveys), almost all clinical laboratories in the United States measure cholesterol enzymatically. This reaction first involves the hydrolysis of cholesterol ester by cholesterol esterase. Free cholesterol is then oxidized in the presence of cholesterol oxidase and hydrogen peroxide is generated. The hydrogen peroxide is coupled with an enzymatic reaction to form a colored oxidation product or a reduced pyridine nucleotide. The intensity of the generated color or the increase in absorbance is proportional to the cholesterol concentration. The cholesterol ester step is critical. Incomplete hydrolysis of cholesterol ester will lead to underestimation of the cholesterol concentration.

According to the NCEP, total cholesterol should be measured until 1992 with bias and imprecision of less than 5%, which corresponds to total allowable error for a single cholesterol measurement of ± 14.2%. Starting in 1992, cholesterol should be determined with bias and imprecision of less than 3%, which corresponds to total allowable error of ± 8.9 percent.[40]

A survey conducted by Children's National Medical Center revealed that 60% of pediatricians in the Washington, D.C., metropolitan area determine cholesterol concentration in their practice using a variety of desktop analyzers. Most of these analyzers perform adequately in the hands of skilled laboratory personnel; however, when used by poorly trained individuals, the results are usually less than desirable.

Since the diagnosis of hypercholesterolemia in children and adolescents will most likely be made in the pediatrician's or family practitioner's office, it is crucial that cholesterol concentration is measured correctly in these settings. At present, cholesterol testing in the physician's office is not as well regulated as that performed in clinical laboratories. State and federal regulatory agencies are beginning to deal with regulatory issues concerning physician's office testing. The NCEP-LSP, however, has recently issued recommendations regarding cholesterol testing outside the clinical laboratories.[38, 41] These recommendations include:

1. the use of accurate and precise analyzers (capable of determining cholesterol concentration within 3% bias of reference values and 3% imprecision);

2. the use of a properly trained operator (ideally, a trained medical technician or technologist);

3. the institution of a quality control system and the participation in proficiency surveys;

4. the use of a system of split-sample analyses to routinely compare cholesterol testing done in the physician's office to that done in a qualified laboratory; and

5. the use of a proper patient preparation procedure to minimize the preanalytical variations.

Such actions will ensure that the quality of testing done in the physician's office is comparable to that of a hospital or reference laboratory.

Measurement of Triglyceride Concentration

Serum triglyceride concentration is determined to establish the triglyceridemic status of an individual as well as to estimate LDL-C concentration (see the section below on estimation of low density lipoprotein cholesterol). Almost all clinical laboratories determine triglyceride concentration enzymatically. Triglycerides are hydrolyzed to glycerol in the presence of lipase. Complete triglyceride hydrolysis is essential for the accurate determination of this analyte. Glycerol is then coupled by one or more enzymatic reactions to generate either a colored dye or an ultraviolet light-absorbing chemical. The intensity of the produced color or the increase in absorbance is proportional to the triglyceride concentration.

Glycerol is a product of normal metabolic processes. Therefore, triglyceride concentration could be overestimated if not corrected for the endogenous glycerol.[42] In normal subjects, endogenous glycerol represents the equivalent of 10–20 mg/dL (0.11–0.22 mmol/L) triglyceride, which is a tolerable bias. However, in certain conditions, such as diabetes mellitus, emotional stress, intravenous administration of drugs or nutrients containing glycerol, contamination of blood collection devices by glycerol, and prolonged storage of whole blood under nonrefrigerated conditions, endogenous glycerol concentrations will be significantly higher and could complicate the interpretation of triglyceride values. In general, clinical chemists feel that the effect of endogenous glycerol will be minimized with careful specimen collection and storage. Furthermore, only minute fractions of samples analyzed in general clinical laboratories contain an appreciable quantity of endogenous glycerol. Therefore, only about 5% of all American clinical laboratories perform blank triglyceride measurements for endogenous glycerol.

Separation of High Density Lipoprotein Fractions

The HDL fractions are separated from the other lipoproteins using precipitation techniques. Several precipitation reagents such as heparin-Mn^{++}, phosphotungstate, and dextran sulfate-Mg^{++} are commonly used to precipitate LDL and VLDL. The cholesterol concentration in the supernate, which represents HDL-C, is then quantitated enzymatically.

The precipitation procedure selected to measure HDL-C should be assessed for analytical performance.[43] Besides assessing the precision and accuracy, the specificity of the assay should be determined. The precipitation techniques used are normally reproducible when performed with a sensitive and reproducible cholesterol assay. The accuracy of the HDL-C assay can be determined by a direct patient specimen comparison with the Centers for Disease Control HDL-C procedure or other equivalent method with well-established accuracy. The specificity of the assay can be determined by the demonstration of complete precipitation of LDL and VLDL and/or no co-precipitation of HDL. This task can be established by:

1. lipoprotein electrophoresis of the supernate and resolubilized precipitate; the supernate should have an HDL or α band only and no β or pre–β band and the precipitate should have no HDL band.

2. measurement of apo A-I and B-100 in the supernate; the supernate should only have apo A-I and not apo B-100.

3. evaluation of the performance of the assay in the presence of high triglyceride concentration.

Estimation of Low Density Lipoprotein Cholesterol

The NCEP guidelines require the use of LDL-C concentration in the diagnosis and management of hypercholesterolemia. LDL-C is not measured in clinical laboratories but is estimated using the Friedewald equation:

LDL-C = Total cholesterol − (HDL-C + VLDL-C)
VLDL-C = Triglyceride/5 (for mg/dL or mg/L LDL-C values), or
VLDL-C = Triglyceride/2.22 (for mmol/L LDL-C values)

It has been shown that LDL-C values derived by the Friedewald formula correlate very highly with those determined by the reference method, the β quantification, when triglyceride concentrations are < 400 mg/dL (4.66 mmol/L).[44] Furthermore, 86% of LDL-C classifications based on NCEP cutpoints were shown to be concordant with those by measured LDL-C when triglyceride concentrations were < 400 mg/dL (4.66 mmol/L).[45]

Fasting specimens are required for the estimation of LDL-C by this formula. High triglyceride concentration can falsely overestimate VLDL-C and therefore underestimate LDL-C. Furthermore, patients with Type III hyperlipoproteinemia have VLDL that are enriched with cholesterol relative to triglyceride. The presence of these abnormal particles can result in an underestimation of VLDL-C and an overestimation of LDL-C. This can be especially problematic since a Type III patient can be misdiagnosed as having Type IIb hyperlipoproteinemia and the treatments for the two disorders are different.[46]

Measurement of Apolipoprotein Concentration

Apo A-I and B-100 are mainly measured in clinical laboratories by turbidimetric or nephelometric immunoassays. Other methods such as radioimmunoassay, radial immunodiffusion, and enzyme-linked immunosorbent assay are used in research settings and some specialized lipid laboratories. At the present time, apolipoprotein testing suffers from three problems: lack of standardization, lack of reference methods, and lack of reference intervals or cutoff values for clinical decisions.[47]

Considerable effort has been expended over the past few years by national and international organizations in overcoming the problems of apo A-I and B-100 standardization. The International Federation of Clinical Chemistry, along with other organizations, embarked on the ambitious pursuit of developing a secondary serum reference material which can be used, without fear of matrix interaction, as a master calibrator for all current commercial assays. This program has been successful and should be completed by the time this text is in print.

When assays for apo A-I and B-100 are standardized and reference methods are developed, dietary and drug intervention trials should be conducted to determine the extent of benefit expected in lowering CHD risk when apo B-100 is decreased and apo A-I is increased. Until this information is available, apolipoprotein measurement in routine patient care to diagnose and manage lipid disorders will be limited.

Management of Children and Adolescents with Hypercholesterolemia

To lower serum cholesterol concentration in children and adolescents, the NCEP adapted a strategy that combines two complementary approaches, a population approach and an individualized approach.[30]

American children and adolescents have relatively high cholesterol concentration and high intake of saturated fatty acids and cholesterol (Table 15–7).[30] The population approach attempts to lower the mean cholesterol concentration by instituting population-wide modification in nutrient intake and eating habits. The AHA Step-One diet is recommended (Table 15–7). Even a modest decrease in mean cholesterol concentration in children and adolescents, if carried into adulthood, could conceivably have a significant impact on lowering CHD incidence. The panel did not recommend any dietary changes for infants from birth to 2 years of age. Toddlers 2 and 3 years of age should start making the transition to the recommended eating pattern. The NCEP also directed recommendations to schools, health professionals, government agencies, the food industry, and the mass media to help influence and modify the eating habits of children and adolescents.

The individualized approach aims to lower cholesterol concentration of children over the age of 2 and adolescents who were identified by the selective screening process and the risk assessment protocol (Figure 15–5).[30] Those with an average LDL-C concentration between 110–129 mg/dL (2.85–3.34 mmol/L) will be placed on the

FIGURE 15–5. Risk Assessment Flowchart as Recommended by the National Cholesterol Education Program/Expert Panel on Blood Cholesterol Levels in Children and Adolescents

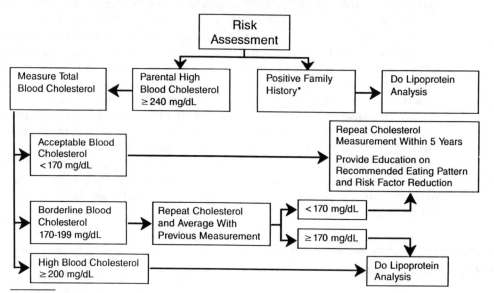

*Defined as a history of premature (before age 55 years) cardiovascular disease in a parent or grandparent

From: National Cholesterol Education Program, Lipid Metabolism Branch, Division of Heart, Lung, and Blood Institute. The Report of the Expert Panel on Blood Cholesterol Levels in Children and Adolescents (Draft), Bethesda, MD: National Institutes of Health, 1991.

AHA Step-One diet, counseled about other CHD risk factors, and reevaluated after 1 year. Those with an average LDL-C concentration ≥ 130 mg/dL (3.37 mmol/L) are also placed on the AHA Step-One diet, evaluated for secondary causes, and their family members are screened. If after 3 months of initiating the dietary therapy the LDL-C concentration remains ≥ 130 mg/dL (3.37 mmol/L), the patient is placed on the AHA Step-Two diet that entails further reduction of the saturated fatty acid and cholesterol intake (Table 15–7).

Drug therapy was recommended by the NCEP in children age 10 years and older if after careful adherence to dietary therapy (6 months to 1 year) the LDL-C concentration remains > 190 mg/dL (4.92 mmol/L) or LDL-C concentration remains > 160 mg/dL (4.14 mmol/L) and the patient has a positive family history of premature CHD or two or more other CHD risk factors. Only bile acid binding resins (cholestyramine and colestipol), which act by binding bile acids in the intestinal lumen, are recommended by the panel for use in children and adolescents. Other cholesterol-lowering drugs have no proven efficacy, relative freedom from side effects, or apparent safety when used in children and adolescents and therefore their use is discouraged in this patient population. Most FH homozygotes are resistant to drug therapy. Plasmapheresis every 2 weeks is a viable alternative to surgery (partial ileal bypass or portacaval shunt) to lower total and LDL cholesterol in these patients.[23]

Management of Children and Adolescents with Hypertriglyceridemia

Patients with primary mild hypertriglyceridemia without hypercholesterolemia are advised to follow a Step-One Diet control their blood glucose, lose weight, and abstain from alcohol intake. Those with primary severe hypertriglyceridemia however are placed on a very low fat diet (10–15 g/day in a child). Since medium-chain triglycerides are absorbed directly from the portal vein, they can replace fat in food preparations for these patients. Drug therapy is seldom used in these patients unless hypertriglyceridemia is accompanied by hypercholesterolemia.[23]

SUMMARY

Atherosclerosis, the cause of CHD, is a process that starts in childhood and develops slowly and silently. The clinical manifestations of CHD usually appear in the fifth or sixth decade of life. Increased serum total and LDL cholesterol and apo B-100 concentrations and/or decreased HDL-C and apo A-I concentrations correlate with increased risk of CHD. Children and adolescents of families with dyslipoproteinemia or premature CHD are at increased risk of developing this disease when they become adults. Therefore, the AAP and the NCEP have recommended screening all children over 2 years of age and adolescents with positive family history for hypercholesterolemia.

The physician must rule out the secondary causes of dyslipoproteinemia before making the diagnosis of a primary dyslipoproteinemia. The incidence, severity, and association with CHD risk vary significantly among the different types of dyslipoproteinemia. These disorders used to be classified according to Fredrickson. However, classification can now be better approached based on lipoprotein metabolic pathways.

Patients with hypercholesterolemia are treated with low-fat diet. Only children over 10 years of age with severe hypercholesterolemia will receive pharmacotherapy. Patients with hypertriglyceridemia are also treated with dietary means and advised to lose weight and abstain from alcoholic intake.

Since only a small fraction of patients with dyslipoproteinemia presents with clinical symptoms, the clinical laboratories are instrumental in making the initial diagnosis as well as monitoring the treatment of these patients.

REFERENCES

1. Gordon T., Kannel WB, Castelli WP, Dawber TR. Lipoproteins, cardiovascular disease, and death: The Framingham Study. Arch Intern Med 1981;141:1128-31.
2. Enos WF, Holmes RH, Beyer JC. Coronary disease among United States soldiers killed in action in Korea. JAMA 1953;152:1090-93.
3. McNamara JS, Molot MA, Stremple JF, et al. Coronary artery disease in combat casualties in Vietnam. JAMA 1971;216:1185-7.
4. Stary HC. The sequence of cell and matrix changes in atherosclerotic lesions of coronary arteries in the first forty years of life. Europ Heart J 1990;11(Supp E):3-19.
5. Strong JP and McGill HC Jr. The pediatric aspects of atherosclerosis. J Atherosclerosis Res 1969;40:37-49.
6. Newman WP, Wattigney W, Berenson GS. Autopsy studies in U.S. children and adolescents. Relationship of risk factors to atherosclerotic lesions. Ann NY Acad Sci 1991;623:16-25.
7. PDAY Research Group. Relationship of atherosclerosis in young men to serum lipoprotein cholesterol concentrations and smoking. A preliminary report from the Pathobiological Determinants of Atherosclerosis in the Youth (PDAY) Research Group. JAMA 1990;264:3018-24.
8. Knuiman JT, Hermus RJ, Hautvast JG. Serum total and high density lipoprotein cholesterol concentrations in rural and urban boys from 13 countries. Atherosclerosis 1980;36:529-37.
9. Lauer RM, Clarke WR. Use of cholesterol measurements in childhood for the prediction of adult hypercholesterolemia: The Muscatine study. JAMA 1990;264:3034-8.
10. Laskarzewski P, Morrison JA, deGroot I, et al. Lipid and lipoprotein tracking in 108 children over a four-year period. Pediatrics 1979;64:584-91.
11. Khoury P, Morrison JA, Kelly K, et al. Clustering and interrelationships of coronary heart disease risk factors on schoolchildren, age 6-19. Am J Epidemiol 1980;112:524-38.
12. Lee J, Lauer RM, Clarke WR. Lipoproteins in the progeny of young men with coronary artery disease: Children with increased risk. Pediatrics 1986;78:330-7.

13. Freedman DS, Srinivasan SR, Shear CL, et al. The relation of apolipoproteins AI and B in children to parental myocardial infarction. N Engl J Med 1986;315:721-6.

14. Rifai N. Lipoproteins and apolipoproteins. Composition, metabolism, and association with coronary heart disease. Arch Path Lab Med 1986;110:694-701.

15. Noble RP. Electrophoretic separation of plasma lipoproteins in agarose gel. J Lipid Res 1968;9:693-700.

16. Kwiterovich PO Jr. Diagnosis and management of familial dyslipoproteinemia in children and adolescents. Pediatr Clin North Am 1990;37:1489-523.

17. Mahley WR, Innerarity TL, Rall SC, et al. Plasma lipoproteins: Apolipoprotein structure and function. J Lipid Res 1984;25:1277-94.

18. Kane JP, Havel RJ. Disorders of the biogenesis and secretion of lipoproteins containing the B apolipoproteins. In: Scriver CR, Beaudet AL, Sly WS, Valle D, eds., The metabolic basis of inherited diseases, 6th ed. New York: McGraw-Hill, 1989:1139-64.

19. Gwynne JT. High density lipoprotein cholesterol levels as a marker of reverse cholesterol transport. Am J Cardiol 1989;64:10G-7.

20. Brown MS, Goldstein JL. A receptor-mediated pathway for cholesterol homeostasis. Science 1986;232:34-47.

21. Patsch JR, Prasad S, Gotto AM Jr, et al. Post prandial lipemia: A key for the conversion of HDL2 into HDL3 by hepatic lipase. J Clin Invest 1984;74:2017-23.

22. Lipid Metabolism Branch, Division of Heart, Lung, and Blood Institute. The Lipid Research Clinics population studies data book. Vol I: The prevalence study. Bethesda, MD: National Institutes of Health, 1980. [NIH Publication No. 80-1527]

23. Diagnosis and treatment of primary hyperlipidemia in childhood. A joint statement for physicians by the Committee on Atherosclerosis and Hypertension in Childhood of the Council on Cardiovascular Disease in the Young and the Nutrition Committee, American Heart Association. Circulation 1986;74:1181A-8.

24. Brunzell JD. Familial lipoprotein lipase deficiency and other causes of the chylomicronemia syndrome. In: Scriver CR, Beaudet AL, Sly WS, Valle D, eds., The metabolic basis of inherited diseases, 6th ed. New York: McGraw-Hill, 1989:1165-80.

25. Kwiterovich PO Jr. HyperapoB: A pleiotropic phenotype characterization by dense low-density lipoproteins and associated with coronary artery disease. Clin Chem 1988;34:B71-7.

26. Mahley RW, Rall SC Jr. Type III hyperlipoproteinemia (Dysbetalipoproteinemia): The role of apolipoprotein E in normal and abnormal lipoprotein metabolism. In: Scriver CR, Beaudet AL, Sly WS, Valle D, eds., The metabolic basis of inherited diseases, 6th ed. New York: McGraw-Hill, 1989:1195-215.

27. Hobbs HA, Leitersdorf E, Goldstein JL, et al. Multiple crm⁻ mutations in familial hypercholesterolemia: Evidence for 3 alleles, including four deletions. J Clin Invest 1988;81:909-17.

28. Karathanasis SK, Ferris E, Haddad IA. DNA inversion within the apolipoprotein AI/CIII/AIV-encoding gene cluster of certain patients with premature atherosclerosis. Proc Natl Acad Sci USA 1987;84:7198-202.

29. Schaefer EJ, Blum CB, Levy RI, et al. Metabolism of high density lipoprotein, apolipoproteins in Tangier disease. N Engl J Med 1978;299:905-10.

30. National Cholesterol Education Program, Lipid Metabolism Branch, Division of Heart, Lung, and Blood Institute. The Report of the Expert Panel on Blood Cholesterol Levels in Children and Adolescents (Draft). Bethesda, MD: National Institutes of Health, 1991.

31. American Academy of Pediatrics Committee on Nutrition. Prudent life-style for children: Dietary fat and cholesterol. Pediatrics 1986;78:521-5.

32. American Academy of Pediatrics Committee on Nutrition. Indication for cholesterol testing in children. Pediatrics 1989;83:141-2.

33. National Cholesterol Education Program Expert Panel. Report of the National Cholesterol Education Program Expert Panel on Detection, Evaluation and Treatment of High Blood Cholesterol in Adults. Arch Intern Med 1988;148:36-69.

34.   Dennison BA, Kikucki DA, Srinivasan SR, et al. Serum total cholesterol screening for the detection of elevated low-density lipoprotein in children and adolescents: The Bogalusa heart study. Pediatrics 1990;85:472-9.

35.   Dennison BA, Kikucki DA, Srinivasan SR, et al. Parental history of cardiovascular disease as an indicator for screening for lipoprotein abnormalities in children. J Pediatr 1989;115:186-94.

36.   Garcia RE, Moodie DS. Routine cholesterol surveillance. Pediatrics 1989;84:751-5.

37.   Griffin TC, Chistoffel KK, Binns HJ, et al. Family history evaluation as a predictive screen for childhood hypercholesterolemia. Pediatrics 1989;84:365-73.

38.   Recommendations for improving cholesterol measurement: A report from the Laboratory Standardization Panel of the National Cholesterol Education Program. Bethesda, MD: National Institutes of Health, 1990 [NIH Publication No. 90-2964]

39.   Myers GL, Henderson LO, Cooper GR, Hassemer DJ. Standardization of lipid and lipoprotein measurements. In: Rifai N, Warnick GW, eds., Methods in clinical laboratory measurement of lipid and lipoprotein risk factor, Washington, DC: AACC Press, 1991:101-26.

40.   Naito HK, Bowers GN Jr, Baillie EE, et al. Current status of blood cholesterol measurement in clinical laboratories in the United States: A report from the Laboratory Standardization Panel of the National Cholesterol Education Program. Clin Chem 1988;34:193-201.

41.   National Heart, Lung, and Blood Institute. Recommendations regarding public screening for measuring blood cholesterol: A summary of a National Heart, Lung, and Blood Institute workshop. Bethesda, MD: National Institutes of Health. 1989. [NIH Publication No. 89-3045]

42.   Cole TG. Glycerol blanking in triglyceride assays: Is it necessary? Clin Chem 1990;36:1267-8.

43.   Wiebe DA, Warnick GR. Measurement of high density lipoprotein cholesterol concentration. In: Rifai N, Warnick GW, eds., Methods in clinical laboratory measurement of lipid and lipoprotein risk factors, Washington, DC: AACC Press, 1991:61-74.

44.   Warnick GR, Knopp RH, Fitzpatrick V, et al. Estimating low density lipoprotein cholesterol by the Friedewald equation is adequate for classifying patients on the basis of nationally recommended cut-points. Clin Chem 1990;36:15-9.

45.   McNamara JR, Cohn JS, Wilson WPF, et al. Calculated values for low density lipoprotein cholesterol in the assessment of lipid abnormalities and coronary disease risk. Clin Chem 1990;36:36-42.

46.   Belcher JD, McNamara JR, Grinstead GF, et al. Measurement of low density lipoprotein cholesterol concentration. In: Rifai N, Warnick GW, eds., Methods in clinical laboratory measurement of lipid and lipoprotein risk factor. Washington, DC: AACC Press, 1991:75-87.

47.   Marcovina SM, Albers JJ. Apolipoprotein assays: Standardization and quality control. Scan J Clin Lab Invest 1990;50:58-65.

Biochemical Tests of Hepatic and Intestinal Disorders

Benny Kerzner, M.D.

INTRODUCTION

The biochemical tests used to evaluate gastrointestinal function are most useful when they are progressively applied to a problem in conjunction with an ongoing dialogue between the clinician and his or her colleagues in the clinical laboratory. For convenience, in this chapter the tests are discussed in three sections: tests of the liver, the GI tract proper, and the pancreas. Emphasis is placed on the physiological principles that underlie the investigations and their application to clinical medicine.

THE LIVER

The battery of tests available to measure the integrity of the liver is frequently referred to as "liver function tests"; however, the liver enzymes are proteins normally confined to hepatocytes, canalicular and duct cells and escape only in response to cell wall injury induced by inflammation or a toxin. They include alanine aminotransferase (ALT), aspartate aminotransferase (AST), alkaline phosphatase, gamma-glutamyl transpeptidase (GGT) and 5'-nucleotidase. More accurate measures of hepatic function are the serum concentrations of proteins produced by the liver, notably serum albumin and the factors that contribute to the coagulation cascade. The organic anions, bilirubin and bile salts, whose secretion is dependent on specific carrier-mediated transport mechanisms, also measure a specific function. The use of these endogenous molecules to define hepatic function has limitations: the pool size is not known and the rate of the chemical's reactions is difficult to control. Exogenous chemicals, i.e., xenobiotics, are therefore increasingly administered at a given point in time, and their clearance and/or the products of their metabolism are measured at a fixed time or at intervals thereafter. The classic example is bromosulfophthalein (BSP), which has fallen out of favor due its side effects. More recently, other xenobiotics such as lidocaine are being employed.

The Aminotransferases

AST and ALT (formerly referred to as SGOT and SGPT) are the enzymes which catalyze the transfer of the amino groups of aspartic acid and alanine. Both are produced in large concentrations in the liver, but AST in particular is also produced in other tissues, notably muscle, kidney, and brain.[1] The serum enzyme activity is normally low, less than 50 U/L in the adult and up to 75 U/L in the newborn, but cell wall damage allows a far greater amount of the protein to enter the bloodstream. To detect the enzyme activity, most laboratories use a spectrophotometric catalytic assay dependent on conversion of NADH to NAD^+. A cofactor for this reaction is pyridoxal phosphate; when it is not present in adequate concentrations, ALT values may be artificially low, prompting some to advocate the routine addition of the vitamin to the assay.[2] Immunoassays allow for the distinction of a mitochondrial and cytosolic AST. The former is present in high concentration after extensive acute tissue damage, but distinction between these isozymes is not made in clinical practice.[3] Enzyme values under 100 U/L can vary by as much as 20%; values above 100 U/L are far more accurate.

Assay of aminotransferases provides a simple, sensitive test which can be used serially to evaluate the progression of hepatic disorders.[4] Only small volumes are needed and the test is readily automated. Some difficulties in interpretation may arise. Not only do low ALT values indicate that pyridoxal phosphate may be deficient, low concentrations also may be due to antibodies evolved against the enzyme in patients with chronic liver disease or may result from difficulties with specimen storage. Patients with chronic renal disease often have disproportionately low concentrations of AST which increase after dialysis; a dialyzable inhibitor is invoked as the cause.[5] Moderate or low concentrations of AST may indicate muscle rather than liver injury. Acute myocardial infarction, myocarditis, pericarditis, myositis, and muscular dystrophy will all cause increased AST values beyond those of ALT. Very high activity of AST can actually exhaust the available substrate, and the study may need to be performed in dilution.

AST is a more sensitive assay of liver injury than ALT, but the latter is more specific. The very high concentrations of the aminotransferases associated with acute hepatic injury reflect the extent of the damage but do not correlate with the outcome. Falling aminotransferase values usually indicate that the pathology is abating, but it must be borne in mind that decreasing aminotransferase values in the face of increasing jaundice and deteriorating neurological status indicate that very few hepatocytes are surviving and that the prognosis is grave.[6] A moderate increase in the values is more common with prolonged injury. When the values remain increased longer than 6 m, a biopsy is needed to determine the cause and offer a prognosis. Massively increased concentrations of the aminotransferases are associated with viral hepatitis and ischemic injury, situations in which cell death is common. However, very high values are also seen in conditions such as Reye's syndrome, in which cell survival is excellent.

Alkaline Phosphatase

Serum contains four major isoforms of these glycoprotein enzymes that demonstrate phosphatase activity at an alkaline pH when zinc is provided as a cofactor. The proteins originate from bone, liver, intestine, and placenta, but the enzyme is also found in kidney and white blood cells.[7] In childhood, 80% of the activity comes from bones, whereas in adults it is reduced to 30%.[8] Alkaline phosphatase has been associated with the microvillous membrane of the intestine and renal tubule, and in hepatocytes both the sinusoidal and canalicular membranes. A smaller amount comes from the cytosol. The precise physiological role of the enzyme remains to be defined.

The values of alkaline phosphatase in serum vary over time. They are highest in the newborn and during periods of growth, particularly puberty.[9] A variety of methods are available to measure alkaline phosphatase activity. They generally rely on detection of the phosphate released or the alcohol product derived from the substrate para-nitrophenol phosphate. When the bone and liver isoenzymes need to be separately defined, electrophoretic techniques are used. Heat inactivation is used to define the presence of the placental variety of the enzyme.[8, 10]

Alkaline phosphatase activity in serum is easily measured and is therefore widely applied to the interpretation of liver injury.[11] Difficulty is encountered because increases in the enzymes need not relate to liver disease; in periods of rapid growth, bone's contribution is high, and bone injuries, ranging from fractures to malignancies, will also increase the values. An isolated increment in alkaline phosphatase unaccompanied by changes in the other biochemical parameters of liver injury is referred to as transient hyperphosphatasia and is probably the result of failed clearance of the enzyme.[12, 13] Such high concentrations have been noted with intrahepatic masses and in children who fail to thrive. There is even a marked increment in alkaline phosphatase after a fatty meal with enzyme of intestinal origin.[14] A parallel situation occurs postprandially in cirrhosis, where the increase in alkaline phosphatase does not reflect obstruction to the biliary tract but rather the delivery of increased quantities of intestinal alkaline phosphatase to the liver, which fails to clear it.[15] Isolated increases in alkaline phosphatase noted during pregnancy are a result of the placental contribution to the serum activity.

Alkaline phosphatase activity is higher in patients with cholestasis than in those with hepatocellular disorders, although there is some overlap. Confirmation that the increase is hepatic in origin is usually readily achieved by considering the clinical situation and whether other indices of cholestasis, increased concentrations of gamma-glutamyl transpeptidase (GGT), 5'-nucleotidase, and bile salts are evident. Low values of alkaline phosphatase can also have clinical application. A transient decrease in alkaline phosphatase during the hemolytic events that characterize Wilson's disease is described. In this situation, copper is thought to displace the zinc necessary for the enzyme's activity.[16] Low values are also noted in hypothyroidism, pernicious anemia, and congenital hypophosphatasia, as well as in situations in which zinc deficiency is prominent, particularly acrodermatitis enteropathica.

Gamma-glutamyl Transpeptidase (GGT)

GGT transfers gamma-glutamyl groups from peptides such as glutathione to other amino acids. The enzyme is ubiquitous, being located in the brain, kidney, pancreas, seminal vesicles, and spleen as well as in the liver.[17] It is found throughout the biliary tract, but the highest concentrations are in the epithelial cells of the ductules. Isoforms do exist, but they have not been applied to clinical practice.

The assay for GGT is relatively easy and depends on the release of chromogenic aniline from gamma-glutamyl paranitroaniline. Values for GGT in the neonate are 5–9 times that of adults. In contrast to alkaline phosphatase, they are not influenced by growth, although they do increase with advancing age. Thus, GGT is very useful in helping interpret increases in alkaline phosphatase.

Greatly increased concentrations of GGT are encountered in conditions primarily affecting the bile canaliculi, and it has been proposed as an assay to help identify patients with biliary atresia and, in adults, primary biliary cirrhosis.[18] Because it is a sensitive index of biliary tract injury, it has also proved to be a useful index of rejection after liver transplantation and a screen for hepatic dysfunction in patients on long-term intravenous feeding. However, some high values may be difficult to interpret, as increases are reported in pancreatic and pulmonary disease and in patients with myocardial infarction, renal failure, and diabetes. Drugs that induce hepatic microsomal hydroxylation systems increase GGT concentrations, notably in patients receiving long-term anticonvulsants, especially phenytoin.[19]

5'-Nucleotidase

5'-nucleotidase releases phosphate from the 5' position of the pentose ring, and, in common with GGT, it is an index of biliary obstruction.[4] This enzyme is also ubiquitous, being located in blood vessels, brain, heart, intestine, and pancreas as well as in the liver. Only the liver, however, seems able to readily release the enzyme into serum. GGT has somewhat displaced this test because the 5'-nucleotidase assay is more difficult to perform and is less sensitive. It can, however, be used to help interpret increased alkaline phosphatase concentrations and isolated increases of GGT.

Serum Albumin

Serum albumin is a good routine test of hepatic function. The albumin pool is normally large and may increase 4–6 times in the face of disease; up to 30 g/d need to be synthesized in the patient with cirrhosis and ascites. Because albumin has a long half-life of approximately 20 d, the serum concentrations tend to be static in acute injury, and a fall in serum albumin therefore can be used to help detect the presence of chronic liver disease.[20, 21]

The advantage of the test relates to its simplicity and reliability. Unfortunately, there are extraneous influences which will cause the serum albumin concentrations to vary. The value is dependent on an adequate supply of amino acids, and malnutrition will ultimately influence the value.[22] In addition, hypoalbuminemia may also be the consequence of renal glomerular disorders or a protein-losing enteropathy. Moreover, conditions that redistribute the body fluid mass and the albumin pool affect serum albumin, as is seen in patients with ascites, where low concentrations may merely reflect fluid shifts.[23] Serum albumin is also an important index of prognosis. In patients with progressive liver disease, a fall in serum albumin helps predict the need for transplantation, because in patients with cirrhosis but no ascites, a fall in serum albumin is directly correlated with a poor outcome.[24]

Prothrombin Time

The liver synthesizes a multitude of factors that contribute to the coagulation cascade, and of these factor I, II (prothrombin), V, VII, IX, and X need to be present for a normal prothrombin time to be recorded.[25] A decreased synthesis of the coagulation factors and fibrinogen is commonly found in severe liver failure. First, circulating levels of factor VII, which has a short half-life, fall. Like factors II, IX, and X, VII is also vitamin K dependent, and vitamin K deficiency is common in liver disease. Factor V is independent of vitamin K, and therefore a fall in its production is not reversed by administration of vitamin K. Furthermore, a prolongation of the prothrombin time based on factor V deficiency is strongly indicative of failed hepatic function.[26]

A major advantage of the prothrombin time is its simplicity and its dependence on the interplay of many hepatic factors. It is a measure of the conversion of prothrombin to thrombin in the presence of thromboplastin and calcium. To exclude a contribution of vitamin K to the coagulation abnormality, it can be remeasured after parenteral administration of 10 mg, or in children as little as 1–2 mg, of vitamin K. The value should improve by at least 30% within 24 h.[27]

There are some difficulties in the interpretation of the result. First, there are a number of other possible explanations for a prolonged prothrombin time: congenital deficiencies of the factors, ingestion of anticoagulants, incomplete clearing of activated factors, impaired plasminogen synthesis, fibrinolysis, and disseminated intravascular coagulation (DIC).[28] Nonetheless, a prolongation of the prothrombin time in the absence of DIC and vitamin K deficiency is strongly indicative of severe hepatic dysfunction. An abnormally prolonged prothrombin time in acute hepatic failure suggests an increasing likelihood of fulminant hepatic failure. When the value falls below 10% of the control, the prognosis is poor.[29] In addition, the test has been effectively used to predict a poor outcome in patients who have taken excessive amounts of acetaminophen and in those having to undergo shunt surgery.[30, 31]

Bilirubin

Jaundice remains a red flag for the identification of hepatic pathology, and measuring total and direct bilirubin in serum is central to the classification of liver disorders into pre-hepatic, hepatocellular, and biliary tract conditions. The infant's liver is immature and is presented with an excess load of hemoglobin consequent to the exchange of fetal hemoglobin for the adult variety after birth. As a result, indirect hyperbilirubinemia is so common that it is considered physiologic. Additionally, hemolysis due to ABO incompatibility and other disorders can increase the concentrations of the fat-soluble indirect portion of bilirubin that has the capacity to enter the brain and raise the specter of kernicterus. The newborn liver is also vulnerable: it is readily injured by infection and metabolic toxins and is subject to congenital bile duct abnormalities including biliary atresia. Screening for hepatocellular and duct abnormalities is best done by measuring the direct fraction of bilirubin in blood.

The diazonium reaction is still widely used to measure bilirubin. The test employs two reactions: one with an accelerator in the medium and the other without the accelerator. In the former, total bilirubin is defined; in the latter, a measure of the direct fraction is given, and the difference represents the indirect fraction. Unfortunately, the results can be interfered with by the products of hemolysis, and precision at low values is poor. Furthermore, bilirubin covalently bound to albumin to form so-called "delta bilirubin" may appear to be direct, causing a false-positive result. Alternative methods based on absorbance are subject to interference by hemoglobin and carotenoids. Transcutaneous spectrophotometric methods, which are obviously of great help in monitoring progression of bilirubin in the neonatal period, are unfortunately less accurate than the chemical means of quantitation and do not distinguish direct from indirect bilirubin.[32, 33, 34]

The examination of stool and urine for bilirubin has application particularly in the newborn. The finding of bilirubin in the urine suggests that the water-soluble conjugated variety is circulating in serum and indicates that an obstructive jaundice is present. A qualitative dipstick test can be done at the bedside, and the Ictotest® is even more sensitive. The failure to find bilirubin in the stool is a strong indication of severe obstruction, necessitating exclusion of biliary atresia. Stool tests should be done with care, as false positives may be a consequence of contamination with urine and, rarely, bilirubin in the mucous content of the stool.

Bile Salts

Bile acids are the end products of cholesterol degradation. The primary bile acids, cholic and chenodeoxycholic acids, are tri- and dihydroxy acids. In the bowel lumen they lose a hydroxyl group to become the secondary bile acids, deoxy- and lithocholic acid. Lithocholic acid is a non-polar toxic chemical which can be sulfated to give sulfolithocholic acid. Bile acids that enter the bowel are reabsorbed, and uptake by the liver and subsequent secretion is extremely efficient. Therefore, in the healthy person, the bulk of the bile acid pool resides in the gall bladder, and small quantities are located in the portal and systemic circulation. The bile salt pool is recycled 4–5 times a day, and minimal defects in the pathway result in increased serum concentrations. Abnormal liver function is usually reflected in both the fasting and postprandial concentrations. In mild liver disease, however, fasting concentrations may be normal, whereas the postprandial values move into the abnormal range because of the increased load presented on re-cycling the pool.[35, 36] As trihydroxy acids are more readily extracted by the liver, in the fasting state, a greater proportion of the bile acids are represented by the dihydroxy component. The ratio of cholic to cheno-deoxycholic acid increases in extrahepatic obstruction due to a prefer-ential sulfation and excretion in urine of the chenodeoxycholate variety.[37]

There are three fundamental ways in which bile salts have been measured, each of which has its own benefits and limitations. A radio-immunoassay for cholylglycine is used most commonly. It is sensitive, precise, and offers the ability to perform the test on large numbers of samples. Radioimmunoassays are available for other bile salts as well, but cholylglycine is used based on the supposition that the relative proportions of the bile acids are constant. Obviously, this is not always true, particularly in pathological circumstances. Furthermore, cross-reactivity can occur, especially with deoxycholylglycine. The second method is a fluorometric enzymatic approach, which depends on oxi-dation of the 3-alpha-hydroxy group common to all bile acids and the concomitant conversion of NAD^+ to NADH. It is sensitive and can be applied to relatively large numbers of samples, but it fails to separate the component bile salts. The most accurate methods are high-perfor-mance liquid and gas-liquid chromatography. They allow separation of the components and definition of the cholic to chenodeoxycholic acid ratio. However, extensive sample preparation is necessary, and only a limited number of samples can be analyzed at any one time. In addi-tion, the value of the ratio of cholic to chenodeoxycholic acid has been questioned in pediatrics.[38-42]

To identify liver disease, bile salts are more sensitive than bilíru-bin and are more specific than the enzyme markers of liver disease. They help confirm that small increases in the value of aminotransfer-ases arise from the liver. However, it is of interest that in some situa-tions AST may be more sensitive than bile salts, because the pathology is extremely patchy as in chronic persistent hepatitis, and liver func-tion is relatively well preserved.[43] Although postprandial concentra-tions might be somewhat more sensitive than fasting ones, it is the fasting concentration that has the greatest clinical application and is almost certainly increased in significant liver disease.

A particularly useful application of serum bile salts is to help dis-tinguish congenital hyperbilirubinemia and hemolysis from hepatobili-ary disease. Since bilirubin and bile salts are handled through entirely separate pathways, a disturbance in the one is not reflected in the other. Bile salt values also have been used to delineate the severity of hepatic disorders. Increased concentrations in chronic active hepatitis are reflective of disease activity. Moreover, they have been applied effectively in predicting survival of cirrhotics.[35]

Xenobiotics or Extraneously Administered Chemicals

Several molecules have been used as probes to assess individual hepatic functions: uptake, secretion, conjugation, acetylation, or hydroxylation. Bromosulfophthalein (BSP) is among the oldest, its clinical application having been reported as early as 1925.[44] BSP was favored because it emulated the transport of bilirubin through the liver, requiring uptake, conjugation to glutathione, and secretion. Serum values 45 min after the administration of a 5 g test dose provided a sensitive indicator of liver disease. Toxicity from the drug has now forced it out of favor, but its use highlighted important considerations relevant to the more general use of other probe molecules or xenobiotics. Not only must the chemicals be safe, but an evaluation of their clearance in unit time must take into account their protein binding and volume of distribution, especially in patients with fluid retention characteristic of chronic liver failure. When uptake is more rapid than excretion, there is intrahepatic concentration of the xenobiotic. Other drugs can substantially interfere with the test by competing for the serum transport proteins and uptake, storage, and conjugation sites, as well as altering hepatic blood flow and inducing liver disease. Other chemicals currently being explored in this regard include indocyanine green, caffeine, galactose, aminopyrine, and para-aminobenzoic acid.

The formation of monoethylglycinexylidide (MEGX) from lidocaine, a conversion mediated by the P450 system of liver enzymes, is now receiving considerable attention in pediatrics. Allergy to lidocaine is rare. The test is simple and results are rapidly obtained. Consequently, the production of MEGX 15 min after IV lidocaine is being used to define the loss of function in chronic liver disease, predict the need for liver transplant, and, of great interest, the functional integrity of donor livers.[45]

The Intestinal Tract

The luminal content of the intestine is separated from the body by an endothelium which has an extensive surface made up of primary folds called the valvulae conniventes, microscopic projections called the villi, and, as seen under the electron microscope, a brush border of microvilli. Transfixed into the microvilli are the digestive enzymes, including oligosaccharidases and peptidases, whose active sites project into the lumen. The brush border is the luminal surface of the enterocytes; these are bound together by so-called "tight junctions" through which a bilateral flow of water is possible.

The passage of food through the intestine is closely regulated to ensure that the luminal content is kept liquid while nutrients are progressively removed. In an adult, it is estimated that in a single day the intestine contributes 7 L of fluid via saliva, gastric, biliary, and intestinal secretions to the 2 L taken by mouth. Water is rapidly assimilated in the relatively permeable upper intestine and the colon removes the last 10% to ensure that the stool is formed and appropriately packaged in anticipation of a bowel movement. The volume is reduced to less than 150 g of stool per day. As digestion proceeds, osmotic tension is maintained close to an isotonic state by fluid entering the lumen.[46, 47] In response to luminal injury, destroyed mature enterocytes on the villous tip are replaced by immature cells from the villous crypt, which has a predictable result: a loss of surface area, a loss of surface digestive and absorptive enzymes, generation of a secretory surface, and decreased permeability of the tight junctions. Moreover, inflammation and/or destruction of the villous lacteal encourage exudation of protein.[48]

The integrity of the intestinal lining can be defined biochemically by measures of surface area and the permeability characteristics of the mucosa. D-xylose, whose absorption is primarily passive and therefore surface-area-dependent, is used to define the former, and probe molecules of varying size, such as polyethylene glycol (PEG), define the latter. Exudation is best measured by detecting serum proteins such as albumin or alpha-1-antitrypsin in the stool. Protein absorption is extremely efficient and it is therefore a poor index of intestinal failure. By contrast, fat, which must be rendered water soluble for assimilation, offers a more rigorous test of GI function. Unfortunately, balance studies done over 3–5 days are required, and therefore simpler methods such as the steatocrit are increasingly used. For carbohydrate absorption, stool testing for reducing substances and pH have merit as screening evaluations, but for more definitive analysis, hydrogen breath testing is preferred.

Stool Tests

In a child too young to cooperate, stool specimens are of value only when care has been taken to ensure that they are fresh and uncontaminated with urine. Rectal stimulation followed by prompt collection, or alternatively, the drainage of stool from the rectum through a short, flexible catheter or into urine bags may be required. Specimens that must be collected over a longer period of time may be retrieved by reversing diapers or lining them with waterproof material such as plastic wrap. More accurate collections may require metabolic beds, but such a stringent technique is rarely warranted in clinical practice.[32]

Stool Electrolytes and Osmolality

It has been suggested that to obtain a true measure of electrolytes in the liquid phase of luminal contents, one should evaluate the fluid from dialysis bags after they have been allowed to pass through the intestine. This technique is too elaborate for practical purposes and is not necessary to determine whether the electrolyte abnormalities are suggestive of secretory or osmotic diarrhea.

Solid stool rarely has significant electrolyte abnormalities, and care should be taken to obtain a representative fresh, liquid specimen. A fresh stool is important because osmolality is artificially increased if complex molecules such as starch are allowed to ferment to short-chain fatty acids. Normal values for stool electrolytes vary considerably between investigators. Values for sodium, potassium, and chloride in adults are approximately 32, 75, and 16 mmol/L and in infants, 22, 54, and 21 mmol/L, respectively.[49]

Stool electrolytes are useful in differentiating secretory, absorptive, and osmotic diarrhea. In absorptive diarrheas caused by viral enteritis, stool sodium is less than 70 mmol/L and the osmotic gap is greater than 100 mOsm. In secretory diarrhea, sodium is greater than 70 mmol/L and the osmotic gap is less than 100 mOsm.[50] In osmotic diarrhea due to an exogenous laxative such as Milk of Magnesia or an endogenous substance such as glucose, an "osmotic gap" develops. Normally, the value of the sodium plus the potassium concentration multiplied by 2 should come within 50 mOsm of 290 mOsm, which is the value for the osmotic tension of serum. Direct measures of stool osmolality are not favored because, as mentioned earlier, the value is often artificially high due to the content of short-chain fatty acids.[51, 52] A very high chloride content is indicative of congenital chloride malabsorption or "chloridorrhea," a rare congenital defect characterized by metabolic alkalosis, in contrast to the acidosis usually associated with dehydration.[53]

Alpha-1-antitrypsin

Under normal circumstances, a small proportion of relatively small proteins such as albumin and alpha-1-antitrypsin escape from the serum into the lumen of the bowel. Conditions which encourage exudation can massively augment this loss and the "protein-losing enteropathy" may result in hypoalbuminemia. The most accurate means of detecting the protein loss is to administer chromium-labelled albumin intravenously and measure the chromium chloride content of the stool over 2–3 days. Unfortunately, this technique is both expensive and cumbersome, and in recent times the preferred method is the detection of alpha-1-antitrypsin losses in stool.[54-57]

Alpha-1-antitrypsin concentrations in stool are determined by immunoassay techniques.[58] The stool is lyophilized (as heat drying lowers the concentration of the protein somewhat) and resuspended in water for the assay. Radioimmune diffusion is commonly used, but a more accurate alternative is immune nephelometry. Normally, stool losses of alpha-1-antitrypsin are low, being less than 4 mg/g dry weight or 1.3 g/L wet volume.[59] Increases can be detected in random stool samples, but a more accurate approach is to express the alpha-1-antitrypsin loss in terms of the amount cleared from serum into stool in a unit of time.

Clearance in mL/d equals F x W/P, where F is the fecal concentration of alpha-1-antitrypsin, W the weight of stool in g/d, and P the plasma concentration of alpha-1-antitrypsin. Clearance studies therefore require a 24 h stool collection and a serum sample. The study of random stool samples offers a much more rapid turnaround time, but clearance tests are more specific and sensitive. Alpha-1-antitrypsin concentrations in stool have been successfully employed to follow the activity of inflammatory bowel disease, celiac disease, and radiation enteritis. Although alpha-1-antitrypsin is resistant to proteases, a proportion is denatured to the point of non-recognition by radioimmune diffusion. For this reason, underestimates of protein loss are especially likely when the pathology involves the stomach, where the denaturing effect of acid is evident. Adding H_2-blocking drugs to the study protocol can help avoid this problem.[60]

Stool Fat Analyses

The assimilation of fat requires an orchestrated interaction of the detergent properties of bile salts, the digestive properties of pancreatic enzymes, and absorption through the mucosa and its lacteals. Consequently, tests for steatorrhea are important measures of intestinal integrity but cannot distinguish between hepatic, intestinal, and pancreatic defects. Evaluation of single stool samples for fat serves as a screen for steatorrhea; however, to overcome variations in the consumption of fat and intestinal transport, the fat content of pooled samples is measured.

An accurate measure of stool fat losses requires the subject to be on a high-fat diet, typically 100 g of fat per day in adults, for a few days before and during the test.[61] The collection lasts 3–5 days. The results are best expressed as a percentage of the fat intake. This requires accurate measurement of the fat eaten over a given period of time, preferably demarcated by the intake of non-absorbed visible markers such as charcoal. The markers also define the beginning and end of the stool collection. The titrimetric method of van de Kamer[62] is used to measure fat content, but if a significant amount of medium-chain triglycerides is consumed, a gravidometric approach is necessary.[63] In adults, more than 7 g/d or 7% of dietary fat in the stool is regarded as abnormal. In infants under age 6 m, up to 15% is considered acceptable.[64]

The 72 h stool fat collection is considered the most definitive for fat malabsorption, and it provides the best evaluation of pancreatic function without duodenal intubation. It is also more sensitive than indirect measures of pancreatic function such as the bentiromide test. Unfortunately, it is aesthetically distasteful and subject to many potential pitfalls: an inadequate record of fat intake, delayed intestinal transport, and incomplete stool collection.

The Steatocrit

This test is a simple semi-quantitative technique used to determine the stool fat content. As the name suggests, it shares the principles of a hematocrit. A homogenate of feces is microcentrifuged at 15,000 rpm for 15 min. The centrifugal forces separate the water phase of stool from the lipid, whose length is readily measured. This technique has proved to be useful in assessing the extent of malabsorption and response to treatment of patients with pancreatic insufficiency. Under these circumstances, neutral fat predominates.[65] In mucosal injuries, where fatty acids and monoglycerides are the dominantly malabsorbed fat, the technique is less likely to be successful because the crystalline fatty acids are to some extent water soluble; nevertheless, excellent correlation with quantitative stool fat losses has been found.[66]

Blood Tests

Xylose Absorption

Absorption of D-xylose has been used as an index of the functional absorptive surface area of the small intestine. This monosaccharide is used for this purpose because it is readily absorbed in the proximal intestine and is considered inert. In fact, there is a weak carrier mechanism encouraging absorption, and to some degree it is metabolized. Nonetheless, experience has confirmed that D-xylose absorption effectively predicts intestinal mucosal integrity.

In adult medicine, an oral loading dose is followed by a 5 h urine collection or a 2 h blood sample. In pediatrics, a 1 h blood value has gained favor. Uniform agreement on an appropriate loading dose has not been reached. The suggestion for adults is 25 g. The recommendation for children is 0.5 g/kg up to 30 kg body weight, or 14.5 g/m^2 to a maximum of 25 g, or a weight adopted dose of 0.35 g/kg.[67-68] A normal 1 h value is strongly predictive of a normal mucosa. Abnormally low values indicate mucosal injury and provide a reasonably sensitive prediction of celiac disease and allergic enteropathy.[67, 69] However, false-positive and false-negative results occur, and the need for definitive biopsy is not necessarily excluded.[70] Conditions which cause patchy mucosal lesions or proximal small bowel involvement with preservation of distal absorption will allow assimilation to normal serum values. False-negative results may be caused by the child's refusing to swallow or vomiting the dose, or by delayed gastric emptying and bacterial overgrowth. Nonetheless, 1 h D-xylose absorption remains an important indicator of mucosal disruption which can be used to monitor recovery and deterioration of intestinal disorders.

Lactulose-Mannitol Ratio and PEG

Tests of intestinal permeability depend on the differential uptake of large and small molecules. Intestinal injury allows large molecular species such as the disaccharide lactulose to enter the bloodstream to be excreted in the urine, whereas the loss of surface area limits assimilation of smaller species such as the monosaccharide mannitol. The ratio of the two in urine therefore expresses the extent of the mucosal injury.[71-73] A similar result is described with the use of an homologous series of molecules such as PEG 200 or 600. The ratio of the larger species to the total PEG concentration in urine serves as the index of the changing permeability.[71, 74] Tests of permeability have been applied to celiac disease and other conditions characterized by mucosal injury, but they are not routinely used in clinical medicine.[75]

The Pancreas

To assess the pancreas with biochemical tests, one depends on the detection of enzymes and peptides such as pancreatic polypeptide that are refluxed into the bloodstream from the organ. Alternatively, a substrate is provided via the bowel lumen which depends on pancreatic digestion to release products into the bowel lumen or bloodstream.

The evaluation of pancreatic exocrine function poses a daunting challenge to the clinician because of the organ's inaccessibility and, ironically, its enormous functional reserve. Pancreatic enzymes are produced in excess, and only when production falls below 2–10% are limits placed on digestion.[76] Therefore, while many tests of pancreatic function accurately detect pancreatic insufficiency, only direct measurements of enzymes produced when the pancreas is stimulated can accurately reflect a progressive fall from normal.

The direct measurement of pancreatic secretions is, however, not a routine laboratory procedure, as it requires intubation of the duodenum and aspiration of contents. This test is therefore uncomfortable and cumbersome, and it has questionable reproducibility. Nevertheless, it is regarded as a gold standard because, when optimally performed, it will detect subnormal function prior to clinical insufficiency.

Detection of the enzymes amylase, lipase, and immunoreactive trypsin in excess in serum is a reflection of organ inflammation. Low concentrations of serum trypsin and pancreatic polypeptide can help screen for pancreatic insufficiency, and they do relate directly to pancreatic mass. Similarly, the presence of the relatively resistant chymotrypsin in stool can also be used to screen for pancreatic insufficiency. However, these values do not assess pancreatic reserves, as they are not measured after the pancreas is stimulated.[77]

Stool Trypsin and Chymotrypsin

Both trypsin and chymotrypsin can be detected in stool, and both are subject to destruction in the bowel; however, chymotrypsin is far more resistant and is therefore preferred.[78] In addition, by including detergents in the assay, chymotrypsin can be separated from the solid waste in stool, and its activity is augmented.[79] The test is valuable for detecting pancreatic insufficiency, and stool concentrations have been correlated with duodenal concentrations after pancreatic stimulation.[80] False negatives can be eliminated by repeating the test on two or three stool specimens.

Serum Amylase, Lipase, and Immunoreactive Trypsinogen

Virtually no amylase is produced by the newborn, and serum values are low in the first year of life.[81] Lipase concentrations follow a similar course over time but trypsinogen, which circulates as a proenzyme, is detected early and is influenced less by age.[82] Increased values are generally the consequence of inflammation, duct obstruction, or poor renal clearance. Low concentrations may indicate pancreatic insufficiency.

Serum amylase serves as a fairly sensitive screen for acute pancreatitis, and persistently increased concentrations are indicative of a pseudocyst.[83] False negatives are common because serum values are often only transiently increased in pancreatitis. False positives occur for a variety of reasons: isoenzymes from the salivary glands may cause an increase, amylase may not be cleared from the serum because of renal disorders, or the enzyme complexes to immunoglobulins to form so-called "macroamylase."[84] Furthermore, other inflammatory lesions in the bowel increase serum amylase activity, e.g., cholecystitis and duodenal ulceration. Pancreatic and salivary isoenzymes can be separated or distinguished by a number of techniques: chromatography, specific enzyme inhibition, differential heat sensitivity, or immunoassay.

The concomitant assay of lipase is also valuable to confirm elevations of amylase suspected to be due to pancreatic inflammation. Lipase concentrations are more consistently increased in the early stages of cystic fibrosis, and low concentrations in the older patient suggest pancreatic insufficiency.

Immunoreactive cationic trypsinogen is even more effective in this regard. Increased values indicate obstructive pancreatic disease, and in the first year of life the test will identify 90% of patients with cystic fibrosis. Values decline steadily, and this trend predicts pancreatic insufficiency. The immunoreactive trypsinogen test is accurate enough to help distinguish pancreatic from intestinal forms of steatorrhea in which serum values are normal.[85-86]

The Bentiromide Test

Bentiromide is a synthetic compound comprising a peptide covalently bound to para-aminobenzoic acid (PABA). It is selectively cleaved by chymotrypsin, the pancreatic enzyme normally responsible for activating trypsinogen. The products of digestion are rapidly absorbed, and the PABA is conjugated in the liver and excreted in the urine. A colorimetric assay is used to detect the PABA in a 1 h blood or a 6 h urine sample. Less than 50% of the administered PABA in urine strongly suggests pancreatic insufficiency. The test is not very useful in the early phases of pancreatic insufficiency, and unfortunately, pathology in the intestine, liver, and kidney can cause a false-negative result.[77] The specificity of the test can be decreased by chymotrypsin-like activity on the brush border or in bacteria. Interference with the test has also occurred from foods emitting aromatic amines.[87-88] Problems with hepatic disease can be overcome by a two-stage test. Following bentiromide, PABA alone is administered to determine whether interference in its excretory pathway has occurred.[89] In severe cases of steatorrhea, the test can help distinguish pancreatic from other intestinal forms of malabsorption.

The biochemical evaluation of intestinal function can be achieved by progressing from simple studies of blood, urine, and stool to loading tests which are of minimal inconvenience to the patient. The discomforts of intubation are increasingly being avoided.

REFERENCES

1. Boyde TRC, Latner AL. Starch gel electrophoresis of transaminase in human tissue extracts and serum. Biochem J 1961;82:52.
2. Lumeng L, Ryan MP, Li T-K. Validation of the diagnostic value of plasma pyridoxal 5' phosphate measurements in vitamin B6 nutrition of the rat. J Nutr 1978;1087:545.
3. Lumeng L. New diagnostic markers of alcohol abuse. Hepatology 1986;6:742.
4. Reichling JJ, Kaplan MM. Clinical use of serum enzymes in liver disease. Dig Dis Sci 1988;33:1601-14.
5. Cohen GA, Goffinet JA, Donabedian RK, et al. Observations of decreased serum glutamic oxaloacetic transaminase (SGOT) activity in azotemic patients. Ann Intern Med 1976;84:275.
6. Patwardhan RV, Smith OJ, Farmelant MH. Serum transaminase levels and cholescintigraphic abnormalities in acute biliary tract obstruction. Arch Intern Med 1987;147:1249.
7. Fishman WH. Perspectives on alkaline phosphatase isoenzymes. Am J Med 1974;56:617.
8. Chapman JF, Woodward LL, Silverman LM. Alkaline phosphatase isoenzymes. In: Kaplan LA, Pesce AJ, eds. Clinical chemistry. 2nd ed. St. Louis: CV Mosby, 1989:902
9. Grausz H, Schmid R. Reciprocal relations between plasma albumin level and hepatic sulfobromophthalein removal. N Engl J Med 1971;284:1403.
10. Meyer-Sabellek W, Sinha P, Kottgen E. Alkaline phosphatase. Laboratory and clinical implications. J Chromatogr 1988;429:419-44.
11. Kaplan MM. Alkaline phosphatase. Gastroenterology 1972;62:452.
12. Schonau E, Herzog KH, Bohles HJ. Transient hyperphosphatasemia of infancy. Eur J Pediatr 1988;148:264-6.
13. Lockitch G, Pudek MR, Halstead AC. Isolated elevation of serum alkaline phosphatase. Clinical and laboratory observations. J Pediatr 1984;105:773-5.
14. Inglis NI, Krant MJ, Fishman WH. Influence of a fat-enriched meal on human serum (L-phenylalanine-sensitive) "intestinal" alkaline phosphatase. Proc Soc Exp Biol Med 1967;124:699.
15. Suzuki H, Yamanaka M, Oda T. Studies on serum alkaline phosphatase isoenzymes. Ann NY Acad Sci 1969;166:811.
16. Shaver WA, Bhatt H, Combes B. Low serum alkaline phosphatase activity in Wilson's disease. Hepatology 1986;6:859.
17. Nemasanszky E, Lott JA. Gamma-glutamyltransferase and its isoenzymes: Progress and problems. Clin Chem 1985;31:797-803.
18. Fung KP, Lau SP. Gamma-glutamyl transpeptidase activity and its serial measurement in differentiation between extrahepatic biliary atresia and neonatal hepatitis. J Pediatr Gastroenterol Nutr 1985;4:208-13.
19. Keeffe EB, Sunderland MC, Gabourel JD. Serum gamma-glutamyl transpeptidase activity in patients receiving chronic phenytoin therapy. Dig Dis Sci 1986;31:1056-61.
20. Rothschild MA, Oratz M, Zimmon D, et al. Albumin synthesis in cirrhotic subjects with ascites studied with carbonate [14] C. J Clin Invest 1969;48:344.
21. Skrede S, Blomhoff JP, Elgyo K, et al. Biochemical tests in evaluation of liver function. Scand J Gastroenterol 1973;(Suppl)8(19):37.
22. Waterlow JC. Observation on the mechanism of adaption to low protein intake. Lancet 1968;ii:1091.
23. Hasch E, Jarnum S, Tygstrup N. Albumin synthesis rate as a measure of liver function in patients with cirrhosis. Arch Intern Med 1967;182:38.
24. Post J, Patek AS. Serum proteins in cirrhosis of the liver. Arch Intern Med 1942;69:67.
25. Suttie JW, Jackson CM. Prothrombin structure, activation and biosynthesis. Physiol Rev 1977;57:1.
26. Spector I, Corn M. Laboratory tests of hemostasis. The relation to hemorrhage in liver disease. Arch Intern Med 1967;119:577.

27.   Lord JW, Andrus W de W. Differentiation of intrahepatic and extrahepatic jaundice. Response of the plasma prothrombin to intramuscular injection of menadione (2-methyl-1, 4-naphthaquinone) as a diagnostic aid. Arch Intern Med 1941;68:199.

28.   Blanchard RA, Furie BC, Jorgensen M, et al. Acquired vitamin K-dependent carboxylation deficiency in liver disease. N Engl J Med 1981;305:242.

29.   Rueff B, Menache D, Sicot C, et al. Acute comatose hepatitis. Minn Med 1971;54:91.

30.   Clarke R, Rake MO, Flute PT, et al. Coagulation abnormalities in acute liver failure: Pathogenetic and therapeutic implications. Scand J Gastroenterol 1973;(Suppl)8(19):63.

31.   Liebowitz HR, Rousselot LM. Bleeding esophageal varices: Portal hypertension. Springfield, IL: Charles C. Thomas, 1959.

32.   St. Louis PJ. Biochemical studies: Liver and intestine. In: Walker WA, Durie PR, Hamilton JR, et al., eds. Pediatric gastrointestinal disease. Philadelphia: B.C. Decker, 1991:1363-74.

33.   Rutledge JC, Ou CN. Bilirubin and the laboratory. Pediatr Clin N Am 1989;36:189-98.

34.   Sherwin JE, Obernolte R. Bilirubin. In Pesce AJ, Kaplan LA, eds. In: Methods in clinical chemistry. St. Louis: CV Mosby, 1987:1105.

35.   Stolz A, Kaplowitz N. Biochemical tests for liver disease. In: Zakim D, Boyer T, eds. Hepatology: A textbook of liver disease, 2nd ed. Philadelphia: W. B. Saunders, 1990:637-66.

36.   LaRusso NF Korman MG, Hoffman NE, et al. Dynamics of the enterohepatic circulation of bile acids: Postprandial serum concentrations of conjugates of cholic acid in healthy, cholecystectomized patients, and patients with bile acid malabsorption. N Eng J Med 1974;292:689.

37.   Berk PD. Javitt NB. Hyperbilirubinemia and cholestasis. Am J Med 1978;64:311.

38.   Blanckaert N, Kabra P, Farina FA, et al. Measurement of bilirubin and its monoconjugates and diconjugates in human serum by alkaline methanolysis and high performance liquid chromatography. J Lab Clin Med 1980;96:198.

39.   Pennington CR, Ross PE, Bouchier IAD. Serum bile acids in the diagnosis of hepatobiliary disease. Gut 1977;18:903.

40.   Siskos PA, Cahill PT, Javitt NB. Serum bile acid analysis: A rapid, direct enzymatic method using dual-beam spectrophotofluorimetry. J Lipid Res 1977;18:666.

41.   Barnes S, Spenney JG. Improved enzymatic assays for bile acids using resazurin and NADH oxidoreductase from Clostridium kluyveri. Clin Chim Acta 1980;102:241.

42.   Simmonds WJ, Korman MG, Go VLW, et al. Radioimmunoassay of conjugated cholyl bile acids in serum. Gastroenterology 1973;65:703.

43.   Ferraris R, Colombatti G, Florentini MT, et al. Diagnostic value of serum bile acids and routine liver function tests in hepatobiliary diseases: Sensitivity, specificity and predictive value. Dig Dis Sci 1983:28:129.

44.   Rosenthal SM, White EC. Clinical application of bromosulfophthalein test for hepatic function. JAMA 1925;84:1112.

45.   Schroeder TJ, Gremse DA, Mansour ME, et al. Lidocaine metabolism as an index of liver function in hepatic transplant donors and recipients. Transplantation Proceedings 1989;21:2299-2301.

46.   Powell DW. Ion and water transport in the intestine. In: Andreoli TE, Hoffman JF, Fanestil DD, Schultz SG, eds. Physiology of membrane disorders. New York: Plenum, 1986:559.

47.   Phillips SF. Diarrhea: A current view of the pathophysiology. Gastroenterology 1972;63:495-518.

48.   Kerzner B, Kelly MH, Gall DG, et al. Transmissible gastroenteritis: Sodium transport and the intestinal epithelium during the course of viral enteritis. Gastroenterology 1977;72:457.

49.   Rhoads JM, Powell DW. Diarrhea. In: Walker WA, Durie PR, Hamilton JR, et al., eds. Pediatric gastrointestinal disease, Philadelphia: B.C. Decker, 1991:62-78.

50.   Ladefoged K, Schaffalitzky de Muckadell OB, Jarnum S. Faecal osmolality and electrolyte concentrations in chronic diarrhoea: Do they provide diagnostic clues? Scand J Gastroenterol 1987;22:813-20.

51.   Krejs GJ, Fordtran JS. Diarrhea. In: Sleisenger MH, Fordtran JS, eds. Gastrointestinal disease: Pathophysiology, diagnosis, management, 3rd ed. Philadelphia: WB Saunders, 1983:257.

52. Read NW, Krejs GJ, Read MG, et al. Chronic diarrhea of unknown origin. Gastroenterology 1980;78:264-71.

53. Holmberg C, Perheentupa J, Launiala K, et al. Congenital chloride diarrhea: Clinical analysis of 21 Finnish patients. Arch Dis Child 1977;52:255-67.

54. Durie PR. Intestinal protein loss and fecal α-1-antitrypsin. J Pediatr Gastroenterol Nutr 1985;4:345-7.

55. Hill R, Hercz A, Corey M, et al. Fecal clearance of α-1-antitrypsin. A reliable measure of enteric protein loss in children. J Pediatr 1981;99:416-8.

56. Crossley J, Elliott R. Simple method for diagnosing protein-losing enteropathies. Br Med J 1977;2:428-9.

57. Bernier J, Florent C, Desmazures C, et al. Diagnosis of protein-losing enteropathy by gastrointestinal clearance of alpha-1-antitrypsin. Lancet 1978;ii:763-4.

58. Wilson CM, McGilligan K, Thomas DW. Determination of fecal α-1-antitrypsin concentration by radial immunodiffusion: Two systems compared. Clin Chem 1988; 34:2268-70.

59. Quigley E, Ross I, Haeney M, et al. Reassessment of faecal α-1-antitrypsin excretion for use as a screening test for intestinal protein loss. J Clin Pathol 1987;40:61-6.

60. Florent C, Vidon N, Flourie A, et al. Gastric clearance of alpha-1-antitrypsin under cimetidine perfusion new test to detect protein-losing gastropathy. Digest Dis Sci 1986;31:12-15.

61. Thompson JB, Su CK, Ringrose RE, et al. Fecal triglycerides. II. Digestive vs. absorptive steatorrhea. J Lab Clin Med 1969;73:521-30.

62. van de Kamer, ten Bokkel Huinink H, Weyers HA. Rapid method for the determination of fat in feces. J Biol Chem 1949;177:347-55.

63. Jeejeebhoy KN, Ahmed S, Kozak G. Determination of fecal fats containing both medium and long chain triglycerides and fatty acids. Clin Biochem 1970;3:157-63.

64. Fomon SJ, Ziegler ER, Thomas LN, et al. Excretion of fat by normal full-term infants fed various milks and formulas. Am J Clin Nutr 1970;23:1299-1313.

65. Columbo C, Maiavacca R, Ronchi M, et al. The steatocrit: A simple method for monitoring fat malabsorption in patients with cystic fibrosis. J Pediatr Gastroenterol Nutr 1987;6:926-30.

66. Guarino A, Terallo L, Greco L, et al. Reference values of the steatocrit and its modifications in diarrheal diseases. J Ped Gastroenterol Nutr 1992;14:268-74.

67. Rolles CJ, Kendall MJ, Nutter S, et al. One-hour blood-xylose screening-test for coeliac children. Lancet 1973;ii:1043-45.

68. Buts J-P, Morin CL, Roy CC, et al. One-hour xylose test: a reliable index of small bowel function. J Pediatr 1978;92:729-33.

69. McNeely MD. D-xylose. In: Pesce AJ, Kaplan LA, eds. Methods in clinical chemistry. St. Louis: CV Mosby, 1987:862.

70. Christie DL. Use of the one-hour blood xylose test as an indicator of small bowel mucosal disease. J Pediatr 1978;92:725-8.

71. Walker-Smith JA. Evaluation of intestinal protein loss and intestinal permeability. Front Gastrointest Res 1989;16:126-34.

72. Juby LD, Rothwell J, Axon ATR. Lactulose/mannitol test: An ideal screen for celiac disease. Gastroenterology 1989;96:79-85.

73. Hamilton I, Hill A, Bose B, et al. Small intestinal permeability in pediatric clinical practice. J Pediatr Gastroenterol Nutr 1987;6:697-701.

74. Lifschitz C, Irving C, Marks L, et al. Polyethylene glycol polymers of low molecular weight as probes of intestinal permeability. II. Application to infants and children with intestinal disease. J Lab Clin Med 1986;108:37-43.

75. Lifschitz C, Shulman R, Langston C, et al. Comparison of the D-xylose and polyethylene glycol absorption tests as indicators of mucosal damage in infants with chronic diarrhea. J Pediatr Gastroenterol Nutr 1989;8:47-50.

76. Di Magno EP, Go VLW, Summerskill WJH. Relations between pancreatic enzyme outputs and malabsorption in severe pancreatic insufficiency. N Engl J Med 1973;288:813-15.

77. Couper R, Durie PR. Pancreatic function tests. In: Walker WA, Durie PR, Hamilton JR, et al., eds. Pediatric gastrointestinal disease, Philadelphia: B.C. Decker, 1991:1363-74.

78. Haverback BJ, Dyce VJ, Gutentag PJ, et al. Measurement of trypsin and chymotrypsin in stool: A diagnostic test for pancreatic exocrine function. Gastroenterology 1963;44:588-97.

79. Kaspar P, Moller G, Wahlefeld A. New photometric assay for chymotrypsin in stool. Clin Chem 1984;30:1753-7.

80. Bonin A, Roy CC, Lasalle R. Fecal chymotrypsin: A reliable index of exocrine pancreatic function in children. J Pediatr 1973;83:594-600.

81. O'Donnell MD, Miller NJ. Plasma pancreatic and salivary type amylase and immunoreactive trypsin concentrations: Variations with age and reference ranges for children. Clin Chim Acta 1980;104:265-73.

82. Lebenthal E, Lee PC. Development of functional response in human exocrine pancreas. Pediatrics 1980;66:556-60.

83. Moosa AR. Diagnostic tests and procedures in acute pancreatitis. N Engl J Med 1984;311:639-43.

84. Johnson SG, Ellis CJ, Levitt MD. Mechanisms of increased renal clearance of amylase: Creatinine in acute pancreatitis. N Engl J Med 1976;295:1214-17.

85. Cleghorn G, Benjamin L, Corey M, et al. Age-related alterations of immunoreactive pancreatic lipase and cationic trypsinogen in young children with cystic fibrosis. J Pediatr 1985;107:377-81.

86. Cleghorn G, Benjamin L, Corey M, et al. Serum immunoreactive pancreatic lipase and cationic trypsinogen for the assessment of exocrine pancreatic function in older patients with cystic fibrosis. Pediatrics 1986;77:301-6.

87. Sterchi EE, Green JR, Lentz MJ. Non pancreatic hydrolysis of N-benzoyl-L-tyrosyl-p-aminobenzoic acid (PABA-peptide) in the human small intestine. Clin Sci 1982;62:557-60.

88. Gyr K, Felsenfeld O, Imondi AR. Chymotrypsin-like activity of some intestinal bacteria. Dig Dis Sci 1978;23:413-416.

89. Mitchell CJ, Humphrey CS, Bullen AW, et al. Improved diagnostic accuracy of a modified oral pancreatic function test. Scand J Gastroenterol 1979;14:737-41.

Diagnosis and Management of Pediatric Tumors

Karen L. Kaucic, M.D.   Gregory H. Reaman, M.D.

INTRODUCTION

Over the past two decades, the clinical laboratory has become increasingly important in the diagnosis and treatment of pediatric malignancies. Not surprisingly, the laboratory's expanding role has paralleled advances in tumor biology, supportive clinical care, and anti-tumor therapy.

Today the clinical laboratory plays a vital role in the diagnosis, treatment, and supportive care of children with malignancies. This chapter focuses on the laboratory's contributions in each of these areas, specifically (1) biological markers in diagnosis and treatment, (2) supportive management, and (3) the clinical pharmacology of anti-neoplastic therapy. The most common pediatric malignancies are summarized in Figure 17–1.

BIOLOGICAL MARKERS

A biological marker can be broadly defined as a molecule, most often a protein or glycoprotein, present in blood, urine, or other body fluid, which is detectable or increased in the presence of a specific tumor or group of tumors. Biological markers may be intracellular or membrane-associated, biologically active or inert. They are frequently detectable in normal tissues, albeit in smaller quantities, and in other

FIGURE 17–1. Relative Incidence of Major Forms of Cancer in Children Younger Than 15 Years of Age, 1973-1976, Based on a 10% Sample of the Entire United States

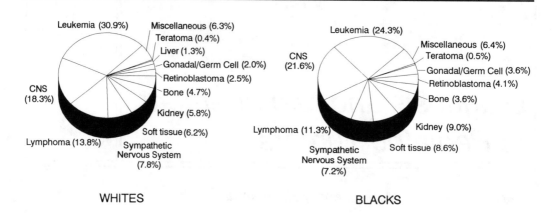

Adapted from Fernbach DJ, Vietti TJ. Clinical pediatric oncology. St. Louis: Mosby Year Book, Inc.

non-malignant disease states, and are thus generally considered to be tumor-associated rather than tumor-specific.[1] Tumor markers are most easily categorized based on their chemical structure or biological function. Five major classes can be identified: carrier/storage proteins, antigens or membrane receptors, enzymes, hormones, and growth factors.[2]

Biological markers theoretically have four major roles in the diagnosis and management of pediatric malignancies: cancer screening, diagnostic confirmation, assessment of response to therapy, and early detection of relapse or recurrence.

With respect to screening, the low incidence of cancer in the pediatric population in general, and the relative lack of specificity of many biological markers for specific tumors, makes screening utilizing biological markers cost ineffective and clinically inefficient. The single exception is infant screening for neuroblastoma by measurement of urinary catecholamine metabolites, which is discussed in greater detail later in this chapter.

Biological markers are useful in the diagnosis of most pediatric malignancies as adjuncts to radiographic imaging and direct microscopic examination of tissue. They often aid in directing more invasive diagnostic testing and provide useful information in difficult diagnostic dilemmas. In addition, the quantitation of tumor markers often provides a means of assessing tumor bulk or the extent of disease. Biological markers are also useful as non-invasive adjuncts to radiographic studies in assessing response to therapy and screening for disease relapse. They are especially useful in situations in which there is no radiographically measurable disease, since detection of increased tumor marker concentrations may provide evidence of microscopic residual disease or microscopic recurrence, before bulk disease is evident on physical examination or radiographic studies. Ideally, baseline concentrations of tumor markers should be determined prior to surgical intervention or the initiation of radiation or chemotherapy, and then measured serially throughout treatment and post-therapy follow-up.

The biological markers relevant to the diagnosis and management of specific pediatric malignancies are discussed individually below. Table 17-1 summarizes the common pediatric tumor markers.

TABLE 17–1. A Summary of the Most Common Biological Markers Grouped by Disease and Their Role(s) in the Diagnosis and Management of Pediatric Malignancies

Disease	Marker	Diagnosis	Prognosis	Screening	Follow-up	Not Defined
ALL	LDH		▲		▲	
	IL–2 Receptor	▲	▲			
	tDT	▲				
	GD3	▲				△
Non-Hodgkin's Lymphoma	LDH		▲			
	IL–2 Receptor	▲	▲			
	β–2–Microglobulin		▲		▲	
	CRP		▲		▲	
	CEA				▲	
Hodgkin's Lymphoma	Ferritin		▲			
	β–2–Microglobulin		▲		▲	
	CRP		▲		▲	
Neuroblastoma	Catecholamines	▲	▲	▲	▲	
	Cystathionine	▲	▲			
	Aminoisobutyric Acid	▲	▲			
	Ferritin		▲			
	NSE		▲		▲	
	CEA				▲	
	GD2	▲				△
Wilm's Tumor	Hyaluronic Acid	▲			▲	
	Erythropoietin	▲			▲	
	CEA				▲	
Hepatoblastoma	AFP	▲			▲	
	HCG	▲			▲	
	Ferritin				▲	
Germ Cell Tumors	AFP	▲			▲	
	HCG	▲			▲	
Soft Tissue Sarcomas	CK					△
	TAA					△
Osteosarcoma	Alkakine Phosphatase		▲		▲	
	TAA					△
Ewing's Sarcoma	LDH		▲			
CNS Tumors	NSE	▲				
	Polyamines	▲			▲	

Carrier and Storage Proteins

α-Fetoprotein

Initially identified in 1944, α-fetoprotein (AFP) was the first circulating tumor-associated marker to be identified.[3] AFP is produced during fetal life by the liver, yolk sac, and gastrointestinal tract and can be detected in high concentrations in fetal serum. A glycosylated protein with structural and functional homology to human albumin, AFP is thought to perform physiological functions in the fetus similar to those of albumin in the adult.[2] Barely detectable in the serum of normal children and adults, its association with human tumors was first described in 1964, when increased concentrations were found in the serum of patients with hepatoma. Subsequently, increased serum concentrations of AFP were well documented in pediatric patients with hepatoblastoma, hepatocellular carcinoma, and gonadal and extragonadal germ cell tumors.[3-7] Other non-malignant conditions, such as hepatitis, cirrhosis, inflammatory bowel disease, ataxia telangiectasia, and tyrosinosis, also have been associated with increased serum concentrations of AFP.[3]

Initially, detection of AFP was accomplished utilizing bidimensional immunodiffusion or counterimmunoelectrophoresis. These detection methods are limited in their sensitivity and have been supplanted by radioimmunoassay[3] and fluorescence polarization immunoassay. Serum AFP concentrations peak during the 13th week of gestation, then decrease to approximately 30 µg/mL by term. By 6 months of age, serum concentrations generally are less than 50 ng/mL, and in normal children and adults rarely exceed 25 ng/mL.[2, 3]

Serum AFP is increased in 70–80% of patients with hepatocellular carcinoma. Available data suggest that increased concentrations are demonstrable in virtually all children with hepatoblastoma. In addition, increased concentrations are observed in children with endodermal sinus (yolk sac) tumors. In patients with hepatic or germ-cell tumors, serum AFP concentrations typically range from 1,000 to 100,000 ng/mL; however, concentrations exceeding 200,000 ng/mL are not uncommon, and concentrations greater than 700,000 ng/mL have been reported.[2] There is evidence to suggest that the extent of AFP glycosylation, which is dependent on the concentration of glycosylase in hepatocytes, may be used in differentiating benign from malignant hepatic tumors. Complete glycosylation of AFP has been observed in benign hepatic neoplasms; however, the extent of glycosylation remains to be determined in patients with malignant tumors.[2]

Serum AFP concentrations decrease dramatically in patients with hepatoblastoma and gonadal germ-cell tumors following tumor resection. Transient post-operative increases (reflecting normal tissue regeneration) are sometimes observed following the resection of hepatic tumors. In patients with recurrent tumors, AFP concentrations often can be detected before clinical disease becomes evident. Hence, serial measurement of serum AFP provides a reliable, non-invasive means of assessing the response to therapy and screening patients for early evidence of disease recurrence.[2] A small subset of children with hepatic malignancies associated with precocious puberty or virilization demonstrate increased concentrations of both AFP and human chorionic gonadotropin (HCG). In these cases, AFP has been found to be a more reliable indicator than HCG of the extent of active disease (see discussion below).[6]

Ferritin

Ferritin is a protein-iron complex consisting of a cluster of 24 polypeptide chains, known as apoferritin, which form an outer shell around variable amounts of ferric hydroxyphosphate. It is found in erythroid progenitors in the bone marrow, hepatic parenchymal cells, and reticuloendothelial cells of the liver, spleen, and bone marrow. There are believed to be at least two structurally different types of polypeptide subunits, which are present in varying proportions in ferritins from different tissues and species, and which impart different electrophoretic mobilities to each of these isoferritins.[2]

In addition to intracellular ferritin, low concentrations of ferritin can be found in the serum of normal children and adults. Normal serum concentrations detected by radioimmunoassay, and more recently by enzyme immunoassay, vary considerably with different detection methods. In pediatric patients the normal range is 6–70 µg/L as determined by enzyme immunoassay.[8]

A sensitive indicator of total body iron stores, ferritin is decreased in the very early stages of iron deficiency. Conversely, it is increased in states of iron overload (hemosiderosis and hemochromatosis), when ferritin-containing hepatocytes undergo necrosis (hepatitis), and in chronic inflammatory conditions (chronic infection, rheumatoid arthritis, chronic renal disease).

In some malignant conditions, ferritin is produced by tumor cells, resulting in an increase in total body ferritin and an increase in serum ferritin. To date, increased concentrations of ferritin have been observed in patients with neuroblastoma, leukemia, Hodgkin's lymphoma, and hepatocellular carcinoma.[2] It is clinically most useful in patients with neuroblastoma, Hodgkin's disease, and hepatic malignancies.

In patients with localized tumors and those with Stage IVS neuroblastoma, serum ferritin concentrations are generally within the normal range, even when active disease is present. In contrast, approximately 50% of patients with advanced-stage disease (III and IV) have increased serum ferritin. In patients with disseminated neuroblastoma, serum ferritin is a reliable indicator of tumor burden and is therefore useful in following response to therapy. In addition, there is some evidence to suggest that ferritin concentrations at diagnosis are of prognostic value in advanced-stage disease. In one series, disease-free survival in patients with Stage III neuroblastoma and normal serum ferritin concentrations at diagnosis was 76%, compared to 23% in patients with increased ferritin concentrations. Survival in patients with Stage IV disease and normal ferritin concentrations was 27%, versus 3% in patients with Stage IV disease and increased ferritin concentrations.[9]

Both acidic and basic isoferritins can be identified in patients with neuroblastoma, and recent evidence suggests that they may have exert inhibitory effects on both T-lymphocytes and granulocytes.[2] In the laboratory, transplantation of neuroblastoma into animal models has resulted in subsequent increase of serum ferritin. Ferritin production by neuroblastoma cells has also been observed *in vitro.*[2]

In patients with Hodgkin's disease, increased serum ferritin at diagnosis appears to be associated with an increased risk of relapse. In addition, the degree of increase correlates directly with disease stage (and therefore tumor burden).[10]

Serum ferritin is also a useful indicator of tumor burden and response to therapy in patients with hepatic malignancies, especially in the subset of patients with normal serum AFP concentrations. However, its utility as a prognostic tool has not been well defined in hepatic tumors.[2]

Enzymes

Alkaline Phosphatase

Alkaline phosphatase is a cell-membrane-associated enzyme present in all tissues. It is present in the greatest quantities in osteoblasts, renal tubular epithelium, intestinal epithelium, liver, and placenta. Several tissue-specific isoenzymes have been identified. Their exact functions have not been clearly elucidated; however, the bone-associated enzyme is thought to have some role in calcium deposition.[11]

Alkaline phosphatase activity is measured spectrophotometrically utilizing a chromogenic substrate. In normal children, maximum serum concentrations range from 100 to 500 U/L, depending on the child's age and the specific methodology employed. Maximum adult concentrations range from 50 to 100 U/L.[8, 11] Isoenzymes can be separated by electrophoresis, heat inactivation analysis, urea or chemical inhibition, or the use of specific antisera.

Alkaline phosphatase is increased in patients with intrahepatic and extrahepatic biliary obstruction, hepatocellular damage, or increased osteoblastic activity.[11] Increased concentrations of alkaline phosphatase can be demonstrated in both the serum and tumor tissue of patients with osteogenic sarcoma. Increased serum concentrations are observed in approximately 40% of patients,[12] although concentrations are not well correlated with tumor bulk, the extent of disease, or, interestingly, the degree of tumor calcification. Hence, measurement is not helpful in monitoring response to therapy.[2, 13] In addition, the clinical utility of serum alkaline phosphatase concentrations is limited in patients with underlying hepatic dysfunction or healing fractures, and in children and adolescents in phases of accelerated growth.

Alkaline phosphatase concentrations may be of prognostic significance in patients with osteogenic sarcoma. Data from several studies have suggested that the risk of disease recurrence is higher among patients with increased serum or tumor tissue concentrations of alkaline phosphatase. In one series, survival in patients with increased serum alkaline phosphatase concentrations was 19%, versus 54% among patients with normal serum alkaline phosphatase. In a study of tissue alkaline phosphatase concentrations in osteosarcoma, 17 of 19 patients (89%) with increased enzyme concentrations in the primary lesion developed recurrent disease, whereas relapse occurred in 1 of 6 patients (17%) with normal tumor alkaline phosphatase concentrations.[13]

Lactate Dehydrogenase

Lactate dehydrogenase (LDH) is a ubiquitous cytosolic enzyme which catalyzes the oxidation of lactate to pyruvate. The highest concentrations are found in cardiac and skeletal muscle, liver, kidney, and red blood cells. A tetrameric enzyme, LDH is composed of four polypeptide subunits. Polypeptide chains are of two types, designated M and H (or A and B). Five isoenzymes have been identified, corresponding to each of the five possible combinations of subunits, and denoted LDH-1 through LDH-5. LDH-1 and LDH-2 are found predominantly in kidney, cardiac muscle, and red blood cells; LDH-3 in a variety of tissues, including endorcine glands, spleen, lung, lymph nodes, and platelets; LDH-4 and LDH-5 in liver and skeletal muscle.[11]

LDH activity is measured spectrophotometrically. Reference values of 200–500 U/L typically are obtained in normal subjects; however reference ranges can vary somewhat depending on the specific methodology employed.[8] Increased serum LDH concentrations have been observed in leukemia, lymphoma, rhabdomyosarcoma, Ewing's sarcoma, neuroblastoma, hepatoma, and germ-cell tumors.[2] Among leukemia patients, it appears that those with lymphoblastic leukemias demonstrate higher serum concentrations of LDH than those with myeloid leukemias.[14] Serum LDH concentrations appear to have prognostic value in acute lymphoblastic leukemia (ALL) and non-lymphoblastic non-Hodgkin's lymphoma, with higher serum concentrations of LDH at diagnosis associated with a poorer prognosis in both cases.[15] Similarly, in patients with non-metastatic Ewing's sarcoma, the rate of disease-free survival is greater among those patients with normal serum LDH concentrations at diagnosis.[16] LDH-1, which is not commonly increased in patients with malignant processes, has been found in increased concentrations in the serum of patients with endodermal sinus tumors.[17]

LDH is also increased in patients with hemolysis, as well as in those with muscle injury, inflammation, or infection. In general, the lack of specificity of LDH limits its usefulness as a diagnostic tool. It can, however, be used prognostically in some malignant processes, and, if increased at diagnosis, can serve as a non-invasive indicator of response to therapy.

Creatine Kinase

The reversible phosphorylation of adenosine diphosphate (ADP) by creatine phosphate to form adenosine triphosphate (ATP) is catalyzed by creatine phosphokinase (CK). CK is present mainly in myocardium, skeletal muscle, and brain, and functions in replenishing cellular stores of ATP following ATP-consuming processes such as muscle contraction. Three dimeric isoenzymes exist, each composed of a combination of M (muscle) and B (brain) subunits. CK-1 (BB) is found mainly in the brain and CK-2 (MB) and CK-3 (MM) in heart and skeletal muscle, with CK-3 the predominant isoenzyme.[11] Measured spectrophotometrically, the normal range in the pediatric population is 40–380 U/L.[8]

Increased concentrations of CK generally are observed in patients with inflammatory or degenerative muscle disorders, myocardial infarction, or damage to brain parenchyma (traumatic, ischemic, or inflammatory).[11] Immunohistochemical studies have demonstrated M and B CK subunits in neuroblastoma and rhabdomyosarcoma cells and B subunits in Ewing's sarcoma. Increased serum concentrations of CK-2 have been demonstrated in patients with rhabdomyosarcoma; however, its usefulness as a biological marker has not been widely explored.[2]

Enolase

Three dimeric forms of enolase, a glycolytic enzyme present in neural tissue, have been identified. Neuron-specific enolase (NSE), composed of two δ subunits, is found primarily in neuronal, endocrine, and neuroendocrine cells. Non-neuronal enolase (NNE), consisting of two α subunits, is found in glial cells. A third hybrid form (α, δ) has also been identified.[2]

Measured by RIA, normal concentrations range from 0 to 15 ng/mL. Presence of the enzyme can be detected in neural tissue by immunohistochemical staining. Increased serum concentrations of NSE have been demonstrated in patients with neuroblastoma, medulloblastoma, and retinoblastoma. Concentrations found in association with the latter two tumors are generally less than 100 ng/mL.[2]

In patients with neuroblastoma, disseminated (Stage III or IV) disease is strongly associated with increased concentrations of NSE. In one large, multi-institutional study, 117 of 121 patients (96%) were found to have increased concentrations of NSE at diagnosis. In this study, serum NSE greater than 100 ng/mL was predictive of a poor outcome in patients less than 2 years of age with Stage III disease, and in those less than 1 year of age with Stage IV disease, but not in older patients or those with lower stage disease.[18] Response to therapy is generally well correlated with a decrease in NSE concentrations;[18, 19] however, the utility of serum NSE as a predictive tool with respect to disease recurrence has not been extensively studied. As is also true of serum ferritin, serum NSE concentrations are not increased in patients with Stage IVS disease.[18]

Terminal Deoxynucleotidyl Transferase

Terminal deoxynucleotidyl transferase (tDT) is a DNA polymerase which is able to form single-stranded DNA from nucleotide monophosphates without a DNA template. It is thought to function in the normal state in immunoglobulin and T-cell receptor gene rearrangement. It can be detected in the nuclei of thymocytes and leukemic lymphoblasts by indirect immunofluorescence. It is not present in mature lymphocytes. Serum concentrations are measurable using quantitative enzyme assays or RIA. Increased concentrations are observed primarily in patients with T-cell and pre-B-cell ALL and CML.[20, 21]

Antigens

Carcinoembryonic Antigen

Carcinoembryonic antigen (CEA) is the best known of the tumor-associated antigens. A glycoprotein, it was initially identified as a cell-surface-associated antigen in patients with adenocarcinoma. It is believed to function in cell-to-cell interaction.[1] CEA is measured by RIA or enzyme immunoassay with normal concentrations ranging from 0 to 10 ng/mL.[22]

Increased concentrations are most often found in the sera of adult patients with gastrointestinal malignancies and can consistently be shown to decrease with successful therapy.[3] CEA has been identified in pediatric patients with a variety of malignancies, including Wilms' tumor, neuroblastoma, lymphoma, germ cell tumors, mesenchymal tumors, and retinoblastoma.[3, 23] The lack of specificity of CEA limits its utility as a diagnostic tool in differentiating pediatric tumors. However, if initially increased, CEA may be useful in monitoring response to therapy or as a non-invasive means of post-therapy follow-up in certain clinical situations.

Tumor-Associated Antigens

Tumor-associated antigens (TAAs) are thought to be normally occurring cellular substances expressed in relatively larger quantities by tumor cells. Proteins, carbohydrates, glycoproteins, and glycolipids have been identified in this structurally heterogeneous group of antigens. TAAs are thought to perform any of a number of cellular functions, including transport and inter- and intracellular signaling.

Utilizing monoclonal antibodies, a number of TAAs have been identified in patients with melanoma and carcinoma. In pediatric patients, TAAs have been detected in the urine of several children with sarcomas of soft tissues and bone. In one series of 50 sarcoma patients, 24 of 25 patients (96%) who developed recurrent disease after initial therapy demonstrated increased urinary TAA titers prior to clinical presentation, whereas 23 of 25 patients (92%) who remained disease-free had no increase of urinary TAAs.[24] While TAAs may be useful in post-therapy follow-up, their utility as biological markers requires further exploration.

β-2-Microglobulin

Considered an acute phase reactant, the peptide β-2-microglobulin (BMG) constitutes the light chain of the human leukocyte antigens (HLA). It is also found freely circulating in the serum. It is measured by RIA with serum reference range of 0.10–0.26 mg/dL.[22] Increased concentrations have been observed in association with advanced stage (III and IV) Hodgkin's and non-Hodgkin's lymphoma and appear to correlate with disease remission and response to therapy.[25]

Gangliosides

Gangliosides are glycolipid molecules containing a lipid core surrounded by sialic acid-containing oligosaccharide moieties. Two distinct gangliosides, GD_2 and GD_3, have been identified on the surfaces of neuroblastoma cells and T-cell ALL lymphoblasts, respectively. GD_2 is shed from cells and can be detected in the serum by HPLC or thin-layer chromatography, and increased concentrations have been demonstrated in patients with neuroblastoma. The utility of GD_2 and GD_3 as diagnostic and prognostic tools remains to be fully defined.[26, 27]

Interleukin-2 Receptor

A soluble form of the interleukin-2 receptor (IL2R), a membrane-associated cellular growth factor receptor, has been demonstrated in the serum by enzyme immunoassay. The reference range in normal children is 400–950 U/mL. Increased concentrations are observed in patients with ALL and non-Hodgkin's lymphoma and appear to correlate with increased LDH concentrations. Serum IL2R appears to correlate inversely with prognosis in both cases.[28, 29]

Hormones

Increased hormone concentrations can be detected in association with a number of malignancies. Tumor-associated hormones can be broadly classified into two groups: those produced by primary endocrine malignancies and those produced by non-endocrine tumors. Primary endocrine malignancies are rare in the pediatric population, representing only 4–5% of all pediatric tumors. The tumors most commonly found are gonadal (45%), thyroid (30%), and pituitary (20%).[30] (The majority of primary endocrine malignancies in children do not secrete hormones.)

Neuroblastoma, germ-cell tumors, and hepatic tumors comprise the non-endocrine tumors that produce hormones in pediatric patients. The hormones most often secreted by these non-endocrine malignancies are human chorionic gonadotropin and the catecholamines.

Human Chorionic Gonadotropin

Human chorionic gonadotropin (HCG), a hetereogeneous glycoprotein dimer, is normally produced by the trophoblastic cells of the placenta. It is structurally similar to the other dimeric gonadotropins produced by the anterior pituitary, follicle-stimulating hormone and luteinizing hormone. Composed of one α and one β subunit, the α subunits are identical among the three hormones. Their unique functional and antigenic properties are imparted by structurally distinct β subunits.[31]

HCG is detected by radioimmunoassay, utilizing an antibody directed against the β subunit. Less than 5 IU/mL is detected in the serum of normal males and non-pregnant females.[2] Increased concentrations are detected in gravid females. In pathologic states, increased concentrations are observed most consistently in association with choriocarcinoma and nonseminomatous germ-cell tumors[31, 32] and, less frequently, in association with seminomatous germ-cell tumors and hepatomas.[2, 4, 6, 31]

The half-life of HCG in the serum is 12–20 h. It is therefore a useful indicator of response to therapy, with a dramatic decrease in serum concentrations often demonstrable within several hours of complete resection of a HCG-secreting tumor.[2] Persistently increased HCG concentrations are reliably associated with residual or recurrent disease, except in children with virilizing hepatic tumors. AFP may be a more reliable indicator of disease status in this small group of patients; however, few patients have been studied extensively.

Catecholamines

The catecholamines epinephrine, norepinephrine, and dopamine are produced by cells of neural crest origin in the adrenal medulla. Epinephrine is secreted in large quantities, and norepinephrine to a much lesser degree, in response to pain, emotional stress, and hypoglycemia. They act primarily on the sympathetic nervous system to increase mean arterial blood pressure and myocardial contractility, and they induce glycogenolysis, resulting in increased serum glucose. Serum concentrations of catecholamines are virtually undetectable in the resting state.

Although rare in children, pheochromocytoma, a malignant transformation of the chromaffin cells of the adrenal medulla, is characterized by high circulating concentrations of epinephrine and norepinephrine, resulting in classical clinical symptoms including tachycardia, hypertension, weight loss, and flushing. Increased concentrations of epinephrine and norepinephrine can be detected in the serum, and their metabolites, vanillylmandelic acid (VMA) and the metanephrines, can be detected in the urine.

Neuroblastoma, one of the most common tumors seen in the pediatric age group, also arises from cells of neural crest origin. In contrast to patients with pheochromocytoma, serum concentrations of epinephrine and norepinephrine are normal or minimally increased in children with neuroblastoma. However, catecholamine metabolites VMA and 3-methoxy-4-hydroxyphenoglycol (MHPG), the major metabolites of norepinephrine, and homovanillic acid (HVA), the major metabolite of dopamine, are excreted in the urine in large amounts.[33]

MHPG is measured by gas-liquid chromatography or high-performance liquid chromatography, with normal urinary excretion of 1–2 mg per day. VMA can be measured spectrophotometrically, and both VMA and HVA by high-performance liquid chromatography (HPLC). Both metabolites can be measured simultaneously utilizing bidirectional paper chromatography.[2, 34] Results generally are reported in terms of urine collection time or urine creatinine. Most commonly, HVA and VMA are measured in 24 h urine collections. Normal urinary excretion is less than 10 mg per day each for HVA and VMA. Reference ranges expressed in terms of creatinine are 1–40 micrograms HVA per mg creatinine and less than 7 micrograms VMA per mg creatinine.[34]

Because they can be measured utilizing less complex methodologies, urinary HVA and VMA are the most frequently assayed metabolites and the laboratory tests of choice in the diagnosis of neural crest tumors.[35] Reported rates of catecholamine metabolite excretion in neuroblastoma patients have ranged from 75 to 95% for VMA and 80 to 95% for HVA.[36, 37] In a recent study employing improved HPLC techniques, no overlap was observed between the reference ranges for urinary VMA and the VMA concentrations in patients with neural crest tumors. Patients with neuroblastoma also had urinary HVA concentrations above the 100th percentile.[38] In one study of 94 patients with neuroblastoma, the absolute value of the urinary VMA concentration and the ratio of VMA to HVA was found to correlate directly with prognosis. That is, patients with higher ratios of VMA to HVA tended to have better prognoses. No correlation was observed between the absolute urinary concentration of HVA and prognosis. The same authors also studied the excretion patterns of three other catecholamine metabolites—vanillactic acid (VLA), normetanephrine (NMN), and vanilglycol (VG)—and found that, in general, the presence of the dopamine metabolite VLA correlated with a poorer prognosis, but the presence of the epinephrine and norepinephrine metabolites NMN and VG did not. They postulated that increased urinary dopamine metabolites (VLA) may be observed in patients with poorly differentiated (and therefore more aggressive) tumors which lack dopamine β-hydroxylase, the enzyme which catalyzes the conversion of dopamine to norepinephrine.[37]

In Japan, mass screening of 6- to 7-month-old infants using a spot test for VMA has resulted in the detection of pre-clinical disease as well as an increase in the number of patients detected earlier in the course of the disease (that is, at a lower clinical stage). The greater proportion of patients detected with localized disease has reportedly resulted in improved outcome since the implementation of mass screening.[39] Verification of these findings is in progress in North America using the Quebec Genetic Screening Program.

Growth Factors

Erythropoietin

Erythropoietin is a hematopoietic growth factor which is produced by the kidney and regulates erythropoiesis. A glycoprotein, it is measured by RIA and ELISA and is normally detectable in minute amounts in the serum and urine.

Erythropoietin has been detected in large amounts in both the serum and urine of patients with Wilms' tumor. Of note, increased concentrations of erythropoietin in these patients is not associated with erythrocytosis, suggesting that the erythropoietin produced by this neoplasm is functionally defective. In one study of 37 patients with Wilms' tumor and increased erythropoietin, concentrations were observed to fall dramatically after resection of the primary mass in patients with localized disease, but to remain persistently increased in patients with metastatic disease.[2]

Thrombopoietin

This glycoprotein is a humoral regulator of thrombopoiesis. It is assayed by measurement of ^{35}S incorporation into platelets. Thrombopoietin concentrations have not been widely studied, either in normal patients or those with malignancies. Increased concentrations of thrombopoietin may account for the thrombocytosis observed in association with some pediatric malignancies such as neuroblastoma, lymphoma, some sarcomas, and hepatoblastoma.[40] Its role as a biological marker, however, will require further investigation, including the development of a more facile assay methodology.

Other Markers

A number of other substances have been identified in increased quantities in children with malignant neoplasms. They include carbohydrate, protein, and nucleic acid constituents or metabolites. Several of these markers are of importance in pediatric patients: C-reactive protein, hyaluronic acid, cystathionine, aminoisobutyric acid, and the polyamines.

C-Reactive Protein

C-reactive protein (CRP) is an acute-phase reactant so named for its ability to react with the C-polysaccharide on the cell wall of *Streptococcus pneumoniae*. It is a pentameric structure consisting of five polypeptide subunits which associate in a ring-like fashion. Functionally, CRP can initiate opsonization and phagocytosis, and the classical complement cascade. It can be measured by RIA, radioimmunodiffusion, and rate nephelometry. The reference range using one of the latter two methods is 80–800 µg/dL.[22] Increased concentrations of CRP are observed in association with infection, inflammation, trauma, and malignancy. Increased concentrations of CRP have been observed in association with advanced-stage lymphomas (Hodgkin's and non-Hodgkin's).[25]

Hyaluronic Acid

The glycosaminoglycan, hyaluronic acid, is a large polysaccharide chain which associates with other glycosaminoglycan and protein subunits to form macromolecules called proteoglycans, the major constituents of cartilage and other connective tissue. It has been detected qualitatively by acetic acid precipitation and quantitatively by hyaluronidase degradation with colorimetric assay of disaccharide degradation products. It has been observed in the serum of several patients with Wilms' tumor, inducing hyperviscosity in some cases. A rapid decrease in serum concentrations has been demonstrated in patients whose tumors are completely resected.[41, 42] While measurement of serum hyaluronic acid concentrations may be of benefit in assessing response to therapy in Wilms' tumor, its utility is currently limited by complex assay methodology and limited patient data and clinical correlation.

Cystathionine and Aminoisobutyric Acid

Cystathionine and aminoisobutyric acid are amino acids that have been found in concentrations in the urine of patients with neuroblastoma. Both can be measured by bidirectional paper chromatography, ion exchange, or HPLC. Increased concentrations of cystathionine have been demonstrated in approximately 60% of all patients with neuroblastoma (Stages I–IV) and in up to 75% of patients with Stage III and IV disease. Comparable rates for aminoisobutyric acid are reported to be 75% and 70%, respectively.[37]

Polyamines

Polyamines such as spermidine, spermine, and putrescine are cationic molecules which function in nucleic acid metabolism. Polyamines are known to be both growth factors and inhibitors of immune function. They can be measured by ion-exchange chromatography and HPLC. Reference values in CSF have been established in patients with nonmalignant neurological disorders and in healthy adults (spermidine 77–293 pmol/mL, putrescine 58–278 pmol/mL). Polyamines are produced in increased quantities by rapidly dividing tumors with high DNA turnover. Increased polyamine concentrations have been demonstrated in the urine, serum, and cerebrospinal fluid (CSF) of patients with central nervous system (CNS) malignancies, especially medulloblastoma. Increased CSF concentrations have been demonstrated in several patients with recurrent CNS tumors before clinical or radiographic evidence of relapse was evident.[43-45]

SUPPORTIVE MANAGEMENT OF PEDIATRIC CANCER PATIENTS

The clinical chemistry laboratory is essential to the diagnosis and appropriate management of patients with biochemical abnormalities resulting from tumor therapy. Metabolic derangements during treatment most commonly result from rapid lysis of tumor cells or the direct effects of chemotherapeutic agents on hepatic, renal, or pancreatic tissues.

Tumor Lysis Syndrome

Acute tumor lysis syndrome (TLS) results from the cytolysis of tumor cells and subsequent release of phosphate and potassium, as well as xanthine, hypoxanthine, and uric acid, the products of nucleic acid degradation.

TLS is observed in association with very large or rapidly dividing tumors and is most often encountered in patients with lymphoma or ALL.[46, 47] Patients particularly at risk are those with Burkitt's lymphoma[48] and T-cell leukemia, both of which have particularly short doubling times. TLS also has been described in association with chronic myelogenous leukemia, recurrent non-Hodgkin's lymphoma,[49] and metastatic medulloblastoma.[50]

The classical metabolic triad of hyperuricemia, hyperphosphatemia, and hyperkalemia characterizes TLS. Phosphate and uric acid are freely filtered by the kidney and, if present in excessive quantities in the serum, can exceed their solubility in urine and precipitate in the renal collecting ducts. In addition, the solubility of uric acid (pKa 5.4) is decreased in the acid environment of the nephron, thus increasing even further the risk of uric acid precipitation. Urate and/or phosphate nephropathy may result in renal dysfunction and oliguria, and ultimately renal failure. Less frequently, excessive uric acid excretion results in the formation of urate stones. Hyperphosphatemia induces hypocalcemia as a result of precipitation of calcium phosphate crystals and sequestration of calcium in bone and other tissues; tetany or seizures may result. Increased serum potassium may induce electrocardiographic abnormalities, including fatal cardiac arrhythmias.

Since it occurs when cellular degeneration is greatest, TLS usually is observed at diagnosis or within the first several days after the initiation of therapy and has been reported to reappear in patients with recurrent tumors (see Figure 17–2). Routine screening of patients at diagnosis, especially those with malignancies in which there is an increased frequency of TLS, is essential in establishing baseline

FIGURE 17-2. A Typical Profile of the Metabolic Derangements Observed in a Patient with ALL and Acute Tumor Lysis Symdrome

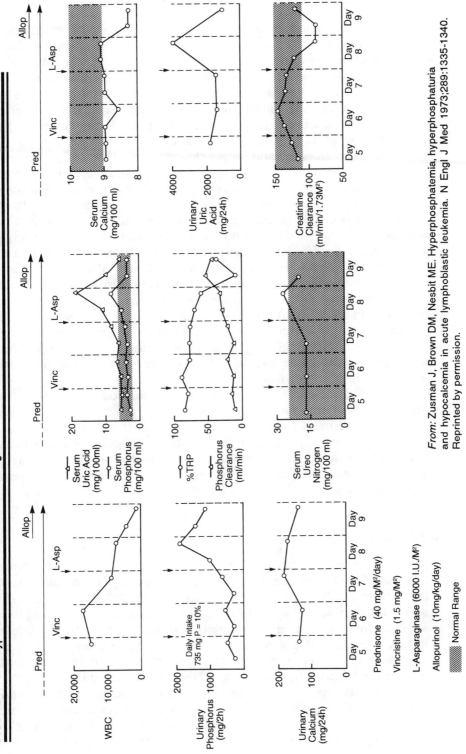

From: Zusman J, Brown DM, Nesbit ME. Hyperphosphatemia, hyperphosphaturia and hypocalcemia in acute lymphoblastic leukemia. N Engl J Med 1973;289:1335-1340. Reprinted by permission.

metabolic parameters and in identifying patients with chemical evidence of TLS without clinical manifestations. The laboratory evaluation should include measurement of electrolyte, calcium, phosphorus, and uric acid concentrations, as well as those of blood urea nitrogen and serum creatinine. Routine measurement of these parameters should continue through the initial phases of therapy, with the frequency of measurement tailored to the degree of metabolic derangement.

Therapy of TLS is aimed at correcting metabolic abnormalities such as hyperkalemia and hypocalcemia and decreasing the risk of renal impairment by minimizing renal deposition of phosphate and urate crystals. The latter is accomplished by vigorous hydration to maintain brisk urinary diuresis; administration of bicarbonate to effect alkalinization of the urine and thereby prevent precipitation of urate and phosphate crystals; and administration of allopurinol, which partially blocks production of uric acid from its oxypurine precursors, xanthine and hypoxanthine, both of which are also excreted in the urine. As a result of allopurinol administration, nucleic acid metabolites are excreted as xanthine, hypoxanthine, and uric acid rather than as uric acid alone, resulting in an increase in the total amount of oxypurine excreted. Urinary pH is maintained between 7.0 and 7.5 in order to prevent precipitation of phosphate in excessively alkaline urine and to minimize the risk of hypocalcemia resulting from excessive systemic alkalinization.

While in most cases TLS can be well controlled with these measures, a small number of patients develop progressive nephropathy and renal failure. In these patients, increased serum potassium induced by tumor cytolysis is exacerbated by poor renal potassium excretion. Dialysis is generally required. Hemodialysis is preferred to peritoneal dialysis in most cases because it affords more precise control of fluid and electrolyte management.

Assessment of Drug Toxicity

Chemotherapeutic agents induce systemic toxicity by one of two mechanisms: (1) interference with cell division in rapidly dividing tissues (gastrointestinal epithelium, bone marrow); or (2) induction of a direct toxic effect on some aspect of cellular function in non-dividing tissues such as liver, kidney, and pancreas. Surveillance for the toxic effects induced by the latter mechanism often can be accomplished by measurement of cellular metabolic products or other metabolic constituents in the serum which are specific for the affected target organ.

Methotrexate, the purine analogues (6-mercaptopurine and 6-thioguanine), *cis*-platinum, L-asparaginase, and corticosteroids are the agents which most frequently induce direct cellular damage which can be assessed using chemical parameters. Routine screening of such parameters facilitates timely treatment of toxic effects and appropriate drug deletions or dose modifications (see Table 17–2).[51-53]

TABLE 17–2. Antineoplastic Agents which Induce Hepatic or Renal Toxicity or Require Dose Modification in Patients with Underlying Hepatic or Renal Dysfunction

	Induces Renal Dysfunction	Induces Hepatic Dysfunction	Altered Pharmacokinetics in Renal Dysfunction	Altered Pharmacokinetics in Hepatic Dysfunction
Anthracyclines				■
Cis–Platinum	□		■	
Methotrexate	□	□	■	
6–Mercaptopurine /6–Thioguanine		□		
5–Fluorouracil				■
Cyclophosphamide	□			■
Ifosfamide	□			■
Melphalan				■
Nitrosoureas	□			
Dacarbazine				■
Etoposide				■
Vincristine	□			■

Methotrexate

This antimetabolite acts by inhibition of the enzyme dihydrofolate reductase, which catalyzes the reduction of oxidized folate to its active reduced form, tetrahydrofolate, ultimately resulting in the cessation of purine synthesis. It is used extensively in the treatment of ALL in children and is also employed in the treatment of osteosarcoma. Methotrexate can be administered orally, intravenously, and intrathecally, and may be used at either conventional or high doses. In the latter case, drug administration is followed by the administration of the leucovorin, a reduced folate analogue which reverses the biochemical effects of methotrexate.

In addition to bone marrow suppression and mucositis, the most commonly observed toxic effect of methotrexate is the induction of acute hepatitis, characterized by an increase of hepatic transaminases. The mechanism of induction of hepatic toxicity is not completely known; however, it is thought to be related to interference with choline synthesis. Older patients and those with underlying liver disease are at greatest risk. High-dose therapy reliably induces an acute increase of hepatic enzymes, with a return to normal concentrations within 1 week. In addition, hyperbilirubinemia is sometimes observed in association with high-dose therapy. Chronic oral administration of lower dose methotrexate, employed in maintenance therapy for ALL, may induce an acute increase of hepatic enzymes, but less predictably than that observed in high-dose therapy. In this situation, temporary suspension of oral therapy or dosage reduction frequently results in return of enzyme concentrations to normal. Chronic hepatic dysfunction is infrequently observed in children. In general, assessment of liver function in patients receiving long-term therapy with methotrexate should be performed monthly and should include measurement of alanine aminotransferase, aspartate aminotransferase, alkaline phosphatase, and bilirubin.

Renal dysfunction, as reflected by blood urea nitrogen (BUN) and creatinine, is induced by the deposition of methotrexate and 7-hydroxymethotrexate in renal tubules. It is observed in association with high-dose therapy. Drug administration in this situation is accompanied by hydration and systemic alkalinization to facilitate renal excretion and reduce precipitation of methotrexate and its metabolites. The assessment of BUN and creatinine is essential prior to therapy and during drug administration.

6-Mercaptopurine and 6-Thioguanine

The purine analogues 6-mercaptopurine and 6-thioguanine (6-TG), which act both by inhibition of *de novo* nucleotide biosynthesis and incorporation into DNA, are important components of ALL and AML therapy in children. 6-MP induces hepatic cholestasis and hepatocellular necrosis, resulting in an increase of hepatic transaminases, alkaline phosphatase, and bilirubin. 6-TG has been associated with similar laboratory findings, albeit much less frequently. The risk of hepatotoxicity is increased in patients receiving concomitant therapy with other hepatotoxic agents such as methotrexate.

Cis-Platinum

Cis-platinum (*cis*-diaminedichloroplatinum or CDDP) is an alkylating agent which acts by induction of DNA crosslinks and interference in DNA synthesis. It is currently used in the treatment of brain tumors, lymphoma, osteosarcoma, and neuroblastoma. Its major non-hematologic side effect is nephrotoxicity, induced by direct cellular damage to the epithelium of the distal tubules and collecting ducts. The major clinical effects are progressive decrease in the glomerular filtration rate and magnesium wasting. The risk of renal damage is decreased with vigorous hydration during CDDP administration.

Routine screening of renal function with BUN and creatinine is essential throughout the duration of therapy and often for several months thereafter. In addition, glomerular function must be assessed prior to the administration of each course of CDDP. The determination of creatinine clearance based on a 24 h urine collection is employed in older children and adolescents who can cooperate with urine collection. Radiologic evaluation utilizing radioisotope renal scanning is necessary in younger children. Dose modification or deletion of CDDP is required with progressive decline in renal function.

Frequent monitoring of serum magnesium concentrations is also necessary during CDDP therapy. Many patients require chronic oral magnesium replacement during and often for several weeks following treatment with repeated courses of CDDP. Asymptomatic hypomagnesemia is most frequently encountered. Rarely, muscle cramping or frank tetany occurs.

L-Asparaginase

The enzyme L-asparaginase is a mainstay of therapy in childhood ALL and lymphoma in children. It acts by catalyzing the conversion of L-asparagine to aspartate, thus depleting cellular stores of L-asparagine and ultimately resulting in the inhibition of protein synthesis. The spectrum of its toxicities include allergic reactions, coagulopathy, acute pancreatitis, and hepatotoxicity. Pancreatic toxicity is manifested by non-ketotic hyperglycemia, requiring assessment of serum and urine glucose concentrations, especially when therapy is initiated. Insulin is occasionally required to control hyperglycemia, especially in those patients also receiving steroid therapy. Death from acute pancreatitis in this setting is rare. Hepatotoxicity, manifested by increased concentrations of hepatic transaminases, is also rarely observed.

Corticosteroids

Although steroid therapy is employed as primary therapy for leukemia and lymphoma in children, its mechanism of action is not well understood. It is also used in patients with central nervous system tumors who have clinical evidence of intracranial pressure. Short courses of steroid therapy, even when administered in high doses, are generally without clinical effects. In contrast, prolonged steroid therapy may have a number of untoward clinical and biochemical effects, including increased appetite, obesity, poor growth, poor wound healing, salt and water retention, hypertension, and hyperglycemia.

Serum glucose must be assessed routinely in patients requiring prolonged steroid therapy and in patients who require concomitant therapy with L-asparaginase, such as those in the initial phases of therapy for ALL or lymphoma.

Miscellaneous Toxicities

A number of other chemotherapeutic agents which induce systemic biochemical toxicity are either less frequently employed in pediatric chemotherapy regimens or less frequently associated with toxicities.

The oxazophosphorine alkylating agents, cyclophosphamide and ifosfamide, are both associated with renal dysfunction. Cyclophosphamide, which is employed in the treatment of lymphoma, leukemia, neuroblastoma, and sarcoma, acts on the renal tubules to induce water retention and secondary hyponatremia in small numbers of patients. Hydration is required during cyclophosphamide administration to minimize morbidity from drug-induced hemorrhagic cystitis. Therefore, frequent assessment of serum electrolytes and urine specific gravity is warranted during cyclophosphamide administration. Ifosfamide, an agent employed in the treatment of sarcomas, has been reported to induce renal insufficiency as a result of direct renal tubular damage.

The alkylating agents, lomustine (CCNU) and carmustine (BCNU), are nitrosoureas which are used in the therapy of lymphomas and central nervous system tumors. High cumulative doses have been associated with the late development of renal dysfunction.

Finally, vincristine, a plant alkaloid which acts by mitotic inhibition, is widely used in the treatment of leukemia, lymphoma, and various solid tumors. Rarely observed in pediatric patients, it has been associated with inappropriate antidiuretic hormone secretion resulting in water retention and hyponatremia.

CLINICAL PHARMACOLOGY AND ANTINEOPLASTIC THERAPY

Therapeutic Drug Monitoring

Therapeutic drug monitoring (TDM) is defined as the measurement of a drug or its metabolite(s) in the serum or another body fluid for the purpose of tailoring systemic drug therapy to provide maximum therapeutic effect and minimal toxicity. The application of TDM to the clinical use of a specific drug requires that (1) its pharmacologic properties are well defined; (2) it can be measured using a reliable, simple, and inexpensive methodology with adequate sensitivity and specificity; and (3) serum or body fluid concentrations can be correlated both with the drug's desired clinical and biological effects and its toxic effects.[53]

The application of TDM to the clinical management of anticonvulsant, antibiotic, and anti-asthmatic therapy is well known. However, despite the extensive use of systemic drug therapy in the treatment of human malignancies, TDM has not been widely implemented with respect to most antineoplastic agents.

Several factors specific to antineoplastic therapy account for the limitations of TDM in this setting.[53] First, the distribution characteristics, metabolic properties, and pharmacokinetics of many neoplastic agents have yet to be fully defined. For some agents, like bleomycin and procarbazine, biologically active metabolites have not been completely identified. For other drugs, such as vincristine, distribution properties are not well characterized.

Secondly, the biological response of tumors to specific chemotherapeutic agents cannot be universally determined. While toxic drug concentrations may be determined with certainty if all active metabolites can be identified and measured, therapeutic concentrations must be assessed for each histologically distinct tumor. The assessment of therapeutic effect is complicated further by the functional heterogeneity of tumors of the same histologic type with respect to their biological response to antineoplastic drugs. This tumor heterogeneity can be subdivided into three subtypes: clonal, cell kinetic, and physical heterogeneity. Clonal heterogeneity refers to the development of genetic mutations within neoplasms, which render tumor cells drug-resistant. Cell-kinetic heterogeneity results from non-synchronous cell division within tumors, which results in non-uniform susceptibility to the effects of a chemotherapeutic agent on a neoplasm. Also, the location of cells within solid tumors relative to their blood supply affects both cellular accessibility and susceptibility to antineoplastic agents. This physical heterogeneity within tumors results in variability in the degree to which individual cells are exposed to both therapeutic drug concentrations and cellular nutrients.

Thirdly, the evaluation of the therapeutic and toxic effects of antineoplastic agents is difficult in the setting of multi-drug or multimodality antineoplastic therapy. While *in vitro* data is essential in assessing a drug's therapeutic effect, *in vivo* drug effects do not always correlate with measurable concentrations. Furthermore, when multidrug therapy is employed clinically, it becomes difficult, if not impossible, to attribute therapeutic or biologic effects to a single agent. Similarly, many drugs used in combination therapy have overlapping toxicities, which limits the clinical correlation between drug concentration and toxicity for individual agents.

Despite current limitations, the utility of TDM in the treatment of malignancies is promising. The potential applications of TDM in antineoplastic therapy include (1) the assessment of compliance; (2) the measurement of bioavailability; (3) the evaluation of efficacy and toxicity in specialized therapy such as high-dose, continuous infusion, regional, and adjuvant chemotherapy; (4) the assessment of dose modifications in patients with underlying organ dysfunction; and (5) the establishment of standard toxic ranges for agents with cumulative dose-limiting toxicities.[53]

Because its pharmacokinetic properties have been well established in both plasma and CSF (see Figure 17–3), TDM in antineoplastic therapy has been most successfully applied to systemic high-dose methotrexate therapy, where lethal doses of methotrexate are administered by continuous infusion over a 6–24 h period, followed by "rescue" therapy with leucovorin. High-dose methotrexate is employed both as a systemic treatment modality (osteosarcoma) or as a means of effecting treatment of or prophylaxis against malignant CNS disease (leukemia and lymphoma). Concentrations can be easily measured in serum and other body fluids by RIA, competitive protein binding, enzyme inhibition assay, immunoassay, or HPLC.[52, 53] The relationship between plasma methotrexate concentration and toxicity has been well established, and the measurement of serum concentrations can be used to tailor leucovorin "rescue" therapy (see Figure 17–4).

More recently, the measurement of serum of 6-mercaptopurine concentrations by HPLC in a small series of children receiving oral maintenance therapy for ALL revealed that patients who relapsed had

FIGURE 17–3. Methotrexate Gradient from Plasma to Cerebrospinal Fluid during Constant Intravenous Infusion

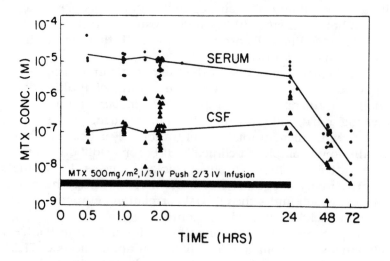

From Freeman AI, Wang JJ, Sinks LF. High-dose methotrexate in acute lymphocytic leukemia. Cancer Treat Rep 1977;61:727-31.

FIGURE 17–4. Methotrexate Plasma Disappearance Curves in Patients Receiving Six-Hour Infusions (50–250 mg/kg), followed by Leucovorin Rescue

Levels for patients who experienced no toxicity are represented by the hatched area.
Non-toxic patients who received additional leucovorin are represented by the solid circles.
Levels for toxic patients are represented by open circles.

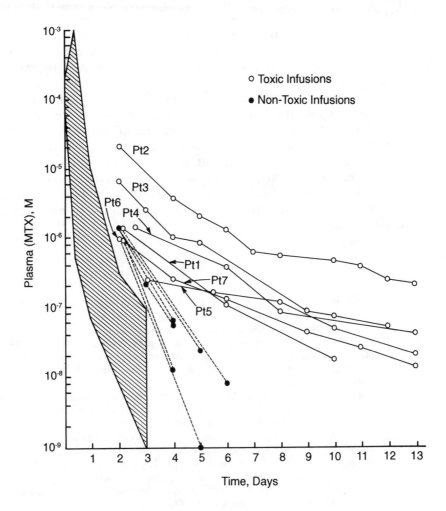

From Stoller RG, Hande KR, Jacobs SA, Rosenberg SA, and Chabner BA. Use of plasma pharmacokinetics to predict and prevent methotrexate toxicity. N Engl J Med 1977;297:630-34. Reprinted by permission.

significantly lower mean systemic exposure to 6-mercaptopurine compared to patients who did not relapse. Although additional prospective data are needed, current evidence suggests that TDM may be useful in optimizing oral therapy with 6-mercaptopurine, thus improving the ultimate clinical outcome in patients with ALL.[54]

CONCLUSION

The clinical laboratory provides rapid identification and measurement of tumor-associated markers in the blood, urine, and other body fluids, assisting the clinician in the diagnosis of many pediatric malignancies. In addition, in many cases the measurement of tumor markers provides a non-invasive means of assessing response to therapy and detecting early disease relapse or recurrence. The toxic effects of antineoplastic agents, specifically renal, hepatic, and pancreatic dysfunction, can be non-invasively detected and monitored in the clinical laboratory. The laboratory is also essential to the diagnosis and clinical management of TLS, a condition characterized by electrolyte and mineral derangements which result from the rapid and massive lysis of tumor cells in the early phases of therapy. Finally, the development of drug monitoring technologies has resulted in their clinical application to antineoplastic therapy. While currently limited to methotrexate and 6-mercaptopurine, the application of TDM to other chemotherapeutic agents is promising.

REFERENCES

1. Herlyn M, Menrad A, Koprowski H. Structure, function, and clinical significance of human tumor antigens. J Natl Cancer Inst 1990;82:1883-89.
2. Ortega JA, Siegel SE. Biological markers in pediatric cancer. In: Pizzo PA, Poplack DG, eds., Principles and practice of pediatric oncology, Philadelphia: Lippincott, 1989:149-62.
3. Mann JR, Lakin GE, Leonard JC, et al. Clinical applications of serum carcinoembryonic antigen and alpha-fetoprotein concentrations in children with solid tumors. Arch Dis Child 1978;53:366-74.
4. Perlin E, Engeler JE, Edson M, Karp D, McIntire KR, Waldmann TA. The value of serial measurement of both human chorionic gonadotropin and alpha-fetoprotein for monitoring germinal cell tumors. Cancer 1976;37:215-19.
5. Talerman A, Haije WG. Alpha-fetoprotein and germ cell tumors: A possible role of yolk sac tumor in production of alpha-fetoprotein. Cancer 1974;34:1722-26.
6. Nakagawara A, Ikeda K, Tsuneyoshi M, et al. Hepatoblastoma producing both alpha-fetoprotein and human chorionic gonadotropin. Cancer 1985;56:1636-42.
7. Tsuchida Y, Saito S, Ishida M. Yolk sac tumor (endodermal sinus tumor) and alpha-fetoprotein: A report of three cases. Cancer 1973;32:917-21.
8. Meites S, Buffone GJ, Cheng MH, et al., eds., Pediatric clinical chemistry, 3rd ed. Washington, DC: AACC Press, 1989.
9. Hann H, Evans A, Seigel S, et al. Prognostic importance of serum ferritin in patients with stage III and IV neuroblastoma: The CCSG experience. Cancer Res 1985;45:2843-48.
10. Hann HL, Lange BJ, Stalhut MW, McGlynn KA. Serum ferritin and prognosis of childhood Hodgkin's disease (abstr). Proc Am Soc Clin Oncol 1987;6:190.

11. Moss DW, Henderson AR, Kachmar JF. Enzymes. In Tietz NW, ed., Textbook of clinical chemistry. Philadelphia: Saunders, 1986:763-74.

12. Scranton PE, DeCicco FA, Totten RS, Yunis RJ. Prognostic factors in osteosarcoma: A review of 20 years' experience at the University of Pittsburgh Health Center Hospitals. Cancer 1975;36:2179-91.

13. Levine AM, Rosenburg SA. Alkaline phosphatase levels in osteosarcoma are related to prognosis. Cancer 1979;44:2291-93.

14. Kornberg A, Polliack A. Serum lactic dehydrogenase (LDH) levels in acute leukemia: Marked elevations in lymphoblastic leukemia. Blood 1980;56:351-55.

15. Pui CH, Dodge RK, Dahl GV, et al. Serum lactic dehydrogenase level has prognostic value in childhood acute lymphoblastic leukemia. Blood 1985;66:778-82.

16. Glaubiger DL, Makuch R, Schwarz J, Levine AS, Johnson RE. Determination of prognostic factors and their influence on therapeutic results in patients with Ewing's sarcoma. Cancer 1980;45:2213-19.

17. Kinumaki H, Takeuche H, Nakamura K. Serum lactate dehydrogenase isoenzyme-1 in children with yolk sac tumor. Cancer 1985;56:178-81.

18. Zeltzer PM, Marangos PJ, Evans AE, Schneider SL. Serum neuron-specific enolase in children with neuroblastoma: Relationship to stage and disease course. Cancer 1986;57:1230-34.

19. Ishiguro Y, Kato K, Ito T, Nagaya M, Yamada N, Sugito T. Nervous system-specific enolase in serum as a marker for neuroblastoma. Pediatrics 1983;72:696-700.

20. Poplack DG. Acute lymphoblastic leukemia. In: Pizzo PA, Poplack DG, eds., Principles and practice of pediatric oncology, Philadelphia: Lippincott, 1989:323-66.

21. Hutton JJ, Coleman MS, Moffitt S, et al. Prognostic significance of terminal transferase activity in childhood acute lymphoblastic leukemia: A prospective analysis of 164 patients. Blood 1982;60:1267-76.

22. Silverman LM, Christenson RH, Grant GH. Amino acids and proteins. In: Tietz NW, ed., Textbook of clinical chemistry. Philadelphia: Saunders, 1986:619-762.

23. Frens DB, Bray PF, Wu JT, Lahey ME. The carcinoembryonic antigen assay: Prognostic value in neural crest tumors. J Pediatr 1976;88:591-94.

24. Huth JF, Gupta RK, Eilber FR, Morton DL. A prospective postoperative evaluation of urinary tumor-associated antigens in sarcoma patients. Cancer 1984;53:1306-10.

25. Child JA, Spati B, Illingworth S, et al. Serum beta 2 microglobulin and c-reactive protein in the monitoring of lymphomas. Cancer 1980;45:318-26.

26. Ladisch S, Wu ZL. Circulating gangliosides as tumor markers. Prog Clin Biol 1985;175:277-84.

27. Schulz G, Cheresh DA, Varki NM, et al. Detection of ganglioside G in tumor tissue and sera of neuroblastoma patients. Cancer Res 1984;44:5914-20.

28. Pui CH, Ip SH, Kung P, et al. High serum interleukin-2 levels are related to advanced disease and a poor outcome in childhood non-Hodgkin's lymphoma. Blood 1987;70:624-28.

29. Pui CH, Ip SH, Behm FG, et al. Serum interleukin 2 receptor levels in childhood acute lymphoblastic leukemia. Blood 1988;71:1135-37.

30. Chrousos GP. Endocrine tumors. In: Pizzo PA, Poplack DG, eds., Principles and practice of pediatric oncology, Philadelphia: Lippincott, 1989:733-57.

31. Altman AJ, Schwartz AD, eds., Malignant diseases of infancy, childhood and adolescence, 2nd ed. Philadelphia: Saunders, 1983.

32. Bosl GJ, Lange PH, Nochomovitz LE. Tumor markers in advanced nonseminomatous testicular cancer. Cancer 1981;47:572-76.

33. Gitlow SE, Dziedzic LB, Strauss L, Greenwood SM, Dziedzic SW. Biochemical and histological determinants in the prognosis of neuroblastoma. Cancer 1973;32:898-905.

34. Chattoraj SC, Watts NB. Endocrinology. In: Tietz NW, ed., Textbook of clinical chemistry. Philadelphia: Saunders, 1986:997-1171.

35. Soldin SJ, Hill JG. Liquid chromatographic analysis for urinary VMA and HVA and its use in the investigation of neural crest tumors. Clin Chem 1981;27:502-3.

36.   Gitlow SE, Bertani LM, Rausen A, Gribetz D, Dziedzic SW. Diagnosis of neuroblastoma by qualitative and quantitative determination of catecholamine metabolites in the urine. Cancer 1970;25:1377-83.

37.   Laug WE, Siegel SE, Shaw KNF, Landing B, Baptista J, Gutenstein M. Initial urinary catecholamine metabolite concentrations and prognosis in neuroblastoma. Pediatrics 1978; 62:77-83.

38.   Soldin SJ. Applications of liquid chromatography in a children's hospital. In: Hawk GE, ed., Biological/biomedical applications of liquid chromatography. M. Dekker, 20:135-44.

39.   Sawada T, Kidowaki T, Sakamoto I, et al. Neuroblastoma: Mass screening for early detection and its prognosis. Cancer 1984;53:2731-35.

40.   Nickerson HJ, Silberman TL, Mc Donald TP. Hepatoblastoma, thrombocytosis, and thrombopoietin. Cancer 1980;45:315-17.

41.   Powars DR, Allerton SE, Beierle J, Butler BB. Wilms' tumor: Clinical correlation with circulating mucin in three cases. Cancer 1972;29:1597-1605.

42.   Wu AHB, Parker OS, Ford, L. Hyperviscosity caused by hyaluronic acid in serum in a case of Wilms' tumor. Clin Chem 1984;30:914-16.

43.   Russell DH, Levy CC, Schimpf SC, Hawk IA. Urinary polyamines in cancer patients. Cancer Res 1971;31:1555-58.

44.   Marton LJ, Hruby O, Levin VA, et al. The relationship of polyamines in cerebrospinal fluid to the presence of central nervous system tumors. Cancer Res 1976;36:973-77.

45.   Marton LJ, Edwards MS, Levin VA, Lubich WP, Wilson CB. Predictive values of cerebrospinal fluid polyamines in medulloblastomas. Cancer Res 1979;39:993-97.

46.   Boles JM, Dutel JL, Briere J, Mialon P, et al. Acute renal failure caused by extreme hyperphosphatemia after chemotherapy of an acute lymphoblastic leukemia. Cancer 1984;53:2425-29.

47.   Zusman J, Brown DM, Nesbit ME. Hyperphosphatemia, hyperphosphaturia and hypocalcemia in acute lymphoblastic leukemia. N Engl J Med 1973;289:1335-40.

48.   Cohen LF, Balow JE, Magrath IT, Poplack DG, Ziegler JL. Acute tumor lysis syndrome: A review of 37 patients with Burkitt's lymphoma. Am J Med 1980;68:486-91.

49.   Boccia RV, Longo DL, Lieber ML. Multiple recurrences of acute tumor lysis syndrome in an indolent non-Hodgkin's lymphoma. Cancer 1985;56:2295-97.

50.   Tomlinson GC, Solberg LA. Acute tumor lysis syndrome with metastatic medulloblastoma: A case report. Cancer 1984;53:1783-85.

51.   Balis FM, Holcenberg JS, Poplack DG. General principles of chemotherapy. In: Pizzo PA, Poplack DG, eds., Principles and practice of pediatric oncology, Philadelphia: Lippincott, 1989:165-205.

52.   Chabner BA. Clinical pharmacokinetics and drug monitoring. In: Chabner BA, ed., Pharmacologic principles of cancer treatment, Philadelphia: Saunders, 1982:100-8.

53.   Moore MJ, Erlichman C. Therapeutic drug monitoring in oncology: Problems and potential in antineoplastic therapy. Clin Pharm 1987;13:205-27.

54.   Koren G, Ferrazini G, Sulh H, et al. Systemic exposure to mercaptopurine as a prognostic factor in acute lymphocytic leukemia in children. N Engl J Med 1990;323:17-21.

Disorders of Porphyrin Metabolism

George H. Elder, B.A., M.D., F.R.C.Path., F.R.C.P.

INTRODUCTION

The porphyrias are a group of disorders of heme biosynthesis in which characteristic clinical features occur in association with specific patterns of overproduction of heme precursors. There are two main types of clinical disease: skin lesions, caused by photosensitization of the skin by accumulated porphyrins, and acute neurovisceral attacks, which typically consist of severe abdominal pain which may be accompanied by peripheral neuropathy, mental disturbances, and convulsions.

The main types of porphyria, their clinical features and prevalence are shown in Table 18–1. Only two of the main types of porphyria, erythropoietic protoporphyria (EPP) and congenital erythropoietic porphyria (CEP), are disorders of childhood. Symptoms in the other types usually do not appear until adult life, even though all porphyrias, except for some forms of porphyria cutanea tarda (PCT), are inherited disorders with biochemical defects present from birth. In particular, the life-threatening acute attacks that occur in acute intermittent porphyria (AIP) and the other acute hepatic porphyrias (see Table 18–1) are very rare before puberty.

TABLE 18–1. The Main Types of Porphyria

Disorder	Acute Attacks	Skin Lesions	Estimated Prevalance of Overt Cases (all ages)
1. PBG-synthase deficiency porphyria	+	−	—
2. Acute intermittent porphyria	+	−	1–2:100,000
3. Congenital erythropoietic porphyria	−	+	Less than $1:10^6$
4. Porphyria cutanea tarda	−	+	1:25,000
5. Hereditary coproporphyria	+	+	Less than 1:250,000
6. Variegate porphyria	+	+	1:250,000
7. Erythropoietic protoporphyria	−	+	1:200,000

In hereditary coproporphyria and variegate porphyria, skin lesions and acute attacks may occur together or separately.

When porphyrias are encountered in pediatric practice, it is usually for one of two different reasons. First, symptoms may suggest a diagnosis of porphyria. Usually these will be dermatological because those types of porphyria that typically present during childhood—CEP, EPP, and rare homozygous variants of the acute porphyrias—mainly affect the skin. Second, advice may be sought about a child who, although asymptomatic, has a family history of porphyria. This chapter focuses on these two aspects, as comprehensive general descriptions of the porphyrias are provided by a number of recent reviews.[1-3]

Abnormalities of porphyrin metabolism occur in several disorders apart from the porphyrias, notably in iron deficiency and some other anemias, in lead poisoning, in cholestasis, and in inherited hyperbilirubinemias.[4, 5] These conditions are not discussed here, except in relation to the differential diagnosis of porphyria.

BIOSYNTHESIS OF HEME

The pathway of heme biosynthesis is outlined in Figure 18–1. Formation of the first committed precursor, 5-aminolevulinate (ALA), from succinyl-CoA and glycine is catalyzed in mitochondria by ALA synthase. A series of condensation reactions then leads to the formation of the linear tetrapyrrole, hydroxymethylbilane, which is then cyclized with reversal of one pyrrolic unit to form the asymmetric tetrapyrrolic macrocycle, uroporphyrinogen III. An alternative fate for hydroxymethylbilane, non-enzymatic cyclisation to the symmetrical porphyrinogen isomer, uroporphyrinogen I, accounts for less than 1% of the metabolism of hydroxymethylbilane in normal circumstances, but may be enhanced in pathological conditions where hydroxymethylbilane accumulates. Uroporphyrinogen is then decarboxylated to coproporphyrinogen by a reaction that is not isomer-specific.

Subsequent side chain modifications and aromatization to form protoporphyrin IX are restricted to the isomer III series. Heme is then formed by enzymatic chelation of ferrous iron (see Figure 18–1). The porphyrinogen intermediates of this pathway are unstable and readily autoxidize to the corresponding porphyrins within tissues and during excretion.

Normal adults synthesize about 7 mol/kg body weight of heme each day, 80–85% of which is used for hemoglobin formation, while the rest is used, mainly in the liver, for the formation of cytochromes and other hemoproteins. At least 50% of the heme made in the liver is incorporated into cytochromes of the P450 series that catalyze the oxidative metabolism of a wide range of endogenous compounds and xenobiotics, including many drugs.

The regulation of the rate of heme biosynthesis in mammalian cells has been studied extensively.[6] The ALA synthases of human liver and erythroid cells are encoded by separate genes on the X chromosome and chromosome 3, respectively, and factors influencing their activities in these tissues are different. In the liver, ALA synthase activity determines the rate of heme synthesis. Activity is controlled by negative feedback regulation by heme of the rate of synthesis of mature mitochondrial enzyme.[7] The short half-life of the enzyme allows the cell to respond rapidly to changes in the demand for heme, for example, in

FIGURE 18–1. The Pathway of Heme Biosynthesis

The reactions are catalyzed by 5-aminolevulinate (ALA) synthase (1), porphobilinogen (PBG) synthase (2), PBG deaminase (3), uroporphyrinogen III synthase (4), uroporphyrinogen decarboxylase (5), coproporphyrinogen oxidase (6), protoporphyrinogen oxidase (7), and ferrochelatase (8.)

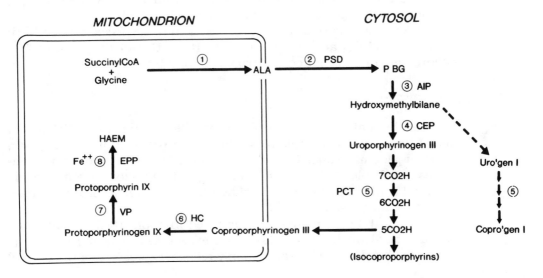

response to administration of a drug that induces cytochrome P450 synthesis.

Heme for the formation of hemoproteins is believed to come from a regulatory heme pool. Depletion of this pool through combination of heme and apoprotein leads to derepression of the synthesis of ALA-synthase and hence to replenishment of the heme pool. This type of mechanism is consistent with an important feature of hepatic heme synthesis: the readiness with which changes in ALA synthase activity occur in response to a wide range of external stimuli, including many drugs that induce cytochrome P450. In contrast, few compounds affect ALA synthase activity in erythroid cells. In these cells, mechanisms for the regulation of heme synthesis are complex and an integral part of the process of progressive differentiation of erythroid cells.[6]

METABOLISM OF HEME PRECURSORS

The close regulation of heme biosynthesis and the kinetics of the inter-mediate reactions ensure that losses from the pathway are normally small. Intermediates that are not converted into heme are not metabo-lized by alternative routes, although hydroxymethylbilane and por-phyrinogens may undergo non-enzymatic conversion to porphyrins, which accumulate in tissues and are excreted unchanged. The route of excretion under normal and pathological conditions is determined by the physicochemical properties of the intermediate.[7] Porphobilinogen (PBG) and ALA are excreted in urine as is the most hydrophilic porphy-rin, the octacarboxylic uroporphyrin. As the number of carboxylic side-chains decreases, biliary excretion increases so that the hydrophobic, dicarboxylic porphyrin, protoporphyrin, is excreted exclusively in the bile. The route of excretion may also be influenced by isomer type, coproporphyrin I being preferentially excreted in the bile.

Reference ranges for heme precursors in urine, feces, and erythro-cytes from adults are shown in Table 18–2. Use of these ranges for children is unlikely to produce diagnostic problems.

BIOCHEMICAL GENETICS

Each of the main types of porphyria results from partial deficiency of one of the enzymes of heme biosynthesis (Table 18-3). In recent years, cDNA or genomic clones have been obtained for all but two of these en-zymes (see Table 18–3), and molecular genetic methods are now being used to identify mutations and define the extent of heterogeneity at the DNA level in these conditions.[8]

Five of the enzyme deficiencies listed in Table 18–3 are inherited as autosomal dominant traits. In all except EPP, enzyme activity is decreased by close to 50% and mainly reflects expression of the normal

TABLE 18–2. Heme Precursor Concentrations

Heme Precursor	Urine		Feces		Erythrocytes
ALA	0–34	µmol/L	–		
PBG	0–8.8	µmol/L	–		
Total porphyrin	20–320	nmol/L	10–200	nmol/g dry wt*	0.4–1-7 µmol/L**
Porphyrin fractions					
Uroporphyrin	0–40	nmol/day			
Coproporphyrin	0–280	nmol/day	0–46	nmol/g dry wt	
Protoporphyrin			0–220	nmol/g dry wt	
Ether-insoluble porphyrin***			0–24	nmo/g dry wt	
Individual porphyrins					
Uroporphyrin	0–24	nmol/L	< 2% total		
Hepta (7C0$_2$H)	0–4	nmol/L	< 2% total		
Hexa (6CO$_2$H)	0–3	nmol/L	< 2% total		
Penta (5CO$_2$H)	0–5	nmol/L	< 2% total		
Isocoproporphyrin			< 0.5% total		
Coproporphyrin	23–115 nmol/L (60–70%)		2–33% total (10–20%)		
Protoporphyrin			60–98% total		

Note: Figures in parentheses give percentage of isomer type III
  * Ether-soluble porphyrin only
  ** More than 90% of total porphyrin erythrocytes is zinc-protoporphyrin
 *** Includes uroporphyrin, heptacarboxylic porphyrin, X-porphyrin
Source: Elder GH, Smith SG, Smyth SJ. Laboratory investigation of the porphyrias.
  Ann Clin Biochem 1990:27;395-412.

TABLE 18–3. The Porphyrias: Enzyme Deficiencies and Inheritance

Disorder	Enzyme Deficiency	Inheritance	Chromosomal Location	Human cDNA/ gDNA Cloned
PBG-synthase deficiency	PBG-synthase	Autosomal recessive	9q34	yes
Acute intermittent porphyria	PBG-deaminase*	Autosomal dominant	11q23-ter	yes
Congenital erythropoietic porphyria	Uroporphyrinogen III synthase	Autosomal recessive	10q25.2–26.3	yes
Porphyria cutanea tarda				
Type I (sporadic)	Uroporphyrinogen decarboxylase			no
Type II (familial)	Uroporphyrinogen decarboxylase	Autosomal dominant	1p34	yes
Toxic	Uroporphyrinogen decarboxylase	Not inherited		no
Hereditary coproporphyria	Coproporphyrinogen oxidase	Autosomal dominant	9	no
Variegate porphyrias	Protoporphyrinogen oxidase	Autosomal dominant	18q22	yes
Protoporphyria	Ferrochelatase	Autosomal dominant		no

*Synonyms: hydroxymethylbilane synthase, uroporphyrinogen-I-synthase.

gene allelic to the mutant gene.[2, 3] In EPP, activity is decreased by 70–80%, which suggests that some additional factor may modify enzyme activity in this disorder. The two remaining porphyrias, CEP and PBG synthase deficiency porphyria, are both autosomal recessive conditions. In all of these conditions, apart from an uncommon form of AIP in which the erythroid isoenzyme of PBG deaminase is unaffected,[8] the inherited enzyme deficiencies are present in all tissues, although the mitochondrial enzyme defects are absent from mature erythrocytes.

In normal cells, the concentrations of the intermediates of heme biosynthesis appear to be lower than the K_ms of the enzymes that metabolize them. A partial enzyme deficiency can therefore be compensated and the rate of formation of heme maintained by increasing the concentration of the substrate of the defective enzyme. This increase is achieved by raising the activity of ALA synthase through operation of the regulatory mechanisms described above. These compensatory changes do not occur to the same extent in all tissues. Thus, in all the autosomal dominant porphyrias except EPP, they are restricted to the liver, whereas in EPP and CEP, ALA synthase activity and tissue porphyrin concentrations are increased in erythroid cells.

There are also wide intra-individual differences between the extent of the compensatory changes. These differences are important clinically because symptomatic porphyria does not occur in the absence of demonstrable overproduction of heme precursors. At least 80% of individuals who inherit one of the autosomal dominant enzyme deficiencies remain asymptomatic throughout life and are considered to have latent porphyria. Many of these persons may show no evidence of heme precursor overproduction. It is not clear why these phenotypic differences in response to the same degree of enzyme deficiency occur. Although drugs and other acquired factors are known to precipitate symptoms in certain types of porphyria, interactions of this type do not provide a full explanation. In general, enzyme activities are lower in the autosomal recessive conditions.[2, 3] Individuals are clinically affected and symptoms tend to start at a young age and persist, although there are some exceptions to this rule which will be described below.

Overproduction of heme precursors can be divided into two main symptom-associated groups. First, acute neurovisceral attacks are always associated with increased excretion of the porphyrin precursor ALA, accompanied by PBG except in the very rare condition, PBG synthase deficiency porphyria.[2] Acute attacks do not occur in porphyrias in which neither PBG nor ALA excretion is increased (see Table 18–1). Possible mechanisms for the neurological basis of the acute attacks have been reviewed.[2] Second, skin lesions in porphyria are the consequence of overproduction of porphyrins, which, except in EPP, are derived from oxidation of accumulated porphyrinogens. They are not seen in the two conditions, AIP and PBG synthase deficiency porphyria (see Table 18–1), in which the enzyme deficiencies do not lead to porphyrin overproduction. The mechanism by which the photodynamic action of porphyrins in light-exposed areas of skin produces photosensitivity and skin lesions has been investigated extensively.[2]

CUTANEOUS PORPHYRIAS IN CHILDREN

Congenital Erythropoietic Porphyria

Congenital erythropoietic porphyria (CEP), or Günther's disease, is an uncommon cutaneous porphyria in which massive overproduction of porphyrins, mainly within the erythropoietic system, produces a severe photodermatosis, hemolytic anemia, and marked porphyrinuria.[9] It was the first of the porphyrias to be described (by Schultz in 1874) and remains the most striking and severe in its cutaneous manifestations.

Clinical Features

CEP occurs worldwide and with equal frequency in both sexes. It usually presents in infancy, where the first symptom is often red discoloration of the diapers that is noticed at or soon after birth. Such infants may be photosensitive and develop erythema in areas of skin exposed to sunlight either directly or through window glass. Severe erythema following phototherapy for hyperbilirubinemia has been reported in CEP. By the second year of life, most affected children have characteristic porphyric lesions on light-exposed skin: subepidermal bullae, hypertrichosis, and superficial erosions resulting from increased mechanical fragility. Rarely, the onset of symptoms is delayed until later in childhood or even adult life.

In older children and adults, there is often extensive scarring of the skin due to repeated infection of blisters and erosions, with atrophy and extensive areas of sclerodermatous change. Together, these lesions may progress to severe photomutilation with atrophy of ears, nose, and digits, while damage around the eyes may lead to corneal ulcerations and blindness.

Almost all patients have erythrodontia, with both the deciduous and permanent teeth being colored reddish-brown due to deposition of porphyrins. The teeth show bright red fluorescence on exposure to long-wave ultraviolet light. Porphyrin also accumulates in erythrocytes, and accelerated destruction of photo-damaged erythrocytes in the spleen probably explains the hemolysis and splenomegaly that is present in many patients, the latter usually appearing as the disease progresses. The hemolytic anemia is characteristically intermittent and is usually mild or moderate in severity, only rarely becoming life-threatening.

Most patients with the classical, childhood-onset form of CEP do not survive beyond age 40. In recent years, careful screening from sunlight and the prevention of secondary infections with antibiotics has been effective in preventing severe photomutilation. It remains to be seen whether the overall prognosis is also improved.

Biochemical Findings

Uroporphyrinogen III synthase activity is decreased by 70–90% in CEP patients and is intermediate between this range and normal in obligatory carriers.[3] At least four point mutations have now been identified in the uroporphyrinogen III synthase gene, for which patients are either homozygous or compound heterozygous.[8, 10] Accumulation of hydroxymethylbilane proximal to the defective enzyme results in the formation of excessive amounts of uroporphyrin I and coproporphyrin I which are excreted in urine and feces and accumulate in erythrocytes (Table 18-4). Protoporphyrin is also increased in erythrocytes, but only to the moderate degree seen both in other homozygous porphyrias and in other hemolytic anemias, and is present mainly as the zinc chelate.

TABLE 18-4. The Porphyrias: Diagnostic Patterns of Overproduction of Heme Precursors

Disorder	Urine PBG/ALA	Porphyrins	Feces Porphyrins	Erythrocytes Porphyrins
PBG-synthase deficiency*	ALA	Copro III	Not increased	Zn-proto
Acute intermittent porphyria	PBG > ALA	(Porphyrin mainly from PBG)	Normal, occas. slight increase (copro, proto)	Not increased
Congenital erythropoietic porphyria	Not increased	Uro I > Copro I	Copro I	Zn-proto,copro, uro
Porphyria cutanea tarda	Not increased	Uro > Hepta***	Isocopro, Hepta***	Not increaed
Hereditary coproporphyria	PBG > ALA**	Copro III (Porphyrin from PBG)	Copro III	Not increased
Variegate porphyria	PBG> ALA	Copro III (Porphyrin from PBG)	Proto IX > Copro III X-porphyrin	Not increased
Protoporphyria	Not increased	Not increased	± Protoporphyrin	Protoporphyrin

*Lead poisoning produces an identical overproduction pattern.
**PBG and ALA excretion may be normal when only skin lesions are present.
***Hexa- and pentacarboxylic prophyrins and coproporphyrin are increased to a smaller extent.

Treatment

Treatment of CEP is unsatisfactory. Skin damage may be lessened by minimizing exposure to sunlight, prompt treatment of secondary infection, and oral carotenoids.[9] Hypertransfusion and intravenous hematin both provide short-term suppression of porphyrin production, but neither is suitable for use over long periods of time. Interruption of the enterohepatic circulation of porphyrins by oral activated charcoal may decrease porphyrin accumulation,[11] but its long-term use requires evaluation. Recently, bone marrow transplantation has been reported to be potentially beneficial,[12] but its use in children who are likely to survive for 30 years or more needs careful consideration. Patients with severe hemolytic anaemia and hypersplenism may benefit from splenectomy.[9]

Prenatal Diagnosis

CEP is probably the only porphyria in which prenatal diagnosis with a view to termination of pregnancy may be justifiable. For this purpose, measurement of porphyrins in amniotic fluid and uroporphyrinogen III synthase in amnion cells[3] is likely to be superseded by recombinant DNA methods for direct detection of mutations.

Uroporphyrinogen Decarboxylase Deficiency Disorders

Two types of cutaneous porphyria result from decreased activity of uroporphyrinogen decarboxylase: porphyria cutanea tarda (PCT) and hepatoerythropoietic porphyria (HEP).[2] PCT is mainly a disease of adults. Its features have been reviewed,[2, 3, 13] and hence it is only discussed briefly here.

Porphyria Cutanea Tarda in Children

Less than 1% of patients with PCT first develop skin lesions during childhood, and these may appear as early as the second year of life. The lesions are much less severe than in CEP and similar to those seen in adults with PCT; skin fragility, sub-epidermal bullae, and hypertrichosis on the backs of the hands, face, and other sun-exposed areas are the usual findings. Photosensitivity is not usually a prominent feature. In contrast to adults with PCT, evidence of co-existent liver disease is uncommon.

Decreased uroporphyrinogen decarboxylase activity in the liver leads to a characteristic pattern of porphyrin overproduction (Table 18–4). Uroporphyrin and other porphyrins with acetic acid substituents (see Figure 18–1) accumulate in the liver and are excreted in excess. In urine, the main porphyrins are uroporphyrin I and III and heptacarboxylic porphyrin III, while isocoproporphyrin and hepta-carboxylic porphyrin are usually the most prominent in feces.[14] Erythrocyte porphyrin concentrations are normal.

PCT is a heterogeneous disorder.[2, 13] It is probable that all affected children have the type II or familial form of PCT in which uroporphyrinogen decarboxylase deficiency is present in all tissues and is inherited in an autosomal dominant fashion (see Table 18–3). Most individuals who inherit the gene for type II PCT are asymptomatic and therefore it is not unusual for patients to be the only clinically affected member of their families. The diagnosis of type II PCT can be established by demonstrating a 50% decrease in erythrocyte uroporphyrinogen decarboxylase.[2, 13]

PCT in children, as in adults, can be treated either by depleting iron stores by repeated venesection or with "low-dose" chloroquine at an appropriately lower dose than for adults.[2, 3] Both treatments produce clinical and biochemical remission which may persist for many years, even throughout life. Remission may also occur without treatment, and if skin lesions are mild, no treatment may be required. In girls, iron depletion following menarche may produce spontaneous remission.

Toxic Cutaneous Porphyria

In the late 1950s, there was a widespread outbreak of cutaneous porphyria in south-eastern Turkey following the consumption of bread made from wheat seed that had been dressed with the fungicide hexachlorobenzene.[15] This compound was later shown to inactivate hepatic uroporphyrinogen decarboxylase and "porphyria turcica" is now regarded as a form of PCT. Many of the affected individuals were children, and hypertrichosis was a prominent clinical feature. Follow-up studies have been published recently.[15]

Hepatoerythropoietic Porphyria

Hepatoerythropoietic porphyria (HEP) is a rare form of cutaneous porphyria that results from severe uroporphyrinogen decarboxylase deficiency.[2, 3, 16, 17] So far, 21 patients have been reported from 18 families. Skin fragility and blisters, often accompanied by hypertrichosis and clinically indistinguishable from the lesions of PCT and CEP, are usually first noticed between the ages of 2 and 5. The skin lesions are usually more severe than in PCT and, with progression, may come to resemble those of CEP with photomutilation. Other clinical features of CEP are usually absent. Porphyrinuria is less marked and may not be sufficient to color the urine; erythrodontia is infrequent and hemolytic anemia with splenomegaly has been reported in only two patients.[16]

Urinary and fecal porphyrin excretion patterns resemble those of PCT. Although small differences have been reported,[16] these are not sufficiently consistent to reliably distinguish HEP from PCT. In contrast to PCT, the erythrocyte porphyrin concentration is invariably raised, largely due to increased zinc-protoporphyrin concentrations.[16]

Differentiation between PCT and HEP depends on measurement of uroporphyrinogen decarboxylase. In erythrocytes, enzyme activity is decreased by at least 70% and usually by close to 90%. These low activities, together with the finding that both parents of affected individuals have enzyme activities around 50% of normal, suggest that patients with HEP may be homozygous for the enzyme defect that causes type II PCT. Immunochemical and molecular genetic investigations have led to the identification of several different mutations in both HEP and type II PCT, but no mutation common to both diseases has yet been identified.[2, 3, 8]

There is no specific treatment for HEP. Both venesection and chloroquine are ineffective. Management of the skin lesions is therefore symptomatic and similar to that recommended for CEP.[9] In theory, oral activated charcoal should decrease porphyrin accumulation.[11]

Other Blistering Cutaneous Porphyrias in Children

Kushner et al[18] have described a patient with partial uroporphyrinogen decarboxylase deficiency, dyserythropoietic anemia, and severe skin lesions, resembling CEP, that started at the age of 4. A similar decrease in enzyme activity was present in asymptomatic relatives, suggesting that interaction between this defect and the dyserythropoietic anemia was responsible for the severe porphyria. Co-existence of two enzyme defects in the heme biosynthetic pathway may also modify the clinical picture, as in an infant with severe photosensitization who was found to have co-existent CEP and hereditary coproporphyria.[19]

Erythropoietic Protoporphyria

Erythropoietic protoporphyria (EPP)[2, 3, 20] is the third most common porphyria (see Table 18–1) and by far the most common form of porphyria in children; indeed, onset of EPP after childhood is uncommon. The condition is produced by accumulation of protoporphyrin IX secondary to decreased ferrochelatase activity with most of the porphyrin coming from the erythropoietic system.[3] Although the mechanism of photosensitization is the same as in other cutaneous porphyrias,[2] the most prominent feature is acute photosensitivity and the condition is clinically distinguishable from all other cutaneous porphyrias. The main diagnostic problem is differentiation of EPP from other causes of acute photosensitivity.

Clinical Features

Patients present with acute photosensitivity that usually starts in early childhood, often before age 2 y.[20] An intense pricking, itching, burning sensation usually occurs within 5 to 30 minutes of exposure to sunlight, but is sometimes delayed for several hours, and blends into burning pain. Erythema and edema with occasional later crusting and petechiae follow, but usually have resolved within a day or two. Uncommonly, small vesicles and acute photo-oncolysis may occur.

Particularly in young children who have had few episodes of photosensitivity, there may be little to suggest EPP apart from the history, and it is probably for this reason that the diagnosis is often delayed. After repeated attacks, the skin may become thickened, waxy, and pitted with small circular or linear scars, especially over the bridge of the nose, around the mouth, and over the knuckles. However, the changes are rarely marked and may be missed on superficial examination. About 25% of patients have a mild hypochromic microcytic anemia that is not caused by iron-deficiency and may result from the enzyme defect. Older patients may develop pigmented protoporphyrin gall stones.

As in other autosomal dominant porphyrias, carriers of the EPP gene are often asymptomatic. Thus, affected individuals often have no relatives with overt EPP, and the risk that a child of a patient with EPP will ever develop symptoms has been estimated at less than 5%.

Progressive hepatic failure is an uncommon but well-recognized complication that appears to result from liver damage caused by accumulation of protoporphyrin in hepatocytes.[21] Onset is usually after age 30 y, but fatal liver damage has been reported in children. Up to 35% of all patients may have biochemical evidence of liver dysfunction at some stage, but not all of these show protoporphyrin deposition or hepatocyte necrosis and fibrosis. In one series, 7 of 55 patients developed cirrhosis over 20 years and two died,[22] but this represents an unusually high incidence.[21] Liver disease does not occur in asymptomatic gene carriers.

Biochemical Findings

The diagnosis of EPP is established by demonstrating an increased concentration of free protoporphyrin in erythrocytes[14] (see Table 18–4). Protoporphyrin concentration may also be increased in plasma and, less frequently, in feces. Urinary porphyrin concentrations are normal, except when liver disease leads to secondary coproporphyrinuria. Ferrochelatase activities are decreased to 10–30% of normal in lymphocytes and other nucleated cells.[3] Detection of asymptomatic gene carriers may require enzyme measurement, as erythrocyte protoporphyrin concentrations are often normal in such individuals. Patients with EPP who are apparently homozygous for ferrochelatase deficiency have been described.[3] cDNA for human ferrochelatase has been cloned recently, and molecular investigations should soon clarify the genetics of this disorder.

Prediction of liver disease is difficult. Liver function should be assessed regularly by standard biochemical tests and persistent abnormalities investigated by biopsy. Very high and increasing erythrocyte porphyrin concentrations (greater than 20–30 µmol/L), high plasma porphyrin concentrations, and relatively low fecal protoporphyrin excretion reflect impaired biliary secretion and thus suggest liver disease.

Treatment

Skin damage may be minimized by avoiding sunlight, by using sunscreen ointments or by building up a protective layer of β-carotene in the skin.[1, 2] Sufficient oral carotene should be given to produce a serum concentration of 6–8 mg/L. At this concentration, the skin turns yellowish-orange and contains sufficient β-carotene to block photo damage by acting as a singlet oxygen trap. In patients with evidence of liver damage, further accumulation of porphyrin may be discouraged either by suppressing synthesis or interrupting the enterohepatic circulation of protoporphyrin. The latter may be achieved by giving oral cholestyramine or activated charcoal. Hypertransfusion or intravenous hematin are impracticable for long-term suppression of heme synthesis, but recent evidence suggests that chenodeoxycholic acid may decrease protoporphyrin concentrations.[21] For hepatic failure, liver transplantation has been successful, although it leads to little decrease in protoporphyrin production and the possibility remains of re-accumulation of porphyrin in the liver.[21]

PEDIATRIC ASPECTS OF ACUTE PORPHYRIA

Episodic acute attacks of neurovisceral dysfunction occur in four types of porphyria (see Table 18–1). Of these, the autosomal recessive disorder, PBG synthase deficiency porphyria, is very rare; one of the four patients reported to date was a child.[3] The autosomal dominant acute hepatic porphyrias—acute intermittent porphyria (AIP), hereditary coproporphyrin (HC), and variegate porphyria (VP)—are essentially adult diseases. In all three disorders, detectable overproduction of heme precursors and symptoms are very uncommon before puberty. The biochemical basis of prepubertal latency is not understood.

Acute illness, clinically similar to acute porphyria and associated with overproduction of ALA, may also occur in children with hereditary tyrosinemia.[23]

Overt Acute Porphyria in Children

Acute attacks of AIP, HC, or VP may occur around the age of puberty but are uncommon earlier in childhood. They are very rare, although a number have been reported, the youngest patient being 4 months old.[24-26] In several cases, the attacks appear to have been precipitated by anticonvulsants. The clinical features and treatment are the same as for adults and have been reviewed in detail.[1, 2] The diagnosis depends on demonstration of excess PBG in urine, followed by analysis of fecal porphyrins to distinguish between AIP, HC, and VP[14] (see Table 18–4). Onset of VP or HC with skin lesions in the absence of acute porphyria does not appear to have been reported in children before puberty.

Detection and Management of Gene Carriers before Puberty

It is important that relatives of patients with AIP, HC, or VP be screened to detect asymptomatic individuals so that they can be advised to avoid various drugs and other factors that can precipitate acute attacks.[1, 2, 3] Screening should be applied to children as well as adults, because, although the risk of an acute attack in children is much less, it does exist. Affected parents are often anxious to know whether their children have inherited porphyria.

Since PBG and porphyrin excretion are invariably normal in children, detection of carriers of the genes for AIP, VP, or HC depends largely on measurement of the activities of the defective enzymes (Table 18–3). Measurement of erythrocyte PBG deaminase will detect gene carriers in the majority of families with AIP, but there is some overlap between enzyme activities in normal and affected individuals and the method has other limitations.[3, 14] In particular, PBG deaminase activity is dependent on the age distribution of circulating erythrocytes, being highest in the least mature cells, which complicates interpretation in young infants and individuals who are not hematologically normal. For this reason, detection of carriers by PBG deaminase measurement should not be attempted until after age 6–8 m. More precise identification of carriers can be obtained by recombinant DNA methods,[8] either by gene tracking using linkage to intragenic DNA polymorphisms or by direct detection of mutations. The former approach requires families that are sufficiently large and contain enough informative individuals to establish linkage, while the latter is made difficult in practice by the extensive molecular heterogeneity of AIP.[8]

Detection of carriers of the VP and HC genes during childhood depends on measurement of protoporphyrinogen and coproporphyrinogen oxidases, respectively. Both measurements require nucleated cells, such as lymphocytes or lymphoblastoid or fibroblast cell lines, are technically difficult, and do not always distinguish between affected and unaffected individuals. DNA methods are not yet available for either gene. At present, it is simplest to manage children of individuals with VP or HC as if they were carriers, in the hope that more precise methods for carrier detection will soon become available.

Children who are known or suspected carriers of the genes for AIP, VP, or HC should be managed in a similar fashion to adult carriers.[1, 2] They or their parents should ensure that drugs known to precipitate acute porphyria are avoided. In addition, they should wear a bracelet or necklace indicating that they have porphyria to prevent, for example, administration of an inappropriate anesthetic after an accident.

Homozygous Forms of the Acute Autosomal Dominant Porphyrias

During recent years, homozygous forms of AIP, VP, or HC have been described.[3, 27, 28] All the affected individuals have been children with enzyme deficiencies of 80% or more and patterns of overproduction of heme precursors resembling those of the corresponding autosomal dominant disorders. Typical acute attacks of porphyria are unusual.[3] None have had an anemia attributable to defective heme biosynthesis, although erythrocyte zinc-protoporphyrin concentrations are increased, as in other homozygous porphyrias.[29] Both parents have the biochemical features of the autosomal dominant counterpart and there is an increased incidence of consanguinity. Either a parent or other close relative may have overt porphyria.

Homozygous AIP

This condition appears to be characterized by excessive excretion of PBG from birth.[27] Three of the four cases had convulsions and different developmental abnormalities of the brain, two had bilateral cataracts, while the fourth is clinically normal at age 2 y.[27] Three of the children, from two families, have been shown to be compound heterozygotes for mutations in exon 10 of the PBG deaminase gene.[27]

Homozygous VP

Six children with this condition have been reported.[28] All developed skin lesions of varying severity early in childhood, usually before the age of 1 year, with blisters, skin fragility, or hypertrichosis as prominent features. Other clinical features that have been present in more than one family, but not in all cases, include mental retardation, convulsions, short stature, and clinodactyly. The combination of short stature and hypertrichosis may provoke extensive endocrine investigation if the other skin changes, which may be minimal, are overlooked. Acute attacks of porphyria have not yet been reported in this condition.

Homozygous HC

Two types of homozygous HC have been described.[3] In two unrelated children, short stature, skin lesions, and attacks of acute porphyria were associated with excessive excretion of coproporphyrin III. The other type has been identified in only one family[3] and is characterized by excretion of harderoporphyrin, a tricarboxylic intermediate of the coproporphyrinogen oxidase reaction (see Figure 18–1). Three siblings had severe hyperbilirubinemia and hemolytic anemia at birth, while one later developed blisters caused by porphyrin-induced photosensitization.

ROLE OF THE LABORATORY IN THE INVESTIGATION OF PORPHYRIA IN CHILDREN

None of the porphyrias have clinical features that are sufficiently distinctive to enable the diagnosis to be made without laboratory investigations. These are essential both to distinguish porphyria from other disorders with similar clinical presentation and to identify the type of porphyria. For most laboratories the former objective is the more important. In adults, and even more so in children, the majority of tests for suspected porphyria will be negative, and it is important not to miss patients at this stage by using inappropriate screening tests. This aspect is discussed below. The second stage in diagnosis—identification of the type of porphyria—requires definition of the pattern of heme precursor overproduction (see Table 18–3). In children, enzyme measurements may also be needed. Methods and diagnostic strategies have been reviewed.[7, 30]

PBG and porphyrins are moderately unstable in biological samples. Fresh, random samples of urine should be used for their measurement and results expressed per liter or per mg/creatinine. Twenty-four-hour collections delay analysis and rarely give additional diagnostic information. Porphyrins in feces should be analyzed as soon as possible after collection. In practice, diagnostically important changes in the PBG or porphyrin content of urine or feces are unlikely to occur in samples kept at room temperature for 24–36 h, provided they are shielded from light. Porphyrins are stable in EDTA-anti-coagulated blood for several days.

Children with Suspected Acute Porphyria

Older children, particularly, may present with the typical features of an attack of acute porphyria, but this is rare. It is much more usual for the laboratory to be asked to exclude AIP, HC, or VP as the cause of unexplained recurrent attacks of abdominal pain or convulsions, perhaps accompanied by behavioral disturbances. The essential investigation is examination of urine for excess PBG. Screening tests, such as the Watson-Schwartz test, which depend on the reaction of PBG with p-dimethylaminobenzaldehyde in acid to form a red color which is insoluble in organic solvents, have been criticized because of poor sensitivity,[30] but if carefully carried out can detect as little as 35–50 μmol PBG/L.[14] If this test is negative while symptoms are present, the child is very unlikely to have an acute porphyria. If doubt remains or if the child is seen between recurrent attacks and the screening test is negative, PBG should be measured by a quantitative method.[14]

A normal concentration excludes AIP. In VP and HC, PBG may return to normal after an acute attack, but fecal porphyrin excretion remains high; these conditions can be excluded by measuring fecal and plasma porphyrins.[14] An increase in fecal porphyrin concentration without any other evidence of heme precursor overproduction is almost always explained by occult gastrointestinal hemorrhage.[14]

Measurement of urinary porphyrins is usually unhelpful. If PBG excretion is increased, it does not differentiate between AIP, VP, or HC; fecal measurements are required for this purpose. If PBG concentration is normal, the most frequent cause of increased urinary porphyrin excretion is coproporphyrinuria.[14] The usual cause is cholestasis, but occasionally lead poisoning or hepatic enzyme induction due, for example, to long-term treatment with anticonvulsants may be responsible.

Children with Suspected Cutaneous Porphyria

Photosensitivity

EPP should be excluded as a possible cause in all children who present with a history of unexplained acute photosensitivity without skin fragility, blisters, or hypertrichosis. The simplest and most reliable method is to measure total erythrocyte porphyrin by a quantitative fluorometric micromethod.[14] Screening tests based on solvent extraction or fluorescence microscopy may give false-negative results and should not be used. A normal erythrocyte porphyrin concentration excludes EPP. If the concentration is increased, the diagnosis of EPP should be confirmed by showing that the increase is caused by free protoporphyrin.[14] In other causes of raised erythrocyte porphyrin concentrations, such as iron deficiency and lead poisoning,[1, 4] zinc-protoporphyrin is increased.

Other Cutaneous Porphyrias

Blisters, skin fragility, and hypertrichosis are features of all the other cutaneous porphyrias of childhood. This is a complex group of rare disorders (Table 18–5). The skin lesions are characteristic of porphyria and detailed investigation of urinary, fecal, plasma, and erythrocyte porphyrins is usually required from the start. Final diagnosis may depend on enzyme measurement. If exclusion of porphyria is required, demonstration of normal total porphyrin concentrations in urine and feces by a spectrophotometric or fluorometric method is adequate.[14]

TABLE 18-5. Porphyrias Presenting in Childhood with Skin Fragility, Blisters, and Hypertrichosis

Condition	Inheritance
Congenital erythropoietic porphyria	Autosomal recessive
Porphyria cutanea tarda (Type II)	Autosomal dominant
Hepatoerythropoietic porphyria	Homozygous UROD defect
Homozygous hereditary coproporphyria	Homozygous for HC gene
Harderoporphyria	(Autosomal recessive?)
Homozygous variegate porphyria	Homozygous for VP gene

REFERENCES

1. Moore MR, McColl KE, Rimington C, Goldberg A. Disorders of porphyrin metabolism. New York: Plenum Press, 1987.
2. Nordmann Y, Deybach J-C. Human hereditary porphyrias. In: Daley H, ed., Biosynthesis of heme and chlorophylls. New York: McGraw-Hill, 1990:491-542.
3. Kappas A, Sassa S, Galbraith RA, Nordmann Y. The porphyrias. In: Scriver CL, Beaudet AL, Sly WS, Valle D, eds., The metabolic basis of inherited disease, 6th ed. New York: McGraw-Hill, 1989:1305-65.
4. McColl KEL, Goldberg A. Abnormal porphyrin metabolism in diseases other than porphyria. Clin Hemeatol 1980;9:427-44.
5. Frank M, Doss MO. Relevance of urinary coproporphyrin isomers in hereditary hyperbilirubinaemias. Clin Biochem 1989;22:221-22.
6. Dierks P. synthase. New York Molecular biology of eukaryotic 5-aminolaevulinate In: Daley H, ed., Biosynthesis of heme and chlorophylls. McGraw-Hill,1990:201-33.
7. Elder GH. The porphyrias: Clinical chemistry, diagnosis and methodology. Clin Hemeatol 1980;9:371-98.
8. Nordmann Y, Verneuil H de, Deybach JC, Delfau M-H, Grandchamp B. Molecular genetics of porphyrias. Annals of Medicine 1990;22:387-91.

9. Nordmann Y, Deybach J-C. Congenital erythropoietic porphyria. Semin Dermatol 5:106-14.

10. Warner CA, Yoo HW, Tsai SF, Roberts AG, Desnick RJ. Congenital erythropoietic por-
    phyria: Characterization of the genomic structure and identification of mutations in the
    uroporphyrinogen III synthase gene. Am J Hum Genet 1990;47:A321.

11. Pimstone NR, Gandhi SN, Mukerji SK. Therapeutic efficacy of oral charcoal in congenital
    erythropoietic porphyria. N Eng J Med 1987:316:390-3.

12. Kauffman L, Evans DIK, Stevens RF, Weinkove C. Bone marrow transplantation for con-
    genital erythropoietic porphyria. Lancet 1991;1:1510-11.

13. Elder GH. Porphyria cutanea tarda: A multifactorial disease. In: Champion RH, Pye RJ,
    eds., Recent advances in Dermatology (Number 8). Edinburgh: Churchill Livingstone,
    1990:55-70.

14. Elder GH, Smith SG, Smyth SJ. Laboratory investigation of the porphyrias. Ann Clin
    Biochem 1990;27:395-412.

15. Cripps DJ, Peters HA, Gocmen A et al. Porphyria turcica due to hexachlorobenzene: A 20
    to 30 year follow-up study on 204 patients. Brit J Dermatol 1984;111:413-22.

16. Smith SG. Hepatoerythropoietic porphyria. Semin Dermatol 1986;5:125-37.

17. Koszo F, Elder GH, Roberts A, Simon N. Uroporphyrinogen decarboxylase deficiency in
    hepatoerythropoietic porphyria: Further evidence for genetic heterogeneity. Brit J Dermatol
    1990;122:365-70.

18. Kushner JP, Pimstone NR, Kjeldsberg CR, Pryor MA, Huntley A. Congenital erythropoietic
    porphyria: Diminished activity of uroporphyrinogen decarboxylase and dyserythropoiesis.
    Blood 1982;59:725-37.

19. Nordmann Y, Amram D, Deybach J-C, Phung LN, Lesbros D. Coexistent hereditary
    coproporphyria and congenital aerythropoietic porphyria (Günther's disease). J Inher Metab
    Dis. 1990;13:687-91.

20. De Leo VA, Poh-Fitzpatrick MB, Matthews-Roth MM, Harberg LC. Erythropoietic pro-
    toporphyria: Ten years experience. Am J Med 1976; 60:8-22.

21. Rank JM, Straka JG, Bloomer JR. Liver in disorders of porphyrin metabolism. J Gastroent
    Hepatol 1990;5:573-85.

22. Doss MO, Frank M. Hepatobiliary implications and complications in protoporphyria: A 20-
    year study. Clin Biochem 1989;22:223-30.

23. Mitchell G, Larochelle J, Lambert M. et al. Neurologic crises in hereditary tyrosinemia. New
    J Med 1990;322:432-37.

24. Barclay N. Acute intermittent porphyria in childhood: A neglected diagnosis? Arch Dis Child
    1974;49:404-5.

25. Beauvais P, Klein M-L, Denave L, Martel C. Porphyria aigue intermittente a l'age de quatre
    mois. Arch Franc Ped 1976;33:987-92.

26. Day RS. Variegate porphyria. Semin Dermatol 1986;5:138-54.

27. Llewellyn DH, Smyth SJ, Elder GH, Hutchesson AC, Rattenbury JM, Smith MF. Homozyg-
    ous acute intermittent porphyria. Hum Genet 1992, in press.

28. Norris PG, Elder GH, Hawk JLM. Homozygous variegate porphyria: A case report. Brit J
    Dermatol 1990;122:253-57.

29. Kordac V, Martasek P, Zaman J, Rubin A. Increased erythrocyte protoporphyrin in
    homozygous variegate porphyria. Photodermatology 1985;2:257-59.

30. Deacon AC. Performance of screening tests for porphyria. Ann Clin Biochem 1988;25:392-
    7.

Therapeutic Drug Monitoring and Clinical Toxicology in a Pediatric Hospital

Steven J. Soldin, Ph.D., F.A.C.B., F.C.A.C.B.
Tai C. Kwong, Ph.D., F.A.C.B.

THERAPEUTIC DRUG MONITORING

General Considerations

Based on theoretical and practical knowledge, a physician attempts to choose the ideal drug for treatment of an identified disease or pathophysiologic process. This search for optimal pharmacotherapy is made more difficult by the growing awareness of immense genetically, environmentally, and age-determined variations in drug response.[1] Some investigators appear biased toward the prediction of pharmacokinetic behavior and the monitoring of drug concentrations in biological fluids as an end in itself. Such measurements in the absence of clinical assessment of pharmacologic or therapeutic effects are likely to prove pointless. Recent indications are that approximately 12% of all drugs prescribed in the United States are for children under age 9 y.[2] A review of drug-dosing habits in neonatal intensive care units has shown that the average number of drugs administered to premature infants under 1000 g varies from institution to institution but is usually in the 15–20 range, while infants over 2500 g usually receive 4–10 drugs during their hospital stay.

Physicians have a responsibility to be informed adequately about the risks, limitations, and use of drugs they prescribe, to acquaint their patients with possible adverse effects, and to ensure that patients are being optimally treated. For certain drugs, this necessitates their measurement in plasma or serum, followed by appropriate dosage adjustments if required.

The use of any drug carries with it a risk that is often not precisely established. When the rate of drug-induced disease is reported as 1 in every 20,000 to 200,000 patients (e.g., the devastating aplastic anemia caused by chloramphenicol); the recognition of a causal relationship is sometimes difficult and delayed.[3]

Some Basic Pharmacokinetic Considerations

An in-depth discussion of pharmacokinetics is beyond the scope of this chapter. However, a brief review of some concepts and definitions is important for a better understanding of therapeutic drug monitoring.

Pharmacokinetics is a tool that serves to describe in quantitative terms what happens to a drug in the body. The primary goal of therapeutic drug monitoring is to optimize drug administration with such information. To reach the required steady-state blood concentrations in a particular patient receiving a drug chronically, it is necessary to establish parameters such as:

- *Apparent Volume of Distribution* (Vd). The volume in which the drug appears to be distributed if it were present throughout the body at the concentration in which it is found in the blood. A very large (greater than the total body water) Vd, e.g., Digoxin (Vd = 5–10 L/Kg), indicates significant tissue binding.

- *Plasma Half-Life:* the time it takes for the plasma drug concentration to decrease by 50% (see Figure 19–1).

- *Total Body Clearance* (Cl): the volume of vascular fluid in which the drug is measured and from which the drug is irreversibly removed per unit of time.

- *Bioavailability* (F): The fraction of the administered dose reaching the systemic circulation intact.

The above parameters can be estimated using average population data, or established more precisely for a patient by analyzing suitably collected blood samples after a trial dose.

When a drug is administered intravenously, it undergoes a distribution phase followed by an elimination phase. The elimination process follows exponential first-order kinetics, i.e., a constant fraction of the drug in the body is eliminated per unit of time (Figure 19–1). The elimination phase half-life is an important parameter often quoted in the literature. If the elimination phase line is extended back to the Y axis, the point of intersection with the Y axis provides the "zero-time" drug concentration. Dividing the dose administered by the zero-time concentration provides the apparent volume of distribution, Vd.

The relationship between elimination half-life, apparent volume of distribution, and clearance is $t_{1/2} = 0.693 \, (Vd/Cl)$.

Based upon the available information, it is possible to recommend the dose (D) and frequency of administration (T) needed to achieve the desired average steady-state blood concentration (C_{ss}) using the relationship in Equation 1, where TBC is the total body clearance.

$$C_{ss} = \frac{F \cdot D}{TBC \cdot T} \qquad \qquad \text{Equation 1}$$

Thus, either the available dosage form is used to calculate the required interval (Equation 2), or a convenient frequency of administration is made to dictate the amount of drug to be administered (Equation 3).

$$T = \frac{F \cdot D}{C_{ss} \cdot TBC} \qquad \qquad \text{Equation 2}$$

$$D = \frac{C_{ss} \cdot TBC \cdot T}{F} \qquad \qquad \text{Equation 3}$$

About 90% of the eventual steady-state concentration will be reached in 3.3 times the $t_{1/2}$ after initiation of the selected dosage regimen, with steady-state concentration being achieved after approximately 5 times the half-life.

FIGURE 19–1. Plasma Drug Concentration versus Time Profile for a Drug Administered Intravenously

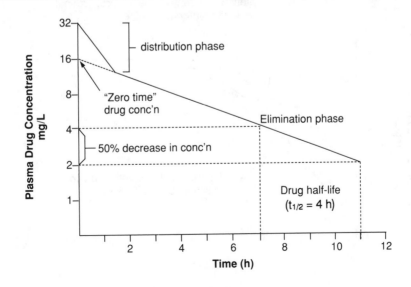

Time of Sampling

The interpretation of drug concentrations depends not only on the dosage regimen, but also on the time of the last dose relative to the time of blood sampling. For a drug administered orally at intervals equal to its half-life (say, 4 h), it takes 4 to 5 times the half-life to achieve steady-state plateau concentrations (Figure 19–2). For most drugs, there is an excellent correlation between the dose and the steady-state serum concentration, e.g., doubling the dose will also double the steady-state concentration. Exceptions to the rule include those drugs undergoing saturation kinetics (e.g., phenytoin, ethanol, and salicylate). Therefore, specimens for analysis should not be drawn until sufficient time has elapsed to enable steady-state concentrations to be achieved (unless, of course, toxicity is suspected at an earlier stage).

For drugs with a long half-life, such as phenobarbital, which are administered at intervals shorter than the half-life, there is little difference between steady-state peak and trough drug concentrations. However, for drugs with a short half-life, such as the aminoglycosides, theophylline, and primidone, differences between peak and trough concentrations may be considerable, and it is often advisable to measure both. As a general rule, however, the ideal sample is one that would provide the steady-state trough serum concentration. This is the sample drawn just before the next dose.

FIGURE 19–2. Plasma Drug Concentration versus Time Profile for a Drug Administered Orally at Intervals Equal to the Drug's Elimination Half-life

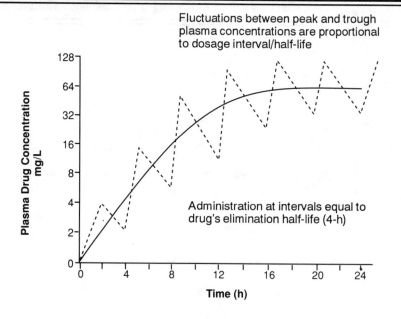

Steady-state drug concentrations can be achieved more rapidly by administering oral, intramuscular, or intravenous loading doses of a drug. Loading doses circumvent the necessity of waiting 5 half-lives to achieve a serum concentration plateau and a maximum therapeutic effect. For a drug administered intravenously (e.g., digoxin), it is necessary to wait a fixed time interval after loading to allow for drug distribution to occur. In the case of digoxin, distribution may take 6 h.

In general, concentration measurements should be made 0.5–1 h after intravenous administration of medication. For example, a specimen representing the "peak" serum concentration for gentamicin is most appropriately drawn 30 min after the end of drug infusion, after distribution is complete.

THE RATIONALE FOR THERAPEUTIC DRUG MONITORING

For most drugs, the intensity and duration of the given pharmacological response is proportional to the drug concentration at the receptor site. This drug concentration depends on many factors, including drug dose and the pharmacokinetic properties of the drug administered. Some of the factors affecting the pharmacokinetics of drugs include genetic differences in drug metabolism, disease, age, drug interactions, and diet. For many drugs, extreme interindividual variation makes it impossible to predict a serum concentration for any given dose based on a weight relationship.

For most drugs, there is a plasma concentration below which the clinical response is unsatisfactory (subtherapeutic). At higher concentrations, the drug elicits a therapeutic effect. At still higher concentrations, unwanted toxic side effects can occur. The aim of drug dosage design is to maintain the plasma concentration in the therapeutic range, as represented in Figure 19–3.

FIGURE 19–3. Relationship between Serum Drug Concentration and Clinical Effect

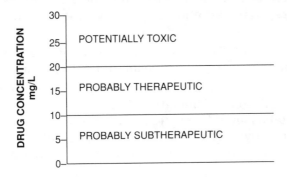

For therapeutic monitoring to be useful in the clinical management of patients, it is necessary that the drugs of interest fulfill certain requirements:

1. The relationship between serum concentration and pharmacological effect must be good. This usually implies a strong correlation between serum concentration and concentration in the target tissue.[4]

2. A reliable and rapid method for drug analysis must be available.

3. A narrow margin should exist between serum concentrations which provide therapeutic effects and those which cause toxic effects, e.g., as observed with digoxin, theophylline, and aminoglycoside antibiotics.

4. There should be a poor correlation between serum concentration and drug dosage due to interindividual differences in drug absorption, metabolism, and excretion. Such poor correlation has been shown with clomipramine used in treatment of enuresis.[5]

5. Pharmacological effects should not be readily measurable, e.g., anticonvulsant drugs in which the suppression of seizure activity is difficult to monitor clinically.

For therapeutic drug monitoring to be regarded as having established value, there should be a better correlation between the plasma drug concentration and the pharmacological effect than between the drug dosage and the pharmacological effect. The need for therapeutic drug monitoring through measurement of serum concentrations also implies the lack of any clear, objective clinical marker of drug effect.

Although the problems listed above pertain to both adult and pediatric populations, there are nevertheless important differences between the two groups:

1. Absorption is altered for many drugs in the neonatal period due to changes in gastric pH and gastric emptying time.

2. There are differences in the apparent volume of distribution due to differences in body composition (the neonate has proportionately less body fat and more body water than children and adults).

3. The clearance of drugs is often low in premature infants and neonates due to immature hepatic and renal function.

4. Biotransformation of many drugs is slow in the premature infant and neonate due to immaturity of the enzymes responsible for drug metabolism (the hepatic microsomal enzyme system). In contrast, the activity of this system is often greater in children than in adults, requiring a higher milligram/kilogram body weight dos-

age in the former to achieve steady-state concentrations comparable to those found in adults. A more detailed discussion of these variables follows.

5. Protein binding may be somewhat decreased in the neonate.

Absorption

Drug absorption is affected by numerous factors, including route of administration, drug formulation, age of recipient, and concomitant administration of other drugs or food. Administration by the intravenous route provides rapid availability, with absorption being quantitative. In contrast, absorption of some drugs, such as phenytoin or diazepam, after intramuscular administration is slower and less complete. Intramuscular dosing with such drugs should be avoided whenever possible. Many drugs are, however, administered orally, and factors that influence the amount of drug absorbed from the gastrointestinal tract (the bioavailability of a drug) include drug formulation, drug solubility and pK, concomitant administration of other drugs, and simultaneous ingestion of food.

Most drugs are absorbed from the gastrointestinal tract by a process of passive diffusion, with absorption occurring primarily in the small intestine. Variables include gastric emptying time, which is considerably prolonged in the neonate and approaches adult values only after age 6 m.[5, 6] Food or any other factor which delays gastric emptying will delay drug absorption. Gastric pH affects the state of ionization of some drugs and hence their absorption across lipid membranes. Erythromycin and ampicillin are acid labile, and delayed retention in the stomach results in decreased absorption. Gastric pH is close to neutral at birth and falls to approximately 2 within several hours; it does, however, return to neutrality by 24 h and remains neutral for 1–2 w. Adult values for gastric acidity are only reached after age 2 y.[7]

For most drugs, the elimination process follows exponential first-order kinetics, i.e., a constant fraction of the drug present in the body is eliminated per unit of time. However, three important drugs undergo dose-dependent or saturation kinetics: phenytoin (discussion follows), salicylate, and ethanol.

Drug Metabolism

Drug metabolism is influenced by genetic and dietary factors, and also by age and the activity of drug-metabolizing enzymes. In addition, altered hepatic, renal, and cardiac function can markedly affect biotransformation and may lead to serious drug accumulation if dosage regimens are not tailored accordingly.

Studies by Vesell and Page[8] indicate the magnitude of genetic control over rates of drug metabolism. In these studies, identical twins were found to have very similar plasma half-lives for antipyrine.

Isoniazid and procainamide are metabolized by acetylation in the liver. The capacity of rapid acetylation occurs in families as a Mendelian dominant gene. Persons lacking the dominant gene for this acetyltransferase display a reduced capacity for metabolism of these drugs, i.e., they are slow acetylators (approximately 50% of the people in North America are slow acetylators), and as a result plasma concentrations of drugs normally acetylated are higher and remain increased longer than in the fast-acetylator group.[9]

Humans are exposed to many chemicals, and some of these have been shown to alter the rates of drug biotransformation by enhancing the activity of the hepatic microsomal enzyme system. For example, the half-life of theophylline is considerably shorter in smokers than in non-smokers.[10, 11] Also, theophylline half-life decreases in patients on long-term theophylline therapy who are fed a charcoal-broiled beef diet.[12] The ratio of protein to carbohydrate in the diet can also affect the rate of drug metabolism. For example, the half-life of both antipyrine and theophylline is markedly reduced when the diet is changed from a low-protein, high-carbohydrate to a high-protein, low-carbohydrate content.[13] Phenobarbital is a well-known inducer of the hepatic microsomal system, while cimetidine inhibits the same system.

The hepatic microsomal enzymes are active at birth, although their titers are considerably reduced in comparison with adult values. Activity increases with advancing fetal and postnatal age and then begins to decrease with the onset of puberty until adult values are reached. Children on chronic drug treatment (e.g., epileptics and asthmatics) should be followed very closely as they progress through puberty, as the drug dose probably will need to be adjusted downward to maintain therapeutic drug concentrations. The theophylline half-life in premature infants has been quoted as 14.4–57.7 h, whereas the half-life in children age 1–4 y has been reported as 1.9–5.5 h.[14] In contrast, theophylline half-life in adults is 3.0–9.5 h.[15]

Protein Binding

The extent of protein binding can significantly affect drug elimination. It is the "free" drug which is pharmacologically active. In disease states characterized by hypoalbuminemia (e.g., hepatic or renal failure, nephrotic syndrome, protein-losing enteropathy), the concentration of the free active drug will be higher at any given total drug concentration. This may give rise to toxicity in patients who nonetheless have a total serum concentration of the drug within the therapeutic range. Since enhanced protein binding slows the elimination of drugs that are removed from the serum by glomerular filtration or diffusion into the liver, it may increase the duration of action of such drugs. Quantitative and qualitative differences in serum proteins in the newborn period frequently alter drug disposition.

In addition to albumin, various blood constituents such as red blood cells and α_1-acid glycoprotein are capable of binding drugs. The concentration in plasma of α_1-acid glycoprotein, a protein which binds many basic drugs,[16] increases with infectious, inflammatory, and malignant diseases and after surgery. Clearly, the binding of drugs such as propranolol and chlorpromazine to α_1-acid glycoprotein is dependent on the concentration of this protein in serum.[16] It is interesting to note that the concentration of α_1-acid glycoprotein in serum is low in the neonate, and consequently a number of drugs show reduced binding in neonatal serum. In a study by Piafsky and Mpamugo,[17] the binding of both lidocaine and propranolol was shown to be significantly reduced in cord serum as compared to binding in serum obtained from 14 healthy adult controls.

Free Drug Concentration

The routine measurement of free drug concentrations may be desirable, but this is still an unrealized ideal. Equilibrium dialysis is time-consuming, and the various membranes available commercially (e.g., Millipore Ultra-Free Membrane System) which allow the free drug concentration to be measured following generation of protein-free ultrafiltrate are costly. Both of the above procedures demand large sample volumes, and this requirement is always a problem in a pediatric population. Nevertheless, in many situations measurement of the non-protein-bound drug should allow a more meaningful evaluation of dosage requirements, and probably will slowly replace the now-accepted correlation of total serum drug concentration with clinical effect.

Knowledge of the free drug concentration is most important in those instances where the drug is strongly protein bound, e.g., phenytoin, valproic acid, and the tricylic antidepressants. For many drugs with a high pKa value (phenytoin, primidone, ethosuximide, carbamazepine, etc.), the concentration in saliva has been shown to approximate the free serum drug concentration. This has led to the suggestion that in many instances saliva should be substituted for the plasma sample. Since saliva is collected by non-invasive techniques,[18] there is further advantage in this approach; it is, however, impractical in neonates and infants.

An in-depth review of free drug measurement has recently been published.[19]

Patient Noncompliance

When a patient fails to follow a prescribed medication regimen, the effectiveness of the therapy is likely to be less than desirable. Unsuspected noncompliance can lead to unnecessary tests, additional medications, or increased and sometimes dangerous dosing. Hospital admissions that might have been prevented can occur. Unused drugs may accumulate in homes and present a risk to others, especially small children.

Noncompliance is particularly problematic in the pediatric population. Bergman and Werner[20] found noncompliance in 82% of children on short-term penicillin therapy. In children, noncompliance is generally due to parental neglect and unwillingness to follow the prescribed regimen. Hence, strategies to improve compliance in children must be directed toward parents.

PRACTICAL ASPECTS OF THERAPEUTIC DRUG MONITORING

Optimal timing for taking of the sample is imperative. For this reason, a service is recommended which includes a venipuncture team or similar personnel whose sole task is to ensure that blood specimens are drawn at appropriate time intervals relative to the drug dose. Also necessary is a special drug-monitoring requisition listing the patient's age, sex, weight, and height; dose, time of last dose, and time of sampling; clinical status, especially with regard to renal, hepatic, and cardiac function; and a list of other medications received by the patient. There must also be a means to convey the sample rapidly to the laboratory for analysis. Shown in Figure 19–4 is the requisition used at Children's Hospital in Washington, D.C., for both therapeutic drug monitoring and requesting a therapeutic drug monitoring consultation.

Selection of Analytical Procedure for Drug Measurement

The ideal analytical procedure chosen for drug measurement would be accurate and precise, rapid, easy to perform, readily automated, and inexpensive. No single analytical technique consistently meets all of these requirements. For example, high-performance liquid chromatography and gas liquid chromatography probably provide the most accurate and precise analysis of many drugs, but they require specialized and expensive equipment and trained personnel, and even today they cannot be regarded as easy to perform. Nevertheless, provided the laboratory workload is sufficiently high, the reagent cost per analysis with

FIGURE 19–4. Therapeutic Drug Monitoring Requisition and Report Form

Date of Requisition:_____

COLLECTION TIMES	DOSE:_____	ROUTE	INFUSION DATA	
□ 1600h	q 4h □	IV □	Start time: _____	
□ 1800h	q 6h □	IM □		
□ 2000h	q 8h □	SC □	Finish time: _____	
□ 2200h	q 12h □	PO □		
□ 2400h	q 24h □		Flush time: _____	
Consultation Requested:	Other:_____	Other:_____		ADDRESSOGRAPH
□ Yes	_____	_____	Initials:___	
□ No				

ANALYSIS WILL NOT BE PERFORMED UNLESS ALL INFORMATION IS PROVIDED

✓	DRUG REQUESTED	RESULT	✓	DRUG REQUESTED	RESULT	✓	DRUG REQUESTED	RESULT
	Amikacin (Amikin) TROUGH	ug/mL		Digoxin (Lanoxin)	ng/mL		Primidone	ug/mL
	Amikacin (Amikin) PEAK	ug/mL		Ethosuximide (Zarontin)	ug/mL		Theophylline	ug/mL
	Caffeine	ug/mL		Gentamicin TROUGH	ug/mL		Tobramycin TROUGH	ug/mL
	Carbamazepine (Tegretol)	ug/mL		Gentamicin PEAK	ug/mL		Tobramycin PEAK	ug/mL
	Chloramphenicol (Chloromycetin) TROUGH	ug/mL		Pentobarbital	ug/mL		Valproic Acid (Depakene)	ug/mL
	Chloramphenicol (Chloromycetin) PEAK	ug/mL		Phenobarbital	ug/mL		Vancomycin TROUGH	ug/mL
	Cyclosporine	ng/mL		Phenytoin (Dilantin)	ug/mL		Vancomycin PEAK	ug/mL

REQUESTING PHYSICIAN:	TIME DRAWN:	OTHER* (please write in):
PRINT:	DRAWN BY:	
BEEPER:		*Interpretation not available

INTERPRETATION AND RECOMMENDATION	PHARMACOKINETIC PARAMETERS
	Volume of Distribution (V_d)
	Elimination Rate Constant (K_e)
	Half-life (t½)
	New Dose
	New Dosing Interval
	Predicted Cp max / Cp min
PHARMACIST INTERPRETATION:	DATE:

THERAPEUTIC RANGES

DRUG REQUESTED	THERAPEUTIC RANGE	DRUG REQUESTED	THERAPEUTIC RANGE	DRUG REQUESTED	THERAPEUTIC RANGE
Amikacin - Send to AML (Amikin) TROUGH	5-10ug/mL	Digoxin (Lanoxin)	0.8-2.0ng/mL	Primidone	5-12ug/mL
Amikacin - Send to AML (Amikin) PEAK	20-35ug/mL	Ethosuximide (Zarontin)	40-100ug/mL	Theophylline	10-20ug/mL
Caffeine	3-15ug/mL	Gentamicin TROUGH	0-2ug/mL	Tobramycin TROUGH	0-2ug/mL
Carbamazepine (Tegretol)	8-12ug/mL	Gentamicin PEAK	5-10ug/mL	Tobramycin PEAK	5-10ug/mL
Chloramphenicol (Chloromycetin) TROUGH	0-10ug/mL	Pentobarbital - Send to AML	1-5ug/mL	Valproic Acid (Depakene)	50-100ug/mL
Chloramphenicol (Chloromycetin) PEAK	10-25ug/mL	Phenobarbital	15-40ug/mL	Vancomycin TROUGH	5-10ug/mL
Cyclosporin (Kidney) (Liver) (Heart) (Bone Marrow)	400-800ng/mL 500-1100ng/mL 600-1200ng/mL 200-450ng/mL	Phenytoin (Dilantin)	10-20ug/mL	Vancomycin PEAK	20-40ug/mL

these techniques is significantly lower than with the alternative methodologies: enzyme immunoassay, fluorescence immunoassay, fluorescence polarization immunoassay, radioimmunoassay, radioenzymatic assay. Furthermore, gas-liquid and high-performance liquid chromatographic techniques often allow for the simultaneous analysis of several drugs or drug metabolites in a single sample, an advantage not offered by any of the immunoassay techniques.

In contrast, drug assays performed by the enzyme multiplied immunoassay system (EMIT, Syva Diagnostics, Palo Alto, CA) and fluorescence polarization immunoassay (FPIA, Abbott Diagnostics, Abbott Park, IL) are straightforward and provide adequate specificity, sensitivity, accuracy, and precision. For smaller laboratories, the increased reagent cost per analysis is offset by the ease of drug quantitation and the ability to provide a fairly comprehensive drug analytic service with minimal technical expertise and equipment cost. Radioreceptor assays may be the method of choice for drugs which are extensively metabolized to both active and inactive metabolites, e.g., digoxin and cyclosporine. This subject was recently reviewed.[21]

Once the analysis has been performed, it is imperative that the results be rapidly conveyed to the requesting physician. Ideally, an interpretative arm of the drug monitoring service would link the laboratory and the wards to ensure that the appropriate adjustments in drug regimen have been made as a result of the analytic service provided. Such a function can best be carried out in a cost-effective fashion by clinical pharmacists supported by a clinical pharmacology service. The official report form should include the drug concentration found, the desired therapeutic concentration range, and recommendations as to how the latter can be achieved. In special instances, it may be desirable to carry out more detailed pharmacokinetic studies to derive parameters necessary to guide dosage adjustment for optimal patient management. At Children's Hospital, the request form is also the report form (Figure 19–4).

Anticonvulsant Drugs

Phenytoin exhibits dose-dependent kinetics, i.e., the concentration of phenytoin increases linearly with dose until a point is reached at which the metabolizing pathways are saturated. Any slight further increase in drug dose can give rise to a large increase in serum concentration and drug toxicity. It is important to note that although phenytoin is effective in suppressing seizures at serum concentrations of 10–20 mg/L (40–80 μmol/L), the drug has been known to produce an exacerbation of seizures at serum concentrations > 40 mg/L (160 μmol/L). Phenytoin is strongly protein bound; therefore, any disease causing a decrease in binding can be associated with a large increase in the free phenytoin concentration, leading to phenytoin toxicity. This is known to occur particularly in patients with renal failure who may have signs of phenytoin toxicity at serum concentrations of 10–20 mg/L (40–80 μmol/L), the usual therapeutic range. In these instances, the measurement of free phenytoin concentrations is recommended, the free concentration being most easily obtained by quantitating the concentration of phenytoin in saliva. The dosage regimen should then be adjusted appropriately to provide a free concentration of 1–2 mg/L (4–8 μmol/L).

Phenobarbital and carbamazepine are potent inducers of the hepatic microsomal enzyme system and can markedly affect the half-life of other drugs metabolized by this route.

The protein binding of valproic acid is variable and dependent on many factors, including the concentration of valproic acid in serum. For example, at 20–60 mg/L (140–420 μmol/L), there is approximately 5% free drug; at 80 mg/L (560 μmol/L), there is approximately 8% free drug; and at 145 mg/L (1015 μmol/L), there is approximately 20% free drug.[22] Furthermore, there is competition for binding sites between valproate and phenytoin, resulting in initial increased free concentrations of both drugs.[23] Removal of phenytoin, carbamazepine, or phenobarbital from a drug regimen including valproic acid has been known to give rise to large increases in valproic acid serum concentrations.[24] Clearly, any change in the drug regimen should be followed shortly thereafter by drug concentration measurement and appropriate adjustment of the drug regimen if required.

Primidone is converted to phenobarbital and phenylethylmalonamide, and anticonvulsant properties have been attributed to all three compounds. Therefore, phenobarbital concentrations should always be measured in patients on primidone therapy. Although the serum primidone concentration is very dependent on the time of sampling relative to the time of drug ingestion, owing to its short half-life, this is not the case for phenobarbital. Hence, adjustments in the primidone dosing schedule are sometimes more appropriately made on the measured phenobarbital concentration.

Finally, the measurement of anticonvulsant drug concentrations is always useful in the detection of patient noncompliance with a prescribed regimen. Table 19-1 lists serum concentrations associated with various toxic signs and symptoms.

Digoxin

Digoxin does not meet many of the criteria for therapeutic drug monitoring. There are major problems in accurately measuring concentrations of digoxin with currently available immunoassays. This is especially so in newborn infants, in hypertensive patients, in states of

TABLE 19–1. Clinical Manifestations of Toxicity for Anticonvulsant Drugs

Drug	Serum Concentration		Clinical Manifestations of Toxicity
Phenobarbital*	40-60 mg/L	(172-258 µmol/L)	Slowness and ataxia
	60-110 mg/L	(258-474 µmol/L)	Comatose, reflexes present
	> 110 mg/L	(474 µmol/L)	No deep tendon reflexes
Phenytoin	20-30 mg/L	(80-120 µmol/L)	Nystagmus
	30-40 mg/L	(120-160 µmol/L)	Nystagmus, ataxia
	> 40 mg/L	(160 µmol/L)	Nystagmus, ataxia, and lethargy
	Chronic use		Gum hypertrophy, hirsutism
Primidone	> 14 mg/L	(64 µmol/L)	Nystagmus, vertigo, ataxia, vomiting, dysarthria
Ethosuximide	> 100 mg/L	(708 µmol/L)	Sedation, nausea, vomiting, pancytopenia
Carbamazepine	> 9 mg/L	(38 µmol/L)	Nystagmus, drowsiness, nausea, vomiting, headache
Valproic acid	> 125 mg/L	(875 µmol/L)	Rare, but include anorexia, nausea, vomiting, and hair loss

*Tolerance to the sedative effect of phenobarbital is marked. Many patients may have serum concentrations as high as 75 mg/L (323 µmol/L) and show no clinical signs of toxicity.

renal and hepatic insufficiency, and in pregnancy, where the existence of endogenous digoxin-like substances (EDLS) may lead to falsely increased values of the glycoside.[25-28]

In a recent study,[30] an association between age and the apparent digoxin readings caused by EDLS was documented in newborn infants. When adding true digoxin to these sera, there was an additive effect upon the measurable digoxin concentration.

There is no accurate definition of a "therapeutic window" for digoxin or digitoxin. Few blind, controlled studies have tried to prove digitalis' efficacy in congestive heart failure. More importantly, sparse information exists on the correlation of serum concentrations of cardiac glycosides with inotropic effects. More information exists on the putative correlation between serum concentrations of digoxin and its antiarrhythmic effects. Some investigators have observed a correlation, whereas others have not.[29-33]

Most authorities regard the therapeutic range of digoxin to be 0.5–2.0 ng/mL (0.6–2.4 nmol/L). At concentrations above 2 ng/mL (2.4 nmol/L), there is an increased risk of digitalis toxicity, presenting as nausea, vomiting, anorexia, yellow vision, malaise, and cardiac arrhythmias. However, there is a wide "gray zone" of concentrations that may be toxic in one individual and nontoxic in another. In a recent study, Koren and Parker[34] demonstrated that even at serum concentrations above 5 ng/mL (6 nmol/L), about one-third of pediatric patients would not show symptoms or signs of toxicity. The risk of toxicity of digitalis glycosides increases in a variety of clinical conditions, including hypokalemia, hypocalcemia, hypomagnesemia, and chronic heart disease.

Despite the limitations outlined above, the therapeutic monitoring of digoxin concentrations is indicated in routine therapy, for several reasons:

1. *To assess patient compliance.* Here, therapeutic drug monitoring may be an important guideline for the assessment of therapeutic failures.

2. *To determine an optimal dosing schedule.* If a patient receives a given dose of digitalis in the hospital, does not respond clinically, and is found to have a steady-state serum concentration of < 1.0 ng/mL (1.2 nmol/L), the clinician can safely increase the dose without achieving potentially toxic concentrations.

3. *To confirm a clinical impression of toxicity.* Many of the symptoms and signs of digitalis toxicity (anorexia, cachexia, nausea, vomiting, arrhythmias) may be caused by the underlying cardiac condition. The only available way to differentiate between these two diagnostic possibilities is by measuring the serum concentration of the glycoside. If the measured concentration is, for example, 0.7 ng/mL (0.8 nmol/L), it is very unlikely that drug toxicity caused the symptoms; if, however, the measured concentration is 3.8 ng/mL (4.6 nmol/L), it is conceivable that drug-related toxicity has occurred.

During the last decade, several drugs that are commonly coadministered with digoxin have been shown to interfere with the disposition of cardiac glycosides and to cause potentially toxic serum concentrations.[35] Quinidine, verapamil, and amiodarone may cause a significant increase in the serum concentration of digoxin, which is often associated with signs of digoxin toxicity. Spironolactone has been shown to decrease digoxin clearance, but no cases of toxicity have been reported.

Digoxin Toxicity. The concept of using hapten-specific antibodies to reverse the toxic effects of a drug has been previously advanced.[36] More recently, digoxin-specific Fab antibody fragments have been purified and used to treat patients with advanced, life-threatening toxicity.[37] In such circumstances, an immunologic approach is feasible, can be lifesaving, and has been used experimentally for over 10 years. Fab antibody fragments recently have become commercially available. The fascinating side of this new approach is that it can neutralize the pharmacologic effects of a drug with a very large distribution volume that cannot be effectively removed by hemodialysis or hemoperfusion. The use of Fab antibody fragments affects the quantitation of digoxin by most immunoassay procedures. These problems can be largely overcome by measurement of "free" digoxin concentrations in a plasma ultrafiltrate.

Theophylline, Caffeine, and Doxapram

Theophylline is used widely in the treatment of bronchial asthma and neonatal apnea. The drug is a smooth muscle relaxant, possibly because of effects on adenosine receptors, and is also an inhibitor of phosphodiesterase, at least *in vitro*. This produces a buildup of intracellular cyclic AMP and consequent smooth muscle relaxation. In addition to its effect on smooth muscle, theophylline is a cardiac muscle stimulant. Theophylline also has a narrow therapeutic index, and progressively more serious side effects have been noted beginning at serum concentrations of 20 mg/L (110 μmol/L). Intersubject variability in theophylline metabolism is large, due to factors such as genetic variation, age, diet, etc., as was already discussed. For this reason, the optimal dosage regimen cannot be readily predicted, and drug monitoring plays a central role in aiding the clinician to optimize therapy. Note that the theophylline half-life is short, and this requires either the use of long-acting theophylline preparations or a regimen in which the drug is administered four times daily. We recommend measurement of trough (predose) and peak (approximately 2 h post-dose) concentrations. Side effects include irritability, insomnia and headache, and gastrointestinal effects such as nausea, vomiting, and gastric irritation. Serum concentrations greater than 40 mg/L (220 μmol/L) have, on occasion, been associated with seizures.

Today, caffeine is preferred over theophylline for the treatment of neonatal apnea. Approximately 30–50% of premature infants suffer from apnea, generally defined as cessation of respiration for more than 20 sec, with or without bradycardia, cyanosis, or both. For infants < 29 w gestational age, the incidence increases to > 90%. Reasons for preferring caffeine to theophylline include its wider therapeutic index, slower excretion, and reduced toxicity, and the fact that, in the neonate, substantial amounts of theophylline are metabolized to caffeine, giving rise to the problem of necessitating monitoring of both drugs. The therapeutic range for caffeine is 5–15 mg/L (25–75 μmol/L).

Doxapram is an effective drug in the treatment of idiopathic apnea of prematurity that is refractory to xanthine (theophylline, caffeine) therapy. In general, infants respond to doxapram at serum concentrations of 1.5–4.0 mg/L (4.0–10.6 μmol/L). Concentrations > 5 mg/L (13.2 μmol/L) are associated with toxicity.

Aminoglycosides

This class of drugs includes gentamicin, tobramycin, and amikacin, which are used for serious gram-negative infection such as pneumonia, meningitis, and UTI. Gentamicin is not a pure chemical substance and consists of several components, all of which appear to have similar antimicrobial activity. These drugs have poor gastrointestinal absorption and are usually administered intravenously. The methods of choice for analysis of gentamicin are enzyme multiplied immunoassay, fluorescence immunoassay, fluorescence polarization immunoassay, and radioimmunoassay. Serum concentration monitoring of aminoglycosides is generally accepted for its clinical utility because these drugs are both nephrotoxic and ototoxic. For gentamicin and tobramycin, peak concentrations (drawn 30 min after the end of an intravenous infusion) should be 5–10 mg/L and trough concentrations (drawn just before the next dose) should be < 2 mg/L. Adverse reactions include allergic reactions, transient agranulocytosis, and increases in serum transaminases in addition to renal and cochlear or vestibular damage. The incidence of these reactions is low. The nephrotoxicity of gentamicin results in proximal tubular damage manifested by rising serum creatinine concentrations, proteinuria, and enzymuria.[38] A rather unique toxic reaction—muscular paralysis and apnea resulting from neuromuscular blockade—has been attributed to various aminoglycosides[39] and is a particular problem in low-birth-weight infants requiring anesthesia.

Antineoplastic Drugs

Progress in this area of therapeutic drug monitoring has been extremely slow, for numerous reasons. Most antineoplastic drugs inhibit the S-phase of the cell cycle, which is that phase in which DNA synthesis/replication occurs. If all tumor cells were in this S-phase, these drugs would be effective; however, the growth fraction or percentage of cells in the tumor that are in the "active" cell cycle varies greatly from one tumor to the next. In general, small tumors tend to have large growth fractions, while larger tumors have a greater number of cells in the quiescent Go (null) phase of the cell cycle. Most antineoplastic drugs are ineffective against cells in the Go phase.

Some cells within the tumors may also become tolerant to the drug being used. This has led to the widespread use of multidrug therapy. Multiple drug resistance (MDR) cells are able to maintain a lowered intracellular drug concentration via the increased activity of an energy-dependent drug efflux mechanism. P-glycoprotein expression correlates with both the decrease in intracellular drug accumulation and the observed degree of drug resistance in many MDR cell lines.[40]

A number of drugs have been found to reverse the MDR effect. These include calcium antagonists such as verapamil and the immunosuppressant cyclosporine.

The time of day that drugs are given can have a profound effect upon their pharmacokinetics and pharmacodynamics, e.g., Rivard et al.[41] showed that the outcome in children with acute lymphocytic leukemia (ALL) who received their maintenance 6-mercaptopurine (6MP) dose at night was better than in those who received their dosage regimen in the morning. Langevin et al.[42] subsequently showed that the area under the serum concentration versus time curve was 1.5 times greater in children with ALL if they received their 6MP dosage at night rather than in the morning. A recent study of the relationship between area under the serum concentration versus time curve for 6MP in children with ALL and outcome[43] indicated that therapeutic drug monitoring may well play an increasing role in the optimization of the drug regimen in these patients. For a review of chronopharmacology, the reader is referred to a recent article by Marks.[44]

The use of methotrexate serum concentrations to identify and treat patients with a high probability of manifesting toxicity when the drug is given at high doses has been a significant contribution to decreasing drug toxicity. The relationship between methotrexate concentrations and clinical toxicity has been well documented.[45] Folinic acid rescue has been used effectively to treat patients and thereby prevent methotrexate toxicity. In many high-dose methotrexate protocols, folinic acid (leucovorin) rescue is continued until methotrexate concentrations drop below 2×10^{-8}M.

Immunosuppressive Drugs

Cyclosporine is currently one of the main drugs used to suppress the immune response in patients receiving a transplanted organ. This drug is extensively metabolized to both active and pharmacologically inactive metabolites. Measurement of the parent drug concentration employing monoclonal immunoassays or high-performance liquid chromatography (HPLC) will not measure the pharmacologically active metabolites, while measurement of cyclosporine blood concentrations employing non-specific polyclonal immunoassays is problematic because it allows measurement of inactive metabolites which cross-react in the assay. Also, the active metabolites do not necessarily cross-react in a manner proportional to their pharmacologic activity. Use of a radioreceptor assay which hypothetically interacts with only "active" metabolites may be the method of choice in the future.[46]

At Children's Hospital, we use the whole blood nonspecific immunoassay (Abbott, TDx) and employ the following therapeutic ranges for the different transplant types.

Liver	500–1100 µg/L
Heart	600–1200 µg/L
Bone Marrow	200–450 µg/L
Kidney	350–875 µg/L

Tables 19-2 and 19-3 provide drug monitoring information for some frequently used drugs, including major active metabolites, bioavailability, protein-binding, recommended dose, therapeutic and toxic concentrations, plasma half-life, time to peak plasma concentration, and apparent volume of distribution.

TABLE 19–2. Drug Monitoring Information

Drug	Major Active Metabolite	Plasma Half-Life of Active Metabolite (h)			Dose Dependent Kinetics
		Neonates	**Children**	**Adults**	
Acetylsalicylic acid	Salicylic acid	4.5–11.5	2–3	2–4.5	Yes (salicylic acid)
Amitriptyline	Nortriptyline			14–93	
Carbamazepine	10,11-Epoxide			5–6	
Desipramine	2-Hydroxydesipramine				
Disopyramide	N-Desisopropyldisopyramide				
Imipramine	Desipramine				
	2-Hydroxyimipramine				
	2-Hydroxydesipramine				
Methotrexate	7-Hydroxymethotrexate				Yes
Phenytoin					
Primidone	Phenobarbital			50–120	
	Phenylethylmalonamide (PEMA)			29–36	
Procainamide	N-Acetylprocainamide			6	
Propranolol	4-Hydroxypropranolol				
Quinidine	3-Hydroxyquinidine				
Theophylline					Yes

TABLE 19–3. Parameters of Interest for Commonly Used Drugs

Drug	% of Oral Dose Absorbed	Route of Administration	% of Protein Bound	Maintenance Dose (mg/kg/d)				Effective Plasma Concentration (mg/L)	Toxic Plasma Concentration (mg/L)	Half-Life (h) of Parent Drug				Time (h) to Peak Plasma Concentration	Apparent Volume of Distribution (L/kg)
				Neonates	Infants	Children	Adults			Neonates	Infants	Children	Adults		
Acetaminophen	100	oral/PR	20–30			20–40	17–34	n/a	>25			2–4	2–4	0.5–1.0	0.8–1.0
Acetylsalicylic acid	80–100	oral/PR	50–80			14–25	30–70	Antipyretic 20–100 Antiinflammatory 100–250	>300			0.25–0.35	0.25–0.35	1.0–2.0	
Amikacin	not absorbed orally	IM/IV	10	10–15		10–15	10–15	15–25	>30 peak, >5 trough	variable		2–3	2–3	0.5–1	0.05–0.7
Carbamazepine	70–80	oral	65–83			15–20	7–15	4–12	>12	8–28		5–30	5–30	3	0.8–1.9
Chloramphenicol	75–90	oral/IV	60–80	25		50	50–100	10–25	>25	8–15	15–22	2.4–3.4	1.5–5.0	2	0.6
Digoxin	50–93	IV/oral	20–40	0.010	0.015	0.01	0.008–0.012	0.8–2.0 µg/L	>2.4 µg/L	20–76	36–180	12–42	33–51	0.5–5.0	5.0–10.0
Disopyramide	80	oral/IV	10–80				8.6	2–5	>5				5–6	0.5–3.0	0.8
Ethosuximide	100	oral	0			15–40	15–30	40–100	>100			30–50	40–60	2–4 capsule, 1–2 syrup	0.7–0.9
Gentamicin	not absorbed orally	IM/IV	0–30			6–7.5	3–5	5–10	>12 peak, >2 trough				2–3	0.5–1	adults, 0.15–0.25; children, 0.07–0.7
Imipramine	29–77	oral/IM					0.7–1.4	0.150–0.250	>0.5			2–3	9–24	0.5–2	10–20
Lidocaine	variable	IM/IV	60–80			0.02–0.05 (per min)	1–3 (per min)	1.5–5.0	>5.0				1–2	0.25–0.5	1.7
Methotrexate	80–100	IV/oral	50–70			variable	variable	Depends on therapeutic regimen	24 h, >10⁻⁵ M; 48 h, >10⁻⁶ M; 72 h, >10⁻⁷ M			variable	variable	1–2	0.75
Phenobarbital	90	IV/IM/oral/PR	45–50	3–5		3–8	2–4	15–40	>40	67–99	40–70	40–70	50–120	6–18	0.7–1 adults
Phenytoin	80–90	IV/IM/oral	87–93	3–5		5–15	5–10	10–20 (adults) 5–20 (children)	>20	17–60*	75±64.5	12–22*	18–30*	4–8	0.5–0.8
Primidone	70–95	oral/IM	0–20		3–5	10–25	10–20	5–12	>12			10–12	10–12	2–4	0.6–1.0
Procainamide	90	IV/oral	15				2.8–3 (per h)	4–10	>10				2–4	1–2 oral, 0.5 IM	1.7–2.4
Propranolol	40–98	oral/IV	85–96			5–30	1.1–9	0.05–0.10	variable				2–6	1–4	2.0–64
Quinidine	95–100	oral/IV	80–90				10–30	2–5	>5				4–7	1–2 sulfate	3±0.25
Theophylline	95–100	PR/oral/IV	55–65			16–24	13–18	10–20	>20	24–30	14.4–57.7	1–10	3.6–12.0	2–3 oral	0.3–0.7
Tobramycin		IM/IV	0–10	3		3–5	3–5	5–10	>12 peak, >2 trough				2–3	1 IM	0.22
Valproic acid	85–100	oral	90–95			15–100	15–45	50–100	>100			6–15	8–15	0.5–4.0	0.15–0.40

*Exhibits saturation kinetics. Half-life therefore dependent on serum concentration.

CLINICAL TOXICOLOGY

Acetaminophen

Acetaminophen (paracetamol in Great Britain) is an effective analgesic and antipyretic drug which lacks anti-inflammatory action. It presents less risk for producing gastrointestinal ulceration and hemorrhage than aspirin and other nonsteroidal anti-inflammatory drugs. With the reported link of Reye's syndrome to aspirin use, usage of over-the-counter acetaminophen medication in recent years has surpassed that of aspirin. Unfortunately, the popularity of acetaminophen and the general belief that the drug is not toxic have made accidental acetaminophen overdose a common toxicological problem. In the United States in 1990, more than 70,000 acetaminophen poisoning cases involving patients age 17 y and younger were reported to poison control centers; 86% of those patients were under age 6 y.[47]

Acetaminophen is available as drops, chewable tablets, and elixir, packaged in child-resistant safety bottles. Acetaminophen is a safe drug when administered in typical pediatric doses of 40-480 mg every 4 h. At higher doses, acetaminophen is hepatotoxic, although the toxic dosage is variable. Single doses of 7.5 g or greater in healthy adults or 150 mg/kg in children are used to define risk for liver damage.[48]

After a therapeutic dose, acetaminophen is more than 90% metabolized by the liver and eliminated as glucuronide and sulfate conjugates. Neither the drug nor these metabolites are toxic. Approximately 4% of the dose is converted by the cytochrome P-450 mixed function oxidase system to a reactive intermediate, N-acetyl-p-benzoquinoneimine (NAPQI). This metabolite, thought to be normally detoxified by endogenous glutathione, is excreted into the urine as mercapturic acid and cysteine conjugates. After an overdose, excessive NAPQI not detoxified by glutathione reacts with and destroys hepatocytes. As hepatocellular damage ensues, hepatic insufficiency and fulminant necrosis may follow.[49]

Acetaminophen is rapidly adsorbed, with peak plasma concentration reached within 30–120 min after therapeutic doses; however, delayed peaks may occur following large doses, due to slower gastric emptying. Clinically, patients overdosed on acetaminophen follow a course that can be divided into four phases.[48] In the initial phase, lasting 0–24 h after ingestion, the patient usually exhibits gastrointestinal irritability, nausea, and vomiting. Some patients may be asymptomatic. Adults who do not develop symptoms within 24 h after ingestion rarely show clinical toxicity, although toxicity in young children (< 6 y) always presents with vomiting within 1 h, regardless of their initial serum concentration.[50] Central nervous system, cardiovascular, respiratory, or metabolic toxicity generally is not present in phase 1. If these symptoms are present, other illnesses or drug ingestion must be suspected.

During the second phase (24–72 h), the patient may feel reasonably well while liver enzymes and bilirubin become abnormal and prothrombin time is prolonged. Oliguria may occur but without increased blood urea nitrogen as a result of decreased hepatic formation. If significant hepatic necrosis has occurred, the third phase (72–96 hours) is characterized by the sequelae of hepatic necrosis including coagulopathy, jaundice, encephalopathy, and renal failure. If the patient survives phase 3 with damage which is not irreversible, complete resolution of hepatic dysfunction will occur within 4 days to 2 weeks.

Children (≤ 12 y) are less susceptible to the hepatotoxic effects of acetaminophen despite concentrations that are toxic in adults. Emesis may also play a role in decreasing toxicity, since children are likely to vomit soon after toxic ingestion.[50]

N-acetylcysteine (NAC) is an effective antidote. In the United States, the standard oral regimen consists of a loading dose of 140 mg/kg followed by 17 doses of 70 mg/kg every 4 h. Protection against hepatotoxicity by NAC is most successful when started within 8 h of ingestion, regardless of the initial plasma acetaminophen concentrations.[51] The effectiveness of oral NAC appears to extend to those high-risk patients who are treated as late as 16–24 h post-ingestion.[51] In Canada and Europe, intravenous administration of 300 mg/kg over a 20 h period is the standard therapy.[52] This protocol of NAC usually has been well tolerated, although anaphylactoid reactions have been reported and it may have no value 16 h post-ingestion.[51] A recent experimental protocol for a 48 h intravenous NAC regimen reportedly was as efficacious as other NAC regimens when treatment was started within 10 h.[53] When treatment was initiated 10–24 h after overdose, it was as effective as the 72 h oral protocol and more effective than the 20 h intravenous treatment.

A nomogram relating time since ingestion and plasma drug concentration has been constructed to predict the risk of hepatotoxicity and is used in evaluating the need for N-acetylcysteine treatment (Figure 19–5).[54] It requires that a blood concentration be obtained at least 4 h after ingestion. Samples drawn before 4 h may not represent peak concentrations. An acetaminophen plasma concentration is in the potentially toxic range if it is above (or to the right of) the toxic line (solid line) of the nomogram which connects 200 µg/mL (1322 µmol/L) at 4 h with 50 ug/mL (330 µmol/L) at 12 h. The nomogram has a lower broken line which is plotted 25% below the solid line to allow for some uncertainty of the time of ingestion. Patients whose plasma concentrations are higher than the broken line are given the entire course of NAC treatment. Since early treatment is critical to a favorable outcome,

FIGURE 19–5. Nomogram Relating Plasma or Serum Acetaminophen Concentration and Time Since Ingestion

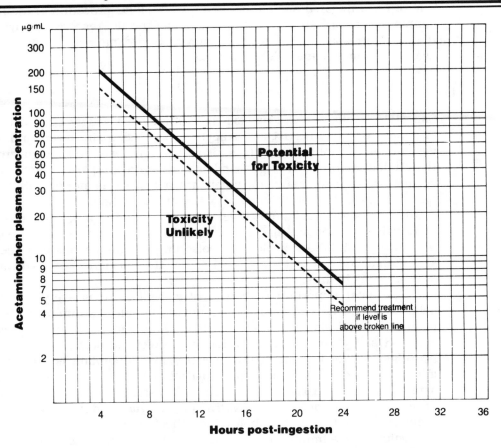

Adapted from: Rumack BH, Matthew H. Acetaminophen poisoning and toxicity. Ped 1975;55:871-6.

the initial plasma drug concentration is a crucial factor in deciding to initiate therapy. Providing prompt and reliable plasma acetaminophen concentrations is an important emergency toxicology service.

Numerous methods are available for the analysis of acetaminophen. Colorimetric tests such as the cresol-ammonia spot test or the quantitative Glynn and Kendal[55] method are fast and sensitive but not specific; the Glynn and Kendal method is interfered with by salicylates. Colorimetric methods based on the prior hydrolysis of acetaminophen *and* its conjugated metabolites to indophenol are not recommended, since the above-mentioned nomogram is based on serum concentration of unconjugated acetaminophen only.[56] HPLC procedures, though simple and rapid, are not as convenient as the fluorescence polarization immunoassay and enzyme immunoassay methods which are available in most clinical laboratories.

Salicylates

Salicylate is one of the least expensive and most widely used drugs. The main therapeutic uses of salicylate to reduce pain, fever, and inflammation are well known. It is also commonly used to treat juvenile rheumatoid arthritis. A large number of different preparations of salicylates are in use, many of which are available as nonprescription medications.[57] The prevalence of salicylate as a household item has resulted in many accidental ingestions. For many years, aspirin and other salicylate-containing over-the-counter medications were the leading cause of childhood accidental poisoning. A number of safety measures enacted resulted in a decline in the incidence of salicylate poisoning in children.[57]

The most important derivative of salicylic acid is acetylsalicylic acid, which is aspirin. Other derivatives include sodium salicylate, magnesium salicylate, choline salicylate, choline magnesium trisalicylate, and salicylsalicylic acid, which is a salicylate derivative that on hydrolysis yields two molecules of salicylate. Benorylate is an acetaminophen ester of aspirin that is hydrolyzed to acetaminophen and aspirin in the gastrointestinal tract. Diflunisal, a recently introduced drug, is a difluorophenyl derivative of salicylic acid that lacks the acetyl group and is not metabolized to salicylate.

After oral administration, salicylate is rapidly adsorbed by the stomach and intestine. Aspirin and other derivatives of salicylic acid are rapidly hydrolyzed to salicylate by esterases, with a plasma half-life of 15–20 min. Serum concentrations peak up to 2 h later following ingestion of enteric-coated aspirin, because the coating is resistant to dissolution in the acidic medium in the stomach and only dissolves after passing into the alkaline medium of the intestine.

The two major metabolic pathways of salicylic acid to salicyluric acid and salicylphenolic glucuronide are saturable and follow Michaelis-Menten kinetics. As the two major pathways become saturated, even after therapeutic doses, the elimination half-life as well as the serum concentrations will increase disproportionately with increasing dosage.[58] Therefore, salicylate in serum can accumulate to toxic concentrations, resulting in chronic intoxication or therapeutic overdose, which is defined as excessive therapeutic administration of salicylate over a period of 12 h or longer.[59] Chronic intoxication is an important cause of salicylate poisoning in children. In one study of pediatric patients hospitalized with salicylate intoxication, therapeutic overdoses were nearly as frequent as acute overdoses.[60]

The toxic severity following an acute overdose is related to the amount of drug ingested.[61] Ingestion of less than 150 mg/kg is unlikely to result in toxic symptoms. Mild to moderate toxic reactions can be expected from an ingested dose of 150–300 mg/kg. Doses in excess of 300 mg/kg lead to severe reactions, and ingestion of more than 500 mg/kg is potentially lethal. The primary pathophysiologic effects of salicylism are complex. They include direct stimulation of the respiratory center, resulting in hyperventilation, respiratory alkalosis, and compensatory excretion of base, uncoupling of oxidative phosphorylation, interference with the Krebs cycle, and accumulation of organic acids leading to metabolic acidosis. In children, respiratory alkalosis is transient, and a late-stage dominant metabolic acidosis is common. Acidemia favors the non-ionized form of salicylic acid and enhances the toxicity of salicylate by increasing tissue uptake of the drug. Thus, neurological symptoms such as confusion, delirium, and coma usually are associated with severe metabolic acidosis.

Acute salicylate intoxication in children is usually not difficult to diagnose. If sufficient quantity of salicylate has been ingested, the typical symptoms of salicylate intoxication will be evident. In addition, children are frequently found ingesting the tablets, and circumstantial evidence such as finding the container nearby often helps in the diagnosis. A diagnosis of salicylate intoxication is readily confirmed by measuring serum salicylate concentration. Thus, the availability of a salicylate assay on an emergency basis is critical.

Diagnosis of chronic salicylate intoxication is much more difficult without a high degree of suspicion. Salicylate is such a common household medication that parents of intoxicated children do not realize the hazard of their seemingly harmless drug therapy and do not typically disclose salicylate intake unless specifically questioned. They may not even be aware that the over-the-counter products being used contain aspirin. This leads to delay in reaching the correct diagnosis, which accounts for the more severe clinical picture that is associated with chronic intoxication. Because of the difficulty in recognizing chronic salicylate intoxication clinically, documentation of increased serum salicylate concentrations becomes very important in the differential diagnosis.

Treatment of salicylate intoxication involves correction of fluid and electrolyte depletion and acid-base imbalance. Alkalinization to enhance urinary excretion of the drug should be considered when the serum salicylate concentrations exceeds 350 µg/mL (2.5 mmol/L), and hemoperfusion or hemodialysis when the serum concentration is 1000 µg/mL (7.2 mmol/L) or greater.[59]

FIGURE 19–6. Done Nomogram for Salicylate Poisoning

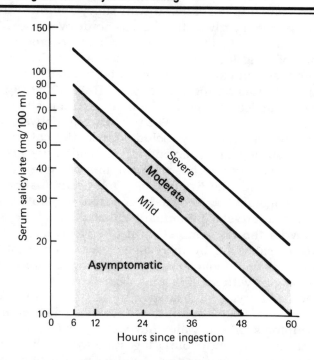

Adapted from: Done AK. Salicylate intoxication: Significance of measurements of salicylate in blood in cases of acute ingestion. Ped 1960;26:800-7.

A nomogram (Done nomogram) is helpful in the interpretation of salicylate concentrations at different times following ingestion to predict the severity of intoxication[62] (Figure 19–6). The greatest clinical value of the nomogram lies in the early estimation of the severity of the intoxication for appropriate patient disposition and in identifying those high-risk patients who may require prompt alkalinization therapy or hemoperfusion. The nomogram is not useful in predicting the rate of salicylate elimination or future serum salicylate concentrations. Furthermore, this nomogram is applicable only to assessment of acute ingestion, not chronic intoxication.

If enteric coated or sustained-release salicylate is ingested, absorption of salicylate and the increase of serum salicylate concentration will be delayed. A patient suspected of ingesting these salicylate formulations should be observed and the serum salicylate determination repeated because the peak salicylate concentration may not be attained until 60–70 h after ingestion. The Done nomogram should not be used, because an ingestion time-serum concentration relationship different from that for regular tablets is involved.

While most clinical chemistry laboratories provide serum salicylate concentrations on a STAT basis, simple qualitative screening tests such as ferric chloride, Trinder's reagent, and Phenistix for urine salicylate are useful for quick confirmation of salicylate overdose if quantitation of serum concentrations is not available immediately.[57] These screening tests are not specific for salicylate; therefore, all positive screening results should be confirmed using quantitative assays and serum samples.

Colorimetric assays based on the reaction of salicylic acid with ferric ion to give a purple color are not specific, and some assays have high serum blanks. Of these assays, Trinder's method with serum blank values less than 10 μg/mL has proved useful in the diagnosis of salicylate intoxication.[63] Fluorescence polarization immunoassay provides a rapid and accurate assay for serum salicylate. Other approaches to salicylate measurement are HPLC and enzymatic; the latter uses the enzyme salicylate hydrolase (EC 1.14.13.1) purified from *Pseudomonas cepacia*.[57]

Alcohols

Ethanol is such a widely used social drug and alcoholic beverages are so readily available at home that there is considerable potential risk for accidental ingestion. Ethanol intoxication among children is common. The ethanol content in beverages ranges from 3.6% in beer, 10-12% in wine, to 40–50% in distilled beverages. The term "proof" means two times the percentage of ethanol by volume. An additional risk for young children is the ingestion of ethanol-containing mouthwashes, cologne, perfume, and aftershaves.[64, 65] These consumer products are commonly available to families, are kept in easily accessible places at home, and are not packaged in child-resistant containers. The ethanol contents of the five leading name-brand mouthwashes range from 14% to 26.9%.[64] A potentially lethal dose of ethanol is approximately 3 mg/kg in a small child, which, for an average 2-year-old, is 6–10 oz of mouthwash. In 1990, The American Association of Poison Control Centers reported 5261 cases of ethanol ingestion in children under age 6 y.[47]

Ethanol is rapidly absorbed from the gastrointestinal tract, 20% in the stomach and 80% in the small intestine. The peak blood ethanol concentration is achieved in 30–60 min, although there is significant inter-subject variability in the peak blood alcohol concentration attained and the time for its achievement due to food intake and physiological variables. Ethanol distributes to total body water with an apparent volume of distribution in children of 0.7 L/kg. The plasma/blood ratio of 1.18 (range of 1.10–1.35), urine/blood ratio of

1.3 (range of 0.3–2.6), and breath/blood ratio of 2180 (range of 1837–2863) have been determined for adults.[66]

Ethanol is metabolized mostly (> 90%) by liver alcohol dehydrogenase to acetaldehyde. The proportion excreted unchanged in breath and urine is relatively small (< 5% at 80 mg/dL [17.4 mmol/L]) but assumes more significance at higher concentrations. Elimination follows first-order kinetics at low concentrations (< 20 mg/dL [4.4 mmol/L]). At higher concentrations and when absorption is essentially completed, metabolism generally is believed to proceed at zero-order kinetics, which is dependent on biological variability, history of use, and dose. In adults, the rate of elimination varies from 8–39 mg/dL/h (1.7–8.6 mmol/L/h),[67] the average being approximately 16 mg/dL/h (3.5 mmol/L/h). In children, elimination may be more rapid; the mean rate has been described as 28.4 mg/dL/h (6.2 mmol/L/h), almost twice that of adults.[68]

Ethanol toxicity in children has been described.[68] Gastrointestinal irritation may result in nausea and vomiting. Ethanol produces central nervous system toxicity, and clinical symptoms are generally consistent with blood ethanol concentrations. Blood alcohol concentrations < 50 mg/dL (11 mmol/L) are unlikely to be associated with symptoms. Exuberance, giddiness, talkativeness, mild incoordination, and visual impairment are noticeable with blood alcohol concentrations up to 150 mg/dL (33 mmol/L). Concentrations of 150–300 mg/dL (33–66 mmol/L) result in verbal confusion, ataxia, exaggerated emotional states, and muscular incoordination. Concentrations in excess of 300 mg/dL (66 mmol/L) are associated with blurred vision, stupor, coma, and compromised cardiorespiratory functions, and death has been reported with concentrations > 400 mg/dL (88 mmol/L).[69]

Other clinical findings include hypothermia secondary to peripheral vasodilatation, CNS depression, and metabolic acidosis in young children. Dehydration may occur because ethanol is a competitor of anti-diuretic hormone, and severe, acute intoxication may result in considerable fluid loss. Hypoglycemia is a serious complication, and the patient may present in a coma or convulsion, with blood alcohol concentrations that may be below 100 mg/dL (22 mmol/L).[70] The hypoglycemic effect of ethanol is the leading cause for childhood hypoglycemic coma. Thus, in the management of a child who has ingested ethanol, the potential for life-threatening hypoglycemia must be considered, and serum glucose concentrations need to be monitored closely.

Many analytical methods for alcohol analysis are in use in clinical laboratories. The most frequently used are assays based on enzymatic oxidation using alcohol dehydrogenase (ADH). The specificity of an enzymatic assay depends on the source of ADH, and interference by methanol and isopropanol varies substantially among kits. Laboratories using the enzymatic assay must be prepared to investigate ingestion of alcohols other than ethanol or the coingestion of ethanol and another alcohol. Gas chromatographic methods can identify ethanol as well as methanol, and isopropanol, and direct inspection of diluted plasma or serum makes it suitable for emergency analysis.

In small hospital laboratories with no facility for either gas chromatographic or enzymatic analysis, the serum osmolarity gap between the measured osmolality and calculated serum osmolarity can serve as an indirect approximation.[71] A formula to calculate serum osmolarity is:

$$1.86 \cdot Na \ (mmol/L) + \frac{Glucose \ (mg/dL)}{18} + \frac{BUN \ (mg/dL)}{2.8}$$

The measured osmolality should be determined by a freezing point depression instrument, not by a vapor pressure osmometer. The expected contribution by ethanol at 100 mg/dL (21.7 mmol/L) is 21 mOsm/kg. Ethanol is the most common cause for elevation of serum osmolarity.

Methanol, Isopropanol, and Ethylene Glycol

Methanol, isopropanol, and ethylene glycol are important industrial chemicals which are also available as household items—methanol and ethylene glycol as a constituent of some antifreeze and windshield washer solutions, and isopropanol as a disinfectant (30–99.9% solution) or as rubbing alcohol (70% solution). Childhood intoxication with methanol and isopropanol due to accidental ingestion is not uncommon, with more than 3600 isopropanol and 350 methanol ingestions reported to poison control centers in 1990.[47]

Methanol, isopropanol, and ethylene glycol are readily absorbed following ingestion, although food in the stomach may delay absorption. They are metabolized by hepatic alcohol dehydrogenase at rates one-tenth or less than that of ethanol and follow zero-order kinetics even at relatively low concentrations.

Methanol is oxidized to highly toxic formaldehyde and its metabolite, formic acid. Formic acid is much more toxic than methanol and accounts for the profound anion gap in metabolic acidosis and ocular toxicity.[72] Single ingestion of as little as 10 mL of methanol has caused permanent blindness in adults, and the fatal dose for children is 1–2 mL/kg. Since methanol is a CNS toxin, symptoms may develop within 20–30 min and may include inebriation, headache, dizziness, seizure, and coma. Nausea, vomiting, stiff neck, abdominal pain, and malaise are also common complaints. There may be a latent period of up to 8–12 h when there is a deceiving lack of severe toxic manifestation until products of metabolism begin to appear, but during which appropriate treatment is critical. Young children are susceptible to hypoglycemia.

Isopropanol is metabolized to acetone, which accounts for the CNS effects and ketonemia. There is no metabolic acidosis. Hemorrhagic tracheobronchitis and gastritis are characteristic findings. An acute, lethal ingested dose of isopropanol has been estimated to be 2–3 mL/kg for a child.[73]

Ethylene glycol is metabolized to glycolaldehyde, glycolic acid, glyoxylic acid, formic acid, and oxalic acid. Clinically, the patient appears drunk 30 min to 12 h post-dose and may have nausea, vomiting, metabolic acidosis, renal failure, muscle paralysis, convulsions, and coma. The presence of oxalic acid crystals in urine is not a very sensitive indicator of ethylene glycol poisoning.

Since the toxicity of methanol, isopropanol, and ethylene glycol is due to their toxic metabolites generated by alcohol dehydrogenase, their treatments are similar.[72, 73] They involve the inhibition of alcohol dehydrogenase activity on methanol, isopropanol, and ethylene glycol with a saturating concentration (100–150 mg/dL) (22–33 mmol/L) of the preferred substance, ethanol. At the same time, hemodialysis is performed to remove these alcohols or ethylene glycol and their toxic metabolites until they reach undetectable levels. Hemodialysis is continued until methanol, isopropanol, or ethylene glycol concentrations are below the level of detection.

Gas chromatography is the method of choice for identification and measurement of methanol, isopropanol, and ethylene glycol. The methods for ethanol are generally applicable to methanol and isopropanol if acetone is adequately resolved from the alcohols.[74]

The popular enzymatic assay for ethanol is not applicable for methanol and isopropanol because of the weak enzyme activity when these alcohols are substrates. However, toxic serum concentrations of these osmotically active substances will result in a significant osmolal gap between measured and calculated serum osmolarity, thus allowing the evaluation of an acute situation when specific assays for methanol, isopropanol, and ethylene glycol are not available.

Lead

The toxic effects of long-term exposure to lead have been known for a long time. Lead poisoning is recognized as a public health problem because its environmental sources are widespread.[75] The greatest risk is posed for young children, as their developing brain and nervous system are particularly susceptible to the deleterious effects of lead.[76] There are many sources and pathways to exposure, but lead-based paint is the most common high-dose source for preschool children, who become poisoned by ingesting paint chips or paint-contaminated dust or soil. A thumbnail-size paint chip may contain 50–200 ug of lead, and ingestion of a few chips a day is a significant toxic dose. Although exterior and interior lead-based paint for residential use has been banned, it has been estimated that 74% of privately owned occupied housing units in the United States built before 1980 contain lead-based paint.[77] Of particular concern is the decrepit housing in economically depressed inner-city areas, where many young children live. Childhood lead poisoning has also resulted from exposure to lead-contaminated dust during renovation or remodeling of older homes.[78] Lead poisoning is not a problem limited to lower socioeconomic families, however; lead in water has been associated with lead poisoning in infants fed home-reconstituted formulas.

Once absorbed, lead is distributed to blood, soft tissues, and bone. It is the lead in blood and soft tissues that causes symptoms of lead poisoning. Chronic exposure results in hypermineralization of bone, which is evident radiographically. Severity of lead intoxication is not directly proportional to total body burden, but to lead concentrations in blood and soft tissues. Doubling of the body burden of lead only increases blood lead concentration by a few ug/dL. Lead is excreted very slowly.

Lead is known to interfere with the various steps of the biosynthetic pathway of heme biosynthesis.[76] Lead produces feedback derepression (stimulation) of delta-aminolevulinic acid (ALA) synthetase and inhibition of ALA dehydratase and coproporphyrin decarboxylase (Figure 19–7). The resulting accumulation of ALA and coproporphyrin

FIGURE 19-7. Effects of Lead on Heme Biosynthesis (X indicates inhibitory action of lead)

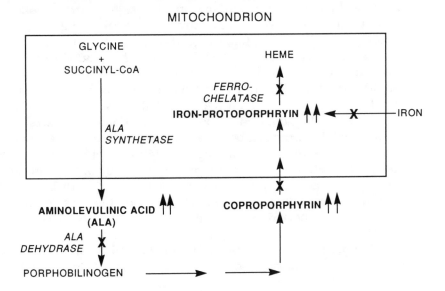

(CP) in urine is evidence of lead poisoning. Lead can also block the insertion of iron into protoporphyrin IX to form heme, causing the accumulation of protoporphyrin and the increase of protoporphyrin in erythrocytes (EP), which also serves as a not-too-sensitive marker for lead poisoning. Since the final step of heme biosynthesis occurs in the mitochondria, the increase in EP not only indicates impaired heme bio-synthesis, but also suggests general mitochondrial injury which may impair a variety of processes, including cellular energetics and calcium homeostasis.[76] The most evident hematological defect is anemia from reduced heme synthesis. Since nutritional iron deficiency is common among children from the lower socioeconomic levels who are also at risk for lead poisoning, childhood anemia is frequently caused by both nutritional iron deficiency and lead poisoning. Anemia caused by lead poisoning alone is quite rare.[79] A finger-stick erythrocyte protoporphyrin and hematocrit are two screening tests for lead poisoning, although the former is no longer recommended due to its lack of sensitivity.[77]

The neurotoxic effect of lead in children is due to the sensitivity of the developing CNS to lead exposure.[76] Chronic exposure to subclinical doses can have a harmful effect on behavioral and intellectual skills in children whose blood lead concentrations are less than "toxic" and do not cause distinctive symptoms.[76, 77, 80] Therefore, the recognized concentration for lead toxicity has progressively shifted downward. The 1985 intervention concentration of 25 ug/dL (1210 nmol/L) recommended by the Centers for Disease Control (CDC) has been revised to 10 ug/dL (480 nmol/L). This has been prompted by a number of recent studies on low-level lead exposure and child development.[77] The CDC has issued a set of recommended guidelines for dealing with children, with blood lead concentrations of 10-25 µg/dL involving scheduled retesting, environmental investigations, and medical follow-up.[77]

Children with blood concentrations of 25-50 ug/dL (1210–2420 nmol/L) may be asymptomatic, although their urinary ALA may be increased. Concentrations of 50-80 ug/dL (2420-3860 nmol/L) may be associated with mild, nonspecific complaints when urinary ALA, CP, and EP are all increased. Symptomatic lead poisoning is characterized by lethargy, anorexia, vomiting, colic and constipation, and is usually associated with increased blood concentrations of at least 70 ug/dL (3380 nmol/L), although occasionally cases have been associated with concentrations as low as 50 ug/dL (2420 nmol/L). Lead encephalopathy, characterized by the above-mentioned symptoms in addition to seizures and coma, is almost always associated with blood lead concentrations exceeding 100 ug/dL (4830 nmol/L). Occasionally, though, it has been reported at concentrations as low as 70 ug/dL (3380 nmol/L).

A child presenting with symptoms of lead poisoning accompanied by an increased blood lead concentration constitutes a medical emergency. The possibility of lead encephalopathy should be considered in the differential diagnosis of children presenting with coma and convulsions of unknown etiology. Damage to the CNS caused by lead is irreversible, and children surviving acute poisoning episodes with or without encephalopathy suffer neurological sequelae.

The blood lead concentration is the most reliable indicator of exposure. The two most frequently used techniques for determination of blood lead concentrations are anodic stripping voltametry and atomic absorption spectrometry.[81] These methods are capable of achieving detection limits of < 2 to 5 ug/dL (97–240 nmol/L), which are below the 10 ug/dL (480 nmol/L) cutoff recommended by CDC. Accuracy and precision in determination of low concentrations of lead, however, will require meticulous attention to the details of analysis. The ubiquity of lead in the environment requires that specimens be collected with care to avoid contamination. Since collection of capillary blood by finger stick is more prone to contamination than venipuncture, a positive result should be confirmed by testing venous blood, which is the preferred specimen.[77] Special lead-free evacuated tubes are available for blood collection, but standard tubes containing EDTA (lavender caps) or heparin (green caps) can be acceptable if each lot of tubes is screened for lead before being put into use.

Blood lead determination is difficult and expensive to perform. Therefore, it is not a screening test. Erythrocyte protoporphyrin (EP) has been used historically as an inexpensive alternate to screening for blood lead. EP is a direct measurement of the toxic effect on heme synthesis. At blood lead concentrations higher than 40 ug/dL (1930 nmol/L), the EP concentration rises exponentially. An increase in a few ug/dL of lead is associated with a much larger increase of EP. Therefore, an increased EP concentration is a sensitive index for identifying children with excessive lead exposure and high blood lead concentrations, and is the basis for further evaluation for lead poisoning.[82] EP concentrations, however, correlate poorly with low blood lead concentrations. Using the current recommended EP cutoff of 35 ug/dL (0.6 µmol/L), EP was shown to be a poor predictor of blood lead concentration ≥ 25 ug/dL (1210 nmol/L); the true positive and false positive rates of EP were 0.23 and 0.04.[83] In another study, the sensitivity of EP (≥ 35 ug/dL) (0.6 µmol/L) dropped from 73% to 37% when the blood lead cutoff was reduced from 25 to 15 ug/dL (1210 to 720 nmol/L). Therefore, screening of children for blood lead concentrations using the most recent recommended cutoff of 10 ug/dL (480 nmol/L) will require direct measurement of blood lead concentration, not EP.[84, 85]

EP concentration can be measured fluorometrically using a hematofluorometer. Most protoporphyrin in erythrocytes (> 90%) is zinc protoporphyrin (ZnP), the fraction measured by hematofluorometers. Methods involving an extraction will strip Zn-protoporphyrin of its zinc and will measure zinc-free erythrocyte protoporphyrin (FEP). On a weight basis, EP, ZnP, and FEP are roughly equivalent. All increased EP results should be followed by a venous blood lead test.

Treatment of lead poisoning is by chelation therapy using BAL (dimercaprol) calcium disodium ethylenediamine tetraacetate ($CaNa_2$-EDTA), and D-penicillamine (not FDA approved, but used in some centers). Succimer (meso-2,3-dimercaptosuccinic acid) was approved by the FDA in 1991.

Symptomatic patients, or those with blood lead > 45 ug/dL (2170 nmol/L) should be treated with chelation therapy immediately. Asymptomatic patients with initial concentrations between 25 and 45 ug/dL (1210–2170 nmol/L) are given the $CaNa_2EDTA$ challenge test to assess the burden of lead. The ratios of lead excreted in urine per dose of $CaNa_2EDTA$ dose (ug Pb/mg $CaNa_2EDTA$) are calculated. An 8 h challenge test is considered positive if the ratio is > 0.6. Children with blood concentrations of 25–44 ug/dL (1210–2130 nmol/L) and a positive challenge test should undergo a 5-day course of chelation. Chelation treatment may be repeated if blood lead remains or rebounds 50 ug/dL (2420 nmol/L) or higher.

Iron

Many iron pills are brightly colored and are attractive to young children. Children under age 6 y accounted for over 80% of the accidental iron ingestions reported.[47]

Many iron salts are available. Ferrous sulfate, the cheapest, is the most frequently involved (Table 19–4). An estimation of the amount of elemental iron in the formulation is important in assessing potential toxicity of an acute ingestion. A dose of less than 20 mg of elemental iron/kg has little risk of toxicity. An ingestion of 20–60 mg/kg can cause mild gastrointestinal distress and poses moderate risk, whereas a dose greater than 80 mg/kg has high risk for toxicity.[86]

TABLE 19–4. Iron Salts and Elemental Iron Equivalents

Iron Salt	% Iron	mg Iron/Tablet*
Sulfate	20	65
Gluconate	12	38
Fumarate	33	106
Lactate	19	—
Chloride	28	—
Ferrocholinate	13	—

*325 mg tablet

Abdominal x-ray may reveal undissolved adult-strength tablets or fragments as long as 6 h or more after ingestion of the tablets. Pediatric preparations, which are chewable iron supplements, dissolve rapidly in 30–60 min and are not always seen.[87] A screening test on gastric fluid is useful in confirming iron ingestion.[88] Addition of deferoxamine causes an immediate color change if iron ingestion has occurred. A negative test obtained within 2 h of ingestion indicates the patient needs no further evaluation. A negative test obtained more than 2 h after ingestion does not rule out iron ingestion because absorption of ingested iron may have been completed.

A qualitative test to predict potential for toxicity is the deferoxamine challenge. A sufficiently large deferoxamine dose is given to bind toxic free iron in plasma to form the reddish feroxamine complex, the appearance of which in urine within 4–6 h post-ingestion implies potential toxicity. This test is useful when measurement of serum iron concentration is not readily available. False-negative results of this test have been reported, and a negative challenge test should not rule out toxicity.[89]

Serum iron concentrations > 350 ug/dL (63 μmol/L) are associated with toxicity, although a lower concentration does not rule out toxicity. Serum iron concentrations within the 350–500 μg/dL (63–90 μmol/L) range may require chelation therapy if these concentrations exceed total iron binding capacity (TIBC) and if the patient is exhibiting signs of systemic toxicity. Serum toxicity and death have been reported in cases with serum concentrations > 500 ug/dL (90 μmol/L). Theoretically, a serum iron value greater than the TIBC implies toxic free-circulating iron is present. TIBC has been reported to rise and remain above serum iron concentrations following the ingestion of a clinically toxic dose, with symptoms of toxicity occurring.[90] Sampling of blood should be 4–6 h post-ingestion of adult formulation and 2 h following ingestion of pediatric preparations. A repeat determination is valuable due to variability in formulation, dissolution, and absorption.

Management of acute iron poisoning includes removal of residual iron in the gastrointestinal tract by emesis or lavage and standard life-support therapy.[86] Deferoxamine chelation therapy is used to chelate free serum iron for excretion and to render the chelated iron unavailable for binding to effect toxicity.

Results from colorimetric methods for serum iron concentrations using bathophenanthroline, ferrozine, tripyridyltriazine (TPTZ), or other proprietary dyes are interfered with by deferoxamine, which functions as a competing chelator to falsely lower results.[91] Therefore, blood should be drawn prior to deferoxamine chelation therapy. Atomic absorption spectroscopy for measurement of serum iron concentrations is impractical, but it is a method that can be used in the presence of deferoxamine.

Drugs of Abuse

At Children's Hospital between 1986 and 1991, the positivity of tetrahydrocannabinol (THC), phencyclidine (PCP), and cocaine/benzoylecgonine was found to be $9.3 \rightarrow 2.2\%$, $9.9 \rightarrow 1.8\%$, and $0.8 \rightarrow 7.7\%$, respectively. All three drugs are first screened in urine employing immunoassay techniques, with all positive screens being confirmed for the presence of the drug in question by gas chromatography / mass spectrometry. Note that while the incidence of urine testing positive for THC and PCP is on the decline in the Washington area, we have witnessed an approximately ten-fold increase in urines testing positive for cocaine/cocaine metabolite between 1986 and 1991.

Cocaine (benzoylmethylecgonine) is an alkaloid extracted from the leaves of the *Erythroxylon coca* plant and is a powerful CNS stimulant. In recent years, the abuse of cocaine has reached epidemic proportions, especially since "crack" became available. "Crack" (so named because of the crackling sound made by the crystals when heated) is a freebase form of cocaine prepared by precipitation from heated cocaine HCl solution made alkaline with baking soda or ammonia. Crack is relatively pure cocaine (80–90%) and is vaporized rather than pyrolysed when heated. Therefore, it can be smoked, unlike cocaine hydrochloride, which is snorted or used intravenously.

Because many cocaine users are women of child-bearing age, many babies are exposed to cocaine *in utero* and could be born with medical, developmental, and behavioral problems.[92] These include low birth weight, microcephaly, pre-term delivery, cerebral infarction, and withdrawal syndrome, which consists of abnormal sleep patterns, visual function disturbances, tremors, poor feeding, hypertonia, and higher pitch crying. Cocaine babies incur significantly higher hospital costs.[93] A study conducted at Children's Hospital found that approximately 13% of the neonates in the Neonatal Intensive Care Unit tested positive for cocaine metabolite in the urine and that clinical suspicion would have detected only about half of those infants.[94]

Clinically, early identification of cocaine-affected infants is not easy. Neither the signs and symptoms of cocaine withdrawal nor the medical problems commonly associated with intrauterine exposure to cocaine are specific. Therefore, testing newborn urines for the cocaine metabolite benzoylecgonine (BE) is an objective means to identify these babies. Urine testing has limitations and is an insensitive test for a number of reasons,[95] including late collection of urine due to delayed appearance of withdrawal symptoms, difficulty in obtaining urine specimens, and low drug concentrations in urine.

Hair or meconium have been proposed as alternative specimens.[96, 97] The limitations of hair analysis of the newborn are as follows:

1. It does not detect exposure that occurs shortly before birth.

2. Low drug concentration in hair means a lot of hair (25 mg and up) is needed. Many newborns do not have enough hair for analysis.

3. Analytical problems such as washing, digestion, sensitivity, and lack of appropriate standards and controls.

Meconium seems promising because it is easy to collect, drug concentration is relatively high and the window of detectability is longer (which is helpful if testing is not done immediately after birth). In a preliminary report of the 15 infants whose meconiums were tested positive for BE by RIA, only five urines were positive by FPIA (at 300 ng/mL cutoff).[97] The disadvantage of meconium is that it is an unfamiliar matrix.

Immunoassays (RIA, EMIT, FPIA) are used routinely to screen urines for drugs of abuse such as benzoylecgonine (BE), cannabinoid metabolites (THC), and phencyclidine (PCP). Typically, the thresholds used in forensic urine drug testing (BE, 300 ng/mL; THC, 100 ng/mL; PCP, 25 ng/mL) for designating a urine as positive are adopted for clinical testing. Lower thresholds are more appropriate for clinical testing, as the number of positive urines is much higher when the thresholds are lowered.[98] An immunoassay positive result is a presumptive result and should be confirmed using one of the chromatographic techniques, preferably by gas chromatography / mass spectrometry.

Other Toxic Agents

Also encountered in pediatric hospitals, although with less frequency, are patients with herbicide, tricyclic antidepressant, amphetamine, barbiturate, ethchlorvynol, and phenothiazine toxicity.

REFERENCES

1. Vesell ES. On the significance of host factors that affect drug disposition. Clin Pharmacol Ther 1982;31:1-7.

2. Kennedy DL, Forbes MB. Pediatric drug prescribing: A preliminary report presented at the American Society of Hospital Pharmacists mid-year clinical meeting, San Francisco, December 1980.

3. Yunis AA. Chloramphenicol toxicity. In: RH Girdwood, ed. Blood disorders due to drugs and other agents. Amsterdam: Exerpta Medica, 1973:107-26.

4. Gorodischer R, Jusko WJ, Yaffe SJ. Tissue and erythrocyte distribution of digoxin in infants. Clin Pharmacol Ther 1976;19:256-63.

5. Smith CA. The physiology of the newborn infant (2nd ed). Springfield: Charles C Thomas 1951:180-198.

6.   Morselli PI. Clinical pharmacokinetics in neonates. Clin Pharmacokinet 1976;1:81-98.
7.   Weber WW, Cohen SN. Aging effects and drugs in man. In: Gillette JR, Mitchell JR, eds. Concepts in biochemical pharmacology, Vol 28. Berlin: Springer 1975:213-33.
8.   Vessell ES, Page JG. Genetic control of the phenobarbital-induced shortening of plasma half-lives in man. J Clin Invest 1969;48:2202-9.
9.   Vessell ES. The role of pharmacogenetics in therapeutic drug monitoring. In: Basic Principles of Therapeutic Drug Monitoring. Presented at the Second Annual Pine Mountain Conference of the American Association for Clinical Chemistry, March 28-April 1, 1976:27-29.
10. Jusko WJ. Influence of cigarette smoking on drug metabolism in man. Drug Metab Rev 1979;9:221-36.
11. Jenne J, Nagasawa H, McHugh R et al. Decreased theophylline half-life in cigarette smokers. Life Sci 1975;17:195-8.
12. Alvares AP, Pantuck EJ, Anderson KE, et al. Regulation of drug metabolism in man by environmental factors. Drug Metab Rev 1979;9:185-205.
13. Kappas A, Anderson KE, Conney AH, et al. Influence of dietary protein and carbohydrate on antipyrine and theophylline metabolism in man. Clin Pharmacol Ther 1976;20:643-53.
14. Aranda JV, Sitar DS, Parson WD, et al. Pharmacokinetic aspects of theophylline in premature newborns. NEJM 1976;295:413-6.
15. Jenne JW, Wyze E, Rood FS, et al. Pharmacokinetics of theophylline: Application to adjustment of the clinical dose of aminophylline. Clin Pharmacol Ther 1972;13:349-60.
16. Piafsky KM, Buda A, MacDonald I, et al. Clinical significance of drug binding to orosomucoid. Reta Pharm Suec 1980;17:99.
17. Piafsky KM, Mpamugo L. Dependence of neonatal drug binding on α-acid glycoprotein concentration. Clin Pharm Ther 1981;29:272.
18. Danhof M, Breimer DD. Therapeutic monitoring in saliva. Clin Pharmacokinet 1978;3:39-57.
19. Kwong TC. Free drug measurements: Methodology and clinical significance. Clin Chem Acta 1985;151:193-216.
20. Bergman A, Werner R. Failure of children to receive penicillin by mouth. NEJM 1963;268:1334-8.
21. Soldin SJ. Drug receptor assays: Quo vadis? Ann Clin Biochem, in press.
22. Cramer JA, Mattson RH. Valproic acid: In vitro plasma protein binding and interaction with phenytoin. Ther Drug Monit 1979;1:105-16.
23. Friel PN, Leal KW, Wilensky AJ. Valproic acid—phenytoin interaction. Ther Drug Monit 1979;1:243-8.
24. Johannessen SI. Antiepileptic drugs: Pharmacokinetic and clinical aspects. Ther Drug Monit 1981;3:17-37.
25. Graves SW, Brown B, Valdes R. An endogenous digoxin-like substance in patients with renal impairment. Ann Int Med 1983;99:604-8.
26. Koren G, Farine D, Maresky D, et al. Significance of the endogenous digoxin-like substance in infants and mothers. Clin Pharmacol Ther 1984;36:759-64.
27. Nanji AA, Greenway RC. Falsely raised plasma digoxin concentrations in liver disease. Br Med J 1985;290:432-3.
28. Soldin SJ. Digoxin: Issues and controversies. Clin Chem 1986;32:5-12.
29. Belz GG, Aust PE, Munkes R. Digoxin plasma concentrations and nifedipine. Lancet 1981;i:844-5.
30. Ford AR, Aronson JK, Grahame-Smith DG, et al. Changes in cardiac receptor sites, 86-Rubidium uptake and intracellular sodium concentrations in the erythrocytes of patients receiving digoxin during the early phases of treatment of cardiac failure in regular rhythm and of atrial fibrillation. Br J Clin Pharmacol 1979;8:125-34.
31. Jogestrand T, Ericsson R, Sundquist K. Skeletal muscle digoxin concentration during digitalization and during withdrawal of digoxin treatment. Eur J Clin Pharmacol 1981;19:97-105.
32. Kim YI, Noble RJ, Zipes DP. Dissociation of inotropic effects of digitalis from its effects on atrioventricular conduction. Am J Cardiol 1975;36:459-67.
33. Shapin W, Narahara K, Taubert K. Relationship of plasma digitoxin and digoxin to cardiac response following intravenous digitalization in man. Circulation 1970;42:1065-72.

34. Koren G, Parker R. Interpretation of excessive serum concentrations of digoxin in children. Am J Cardiol 1985;55:1210-4.

35. Koren G. Interaction between digoxin and commonly coadministered drugs in children. Pediatrics 1985;75:1032-7.

36. Butler VP Jr, Chen JP. Digoxin-specific antibodies. Proc Natl Acad Sci USA 1967;57:71-8.

37. Smith TW, Butler VP Jr, Haber E, et al. Treatment of life-threatening digitalis intoxication with digoxin-specific Fab antibody fragments. NEJM 1982;307:1357-62.

38. Kumin GD. Clinical nephrotoxicity of tobramycin and gentamicin: A prospective study. JAMA 1980;224:1808-10.

39. Pittinger CB, Eryasa Y, Adamson R. Antibiotic-induced paralysis. Anesth Analg 1970;49:487-501.

40. Endicott JA, Ling V. The biochemistry of p-glycoprotein-mediated multidrug resistance. Ann Rev Biochem 1989;58:137-71.

41. Rivard GE, Hoyoux C, Infante-Rivard C, Champagne J. Maintenance chemotherapy for childhood acute lymphoblastic leukemia: Better in the evening. Lancet 1985;ii:1264-6.

42. Langevin AM, Koren G, Soldin SJ, Greenberg M. Pharmacokinetic case for giving 6-mercaptopurine maintenance doses at night. Lancet 1987;ii:505-6.

43. Koren G, Ferrazini G, Sulh H, et al. Systemic exposure to mercaptopurine and a prognostic factor in acute lymphocytic leukemia in children. NEJM 1990;323:17-21.

44. Marks V, English J, Aherne W, Arendt J. Chronopharmacology. Clin Biochem 1985;18:154-7.

45. Stoller RG, Hande KR, Jacobs SA, et al. Use of plasma pharmacokinetics to predict and prevent methotrexate toxicity. NEJM 1977;297:630-4.

46. Russell R, Donnelly J, Palaszynski E, Chan M, Soldin SJ. A preliminary study to evaluate an in vitro assay for determining patient whole blood immunosuppressive cyclosporine A and metabolite activity: Comparison with cytosolic binding assays using cyclophilin, a 50KDa binding protein, and the Abbott TDx™ cyclosporine A parent and parent and metabolites assays. Ther Drug Monit 1991;13:32-6.

47. Litovitz TL, Bailey KM, Schmitz BF, Holm KA, Klein-Schwartz W. 1990 Annual Report of the American Association of Poison Control Centers National Data Collection System. Am J Emerg Med 1991;10:461-509.

48. Linden CH, Rumack BH. Acetaminophen overdose. Emerg Med Clin North Am 1984;2:103-19.

49. Cocoran GB, Mitchell JR, Vaishnav YN, Horning EC. Evidence that acetaminophen and N-hydroxyacetaminophen form a common arylating intermediate, N-acetyl-p-benzoquinoneimine. Mol Pharmacol 1980;18:536-42.

50. Rumack BH. Acetaminophen overdose in young children. Treatment and effects of alcohol and other additional ingestant in 417 cases. Am J Dis Child 1984;138:428-33.

51. Smilkstein MJ, Knapp GL, Kulig KW, Rumack BH. Efficacy of oral N-acetylcysteine in the treatment of acetaminophen overdose. N Engl J Med 1988;319:1557-62.

52. Prescott LF, Illingwork RN, Critchley JA, et al. Intravenous N-acetylcysteine: The treatment of choice for paracetamol poisoning. Br Med J 1979;2:1097-100.

53. Smilkstein MJ, Bronstein AC, Linden C, Angenstein WL, Kulig KW, Rumack BH. Acetaminophen overdose: A 48-hour intravenous N-acetylcysteine treatment protocol. Ann Emerg Med 1991;20:1058-63.

54. Rumack BH, Matthew H. Acetaminophen poisoning and toxicity. Ped 1975;55:871-6.

55. Glynn JR, Kendal SE. Paracetamol measurement. Lancet 1975;i:1147-8.

56. Stewart MJ, Chambers AM, Watson ID. Letter to the Editor. Clin Chem 1984;30:1885.

57. Kwong TC. Salicylate measurement: Clinical usefulness and methodology. CRC Critical Reviews in Clin Lab Med 1987;25:137-59.

58. Paulus HE, Siegel M, Morgan E et al. Variations of serum concentrations and half-life of salicylate in patients with rheumatoid arthritis. Arthritis Rheum 1971;14:527-32.

59. Proudfoot AT. Toxicity of salicylates. Am J Med 1983;75(suppl 5A):99-103.

60. Gaudreault PI, Temple AR, Lovejoy FH. The relative severity of acute versus chronic salicylate poisoning in children: A clinical comparison. Ped 1982;70:566-9.

61. Temple AR. Acute and chronic effects of aspirin toxicity and their treatment. Arch Int Med 1981;14:354-9.

62. Done AK. Salicylate intoxication: Significance of measurements of salicylate in blood in cases of acute ingestion. Ped 1960;26:800-7.

63. Trinder P. Rapid determination of salicylate in biological material. Biochem J 1954;57:301-3.

64. Weller-Fahy ER, Berger LR. Mouthwash: A source of acute ethanol intoxication. Ped 1980;66:302-5.

65. Scherger DL, Wsuk KM, Kulig KW, Rumack BH. Ethyl alcohol (ethanol)-containing cologne, perfume, and aftershave ingestions in children. Am J Dis Child 1988;142:630-2.

66. Basalt RC, Cravey RH. Disposition of toxic drugs and chemicals in man.(3rd ed.). Chicago: Year Book Medical Publishers 1989;322-6.

67. Forrest ARW. Non-linear kinetics of ethyl alcohol metabolism. J Forensic Sci Soc 1986;26:121-3.

68. Leung AKC. Ethyl alcohol ingestion in children. Clin Ped 1986;25:617-9.

69. Lovejoy FH. Ethanol intoxication. Clin Tox Rev 1981;4:1-2.

70. Ricci LR, Hoffman SA. Ethanol-induced hypoglycemic coma in a child. Ann Emerg Med 1982;11:202-4.

71. Geller RJ, Spyker DA, Herold DA, Bruns DE. Serum osmolal gap and ethanol concentration: A simple and accurate formula. Clin Toxicol 1986;24:77-84.

72. McCoy HG, Cipolle RJ, Ehlers SM, et al. Severe methanol poisoning. Am J Med 1979;67:804-7.

73. Lacouture PG, Wason S, Abrams A, Lovejoy, Jr FH. Acute isopropyl alcohol intoxication: Diagnosis and management. Am J Med 1988;75:680-6.

74. Gadsden RH, Terry CS, Thompson BC. Alcohols in biological fluids by gas chromatography (automated head-space method). In: Frings CS, Faulkner WR, eds. Selected Methods of Emergency Toxicology. Washington: AACC Press 1986:40-43.

75. Mushak P, Crocetti AF. Determination of number of lead-exposed American children as a function of lead source: Integrated summary of a report to the U.S. Congress on childhood lead poisoning. Environ Res 1989;50:210-29.

76. Muschak P, Davis JM, Crocetti AF, Grant LD. Prenatal and postnatal effects of low-level lead exposure: Integrated summary of a report to the U.S. Congress in childhood lead poisoning. Environ Res 1989;50:11-36.

77. Centers for Disease Control. Preventing lead poisoning in young children: A statement by the Centers for Disease Control. Atlanta, Georgia, U.S. Health and Human Services 1991.

78. Friedman JA, Weinberger HL. Six children with lead poisoning. Am J Dis Child 1990;144:1039-44.

79. Mahaffey KR, Annest JL, Roberts J, Murphy RS. National estimates of blood lead levels, United States, 1976-1980: Association with selected demographic and socioeconomic factors. N Engl J Med 1982;207:573-9.

80. Agency for Toxic Substances and Disease Registry. The nature and extent of lead poisoning in children in the United States: A report to Congress. Atlanta, Georgia, U.S. Health and Human Services 1988.

81. Tabor MW. Lead. In: Pesce A, Kaplan LA, eds. Methods in clinical chemistry. St. Louis: CV Mosby 1987;394-404.

82. Piomelli S, Davidow B, Guinee V, Young P, Giselle G. The FEP (free erythrocyte porphyrin) test: A screening micromethod for lead poisoning. Ped 1973;51:254-9.

83. DeBaum MR, Sox HC Jr. Setting the optional erythrocyte protoporphyrin screening decision threshold for lead poisoning: A decision analytical approach. Ped 1991;88:121-31.

84. McElvaine MD, Orbach HG, Binder S, Blanksma LA, Macs EF, Kreig RM. Elevation of the erythrocyte protoporphyrin test as a screen for elevated blood lead levels. Ped 1991;119:548-50.

85. Turk DS, Schonfeld DJ, Cullen J, Rainey P. Sensitivity of erythrocyte protoporphyrin as a screening for lead poisoning. N Engl J Med 1992;326:137-8.

86. Schauben JL, Augenstein WL, Cox J, Sato R. Iron poisoning: Report of three cases and a review of therapeutic intervention. J Emerg Med 1990;8:309-19.

87. Everson GW, Oudjhane K, Young LW, Krenzelock EP. Effectiveness of abdominal radiographs in visualizing chewable iron supplements following overdose. Am J Emerg Med 1989;7:459-63.
88. McGuigan MA, Lovejoy FH, Marino SK, Propper RP, Goldman R. Qualitative deferoxamine color test for iron ingestion. J Ped 1979;94:940-2.
89. Proudfoot AT, Simpson D, Dyson EH. Management of acute iron poisoning. Med Toxicol 1986;1:83-100.
90. Burkhart KE, Kulig KW, Hammond KB, Piearson JR, Ambruso, Rumack BH. The rise in the total iron binding capacity after iron overdose. Am Emerg Med 1991;20:532-5.
91. Helfer RE, Rodgerson DO. The effects of deferoxamine on determination of serum and iron binding capacity. J Ped 1966;68:804-6.
92. Giacola GP. Cocaine in the cradle: A hidden epidemic. South Med J 1990;83:947-51.
93. Phibbs CS, Bateman DA, Schwartz RM. The neonatal costs of maternal cocaine use. JAMA 1991;266;1521-6.
94. Rifai N, Morales A, MacDonald MG, Soldin SJ. Prevalence of cocaine in a neonatal intensive care unit: The impact of staff education. Pediatric AIDS and HIV infection: Fetus to Adolescent, 1991;2:137-8.
95. Osterlolh JD, Lee BL. Urine drug screening in mothers and newborns. Am J Dis Child 1989;143:791-3.
96. Graham K, Koren G, Klein J, Schneiderman J, Greenwald M. Determination of gestational cocaine exposure by hair analysis. JAMA 1989;262:3328-30.
97. Ostrea EM, Brady MJ, Panks PM, Asenio DC, Naluz A. Drug screening of meconium in infants of drug-dependent mothers: An alternative to urine testing. J Ped 1989;115:474-7.
98. Hicks JM, Morales A, Soldin SJ. Drugs of abuse in a pediatric outpatient population. Clin Chem 1990;36:1256-7.

Pediatric Clinical Biochemistry: Why Is It Different?

Jocelyn M.B. Hicks, Ph.D., F.A.C.B.

INTRODUCTION

The big difference between a pediatric hospital laboratory and a general hospital is in the type of service provided. In the general hospital, the patient population is relatively similar, with a typical mix of surgical, medical, and critical care cases. The pediatric hospital has, in addition to the same types of cases that are found in an adult facility, a patient population that includes premature infants, newborns, and children at all stages of development, including adolescents and young adults. In fact, pediatrics is characterized by infant growth and development, upon which disease entities are superimposed. Issues that are of particular concern in a pediatric laboratory include the correct collection of specimens and the choice of appropriate instrumentation and methods whereby only a small volume of sample is used. The methods should not be subject to common interferences such as bilirubin, hemoglobin, and lipids. It is also important to have a knowledge of reference ranges by age. The diagnosis of metabolic diseases and an understanding of the pharmacokinetics of therapeutic drugs is a must for the pediatric laboratory. Other important aspects of pediatric laboratory practice include rapid turnaround time for results and a good quality assurance program.

BLOOD COLLECTION

Blood drawing is a major problem in pediatric medicine, especially from premature infants and neonates. In the Middle Ages, blood letting using blood cups or leeches was considered as a cure for patients. Today, the collection of blood or other body fluids is used as a key to the diagnosis and therapy of disease.

Skin Puncture

Although venipunctures are practical and even preferred for older children, finger or heel sticks are better and less traumatic for young children and neonates. Other possible, although less desirable, sites are the great toe or the ear lobe. The lateral or medial portion of the plantar surface of the heel is the preferred site in neonates, but the finger is preferable for infants and young children.

Blumenfeld et al. described the preferred way of collecting skin puncture specimens.[1] A possible complication of heel punctures is the development of calcaneal osteomyelitis. In his article, Blumenfeld showed that this can be avoided if the calcaneus is not penetrated during blood collection. The risk of puncturing the calcaneus is greater in premature infants before the distance between the dermal subcutaneous junction and the periosteum increases as the infant gains weight. If the puncture is less deep than 2.4 mm, there is no risk of puncturing the perichondrium, even in tiny premature infants. Since the distance from skin surface to the perichondrium is least at the posterior curvative of the heel, it is strongly advised not to use this position to draw blood. Figure 20–1 illustrates the best area from which to obtain blood from an infant's heel.

FIGURE 20–1. Sites of Collection from an Infant's Heel

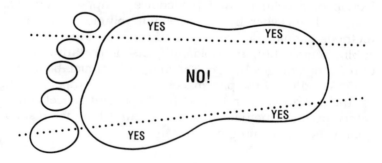

From: Blumenfeld, TA, Turi, GK, and Blanc, WA: Lancet 1979; 1:231. Reprinted with permission.

Procedure

In 1986, the National Committee for Clinical Laboratory Standards (NCCLS) published *Procedures for the Collection of Diagnostic Blood Specimens by Skin Puncture*.[2] Since skin-puncture blood is a mixture of blood from arterioles, venules, and capillaries and contains interstitial and intracellular fluids, it is important that the skin site be warmed prior to puncture, especially for specimens for blood gas analysis. The most practical approach is to use a washcloth or towel that has been soaked in hot running water (38–42° C). It has been demonstrated that warming the skin puncture site can increase blood flow sevenfold, and that it primarily increases the arterial blood flow.[3]

To prevent nosocomial infections, the person drawing the blood should remove all jewelry and wash his or her hands and forearms thoroughly up to the elbows. After the infant's skin has been warmed, the site should be cleaned with a 75% aqueous solution of isopropanol (75% w/v). The site should then be thoroughly dried with a sterile gauze pad so that residual alcohol does not cause hemolysis. Betadine should not be used, as it can increase concentrations of potassium, phosphorus, or uric acid.[4]

A short-tipped, sterile lancet or an automated device that does not cause a puncture of more than 2.4 mm should be used. After the site has been chosen and punctured, the first drop of blood should be wiped away, since it is most likely to contain excess tissue fluid.

After blood has been collected from an infant's heel or finger, the limb should be raised above the level of the heart and a sterile gauze pad pressed against the puncture site until the bleeding stops. It is not advisable to use adhesive bandages for small infants, as their skin is sensitive. Also, there is a danger with infants that the bandage will be pulled off, placed in the mouth, and aspirated.

The Pediatric Committee of the American Association for Clinical Chemistry made recommendations regarding the actual technique for obtaining the blood.[5] The infant's heel should be grasped with a moderately firm grip, placing one's forefinger at the arch of the foot and one's thumb well below the puncture site, at the ankle. The puncture should be made in a continuous, deliberate motion, in a direction perpendicular to the puncture site. The pressure with the thumb should be eased and reapplied as drops of blood form and flow into the collection device. Strong massage or "milking" should be avoided, since this can cause hemolysis or introduce interstitial fluid into the specimen, which could cause falsely increased values for analytes such as potassium and magnesium. There are also differences between skin puncture values and venipuncture values for certain analytes, such as glucose, where the skin puncture value can be up to 10% higher than the venipuncture value.

Venipuncture

This is the technique of choice with older children, as they have larger and firmer veins and are less likely to be psychologically affected by the sight of a needle. Generally speaking, the median cubital vein is used for obtaining blood. A tourniquet should be applied midway between the child's elbow and shoulder, with enough pressure to compress the vein but not the artery. A syringe with a needle attached or a vacutainer system may be used. In our experience, however, the needle of a 23-gauge butterfly works well. This should be inserted in line with the vein at a 15° angle to the skin. Once the blood is flowing through the butterfly and into the collection tube, the tourniquet should be removed. When the needle has been removed, a sterile cotton gauze should be applied with pressure until the bleeding has stopped (about three minutes) and then an adhesive bandage applied.

Arterial Puncture

This is the technique of choice for blood-gas analysis. It should be done by an experienced physician.

SPECIMEN CONSIDERATIONS

Specimen Volume

Even though much modern instrumentation uses small volumes of specimens, specimen size remains of prime concern to the pediatric laboratory. This is because the number of very premature babies cared for in neonatal nurseries increases year by year. In our nursery, the number of babies under 1000 g ten years ago was approximately 9–10 per year; now there are more than 50.

Although the total blood volume of a healthy newborn is approximately 85 µL, that of a premature infant can be much less. Figure 20-2 shows how total blood volume can be estimated according to the age and size of the infant. Since the hematocrit in a newborn infant can be 60% or more, the yield of serum or plasma is often less than can be expected from the volume of blood collected.[2] Table 20–1 shows hematocrit by age. An infant's hematocrit reaches adult values by approximately three months of age.

In the premature infant, good planning of required laboratory tests should be done to avoid excessive blood drawing. The blood hematocrit and hemoglobin should be monitored and a replacement blood transfusion should be given if essential.

FIGURE 20–2. Infant Blood Volume

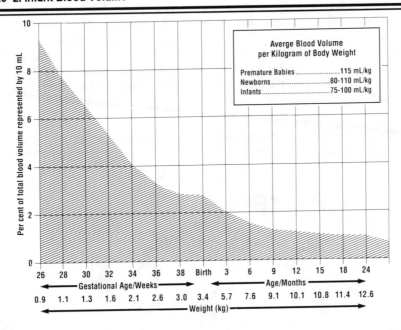

Averge Blood Volume
per Kilogram of Body Weight

Premature Babies ....115 mL/kg
Newborns ....80-110 mL/kg
Infants ....75-100 mL/kg

From: Werner, M, ed. Microtechniques for the clinical laboratory. New York: Wiley, 1976:2. Reprinted with permission.

TABLE 20-1. Hematocrit By Age

Age	Hct (%) + S.D.
1d	61 ± 7.4
2d	60 ± 6.4
3d	62 ± 9.3
4d	57 ± 8.1
5d	57 ± 7.3
6d	54 ± 7.2
7d	56 ± 9.4
1–2w	54 ± 7.3
2–3w	43 ± 5.7
3–4w	36 ± 4.8
4–5w	36 ± 6.2
5–6w	36 ± 5.8
6–7w	36 ± 4.8
7–8w	33 ± 3.7
8–9w	31 ± 2.5
9–10w	32 ± 2.7
10–11w	34 ± 2.1
11–12w	33 ± 3.3

From: Matoth Y, Zaizov R, Varsaro I. Acta Paed. Scand 1971;60:318. Reproduced with permission.

Evaporation

Specimen evaporation can be a major problem with small specimens. Rifai[14] has shown the effects of leaving serum samples uncovered for a period of 30–240 min (see Figure 20-3). It can be seen that in an hour, values can change by as much as 10% if the sample is 0.1 mL in size, whereas it is much less if the sample is larger, i.e., 5 mL (see Figure 20–4).

FIGURE 20–3. Evaporation Effects on Serum Samples (sample volume 0.1 mL)

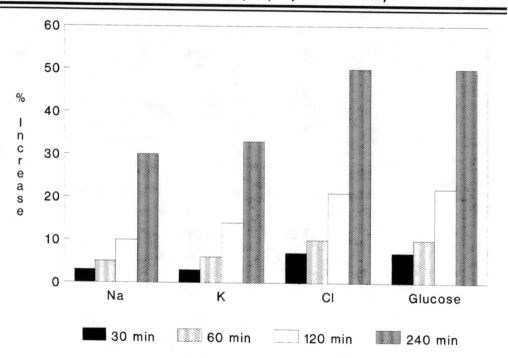

Interferences

Hemolysis

Several analytes in serum or plasma will yield erroneous results if they are measured in hemolyzed specimens. Potassium, magnesium, lactate dehydrogenase, and other constituents are present in higher concentrations in red blood cells than in extracellular fluid. Hemolysis will therefore cause increased concentrations of these analytes in serum or plasma (see Table 20–2). Hemoglobin can also interfere in the technical procedure; for example, the presence of hemolysis can cause a decrease in the measured bilirubin concentration. It is therefore important to avoid hemolysis when drawing specimens.

FIGURE 20–4. Evaporation Effects on Serum Samples (sample volume 5mL)

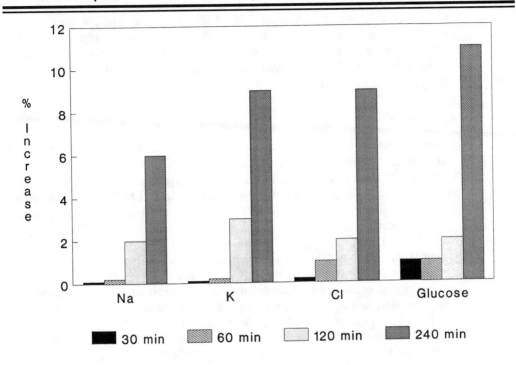

TABLE 20–2. The Effect of Hemolysis on Some Commonly Measured Analytes (↑ = increased , ↓ = decreased)

Analyte	Result
Acid Phosphatase	↑
Amino Acids	↑
Ammonia	↑
Aspartate aminotransferase	↑
Alanine aminotransferase	↑
Bilirubin	↓
Creatinine Kinase	↑
Iron	↑
Lactate dehydrogenase	↑
Magnesium	↑
Phosphorus	↑
Potassium	↑
Total Protein	↑

Lipemia

Premature infants receiving Intralipid (Kabi Vitrum Inc., Alameda, CA 94501) may sometimes have lipemic blood specimens. Lipemia, especially if severe, can interfere with any analysis performed by spectrophotometric techniques or with sodium and potassium measurements using a flame photometer.

Bilirubinemia

Many premature and some term infants will exhibit bilirubinemia in the first few days of life. Bilirubin may interfere with certain analyses using particular instrumentation. For example, bilirubin will produce spuriously low cholesterol values when using the Cobas Mira (One Sunset Avenue, Montclair, NJ 07042), and will also significantly lower the creatinine values obtained using the Hitachi 705 (Boehringer-Mannheim Diagnostics, Inc., Indianapolis IN 46250). The Cobas Mira using Roche creatinine reagents employs a kinetic modification of the Jaffe reaction, with creatinine and picric acid at alkaline pH forming a red complex measured at 520 nm. The Hitachi also uses a modified Jaffe method using picric acid in alkaline medium. The color intensity is measured photometrically at 505 and 507 nm. The Ektachem systems (Eastman Kodak Co., Rochester, NY 14560), which show no interference of bilirubin with the creatinine method, measure creatinine by its enzymatic hydrolysis to produce ammonia. The reflectance is measured at 600 nm. An excellent guide to interferences in clinical chemistry instruments was published in 1987 by Glick and Ryder.[6]

Labelling the Specimen

Small tubes can be very difficult to label adequately. It is, however, essential to include the last and first name of the patient, the hospital identification number, the location of the patient (floor or clinic), and the date the specimen was obtained. The tube label should also be signed by the person obtaining the specimen. Since micro tubes are so small, it is generally not possible to take advantage of the patient identification bar coding that is available on certain equipment.

Collection Devices

Capillary tubes are needed for the collection of blood gases. These can hold up to 140 µL blood (Ciba-Corning, Medfield, MA 02052). These are heparinized with $Na^+/Li^+/Ca^{++}$ heparin. Specimens for blood gases should be mixed using "metal fleas." All blood-gas analyses should be performed immediately after the blood is obtained. The specimens should be received on ice.

Although somewhat expensive, the Microtainer (Becton Dickinson, Rutherford, NJ 07070) is preferred for serum collection. These tubes have a serum separator and hold 600 µL blood. The tubes are easy to label and separation of the serum from the cells occurs after a single short centrifugation. In addition, the serum separator does not affect the values of most common analytes.[7] Plasma may be obtained by using a green topped (lithium heparin) microtainer tube. Common practice in our institution is to draw the blood using a Butterfly (Abbott Diagnostics, N. Chicago, IL 60064) attached to a syringe. If larger volumes of blood are required for certain assays, such as hormones, the 3 or 5 mL vacutainers (Becton-Dickinson, Mountain View, CA 94039) may be used as collection devices. We do not use the vacutainer method of drawing, since the veins collapse easily in young children.

Choice of Anticoagulant

Although most laboratories in the United States use serum for the majority of clinical chemistry analyses, we recommend the use of plasma. This is because it speeds up the turnaround time, since one does not have to wait for clotting to occur, and there is generally less hemolysis. Also, there is good evidence that plasma should be used for the measurement of potassium.[8] This is particularly the case in those patients who have high platelet or white blood cell counts. It is important to ensure that the anticoagulant used does not directly influence the analyte to be measured.

Heparin

The ammonium, sodium, or lithium salts of heparin may be used. We generally prefer the lithium salt, except in the measurement of lithium, wherein falsely increased values will be obtained. This is not the case, however, with the measurement of sodium using sodium heparin tubes, because the concentration of sodium is very small compared to the concentration in serum or plasma.

Sodium Fluoride

This is the preservative of choice for glucose analyses. The fluoride prevents glycolysis and therefore stops the usual decrease in glucose that occurs if the specimen is left unseparated for a period of time. If the serum is not separated from the red cells immediately after collection, one sees a decrease of serum glucose of 7% in the first hour.[9]

Ethylenediamine Tetraacetric Acid (EDTA)

EDTA is used for the collection of whole blood for lead analysis. It is also used for the collection of hematologic specimens, as it does not destroy the cellular components of blood. The ratio of EDTA to blood is important for hematologic specimens. It is imperative that the tube be filled with blood.

Centrifugation of Microspecimens

Any small table-top centrifuge that can attain speeds of 10,000 to 13,000 g may be used. Serum or plasma separation can then be effected in 1–2 minutes.

Environment

When drawing specimens from children, it is important to have a pleasant atmosphere. It is advisable that phlebotomists wear colored uniforms rather than white. The rooms should be colorful as well. The phlebotomist should have a positive, pleasant attitude and should spend the time to put the patient at ease and gain his or her confidence. The child should be told what is going to happen, that it is going to hurt a little, and that it will soon be finished. It is very important to identify the patient correctly. With an inpatient, the armband should be checked carefully. With an outpatient, the parent, or the child, if old enough, should be asked for his or her name.

Collection of Cerebrospinal Fluid (CSF)

CSF should be collected by lumbar puncture by an experienced and qualified physician. Four separate sterile tubes are used for collecting the specimens. The first tube should be saved for future studies; the second tube should be used for microbiology and virology studies, the third tube for clinical chemistry studies, and the fourth tube for hematology studies. Protein analysis should not be done on a bloody specimen, because the contribution of protein from lysed blood cells and plasma cannot be assessed accurately. Specimens for glucose should be refrigerated.

Collection of Other Specimens

Fluids such as knee-joint aspirates and peritoneal, pericardial, and ascitic fluids should be collected into plain, sterile tubes by a qualified physician.

Urine Collection

It is frequently preferable to collect a 24-hour specimen, since urine specimens can be more or less concentrated at different times of the day. There can also be significant diurnal variation in the excretion of certain analytes. To collect a good 24-hour specimen, the bladder should be emptied and the specimen discarded, the time noted, and all urine specimens in the following 24 hours should be collected, including one at the same time of day as when the collection was started. The specimens should be pooled and mixed thoroughly. The laboratory should provide the appropriate container. Table 20-3 shows the correct preservatives to use. It is very difficult to collect specimens from neonates and young babies. It is recommended to collect specimens using a plastic bag designed for the purpose (U bag, Hollister Inc., Chicago, IL 60048).

Since 24-hour urinary collections can be notoriously inaccurate, it is of value to know the expected urine volume from children of different ages so as to have some idea of the appproriate volume. Figure 1-5 shows expected urine volumes in the normal pediatric population. Specimens for urinalysis should be kept refrigerated. Early-morning specimens are also the specimens of choice for pregnancy testing and screening for metabolic disorders.

TABLE 20-3. Preservation of Urine

Test	Instructions	Preservative and Amount to be Used		
		< 6 mo.	*6 mo to 5 y*	*5 to 18 y*
Amino levulinic acid	Protect from light	8 mL 6N HCl	15mL 6N HCl	30mL 6N HCl
Aldosterone	Add boric acid	2–5g H_3BO_3	5g H_3BO_3	10g H_3BO_3
Arylsulfatase A	Freeze			
Calcium	Verify pH is < 7	8 mL 6N HCl	15 mL 6N HCl	30 mL 6N HCl
Catecholamines		1–3g Na_2CO_3	2–5g Na_2CO_3	5g Na_2CO_3
Coproporphyrin	Protect from light	—	—	—
Cortisol (free)	1g boric acid per 100 mL urine	—	—	—
Heavy metals	Adjust pH	8 mL 6N HCl	15 mL 6N HCl	30 mL 6N HCl
5-HIAAA	Adjust pH	8 mL 6N HCl	8 mL 6N HCl	30 mL 6N HCl
HVA		5 mL 50% HAC*	12 mL 50% HAC*	25 mL 50% HAC*
17-OH-Corticosteroid	Add 1 g boric acid per 100 mL urine	—	—	—
17-Ketosteroids	Adjust pH	8 mL 6N HCl	15 mL 6N HCl	30 mL 6N HCl
Lead	Lead-free container	—	—	—
Metanephrines		8 mL 6N HCl	12 mL 6N HCl	30 mL 6N HCl
Oxalate	Adjust pH	8 mL 6N HCl	15 mL 6N HCl	30 mL 6N HCl

*Acetic acid

Continued

TABLE 20–3 Continued

Test	Instructions	Preservative and Amount To Be Used		
		< 6 mo.	*6 mo to 5 y*	*5 to 18 y*
Phosphorus	Adjust pH	8 mL 6N HCl	15 mL 6N HCl	30 mL 6N HCl
Porphobilinogen	Protect from light; *freeze*	—	—	—
Porphyrins	Protect from light; refrigerate	1–3 g Na₂CO₃	2–5 g Na₂CO₃	5 g Na₂CO₃
Pregnanetriol	No preservative	—	—	—
Urea nitrogen	Refigerate; no preservative	—	—	—
Uric Acid	No preservative	—	—	—
Urobilinogen	2 h timed specimen; *freeze* immediately; protect from light	1–3 g Na₂CO₃	2–5 g Na₂CO₃	5 g Na₂CO₃

FIGURE 20–5. Expected Urine Volumes in the Normal Pediatric Population

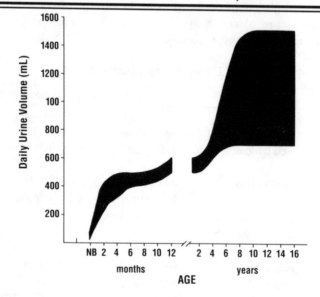

Fecal Collection

It is sometimes necessary to collect fecal specimens for specialized tests, such as fecal fat determinations for the diagnosis of pancreatic insufficiency, fecal trypsin for the diagnosis of cystic fibrosis, reducing substances for the diagnosis of sucrose intolerance, and fecal electrolytes to assess severe electrolyte losses. Stools may also be examined for the presence of occult blood. When collecting fecal specimens, the patient should be told not to contaminate the specimen with urine. A well-cleaned and boiled glass container or a plastic container may be used.

Specimen Transport

A general rule is that all specimens should be transported to the laboratory as soon as possible. This is particularly important for some analyses, such as blood gases and ammonia; these specimens should be transported on ice. Blood for a complete blood count and differential and urines should also be transported quickly, since cellular elements can disintegrate.

UNIVERSAL PRECAUTIONS

Because the potential *infectivity* of any patient's blood or body fluids cannot be known with certainty, it is important that the blood and body fluid precautions recommended by the CDC[10] be followed for all patients. NCCLS recommends that gloves be worn at all times when handling laboratory specimens.[11] It is also important for phlebotomists to wear gloves when drawing blood or obtaining specimens from patients. Laboratory coats should not be worn outside of the laboratory, but should be removed before going home, out for lunch, etc.

REFERENCE RANGES

Correct interpretation of laboratory data depends on the availability of appropriate reference ranges (normal values) for the age and development of the child. Laboratory data obtained from cord blood serum are often close to those of the mother's serum. Thereafter, they may change rapidly. For example, cord blood T_4 was reported by Walfish to be 6.6–17.5 ng/dL (85–225 nmol/L) and to rise at 1–3 days of age to 10.0–21.5 ng/dL (142–278 nmol/L).[12] Serum proteins, especially immunoglobulins, also undergo changes during the maturation of the neonate to an adolescent. The analyte that shows marked changes with age is alkaline phosphatase. During the growth spurts in infancy and adolescence, the serum alkaline phosphatase increases greatly to values which would be considered pathological in an adult. For example, the reference range on the Ektachem 700 for a female aged 12–13 y is 105–420 U/L and at age 16–19 y is 50–130 U/L.[13] These reference ranges are also different for males and females. For example, at the same ages, the reference ranges for males are 200–495 U/L and 65–260 U/L, respectively.

LABORATORY INSTRUMENTATION AND METHODOLOGY

In the pediatric laboratory, both methods and instruments should be chosen with the sample size in mind. For automated equipment, the sample size should probably be no bigger than 10 μL. Methods should be chosen that are not subject to interference from endogenous or exogenous substances. In particular, the common interferents bilirubin, hemoglobin, and lipids should not affect the results. As mentioned earlier, there is an excellent monograph by Glick[6] which shows the effect of common interferents on analyses using a variety of clinical chemistry analyzers.

Certain requirements are basic in the pediatric laboratory:

(a) Care must be taken to minimize the evaporation of the sample, which can be considerable if specimens and samples are not kept covered at all times. The use of narrow, deep containers is recommended to reduce the area from which evaporation can occur.

(b) Precise pipetting of small-volume specimens is essential.

(c) A well-defined list of those tests which can be ordered on a stat basis should be developed in conjunction with the medical staff.

An important consideration that is often overlooked is the dead volume, i.e., the amount of sample that must remain in the sample cup after the samples are aspirated for analysis. There is no point to having a 5 μL sample requirement if the dead volume is 300 μL (see Table 20–4).

TABLE 20–4. Dead Volume Requirements for Certain Analyzers

Analyzer	Sample Volume (μL)	Dead Volume (μL)
Ektachem (Kodak)	10	30
TDx (Abbott)	50	10–20
ADx (Abbott)	50	10–20
IMx (Abbott)	150	50
System 6300 (Beckman)	100	250 (Extraction)
HPLC (Hewlett-Packard)	100	N/A
BGS 288 (Corning)	100	N/A
SpectrAA (Varian)	200	N/A

N/A = not applicable

SERVICES OFFERED

In a comprehensive pediatric clinical chemistry laboratory, there should be a wide variety of services and a large armamentarium of tests. It is necessary to provide services in the following areas: routine clinical chemistry tests, endocrinology, trace metals, therapeutic drug monitoring, toxicology, urinalysis, and, if there is no separate immunology section in the laboratory, specific proteins. It is also often advantageous to have satellite operations overseen by the main laboratory; these could include laboratories for blood gases, electrolytes, and glucoses in the neonatal unit and intensive care areas; an emergency room laboratory for stat chemistry, hematology, and blood gases; and whole-blood electrolytes and blood gases in the operating room.

As the diagnosis and therapy of disease is the *raison d'être* of the clinical pathology laboratory, it is essential to staff the laboratory with a skilled technical staff and directors at the M.D. and Ph.D. level. These directors must be available 24 hours a day, seven days a week, through an "on-call" system. It is through good planning and goal setting that an excellent service can be provided to allow the laboratory to assist the physician in his or her task of patient care. The quality of the work must be assessed constantly through good quality-control and quality-assurance programs.

REFERENCES

1. Blumenfeld TA, Turi GK, Blanc WA. Recommended site and depth of newborn heel skin punctures based on anatomical measurements and histopathology. Lancet 1979;1:230-33.
2. Procedures for the collection of diagnostic blood specimens by skin puncture, 2nd ed. NCCLS Approved Standard, 1986.
3. Wilkinson RH. Chemical micromethods in clinical medicine. Springfield, IL: Charles C Thomas, 1960:19-25.
4. Van Steirteghem AC, Young DS. Povidone-iodine (betadine) disinfectant as a source of error. Clin Chem 1977;23:1512-6.
5. Meites S, Levitt MJ. Skin puncture and blood collecting techniques for infants. Clin Chem 1979;25:183-89.
6. Glick MR, Ryder K. Interferographs: User's guide to interferences in clinical chemistry instruments. Indianapolis: Science Enterprises, Inc., 1987.
7. Hicks JM, Rowland GL, Buffone GJ. Evaluation of a new blood collecting device ("Microtainer") that is suited for pediatric use. Clin Chem 1976;22:2034-6.
8. Oski FA. Hematological problems in neonatology. In: Neonatology: Pathophysiology and management of the of the newborn, 2nd ed. G.B. Avery, Ed. Philadephia: J.B. Lippincott Co., 1981:545.
9. Weissman M, Klein B. Evaluation of glucose determinations in untreated serum samples. Clin Chem 1958;4:420-4.
10. CDC update: Universal precautions for prevention of transmission of human immunodeficiency virus, hepatitis B virus, and other bloodborne pathogens in health-care settings. MMWR 37:377-87, 1988.
11. Protection of laboratory workers from infectious disease transmitted by blood, body fluids and tissue. NCCLS Document M29-T, 1989, pp. 18.
12. Walfish PG. Thyroid function in pediatrics. In: Hicks JM, Boeckx RL., eds., Pediatric clinical chemistry. Philadelphia: Saunders, 1984:170-239.
13. Lockitch G, Halstead AC In: Meites S, Ed., Pediatric clinical chemistry: Reference (normal) values, Washington, DC: AACC Press, 1988:209.
14. Rifai N. Personal communication.

Some of this text is taken from Hicks JM, Boeckx, RL, in Pediatric Clinical Chemistry, W. B. Saunders Company, Philadelphia, PA, with permission from the publisher.

Index

552

Neurofibromatosis, 182
Neuroimaging, 294
Neuroleptic medications, 308
Neurologic and psychiatric
  disorders, 291
  attention-deficit hyperactivity
    disorder, 312-14
  in bronchopulmonary
    dysplasia, 63
  epilepsy, 293-302, See also
    Epilepsy
  major depressive disorder,
    315-17
  migraine headache, 304-6
  movement disorders, 306-7
  obsessive-compulsive
    disorder, 309-11
  Tourette's syndrome, 307-9
  Wilson's disease and, 15
Neuromuscular disorders, 119
Neuropathy, diabetic, 275
Neurotoxicity, lead-related, 526
Neurotransmitters, 295, 297,
  304, 306
Neurovisceral attacks, 480
Neutrophil, leucocyte esterase
  in, 93
Newborn
  ambiguous genitalia in,
    173-77, 178f
  calcium and phosphorus
    levels in, 249-50
  hypoglycemia in, 277
  lupus syndrome in, 323
  respiratory disorders in, See
    Respiratory disorders
  thyroxine concentrations in,
    199-200
  tyrosinemia in, 383
  vitamin deficiency in, 23, 28
Niacin (nicotinic acid), 32-34
Nicotinamide adenine
  dinucleotide (NAD), 33, 34,
    428, 434
  phosphate (NADP), 33, 34
Nicotinic acid, See Niacin
Niemann-Pick disease, 117
Nitrite, urinary, 93
Nitrogen balance, 5
Nitrogenous wastes, 101
Nitroprusside, See Sodium
  nitroprusside
Non-Hodgkin's lymphoma, 454,
  455, 561
Noonan's syndrome, 189
Norepinephrine (Noradrenaline),
  234, 458
Normoglycemia, achievement
  of, 269-70
Nortriptyline, 316-17
Nose-breather, 65
Nosocomial infection, 539

Nucleic acid, 464
5-Nucleotidase, 430, 431
Nutrition, 1-3, 4, See also
  Malnutrition
  calcium and phosphorus
    disorders and, 257-58
  and diabetic ketoacidosis, 268
  growth effects, 141, 148-49
  lipids, 8-9
  neonatal, monitoring, 65
  parenteral, 42-45, See also
    Parenteral nutrition
  protein-energy, 3-8, 21
  trace elements, 3, 9-20, See
    also specific trace element
  vitamins, 20-42, See also
    specific vitamin

Obesity, and cholesterol, 129
Obsessive-compulsive disorder
  (OCD), 309-11
  Tourette's syndrome and, 307,
    308, 309
Oculocutaneous tyrosinemia,
  383
Oligomenorrhea, 345
Ophthalmologic examination, in
  diabetes, 271
Organic acid disorders, 387-92
Organomegaly, 363
Ornithine carbamoyl
  transferase, 385-86
Orotic acid, 386
Orotidine, 386
Orthostatic proteinuria, 96
Osmolal gap, urine, 89
Osmotic diuresis, 266
Osmotic tension, 436
Osteoblasts/Osteoclasts, 248
Osteodystrophy, 103-4
Osteogenic sarcoma, 453
Osteomalacia, 23
Osteomyelitis, 331
Osteoporosis, 349
Osteosarcoma, 465
Ototoxicity, aminoglycoside, 511
Ova, 166
Ovarian cancer, 349-50
Ovarian cyst, 181
Ovarian failure, 344, premature,
  345
Ovary(ies), 166, 168, 187
Oxalate, 39
Oxazophosphorine, 468
Oxidation, vitamin C effects on,
  39
Oxidative changes, low density
  lipoprotein uptake and, 130
Oxosteroid isomerase, 230
Oxygen
  and adult respiratory distress
    syndrome, 71

  in bronchopulmonary
    dysplasia, 63
  extracorporeal membrane
    oxygenation, 72-76
  and myocardial ischemia, 131

p-dimethylaminobenzaldehyde,
  491
P-glycoprotein, 511
Paint, lead poisoning from,
  524-25
Palmitic acid, 9
Pancreas, 280, 440-42
Pancreatic toxicity,
  L-asparaginase-related, 467
Pancreatitis, 136, 411
Pantothenic acid, 41-42
Papanicolaou smear (Pap
  smear), 350
Para-aminbenzoic acid, 442
Parainfluenza virus, 68
Parathyroid gland, removal of,
  256
Parathyroid hormone, 246, 247f,
  249, 250
Parenteral nutrition
  complications of, 1, 42-45
  evaluation of, 45
  manganese deficiency and, 18
  selenium deficiency and, 16
  zinc deficiency and, 12
Patent ductus arteriosus, 56,
  120, 122-24, 137
PCO2, 54, 89
PEG, intestinal function testing
  and, 440
Pellagra, 33
Pelvic examination, 344, 352
Pelvic masses, in adolescents,
  349-50
Pema, See
  Phenylethylmalonamide
Penicillin V, 342
Penis, formation of, 170
Pentane, 27
Perichondrium, 538
Perimenarcheal cycles, 344
Peripheral polyneuropathy, 30
Peroxidase antibodies, 204
Peroxisomal disorders, 363,
  371-72, 394
Persistent pulmonary
  hypertension of the newborn
  (PPHN), 56-58
pH, 3
  urinary, 88, 339
Pharmacokinetics, 495, 496-97,
  499, 512
Pharmacotherapy, 495
Pharyngeal tone, in preterm
  infants, 60
Phencyclidine, 530

Phenobarbital, 300, 502
  for epilepsy, 299-300, 303
  for migraine headache, 305
  side effects, 300, 303
  therapeutic drug monitoring,
    507
Phenostix, 521
Phenothiazine, 32, 306
Phensuximide, 302
Phenylalanine, 376
Phenylethylmalonamide
  (Pema), 300
Phenylketonuria (PKU), 360,
  376
Phenylethylmalonamide, 507
Phenytoin (Dilantin), 430, 498,
  503
  for epilepsy, 297-98, 303
  for migraine headache, 305
  therapeutic drug monitoring,
    506-7
  thyroid hormone effects, 209
Pheochromocytoma, 106,
  238-39
  catecholamine concentrations
    in, 458, 459
Phosphate, 87, 88
Phosphatidylglycerol, 56, 355
Phosphaturia, 248
Phospholipids, 399
Phosphorus
  biochemistry and physiology,
    246-49
  intrauterine accretion, 249
  metabolism, disorders of,
    250-58
  supplementation, 253
Phosphorylase kinase, 118, 373
Photosensitivity, 8, 486, 491-92
Phototherapy, 42
Phylloquinone (vitamin K1), 27,
  29
Picric acid, 544
Pimozide, 308, 309
pKa value, 503
Placenta, premature separation
  of, 356
Plaque, atherosclerotic, 130
Plasma
  amino acids in, 375-76
  catecholamine levels in, 237,
    238
  collection, 545
  fatty acid concentrations in, 9
  growth hormone
    concentrations in, 144-45
  half-life, of drug, 496
  nutrient concentrations, 2-3
  proteins, assessment of, 5-7
Plasmapheresis, 423
Plateau, 126
Platelet, 76, 123

Respiratory disorders *Continued*
persistent pulmonary
hypertension, 56-58
pneumonia, 58-59
respiratory distress syndrome,
53, 54-56
special needs of newborn,
64-65
syncytial virus, 58, 68
Resting membrane potential
(RMP), 124-25
Restriction fragment length
polymorphism (RFLP), 361
Retinol, *See* Vitamin A
Retinol-binding protein, 6, 20
Retinopathy of prematurity, 63
Retrotransmitter system,
abnormality of, 308
Reverse genetics, 359
Reye's syndrome, 284, 285, 515
Rh-negative mothers, 351, 356
Rheumatic disorders, 321-34
acute phase reactants in,
332-33
acute rheumatic fever, 331-32
inflammatory bowel disease,
328-29
juvenile dermatomyositis,
323-25
juvenile rheumatoid arthritis,
322, 327, 328t, 329
Lyme disease, 332
neonatal lupus syndrome, 323
progressive systemic
sclerosis, 329
spondyloarthropathies, 325-28t
juvenile ankylosing
spondylitis, 325-27
juvenile psoriatic arthritis, 327
Reiter's syndrome, 327-28
systemic and joint disorders,
330-31
systemic lupus
erythematosus, 322-23
vasculitis, 329-30
Rhinovirus, 68
Rhizomelic chondrodysplasia
punctata, 372
Riboflavin, 31-33
Rickets, 23, 24, 25, 252, 258
Rifampin, 209
Ritalinic acid, 313
Ritodrine hydrochloride, 355
Rituals, 309, 310
Rouleaux, 333
Rubella, 351

Safflower oil, 43
Salbutamol (albuterol), 70
Salicylates, 498
enteric coated or sustained
release, 520

hypoglycemia from, 285
thyroid hormone binding
effects, 200
toxicity, 518-21
Salicylphenolic glucuronide, 518
Salicyluric acid, 518
Saliva, 219, 503
Salt, *See* Sodium
Sarcoma
Ewing's, 454
osteogenic, 453
Saturation kinetics, 498
Scarring, in porphyria, 481, 486
Scheie's syndrome, 116, 117
Schilling test, 39
Scintiscanning, 204
Sclerosis, progressive systemic,
329
Scurvy, 40
Sediment, in obstructive
uropathy, 102
Seizures, 293-95, *See also*
Epilepsy
absence, 295
exacerbation of, 506
generalized, 297-300
lead-induced, 526
pyridoxine dependency in, 35
Selenium, 16-17
Sensitive thyroid-stimulating
hormone (sTSH),196, 205,
207, 208
Septic arthritis, 330
Serologic testing, in Lyme
disease, 332
Serotonin, 304, 310, 311
Serotonin reuptake blockers,
309, 310-11
Serratia, 58
Sertoli cells, 168
Serum, 545
collection, 545
insulin-like growth factor in,
158
osmolarity, calculation of, 523
samples, evaporation effects
on, 542, 542f, 543f
sickness, 330
Sex chromosome, in delayed
puberty, 190
Sex determining region (SRY),
167, 167f, 168, 174
Sex steroids, pubertal growth
and, 148
Sexual development, stages of,
179, 179t
Sexual differentiation, 165-70
abnormal, 170-77, 178f
Sexual organs, formation of,
166-70
Sexually transmitted disease,
screening for

in adolescent male, 342-44
during pregnancy, 350-51, 354
Shigella, 343
Short stature, *See* Growth
Shunting, in persistent
pulmonary hypertension of
the newborn, 56, 57
Sickle cell anemia, 39, 333, 336
Silicone membrane lung, 72, 73f
Single photon emission
computed tomography
(SPECT), 294
Skeletal growth, 141, 143f
Skeletal muscle, 118
Skin
dermatomyositis of, 324
in porphyria, 480, 492, 492t,
See also Porphyria,
cutaneous
in progressive systemic
sclerosis, 329
lesions, essential fatty acid
deficiency in, 8
puncture, for blood collection,
538-39
vitamin D formation in, 248
Small-for-gestational-age (SGA)
infants
hypoglycemia in, 285
serum thyroid hormone levels
in, 195
thyroxine serum
concentrations in, 199-200
Smooth muscle, relaxation,
510
Sodium (Na+), 89 *See also*
Hypernatremia;
Hyponatremia
in acute renal failure, 103
cardiopulmonary bypass
effects on, 133-34
current, 125
in diabetic ketoacidosis, 267
extracellular fluid, 108
in kidney disease, 82
loss, 108, 187
in 21-hydroxylase deficiency,
226, 228
reabsorption, heart failure and,
121
renal tubular function testing
and, 85-88
replacement, in extracorporeal
membrane oxygenation, 76
restriction, mineralocorticoid
measurement by, 224-25
retention, heart failure and, 122
stool, 437
wasting, 110, 227
Sodium-EDTA test, 254
Sodium fluoride, in glucose
analysis, 545

Sodium nitroprusside, 108
Soft signs, in
obsessive-compulsive
disorder, 310
Somatomedin, *See* Insulin-like
growth factor I
Somatomedin-C, measurement
of, 157
Somatostatin, 144, 280, 282
Soy, 43
Specimen
centrifugation of, 546
collection, 546
of cerebrospinal fluid, 546
choice of anticoagulants,
545-46
devices for, 544-45
environment for, 546
fecal, 548-49
urine, 547-48f
evaporation, 542, 542f, 543f
interferences, 542-44
labeling, 544
transport, 549
volume, 540-41f
Spectrophotometric methods,
433
Spermatogonia, 166
Sphingomyelin:lecithin ratio, 56,
355
Spironolactone, 97, 509
Spondylitis, 328
ankylosing, 325, 327, 330
Spondyloarthropathies (SAS),
144, 325, 327-29
SRIF, growth hormone secretion
effects, 144
Stamey test, 94
Staphylococcus, 93, 330
saprophyticus, 340
Starling mechanism, 121-22
Status asthmaticus, 70
Status epilepticus, treatment of,
303
Steady-state drug
concentration, 497, 498,
499
Steatocrit, 436, 439
Steatorrhea, tests for, 438
Steely hair syndrome, 14-15
Steroid(s)
adrenal, 213-20, 221t
decreased production of,
233
tumors producing, 231-32
gonadal, secretion of, 181
sex, 148, 168
Steroid enzyme deficiency, 187,
188
Steroid hormone precursors,
220, 222
Steroid sulfates, 176